Method Development and Validation in Food and Pharmaceutical Analysis

Method Development and Validation in Food and Pharmaceutical Analysis

Editors

In-Soo Yoon
Hyun-Jong Cho

MDPI • Basel • Beijing • Wuhan • Barcelona • Belgrade • Manchester • Tokyo • Cluj • Tianjin

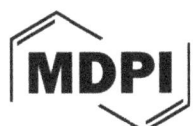

Editors

In-Soo Yoon
Pusan National University
Republic of Korea

Hyun-Jong Cho
Kangwon National University
Republic of Korea

Editorial Office
MDPI
St. Alban-Anlage 66
4052 Basel, Switzerland

This is a reprint of articles from the Special Issue published online in the open access journal *Molecules* (ISSN 1420-3049) (available at: https://www.mdpi.com/journal/molecules/special_issues/method_development_validatioin_analysis).

For citation purposes, cite each article independently as indicated on the article page online and as indicated below:

LastName, A.A.; LastName, B.B.; LastName, C.C. Article Title. *Journal Name* **Year**, *Volume Number*, Page Range.

ISBN 978-3-0365-6330-5 (Hbk)
ISBN 978-3-0365-6331-2 (PDF)

© 2023 by the authors. Articles in this book are Open Access and distributed under the Creative Commons Attribution (CC BY) license, which allows users to download, copy and build upon published articles, as long as the author and publisher are properly credited, which ensures maximum dissemination and a wider impact of our publications.

The book as a whole is distributed by MDPI under the terms and conditions of the Creative Commons license CC BY-NC-ND.

Contents

About the Editors ix

Preface to "Method Development and Validation in Food and Pharmaceutical Analysis" ... xi

Mei-Jun Chu, Xin-Min Liu, Ning Yan, Feng-Zhong Wang, Yong-Mei Du and Zhong-Feng Zhang
Partial Purification, Identification, and Quantitation of Antioxidants from Wild Rice (*Zizania latifolia*)
Reprinted from: *Molecules* **2018**, *23*, 2782, doi:10.3390/molecules23112782 1

Song-Tao Dong, Ying Li, Hao-Tian Yang, Yin Wu, Ya-Jing Li, Cong-Yang Ding, Lu Meng, et al.
An Accurate and Effective Method for Measuring Osimertinib by UPLC-TOF-MS and Its Pharmacokinetic Study in Rats
Reprinted from: *Molecules* **2018**, *23*, 2894, doi:10.3390/molecules23112894 17

Stefan Fritzsche, Susan Billig, Robby Rynek, Ramarao Abburi, Elena Tarakhovskaya, Olga Leuner, Andrej Frolov, et al.
Derivatization of Methylglyoxal for LC-ESI-MS Analysis—Stability and Relative Sensitivity of Different Derivatives
Reprinted from: *Molecules* **2018**, *23*, 2994, doi:10.3390/molecules23112994 27

Shenghua Gao, Lili Meng, Chunjie Zhao, Tao Zhang, Pengcheng Qiu and Fuli Zhang
Identification, Characterization and Quantification of Process-Related and Degradation Impurities in Lisdexamfetamine Dimesylate: Identifiction of Two New Compounds
Reprinted from: *Molecules* **2018**, *23*, 3125, doi:10.3390/molecules23123125 47

Jia Zhou, Hao Cai, Sicong Tu, Yu Duan, Ke Pei, Yangyang Xu, Jing Liu, et al.
Identification and Analysis of Compound Profiles of Sinisan Based on 'Individual Herb, Herb-Pair, Herbal Formula' before and after Processing Using UHPLC-Q-TOF/MS Coupled with Multiple Statistical Strategy
Reprinted from: *Molecules* **2018**, *23*, 3128, doi:10.3390/molecules23123128 63

Seung-Sik Cho, Seung-Hui Song, Chul-Yung Choi, Kyung Mok Park, Jung-Hyun Shim and Dae-Hun Park
Optimization of the Extraction Conditions and Biological Evaluation of *Dendropanax morbifera* H. Lev as an Anti-Hyperuricemic Source
Reprinted from: *Molecules* **2018**, *23*, 3313, doi:10.3390/molecules23123313 79

Rui-ze Gong, Yan-hua Wang, Yu-fang Wang, Bao Chen, Kun Gao and Yin-shi Sun
Simultaneous Determination of N^{ε}-(carboxymethyl) Lysine and N^{ε}-(carboxyethyl) Lysine in Different Sections of Antler Velvet after Various Processing Methods by UPLC-MS/MS
Reprinted from: *Molecules* **2018**, *23*, 3316, doi:10.3390/molecules23123316 87

Seung-Yub Song, Seung-Hui Song, Min-Suk Bae and Seung-Sik Cho
Phytochemical Constituents and the Evaluation Biological Effect of *Cinnamomum yabunikkei* H.Ohba Leaf
Reprinted from: *Molecules* **2019**, *24*, 81, doi:10.3390/molecules24010081 101

Jung-hyun Shim, Jung-il Chae and Seung-sik Cho
Identification and Extraction Optimization of Active Constituents in *Citrus junos* Seib ex TANAKA Peel and Its Biological Evaluation
Reprinted from: *Molecules* **2019**, *24*, 680, doi:10.3390/molecules24040680 109

Wenrong Yao, Ying Guo, Xi Qin, Lei Yu, Xinchang Shi, Lan Liu, Yong Zhou, Jinpan Hu, Chunming Rao and Junzhi Wang
Bioactivity Determination of a Therapeutic Recombinant Human Keratinocyte Growth Factor by a Validated Cell-based Bioassay
Reprinted from: *Molecules* 2019, 24, 699, doi:10.3390/molecules24040699 119

Yin-Ling Ma, Feng Zhao, Jin-Tuo Yin, Cai-Juan Liang, Xiao-Li Niu, Zhi-Hong Qiu and Lan-Tong Zhang
Two Approaches for Evaluating the Effects of Galangin on the Activities and mRNA Expression of Seven CYP450
Reprinted from: *Molecules* 2019, 24, 1171, doi:10.3390/molecules24061171 133

Rui-ze Gong, Yan-hua Wang, Kun Gao, Lei Zhang, Chang Liu, Ze-shuai Wang, Yu-fang Wang and Yin-shi Sun
Quantification of Furosine (N^{ε}-(2-Furoylmethyl)-L-lysine) in Different Parts of Velvet Antler with Various Processing Methods and Factors Affecting Its Formation
Reprinted from: *Molecules* 2019, 24, 1255, doi:10.3390/molecules24071255 149

Shengwei Sun, Meijuan Liu, Jian He, Kunping Li, Xuguang Zhang and Guangling Yin
Identification and Determination of Seven Phenolic Acids in Brazilian Green Propolis by UPLC-ESI-QTOF-MS and HPLC
Reprinted from: *Molecules* 2019, 24, 1791, doi:10.3390/molecules24091791 163

You Jin Han, Bitna Kang, Eun-Ju Yang, Min-Koo Choi and Im-Sook Song
Simultaneous Determination and Pharmacokinetic Characterization of Glycyrrhizin, Isoliquiritigenin, Liquiritigenin, and Liquiritin in Rat Plasma Following Oral Administration of Glycyrrhizae Radix Extract
Reprinted from: *Molecules* 2019, 24, 1816, doi:10.3390/molecules24091816 177

Subindra Kazi Thapa, Mahesh Upadhyay, Tae Hwan Kim, Soyoung Shin, Sung-Joo Park and Beom Soo Shin
Liquid Chromatography-Tandem Mass Spectrometry of Desoxo-Narchinol a and Its Pharmacokinetics and Oral Bioavailability in Rats and Mice
Reprinted from: *Molecules* 2019, 24, 2037, doi:10.3390/molecules24112037 191

Eun-Sol Ha, Dong-Gyun Han, Seong-Wook Seo, Ji-Min Kim, Seon-Kwang Lee, Woo-Yong Sim, In-Soo Yoon, et al.
A Simple HPLC Method for the Quantitative Determination of Silybin in Rat Plasma: Application to a Comparative Pharmacokinetic Study on Commercial Silymarin Products
Reprinted from: *Molecules* 2019, 24, 2180, doi:10.3390/molecules24112180 203

Sojeong Jin, Ji-Hyeon Jeon, Sowon Lee, Woo Youl Kang, Sook Jin Seong, Young-Ran Yoon, Min-Koo Choi, et al.
Detection of 13 Ginsenosides (Rb1, Rb2, Rc, Rd, Re, Rf, Rg1, Rg3, Rh2, F1, Compound K, 20(S)-Protopanaxadiol, and 20(S)-Protopanaxatriol) in Human Plasma and Application of the Analytical Method to Human Pharmacokinetic Studies Following Two Week-Repeated Administration of Red Ginseng Extract
Reprinted from: *Molecules* 2019, 24, 2618, doi:10.3390/molecules24142618 211

Mengqi Zhang, Xia Ren, Shijun Yue, Qing Zhao, Changlun Shao and Changyun Wang
Simultaneous Quantification of Four Phenylethanoid Glycosides in Rat Plasma by UPLC-MS/MS and Its Application to a Pharmacokinetic Study of Acanthus Ilicifolius Herb
Reprinted from: *Molecules* 2019, 24, 3117, doi:10.3390/molecules24173117 229

Ha-Na Oh, Dae-Hun Park, Ji-Yeon Park, Seung-Yub Song, Sung-Ho Lee, Goo Yoon, Hong-Seop Moon, et al.
Tyrosinase Inhibition Antioxidant Effect and Cytotoxicity Studies of the Extracts of *Cudrania tricuspidata* Fruit Standardized in Chlorogenic Acid
Reprinted from: *Molecules* **2019**, *24*, 3266, doi:10.3390/molecules24183266 . . . . **241**

Gregorio Carballo-Uicab, José E. Linares-Trejo, Gabriela Mellado-Sánchez, Carlos A. López-Morales, Marco Velasco-Velázquez, Lenin Pavón, Sergio Estrada-Parra, et al.
Validation of a Cell Proliferation Assay to Assess the Potency of a Dialyzable Leukocyte Extract Intended for Batch Release
Reprinted from: *Molecules* **2019**, *24*, 3426, doi:10.3390/molecules24193426 . . . . **251**

Joo Tae Hwang, Ki-Sun Park, Jin Ah Ryuk, Hye Jin Kim and Byoung Seob Ko
Development of an Oriental Medicine Discrimination Method through Analysis of Steroidal Saponins in *Dioscorea nipponica* Makino and Their Anti-Osteosarcoma Effects
Reprinted from: *Molecules* **2019**, *24*, 4022, doi:10.3390/molecules24224022 . . . . **261**

Seung-Hyun Jeong, Ji-Hun Jang, Hea-Young Cho and Yong-Bok Lee
Pharmacokinetic Comparison of Epinastine Using Developed Human Plasma Assays
Reprinted from: *Molecules* **2019**, *25*, 209, doi:10.3390/molecules25010209 . . . . **277**

Yoo-Seong Jeong, Minjeong Baek, Seungbeom Lee, Min-Soo Kim, Han-Joo Maeng, Jong-Hwa Lee, Young-Ger Suh, et al.
Development and Validation of Analytical Method for SH-1242 in the Rat and Mouse Plasma by Liquid Chromatography/Tandem Mass Spectrometry
Reprinted from: *Molecules* **2019**, *25*, 531, doi:10.3390/molecules25030531 . . . . **297**

About the Editors

In-Soo Yoon

In-Soo Yoon is currently working as a Professor in College of Pharmacy Pusan National University (Busan, Republic of Korea). He has authored and co-authored > 140 peer-reviewed journal articles (H-index = 32). At present, he is a member of the Editorial Board for Molecules (MDPI, eISSN 1420-3049) and Drug Development Research (WILEY, ISSN 0272-4391). His areas of expertise are biopharmaceutics, the study of the fate of drugs in biological systems after administration (i.e., absorption, distribution, metabolism, and excretion; ADME), and pharmacokinetics, the science of the kinetics of drug ADME. He is mainly working on the following research topics through various in vitro/in vivo experimental and in silico kinetic modeling approaches.
- Drug-metabolizing enzyme- and transporter-mediated ADME of xenobiotics;
- Drug interactions with drugs, foods, and natural products;
- Bioanalytical method development;
- Physiologically based pharmacokinetic/pharmacodynamic modeling;
- Drug formulations for oral and transdermal bioavailability enhancement.

Hyun-Jong Cho

Hyun-Jong Cho is currently working as a Professor in the College of Pharmacy Kangwon National University (Chuncheon, Republic of Korea). He has authored and co-authored > 165 peer-reviewed journal articles (H-index = 40). At present, he serves as an Associate Editor of the Journal of Pharmaceutical Investigation and Editorial Board Member of Molecules and Pharmaceutics. His research areas cover the development of oral, intravenous, intraarterial, subcutaneous, and intra(peri)tumoral formulations and their in vitro/in vivo evaluations. For in vitro/in vivo assessments of developed drug delivery systems, several analytical techniques, from chromatographic to imaging analyses, have been adopted.
- Disease-targeted drug delivery systems;
- Pharmacokinetic study following formulation administration;
- Bioimaging analysis for monitoring the in vivo fate of drug cargos and their delivery systems.

Preface to "Method Development and Validation in Food and Pharmaceutical Analysis"

Prior to the commercialization of foods and pharmaceuticals, the analytical methods for those substances should be developed and further validated. The appearance and discovery of diverse ingredients in foods and medicines create the necessity for new and exquisite analytical methodologies. Advanced and integrated analytical techniques are required for the various physicochemical and biological characteristics of analytes, from small chemicals to biomacromolecules (including nucleic acids, peptides, and proteins). Given the human intake of foods and medicines, those substances should be selectively analyzed in biological samples, as well as in in vitro test specimens. Rapid, specific, accurate, precise, sensitive, economic, eco-friendly, user-friendly, robust, and versatile analytical methods can be widely applied to the growth of the food and pharmaceutical industries, and they can contribute to their efficient and safe clinical application. The Special Issue "Method Development and Validation in Food and Pharmaceutical Analysis", gathered in this book, was proposed by two Guest Editors, all of whom are professors conducting research and teaching in the fields of pharmaceutics, analytical chemistry, pharmacokinetics/pharmacodynamics, and physical pharmacy. This book covers a wide range of topics, including, but not limited to, new analytical and bioanalytical methods relevant to the separation, identification, and determination of substances in pharmaceutics, pharmacokinetics, nanobiotechnology, clinical chemistry, biomedical engineering, and related disciplines. The papers (18 articles and 5 communications) presented in this book were submitted by research groups from different countries that fit the aims and scopes of our Special Issue. We would like to thank all contributors and colleagues who chose to publish their works here, as well as the reviewers who dedicated their time, effort, and expertise to evaluating the submissions and assuring the high quality of the published work. We would also like to thank the publisher MDPI and the editorial staff of the journal for their professional support. Finally, we hope that the content of this book will offer new perspectives and ideas to initiate and continue further research.

In-Soo Yoon and Hyun-Jong Cho
Editors

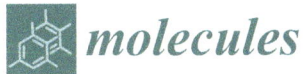

Article

Partial Purification, Identification, and Quantitation of Antioxidants from Wild Rice (*Zizania latifolia*)

Mei-Jun Chu [1], Xin-Min Liu [1], Ning Yan [1], Feng-Zhong Wang [2], Yong-Mei Du [1,*] and Zhong-Feng Zhang [1,*]

1. Tobacco Research Institute, Chinese Academy of Agricultural Sciences, Qingdao 266101, China; chumjun@163.com (M.-J.C.); liuxinmin@caas.cn (X.-M.L.); yanning@caas.cn (N.Y.)
2. Institute of Food Science and Technology, Chinese Academy of Agricultural Sciences, Beijing 100193, China; wangfengzhong@caas.cn
* Correspondence: duyongmei@caas.cn (Y.-M.D.); zhangzfng@163.com (Z.-F.Z.); Tel.: +86-532-88702239 (Z.-F.Z.)

Received: 15 September 2018; Accepted: 23 October 2018; Published: 26 October 2018

Abstract: To provide further insights into the potential health-promoting antioxidants from wild rice (*Zizania latifolia*), which is an abundant but underutilized whole grain resource in East Asia, a partial purification based on D101 macroporous resin was carried out for the purification and enrichment of the antioxidants from the bioactive ethanol extracts of wild rice. On that basis, 34 phenolic compounds in the antioxidant fractions were identified by a high-performance liquid chromatography-linear ion trap quadrupole-Orbitrap-mass spectrometry (HPLC-LTQ-Orbitrap-MS^n). The results suggested that phenolic acids could be enriched in the 10% ethanol-eluted fraction whereas flavonoids (including procyanidins and flavonoid glycosides) could be enriched in 20–30% ethanol-eluted fractions. A quantitative analysis determined by the multiple reaction monitoring mode of the ultra-performance liquid chromatography-triple quadrupole-tandem mass spectrometry (UPLC-QqQ-MS/MS) revealed a high content of procyanidins in wild rice. Compared with phenolic acids, flavonoids may contribute more to the potent antioxidant activity of wild rice. This is the first study on the antioxidants from wild rice *Z. latifolia*. These findings provide novel information on the functional components of wild rice, and will be of value to further research and development on *Z. latifolia*.

Keywords: wild rice; antioxidant; macroporous resins; LC-MS/MS; phenolics; procyanidins

1. Introduction

Wild rice is the seed of an aquatic plant belonging to the genus *Zizania*, family Poaceae. Among the four species of genus *Zizania* around the world, *Z. aquatica*, *Z. palustris*, and *Z. texana* are indigenous to North America, whereas *Z. latifolia* is native to East Asia [1]. In China, *Z. latifolia* is widely distributed in areas along the Yangtze and Huai Rivers without any cultivation and domestication [2]. Wild rice is an age-old grain that has been used to treat diabetes and other diseases associated with nutrition, in Chinese medicinal practice, with a recorded history of over three thousand years of use in China. Today its use as a grain has almost disappeared, owing to the very different ripening times and easy seed shattering of the cereal [3–5]. In North America, dehulled but unpolished wild rice was historically consumed by Native Americans as a staple food [6]. Since the late 20th century, a growing commercialization of wild rice has been emerged to meet the increased demand for health-promoting cereals. In recent years, North American wild rice has been widely used in gourmet food products because of its unique flavor, color, and texture [7].

With its nutritional quality characterized by a high content of proteins, dietary fiber, minerals, vitamins, and other bioactive phytochemicals (such as phenolics and γ-oryzanols), and a low fat content, wild rice was recognized as a whole grain by the U.S. Food and Drug Administration (FDA) in 2006 [4,7–9]. Epidemiological studies have demonstrated that the regular consumption of whole grains is beneficial to human health and can reduce the risk of non-communicable diseases such as obesity, diabetes, and cardiovascular diseases [10,11].

Most of the reports on wild rice have focused on its nutrients and health benefits [4,12]. Phytochemicals are key contributors to the health benefits of whole grains, due to their bioactivities, especially antioxidant capacities [10]. Phytochemicals in wild rice have been investigated to a much lesser degree in comparison with those in other cereal grains. To date, there have been only three reports on the characterization of antioxidants from wild rice. Specifically, Qiu et al. identified eight soluble and insoluble monomeric phenolic acids, four ferulate dehydrodimers, and two sinapate dehydrodimers from wild rice Z. aquatica by HPLC-MS/MS [7]. Fourteen phenolic acids and six flavonoids (including catechin, epicatechin, epigallocatechin, rutin, quercetin, and kaempferol) in free and bound phenolic fractions of wild rice Z. aquatica were determined using HPLC, by Sumczynski et al. [8]. Moreover, Qiu et al. identified three flavonoid glycosides (including diglucosyl apigenin, glucosyl-arabinosyl apigenin, and diarabinosyl apigenin) and six flavan-3-ols (including catechin, epicatechin, and four oligomeric procyanidins) from wild rice Z. palustris and Z. aquatica, via HPLC-MS/MS [13]. Earlier studies have shown that the other wild rice species Z. latifolia, native to East Asia, has a high nutritional value [14,15], and was effective in suppressing hyperlipidemia and oxidative stress, preventing obesity and liver lipotoxicity, and alleviating insulin resistance induced by a high-fat/cholesterol diet in rats [3,5,16]. However, no investigation on the antioxidant activities and bioactive compounds from East Asian wild rice Z. latifolia has been reported.

It is well-known that unpurified crude plant extracts always contain carbohydrates, proteins, and other impurities, which may limit further identification and even the application of the bioactive substances [13,17]. Therefore, it is of great importance to purify antioxidants from wild rice. Purification of phytochemicals from wild rice has been little studied apart from one preliminary report by Qiu et al., who fractionated crude extracts of North American wild rice on a Sephadex LH-20 column to improve the detection of procyanidins [13]. As an efficient and practical adsorption material, macroporous resins have been widely used in the purification and separation of phytochemicals, for their many advantages, including suitable adsorption and desorption capacities, high adsorption selectivity, low cost, easy recycling, lower pollution, and suitability for large-scale production [18]. Nevertheless, no studies have been conducted to investigate the use of macroporous resin for the purification of phytochemicals from wild rice.

In order to exploit the whole grain Z. latifolia resources and obtain further insights into the potential health-promoting antioxidants from wild rice, an activity-guided study was carried out to evaluate the in vitro antioxidant activity of wild rice Z. latifolia, partially purify and separate the antioxidant constituents using a macroporous resin column, and identify and quantify individual compounds by the high-performance liquid chromatography-linear ion trap quadrupole-Orbitrap-mass spectrometry (HPLC-LTQ-Orbitrap-MS^n) and ultra-performance liquid chromatography-triple quadrupole-tandem mass spectrometry (UPLC-QqQ-MS/MS).

2. Results and Discussion

2.1. Selection of Extraction Solvent

Considering the significant effect of the extraction solvent on the antioxidants extracted from plants [19–21], twelve different types of solvents were used to select the suitable solvent to get the maximum extraction of antioxidants from wild rice, since they were the most common ones for the extraction of antioxidants from plants [7,13,19,22]. The antioxidant activities, total flavonoid content (TFC), and total phenolic content (TPC) of each solvent extract were determined (Figure S1 in the Supplementary Materials). The results displayed that the extracts derived from ethanol, methanol, and acetone showed equivalent antioxidant activities, TFC, and TPC, which were higher than those of the other solvent extracts. Therefore, the biocompatible ethanol, with a lower cost and being less polluting, was selected as the optimal extraction solvent [22].

2.2. Antioxidant Activities, TFC and TPC of Ethanol Crude Extracts

Owing to the fact that pigmented rice has higher amounts of antioxidants than those of non-pigmented rice [23], and red rice *Oryza sativa* is recognized as a functional ingredient for nutraceuticals and functional foods [24], both the red and white rice *O. sativa* were used as control samples in this study. According to the results shown in Table 1, wild rice collected from Jingzhou showed the highest DPPH radical scavenging activity (45.4 ± 0.2 μmol AAE/g), followed by wild rice collected from Huai'an (20.8 ± 0.1 μmol AAE/g). The relative low DPPH radical scavenging activities of the red and white rice *O. sativa* were observed (10.0 ± 0.0 and 1.4 ± 0.0 μmol AAE/g, respectively) ($p < 0.05$). The ABTS radical scavenging activities of Jingzhou and Huai'an wild rice (24.9 ± 0.1 and 17.0 ± 0.1 μmol AAE/g, respectively) were significantly higher than those of the control samples (red rice, 9.9 ± 0.1 μmol AAE/g; white rice, 1.8 ± 0.0 μmol AAE/g) ($p < 0.05$). In the reducing power assay, Jingzhou and Huai'an wild rice exhibited reducing powers of 63.7 ± 0.3 and 40.3 ± 0.2 μmol AAE/g, respectively, which were obviously higher than those of the control samples (21.5 ± 0.1 μmol AAE/g for red rice and 3.5 ± 0.0 μmol AAE/g for white rice) ($p < 0.05$).

Table 1. Antioxidant activities, total flavonoid content (TFC), and total phenolic content (TPC) of ethanol crude extracts from wild rice and control samples.

Sample	DPPH (μmol AAE/g)	ABTS (μmol AAE/g)	Reducing Power (μmol AAE/g)	TFC (mg QE/g)	TPC (mg GAE/g)
Wild rice (Jingzhou)	45.4 ± 0.2 [a]	24.9 ± 0.1 [a]	63.7 ± 0.3 [a]	16.6 ± 0.2 [a]	4.8 ± 0.2 [a]
Wild rice (Huai'an)	20.8 ± 0.1 [b]	17.0 ± 0.1 [b]	40.3 ± 0.2 [b]	12.6 ± 0.1 [b]	2.1 ± 0.0 [b]
Red rice (*O. sativa*)	10.0 ± 0.0 [c]	9.9 ± 0.1 [c]	21.5 ± 0.1 [c]	6.5 ± 0.1 [c]	1.4 ± 0.0 [c]
White rice (*O. sativa*)	1.4 ± 0.0 [d]	1.8 ± 0.0 [d]	3.5 ± 0.0 [d]	3.2 ± 0.0 [d]	1.3 ± 0.0 [c]

Values are expressed as mean $\pm$ standard error ($n = 3$). Values with different letters in the same column indicate significant differences ($p < 0.05$). AAE, ascorbic acid equivalents; QE, quercetin equivalents; GAE, gallic acid equivalents.

The TFC and TPC of the ethanol crude extracts of wild rice and the control samples were also determined, since most antioxidant activities of plant sources correlate with the phenolic contents [21,25]. The results showed that the TFC (16.6 ± 0.2 mg QE/g) and TPC (4.8 ± 0.2 mg GAE/g) of Jingzhou wild rice were higher than those of Huai'an wild rice (12.6 ± 0.1 mg QE/g and 2.1 ± 0.0 mg GAE/g, respectively). The TFC and TPC of red rice control were 6.5 ± 0.1 mg QE/g and 1.4 ± 0.0 mg GAE/g, respectively. The white rice control contained the lowest levels of TFC (3.2 ± 0.0 mg QE/g) and TPC (1.3 ± 0.0 mg GAE/g) (Table 1) ($p < 0.05$).

These results verified that the antioxidant activity, TFC, and TPC were much higher for wild rice than for red and white rice *O. sativa*, indicating more abundant antioxidants in the former than in the latter. Furthermore, it was observed that the antioxidant profile of Jingzhou wild rice was better than that of Huai'an wild rice. This is probably attributable to the different ecological environments of the two samples, which belong to the Yangtze and Huai River basins, respectively. The level of antioxidants in the plants was influenced by various factors, such as climate, growing conditions, and ripening process. Moreover, stress conditions, such as infection by parasites and pathogens, and air pollution, may have accelerated the increase in some antioxidant metabolites [8].

2.3. Purification and Separation of Antioxidants

2.3.1. Screening of Macroporous Resins

Six different resins were used in the study, to compare their adsorption and desorption performances for antioxidants from wild rice. Figure 1 shows that although the adsorption capacity of D101 resin (17.8 μmol AAE/g) was slightly lower than that of HPD600 resin (19.1 μmol AAE/g), which was the highest among the tested resins, the desorption ratio of D101 resin (90.4%) was higher than that of the other resins. Therefore, D101 resin was selected for further purification and separation. D101 resin exhibited high adsorption and desorption capacities not only because of its appropriate polarity, but also because of its large surface area and ideal average pore diameter, which correlate with the chemical feature of the adsorbate molecules [18]. If the pore diameter is too small, it can restrict the diffusion of adsorbate molecules. On the other hand, if the pore diameter is too large, the adsorbed molecules will be prone to simultaneous desorption [26]. In addition, the low desorption ratios of the polar resins HPD600 and NAK-9 indicated that some antioxidants were irreversibly adsorbed on the resins, which might be due to a strong interaction between the polar hydroxyl groups of the antioxidants and the resins [27].

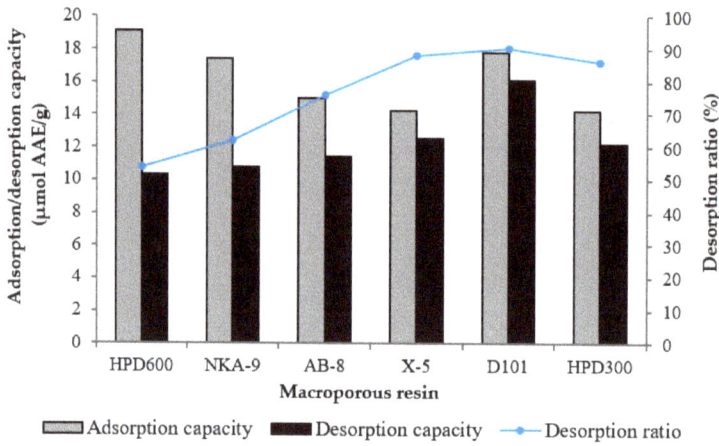

Figure 1. Adsorption, desorption capacities and desorption ratios of the antioxidants on different resins.

2.3.2. Determination of Dynamic Breakthrough Curve

To avoid losses of target compounds during the loading process on the resin column and to make the purification efficient, a dynamic breakthrough curve of the antioxidants on D101 resin was constructed. The antioxidants were almost undetectable in the effluent before 32 mL; then, the antioxidants content in the effluent increased rapidly until it reached a steady plateau at 110 mL (Figure S2 in the Supplementary Materials). According to the standard that a 10% ratio of the exit to the inlet solute concentration is defined as the breakthrough point [18], 44 mL of crude extract solution was determined as the saturated adsorption volume for the D101 resin column.

2.3.3. Antioxidant Activities of Fractions 1–4

The crude extract of Jingzhou wild rice was subjected to a D101 resin column to obtain four fractions (Frs. 1–4). The antioxidant activities of Frs. 1–4 (at a concentration of 0.5 mg/mL) were determined (Figure 2). The percentage scavenging of DPPH and ABTS radicals and the reducing power were highest for Fr. 2, followed by Fr. 1. Frs. 3 and 4 displayed low antioxidant activities. To identify the specific compounds in the bioactive constituents of wild rice, the active Frs. 1 and 2 were analyzed by the HPLC-LTQ-Orbitrap-MS^n.

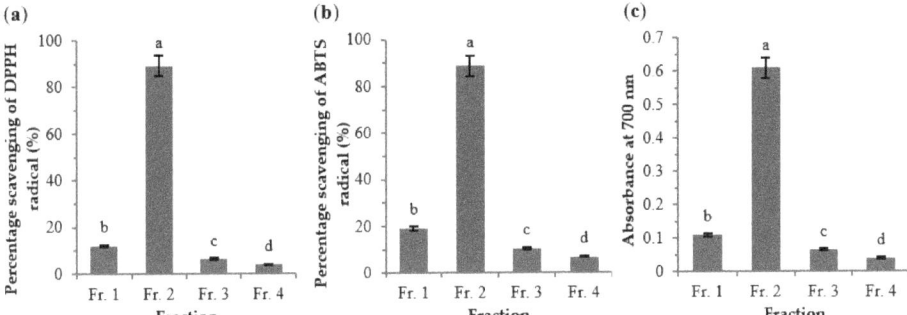

Figure 2. Antioxidant activities of the four fractions (c = 0.5 mg/mL) eluted from D101 resin column by DPPH radical (**a**), ABTS radical (**b**), and reducing power assay (**c**). The results are expressed as mean ± standard deviation (n = 3). Different letters above each bar within the same figure indicate significant differences ($p < 0.05$).

2.4. Identification of Phenolic Acids and Their Derivatives in Fr. 1

Natural phenolic acids are distinguished by hydroxybenzoic acids and hydroxycinnamic acids structures [7]. In this study, eight hydroxybenzoic acids and their derivatives (**A1–7** and **A12**) and four hydroxycinnamic acids (**A8–11**) (the structures are shown in Figure S3 in the Supplementary Materials) were identified from Fr. 1. Table 2 presents the retention times, molecular formulas, measured and calculated deprotonated molecular ions (m/z), mass errors, and major fragment ions (m/z) for the twelve peaks in the base peak chromatogram of Fr. 1 (Figure S4A in the Supplementary Materials). According to the molecular formulas indicated by accurate molecular masses and major fragment ions from losses of molecules of CO_2 (44 Da) and CO (28 Da) in the MS spectra, peaks **A1–12** were identified as gallic acid, protocatechuic acid, p-hydroxybenzoic acid, vanillic acid, p-hydroxybenzaldehyde, syringic acid, vanillin, p-coumaric acid, o-coumaric acid, ferulic acid, sinapic acid, and protocatechuic acid ethyl ester, respectively, which were confirmed by their standards.

Table 2. Identification of phenolic acids and their derivatives in Fr. 1.

Peak [a]	Compound [b]	t_R (min)	Formula	[M − H]⁻ (m/z) Measured	[M − H]⁻ (m/z) Calculated	Error (ppm)	Fragment Ion (m/z)
	Hydroxybenzoic acids and their derivatives						
A1	Gallic acid	3.07	$C_7H_6O_5$	169.0141	169.0142	−0.86	125.0244
A2	Protocatechuic acid	5.70	$C_7H_6O_4$	153.0190	153.0193	−2.15	109.0129
A3	p-Hydroxybenzoic acid	9.08	$C_7H_6O_3$	137.0243	137.0244	−0.59	93.0340, 65.0394
A4	Vanillic acid	11.82	$C_8H_8O_4$	167.0346	167.0350	−2.31	123.0450
A5	p-Hydroxybenzaldehyde	12.00	$C_7H_6O_2$	121.0291	121.0295	−3.51	-
A6	Syringic acid	13.76	$C_9H_{10}O_5$	197.0447	197.0455	−3.94	153.0551, 123.0449
A7	Vanillin	15.19	$C_8H_8O_3$	151.0398	151.0401	−1.83	136.0163, 107.0500
A12	Protocatechuic acid ethyl ester	26.25	$C_9H_{10}O_4$	181.0504	181.0506	−0.98	153.0553
	Hydroxycinnamic acids						
A8	p-Coumaric acid	19.93	$C_9H_8O_3$	163.0397	163.0401	−2.39	119.0500
A9	o-Coumaric acid	20.82	$C_9H_8O_3$	163.0396	163.0401	−2.87	119.0500
A10	Ferulic acid	23.91	$C_{10}H_{10}O_4$	193.0503	193.0506	−2.05	149.0602
A11	Sinapic acid	25.11	$C_{11}H_{12}O_5$	223.0603	223.0612	−4.08	179.0709, 164.0471

[a] Peaks were numbered according to their order of elution from the lowest to the highest retention times.
[b] Identification of the compounds was confirmed by authentic standards. t_R, retention time.

2.5. Identification of Flavonoids and Phenolic Acids in Fr. 2

As one of the most important antioxidants in plants, flavonoids can be classified into different subclasses according to the substitution patterns and degrees of oxidation.

In this study, 22 compounds belonging to various metabolite families that include procyanidins (**B1–8, B11, B13, B18,** and **B19**), flavonoid glycosides (**B9, B10, B12, B15–17**), hydroxycinnamic acid derivatives (**B14** and **B21**), flavonols (**B20**), and flavones (**B22**) were identified from Fr. 2 (Table 3). The structures of the compounds and the base peak chromatogram of Fr. 2 are provided in Figures S3 and S4B in the Supplementary Materials, respectively.

Table 3. Identification of flavonoids and phenolic acids in Fr. 2.

Peak [a]	Compound	t_R (min)	Formula	[M + H]⁺ (m/z) Measured	[M + H]⁺ (m/z) Calculated	Error (ppm)	Fragment Ion (m/z)
	Procyanidins						
B1	Procyanidin B1 [b]	7.63	$C_{30}H_{26}O_{12}$	579.1480	579.1497	−2.87	561.1380, 453.1170, 427.1016, 409.0912, 291.0862, 289.0705
B2	Procyanidin B2 [b]	8.34	$C_{30}H_{26}O_{12}$	579.1480	579.1497	−2.87	561.1380, 453.1170, 427.1016, 409.0912, 291.0862, 289.0705
B3	Procyanidin B3 [b]	9.55	$C_{30}H_{26}O_{12}$	579.1481	579.1497	−2.69	561.1380, 453.1170, 427.1016, 409.0912, 291.0862, 289.0705
B4	Epigallocatechin [b]	10.10	$C_{15}H_{14}O_7$	307.0818	307.0812	1.89	181.0490
B5	Catechin [b]	11.01	$C_{15}H_{14}O_6$	291.0862	291.0863	−0.56	273.0747, 165.0544, 139.0836
B6	Epicatechin [b]	11.08	$C_{15}H_{14}O_6$	291.0862	291.0863	−0.56	273.0347, 165.0544, 139.0836
B7	A-type procyanidin tetramer [c]	12.97	$C_{60}H_{48}O_{24}$	1153.2559	1153.2608	−4.30	865.1963, 713.1592, 577.1334
B8	A-type procyanidin dimer [c]	15.79	$C_{30}H_{24}O_{12}$	577.1326	577.1341	−2.86	559.1220, 451.1013, 425.0858
B11	B-type procyanidin tetramer [c]	17.07	$C_{60}H_{50}O_{24}$	1155.2715	1155.2765	−4.41	1029.2438, 1003.2283, 867.2122
B13	A-type procyanidin trimer [c]	17.96	$C_{45}H_{36}O_{18}$	865.1955	865.1974	−2.27	713.1488, 695.1382, 577.1543
B18	A-type procyanidin trimer [c]	21.07	$C_{45}H_{34}O_{18}$	863.1792	863.1818	−2.95	845.1689, 711.1322, 693.1221
B19	Procyanidin C1 [b]	22.15	$C_{45}H_{38}O_{18}$	867.2138	867.2131	0.92	715.1660, 697.1447
	Flavonoid glycosides						
B9	Rutin [b]	16.10	$C_{27}H_{30}O_{16}$	611.1597	611.1607	−1.69	303.0485
B10	Eriodyctyol 7-O-hexoside [c]	16.81	$C_{21}H_{22}O_{11}$	451.1222	451.1235	−2.91	289.0714, 271.0608, 245.0818
B12	6,8-di-C-hexosyl apigenin [c]	17.36	$C_{27}H_{30}O_{15}$	595.1647	595.1657	−1.80	577.1543, 559.1436, 475.1226, 355.0808
B15	6-C-hexosyl-8-C-pentosyl apigenin [c]	18.79	$C_{26}H_{28}O_{14}$	565.1534	565.1552	−3.13	547.1437, 529.1331, 475.1123, 445.1124, 415.1020, 355.0808
B16	6-C-pentosyl-8-C-hexosyl apigenin [c]	19.35	$C_{26}H_{28}O_{14}$	565.1544	565.1552	−1.39	547.1437, 529.1331, 475.1123, 445.1124, 415.1020, 355.0808
B17	6,8-di-C-pentosyl apigenin [c]	20.69	$C_{25}H_{26}O_{13}$	535.1431	535.1446	−3.86	517.1345, 499.1221, 475.1225, 445.1123, 355.0810
	Others						
B14	Dihydroferulic acid 4-O-glucuronide [c]	18.28	$C_{16}H_{20}O_{10}$	373.1134	373.1129	1.33	355.1022, 197.0807
B20	Quercetin [b]	24.09	$C_{15}H_{10}O_7$	303.0494	303.0499	−1.61	181.0128, 153.0178
B21	3,4,5-Trimethoxycinnamic acid [c]	26.13	$C_{12}H_{14}O_5$	239.0915	239.0914	0.26	224.0684, 195.1019
B22	Tricin [c]	28.05	$C_{17}H_{14}O_7$	331.0796	331.0812	−4.90	316.0568, 301.0340

[a] Peaks were numbered according to their order of elution from the lowest to the highest retention times. [b] Identification of the compound was confirmed by authentic standard. [c] Compound was tentatively identified by comparison with literature data. t_R, retention time.

2.5.1. Procyanidins

Procyanidins, the oligomers and polymers of catechin and epicatechin, can be divided into two different structure types. In the more common B-type procyanidins, the (epi)catechin units are connected through a single bond between C-4 of the upper unit and C-6 or C-8 of the lower unit. The A-type procyanidins differ from the B-type by having an additional bond between adjacent (epi)catechin units that connects C-2 of the upper unit via an oxygen atom to C-7 or the less abundant C-5 of the lower unit [28].

Red rice *O. sativa* has been demonstrated to be a natural source of procyanidins [25]. However, procyanidins from wild rice have not been well studied with the exception of one primary research on North American wild rice, in which only catechin, epicatechin, and four procyanidin oligomers were identified [13].

Twelve procyanidins were identified from Fr. 2. Peaks **B1–3** showed a protonated molecular ion at m/z 579.1480 $[M + H]^+$ with fragment ions at m/z 291.0862 $[M + H - 288]^+$ generated by the loss of an (epi)catechin unit through quinone methide (QM) cleavage of the interflavan bond, and 561.1380 $[M + H - 18]^+$ from the loss a water molecular [28], and three noticeable fragment ions of B-type procyanidin dimers formed by losses of 126, 152, and 170 Da [29]. As is shown in Figure 3, the fragment at m/z 453.1170 $[M + H - 126]^+$ corresponded to the elimination of a phloroglucinol molecule through heterocyclic ring fission (HRF). The fragments at m/z 427.1016 $[M + H - 152]^+$ and 409.0912 $[M + H - 170]^+$ originated from a retro-Diels–Alder (RDA) reaction, and the latter eliminated a water molecule. The fragment at m/z 289.0705 $[M + H - 290]^+$ was generated by QM cleavage of the interflavan bond [28,30]. Accordingly, peaks **B1–3** were respectively identified as procyanidins B1, B2, and B3, based on the standards. Peaks **B4** (m/z 307.0818 $[M + H]^+$), **B5** and **B6** (m/z 291.0862 $[M + H]^+$) were respectively identified as epigallocatechin, catechin, and epicatechin, using the standards. Peak **B7** (m/z 1153.2559 $[M + H]^+$) exhibited fragments at m/z 865.1963 $[M + H - 288]^+$, 713.1592 $[M + H - 288 - 152]^+$, and 577.1334 $[M + H - 288 - 288]^+$ (from QM cleavage and RDA reaction), being identified as an A-type procyanidin tetramer [30]. The protonated molecular ion at m/z 577.1326 $[M + H]^+$ and fragments at m/z 559.1220 $[M + H - 18]^+$ (loss of a water molecule), 451.1013 $[M + H - 126]^+$ (loss of a phloroglucinol molecule), and 425.0858 $[M + H - 152]^+$ (from RDA reaction) led to the assignment of peak **B8** as an A-type procyanidin dimer [29]. Furthermore, a B-type procyanidin tetramer (peak **B11**, m/z 1155.2715 $[M + H]^+$) showing fragments at m/z 1029.2438 $[M + H - 126]^+$ (loss of a phloroglucinol molecule), 1003.2283 $[M + H - 152]^+$ (from RDA reaction), and 867.2122 $[M + H - 288]^+$ (loss of an (epi)catechin unit) was identified [31]. In addition, peaks **B13** (m/z 865.1955 $[M + H]^+$) and **B18** (m/z 863.1792 $[M + H]^+$), with the typical fragment ions of procyanidin oligomers (Table 3), were assigned as A-type procyanidin trimers, on the basis of literature data [30,32]. Peak **B19** (m/z 867.2138 $[M + H]^+$) was identified as procyanidin C1 using the standard.

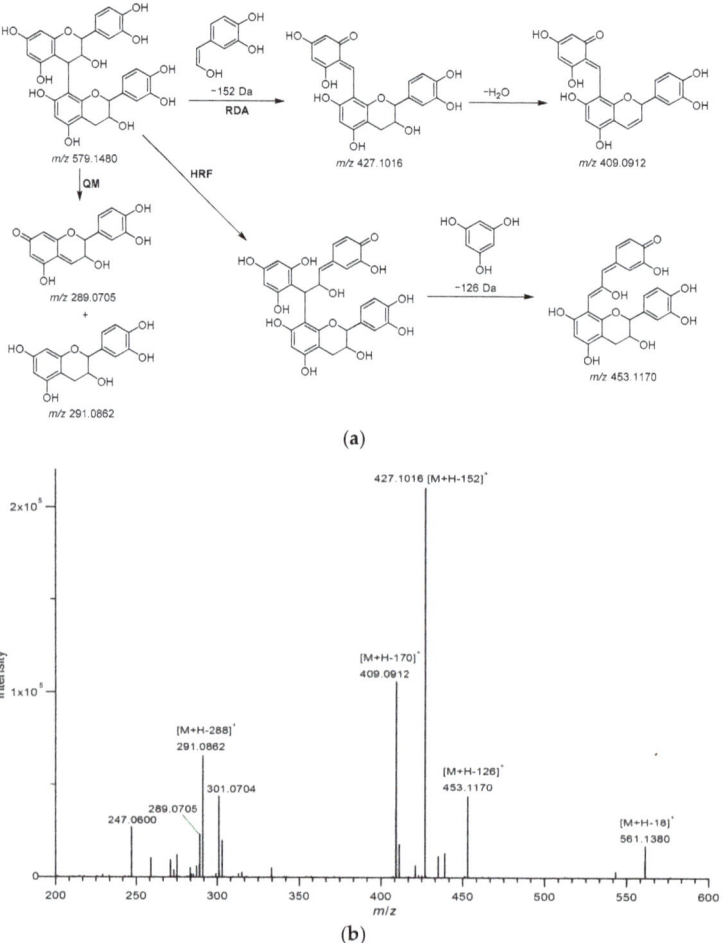

Figure 3. Fragmentation pathway (**a**) and MS^2 spectrum (**b**) of B-type procyanidin dimers. The fragment mechanisms are RDA (retro-Diels-Alder), HRF (heterocyclic ring fission), and QM (quinone methide) cleavage.

2.5.2. Flavonoid Glycosides

Natural flavonoids are usually found in *O*-glycoside and *C*-glycoside forms. Six flavonoid glycosides were identified from Fr. 2. Peak **B9** (*m*/*z* 611.1597 [M + H]$^+$) with a major fragment at *m*/*z* 303.0485 [M + H − 308]$^+$ (loss of a rutinose moiety) was identified as rutin, based on the standard. Peak **B10** had a protonated molecular ion at *m*/*z* 451.1222 [M + H]$^+$, dissociating to yield fragments at *m*/*z* 289.0714 [M + H − 162]$^+$ (loss of a hexose moiety), 271.0608 [M + H − 162 − 18]$^+$ and 245.0818 [M + H − 162 − 44]$^+$ (for the presence of eriodictyol), and was identified as eriodictyol 7-*O*-hexoside [33]. Generally, in the MS spectrum, the characteristic losses for *O*-glycosides are 162 (hexose), 146 (deoxyhexose), and 132 Da (pentose), which correspond to the complete losses of the sugar moieties produced by cleavage at *O*-glycosidic bonds. In contrast to *O*-glycosides, the losses of 120, 90, and 60 Da, formed by cross-cleavages within sugar moieties, and an additional 18 Da representing a water molecule loss, could be diagnostic for *C*-glycosides. In most cases, *C*-glycosylation was found at C-6 and C-8 positions of the flavonoid aglycone [13]. Figure 4 illustrates the fragmentation pattern of the *C*-glycosylated flavonoids (peaks **B12**, **B15–17**) identified from Fr. 2. Peak **B12** (*m*/*z* 595.1647

[M + H]$^+$) produced fragments from losses of water molecules (m/z 577.1543 [M + H − 18]$^+$ and 559.1436 [M + H − 36]$^+$), and 475.1226 [M + H − 120]$^+$ (formed by cross-ring cleavage of the hexose moiety), indicating the presence of a C-diglycosylated flavonoid [34]. The aglycone of apigenin was deduced from the occurrence of a fragment at m/z 355.0808 [M + H − 120 − 120]$^+$ [13]. Therefore peak **B12** was identified as 6,8-di-C-hexosyl apigenin. Peaks **B15** (m/z 565.1534 [M + H]$^+$) and **B16** (m/z 565.1544 [M + H]$^+$) produced fragments at m/z 475.1123 [M + H − 90]$^+$, 445.1124 [M + H − 120]$^+$, 415.1020 [M + H − 60 − 90]$^+$, 547.1437 [M + H − 18]$^+$, and 529.1331 [M + H − 36]$^+$, which suggested that the two compounds were C-glycoside comprising one hexosyl and one pentosyl moiety. Furthermore, a fragment of peaks **B15** and **B16** at m/z 355.0808 [M + H − 120 − 90]$^+$ representing apigenin was also observed. Accordingly, the two compounds were assigned as hexosyl-pentosyl apigenin. According to earlier reports [13,34], in the MS^2 spectrum of 6-C-hexosyl-8-C-pentosyl apigenin, the ion [M + H − 120]$^+$ formed by cross-ring cleavage of the hexose moiety, has a higher relative intensity than that of the ion [M + H − 90]$^+$ from the cross-ring cleavages of both the hexose and pentose moieties, and an opposite result should be obtained for 6-C-pentosyl-8-C-hexosyl apigenin; hence, peaks **B15** and **B16** were concluded to be 6-C-hexosyl-8-C-pentosyl apigenin and 6-C-pentosyl-8-C-hexosyl apigenin, respectively, because higher relative intensities of 445.1124 [M + H − 120]$^+$ for peak 15 and 475.1123 [M + H − 90]$^+$ for peak 16 were observed. Peak **B17** (m/z 535.1431 [M + H]$^+$) exhibited fragments from losses of water molecules (m/z 517.1345 [M + H − 18]$^+$ and 499.1221 [M + H − 36]$^+$), from cross-ring cleavage of the pentose moiety (m/z 475.1225 [M + H − 60]$^+$ and 445.1123 [M + H − 90]$^+$), and for the presence of apigenin (m/z 355.0810 [M + H − 90 − 90]$^+$), and was hence identified as 6,8-di-C-pentosyl apigenin [34].

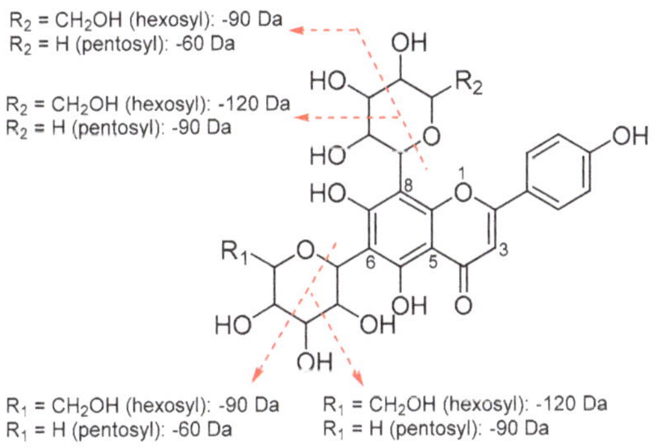

Figure 4. Fragmentation pattern of 6,8-di-C-diglycosylated apigenins.

2.5.3. Others

Peak **B14** (m/z 373.1134 [M + H]$^+$) was identified as hydroferulic acid 4-O-glucuronide, on the basis of the fragments at m/z 355.1022 [M + H − 18]$^+$ (loss of a water molecule) and 197.0807 [M + H − 176]$^+$ (loss of a glucuronic acid moiety) [35]. Peak **B20** (m/z 303.0494 [M + H]$^+$) was identified as quercetin, using the standard. 3,4,5-Trimethoxycinnamic acid (Peak **B21**, m/z 239.0915 [M + H]$^+$), exhibiting fragments at m/z 224.0684 [M + H − 15]$^+$ (loss of a methyl) and 195.1019 [M + H − 44]$^+$ (loss of a CO$_2$ molecule), was identified based on the literature [36]. Peak **B22** (m/z 331.0796 [M + H]$^+$), with fragments at m/z 316.0568 [M + H − 15]$^+$ (loss of a methyl) and 301.0340 [M + H − 30]$^+$ (loss of two methyls), was tentatively assigned as tricin [37].

A total of 34 phenolic compounds were identified from Fr. 1 (mainly low molecular weight phenolic acids) and Fr. 2 (mainly flavonoids). Strong and positive correlations between the phenolics content and antioxidant activities of wild rice measured by DPPH and ABTS radical methods, have been revealed in an earlier report [8]. To the best of our knowledge, 14 compounds, including nine procyanidins (**B1–3**, **B7**, **B8**, **B11**, **B13**, **B18**, and **B19**), two flavonoid glycosides (**B10** and **B16**), two hydroxycinnamic acid derivatives (**B14** and **B21**), and one flavone (**B22**), have been identified from wild rice for the first time, in this study. All the phenolic acids and flavonoids from wild rice, reported previously, are summarized in Table S1 in the Supplementary Materials.

2.6. Quantification of Antioxidants

The contents of the compounds in two wild rice and control samples were determined using the multiple reaction monitoring (MRM) mode of UPLC-QqQ-MS/MS. Due to the lack of available standards, only 21 compounds were quantified. The representative MRM chromatograms of Jingzhou wild rice are shown in Figure 5. The results (Table 4) revealed that significantly higher concentrations of phenolic acids and flavonoids were detected in wild rice than in the control samples. Ferulic acid, followed by gallic acid and sinapic acid, was the most abundant phenolic in both the wild rice samples. Huai'an wild rice had higher amounts of ferulic acid (189.7 ± 1.0 µg/g) and gallic acid (167.1 ± 0.6 µg/g) than those of Jingzhou wild rice (121.1 ± 0.8 and 64.6 ± 0.4 µg/g, respectively), whereas a smaller amount of sinapic acid was detected in Huai'an wild rice (26.8 ± 0.3 µg/g) than in Jingzhou wild rice (59.4 ± 0.4 µg/g). As for the content of total phenolic acids, a higher value of 472.5 µg/g was assessed in Huai'an wild rice than in Jingzhou wild rice (349.3 µg/g). A high content of procyanidins was detected in both the wild rice samples. The results established the following order of procyanidin content in wild rice: epicatechin > procyanidin C1 > catechin > procyanidin B1 > epigallocatechin > procyanidin B3 > procyanidin B2. It was worth noting that, in contrast to total phenolic acids content, the total procyanidins content was higher in Jingzhou wild rice (126.2 µg/g) than in Huai'an wild rice (86.4 µg/g). The control sample red rice contained a total procyanidins content of 28.9 µg/g. No procyanidins were detected in the white rice control. The aforementioned information together with the order of the antioxidant activities of the three samples (Jingzhou wild rice > Huai'an wild rice > red rice > white rice) implied that the antioxidant activity of wild rice may mainly be associated with the accumulation of flavonoids, especially procyanidins, which were found in Fr. 2, the most active fraction. Supporting the aforementioned speculation, an earlier study reported that phenolic acids only constitute a small portion of antioxidant compounds in wild rice, and flavonoids and other phytochemicals may contribute to the bulk of its antioxidant capacity [7].

Table 4. Quantification results (µg/g rice) of phenolic compounds in wild rice and control samples.

Compound	Wild Rice (Jingzhou)	Wild Rice (Huai'an)	Rice (O. sativa) Red	Rice (O. sativa) White
Phenolic acids				
Gallic acid	64.6 ± 0.4 [b]	167.1 ± 0.6 [a]	1.1 ± 0.0 [c]	0.2 ± 0.0 [d]
Protocatechuic acid	15.6 ± 0.2 [a]	12.9 ± 0.1 [b]	7.8 ± 0.1 [c]	nd
p-Hydroxybenzoic acid	11.1 ± 0.1 [a]	7.1 ± 0.1 [b]	nd	0.8 ± 0.0 [c]
Vanillic acid	17.8 ± 0.2 [a]	6.3 ± 0.1 [b]	nd	1.3 ± 0.0 [c]
p-Hydroxybenzaldehyde	15.6 ± 0.1 [a]	12.1 ± 0.1 [b]	nd	nd
Syringic acid	19.5 ± 0.2 [a]	5.1 ± 0.0 [b]	nd	0.9 ± 0.0 [c]
Vanillin	13.0 ± 0.1 [b]	22.3 ± 0.2 [a]	1.0 ± 0.0 [c]	nd
Protocatechuic acid ethyl ester	2.0 ± 0.0 [b]	6.1 ± 0.0 [a]	nd	nd
p-Coumaric acid	6.7 ± 0.0 [a]	7.0 ± 0.1 [a]	1.1 ± 0.0 [b]	1.2 ± 0.0 [b]
o-Coumaric acid	2.9 ± 0.0 [b]	10.0 ± 0.1 [a]	nd	nd
Ferulic acid	121.1 ± 0.8 [b]	189.7 ± 1.0 [a]	12.4 ± 0.3 [c]	10.9 ± 0.1 [d]
Sinapic acid	59.4 ± 0.4 [a]	26.8 ± 0.3 [b]	3.2 ± 0.0 [d]	4.6 ± 0.0 [c]
Total phenolic acids	**349.3**	**472.5**	**26.6**	**19.9**
Flavonoids				
Catechin	21.3 ± 0.3 [a]	15.6 ± 0.2 [b]	6.6 ± 0.1 [c]	nd
Epicatechin	43.3 ± 0.5 [a]	24.3 ± 0.3 [b]	3.5 ± 0.0 [c]	nd
Epigallocatechin	10.0 ± 0.2 [a]	7.5 ± 0.2 [b]	nd	nd
Procyanidin B1	13.0 ± 0.2 [a]	10.2 ± 0.1 [b]	7.0 ± 0.1 [c]	nd
Procyanidin B2	5.0 ± 0.1 [a]	5.5 ± 0.1 [a]	2.4 ± 0.0 [c]	nd
Procyanidin B3	9.4 ± 0.1 [a]	6.3 ± 0.1 [b]	3.4 ± 0.0 [c]	nd
Procyanidin C1	24.2 ± 0.1 [a]	17.0 ± 0.2 [b]	6.0 ± 0.1 [c]	nd
Total procyanidins	**126.2**	**86.4**	**28.9**	**-**
Rutin	103.7 ± 0.7 [a]	83.6 ± 0.5 [b]	20.8 ± 0.2 [c]	15.7 ± 0.2 [d]
Quercetin	15.4 ± 0.1 [b]	44.1 ± 0.2 [a]	16.6 ± 0.2 [c]	nd

Values are mean ± standard error ($n = 5$). Values with different letters in the same row indicate significant differences ($p < 0.05$). nd, not detected.

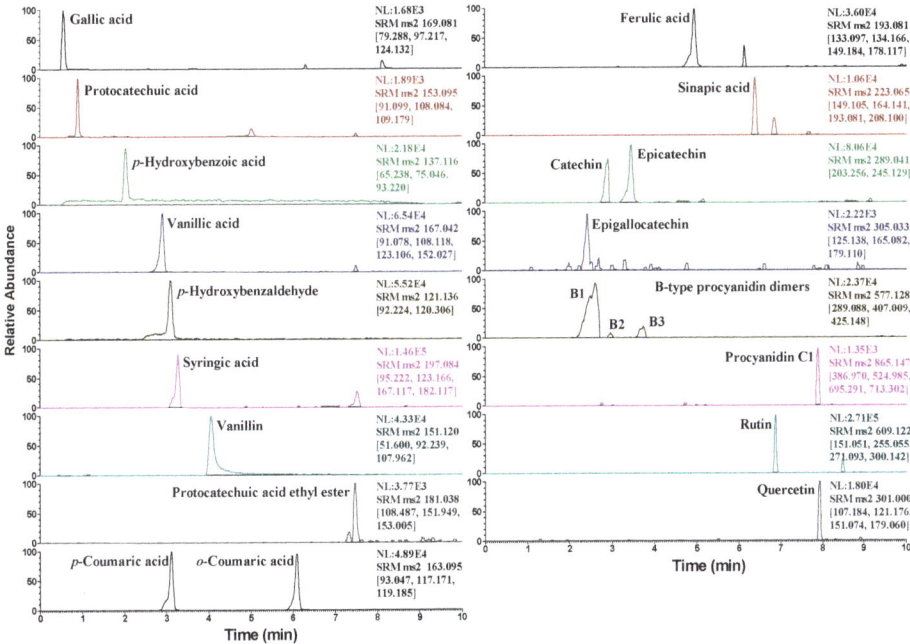

Figure 5. MRM chromatograms of Jingzhou wild rice containing 21 target compounds.

3. Materials and Methods

3.1. Plant Materials and Chemicals

Whole grains of wild rice (*Z. latifolia*) were hand-harvested from Jingzhou (Hubei Province, China) and Huai'an (Jiangsu Province, China) in September 2017. The whole grains of red and white rice *O. sativa* collected from Huai'an was used as control samples. All the freeze-dried rice grains were ground to a fine powder in a mechanical grinder and sieved through a 0.45 mm sifter.

Folin-Ciocalteu reagent, DPPH (2,2-diphenyl-1-picrylhydrazyl) (97% purity), ABTS (2,2′-azino-bis(3-ethylbenothiazoline-6-sulfonic acid) diammonium salt (98% purity), and all the phenolic acid and flavonoid standards (≥99% purity) were purchased from Sigma-Aldrich Chemical Co. (St. Louis, MO, USA). Precoated silica gel plates GF254 purchased from Qingdao Haiyang Chemical Co. Ltd. (Qingdao, China) were used for thin layer chromatography analyses. The LC-MS grade solvents (99.9% purity) were purchased from Sigma-Aldrich Chemical Co (St. Louis, MO, USA). Six macroporous resins, including HPD600, NKA-9, AB-8, X-5, D101, and HPD300, with different physical properties (Table S2 in the Supplementary Materials), were purchased from Solarbio Science & Technology Co. Ltd. (Beijing, China). Before the experiments, the resins were pretreated as previously reported [38].

3.2. Extraction

Twelve different solvents, including six native solvents (ethanol, methanol, acetone, 70% aqueous ethanol, 70% aqueous methanol, and 70% aqueous acetone) alone and acidified with 1% (v/v) acetic acid, were used to obtain antioxidants from wild rice. The rice flour was extracted twice with the solvent in an ultrasonic cleaner for 1 h, at 40 °C and a ratio of liquid to solid of 50 mL/g [7,13]. The mixture was centrifuged at 5000 rpm for 20 min. The supernatants were combined and used as the crude extract to determine the antioxidant activities, TFC, and TPC. The crude extract derived from ethanol, which was concentrated in vacuum, was stored at −20 °C for further purification and identification.

3.3. Evaluation of Antioxidant Activities

The in vitro antioxidant activities were evaluated by DPPH [39] and ABTS radical [40], and reducing power [39] methods, with ascorbic acid as the reference. The results were expressed as micromoles of ascorbic acid equivalents (AAE) per g of rice on a dry weight basis (μmol AAE/g). The antioxidants content measured by the DPPH radical method was expressed as micromoles of ascorbic acid equivalents per mL of the sample solution (μmol AAE/mL).

3.4. Determination of TFC and TPC

The TFC and TPC were measured according to previously described methods [41]. TFC was calculated using a standard quercetin curve and expressed as mg of quercetin equivalents (QE) per g of rice (mg QE/g). TPC was expressed as mg of gallic acid equivalents (GAE) per g of rice (mg GAE/g).

3.5. Screening of Macroporous Resins

Macroporous resins were screened by static adsorption and desorption tests, according to a previously described method [17], with minor modifications. The ethanol crude extract of wild rice was dissolved in distilled water to give a crude extract solution (antioxidants content, 0.50 μmol AAE/mL). 1.0 g of the pretreated resin was put into a 200 mL flask and then 50 mL of the crude extract solution was added. After shaken on an immersion oscillator (120 rpm), at room temperature for 24 h to reach adsorption equilibrium, the resins were washed with deionized water and then desorbed with 50 mL of 70% (v/v) aqueous ethanol in the flask, which was continually shaken (120 rpm) at room temperature for 24 h. The screening of resins was based on the capacities of adsorption and desorption, and the desorption ratio, which were quantified according to Equations (1)–(3):

$$Q_a = (C_0 - C_a) \times V_0/m \tag{1}$$

$$Q_d = C_d \times V_d/m \tag{2}$$

$$D = C_d \times V_d/[(C_0 - C_a) \times V_0] \times 100 \tag{3}$$

where Q_a is the adsorption capacity at adsorption equilibrium (μmol AAE/g dry resin); Q_d is the desorption capacity after adsorption equilibrium (μmol AAE/g dry resin); C_0, C_a, and C_d represent the antioxidants contents of the solution at initial, absorption equilibrium, and desorption status, respectively (μmol AAE/mL); V_0 and V_d are the volumes of the initial sample and desorption solution (mL), respectively; m is the dry weight of resin (g); and D means the desorption ratio (%).

3.6. Determination of Dynamic Breakthrough Curve

The dynamic breakthrough curve of antioxidants on the D101 resin column was constructed using a dynamic adsorption test, which was performed on a glass column (16 × 300 mm) wet-packed with 15.0 g of D101 resin. The bed volume (BV) of the resin was 20 mL. The adsorption process was carried out by overloading the column with the crude extract solution (antioxidants content, 0.50 μmol AAE/mL) at a flow rate of 2 BV/h. The effluent liquids were collected by an automatic fraction collector (4 mL for each tube) and the antioxidants content for each tube was analyzed.

3.7. D101 Macroporous Resin Column Chromatography

The crude extract solution (44 mL) was subjected to a glass column (16 × 300 mm) wet-packed with 15.0 g of D101 resin. After reaching adsorption equilibrium, the resins adsorbed with the sample were initially washed with deionized water (2 BV), and then eluted successively with 10%, 20%, 30%, 40%, 50%, 60%, 70%, 80%, 90%, and 100% (v/v) aqueous ethanol (5 BV for each, 2 BV/h).

In sequence, the effluents of the different eluents were collected and then concentrated and pooled to obtain four fractions (Frs. 1–4) based on their TLC and HPLC fingerprint chromatograms (Figure S5 in the Supplementary Materials). In general, the 10% ethanol eluent was collected as Fr. 1. The 20–30% ethanol eluents were combined as Fr. 2. The eluents of 40–60% ethanol gave Fr. 3. Lastly, the eluents of 70–100% ethanol produced Fr. 4.

3.8. HPLC-LTQ-Orbitrap-MS^n Analysis

An Accella HPLC instrument with a diode-array detector and an autosampler, coupled with an linear ion trap quadrupole Orbitrap XL mass spectrometer (Thermo Scientific, San Jose, CA, USA), was used for the compounds identification. During the analysis, 5 μL of sample was injected and eluted through an Agilent poroshell 120 EC-C18 column (2.7 μm, 4.6 × 150 mm) with a gradient mobile phase consisting of 0.1% (v/v) acetic acid in acetonitrile (solvent A) and 0.1% (v/v) acetic acid in water (solvent B) at a flow rate of 0.3 mL/min. The solvent system used for Fr. 1 was as follows: 0–15 min, 5–10% A; 15–20 min, 10–15% A; 20–25 min, 15–20% A; 25–30 min, 20–5% A. The solvent system used for Fr. 2 was as follows: 0–10 min, 5–10% A; 10–25 min, 10–15% A; 25–30 min, 15–40% A; 30–35 min, 40–5% A.

For mass detection, an electrospray ionization (ESI) source was operated in negative mode with a scan range from m/z 50 to 1000 for Fr. 1, and positive mode with a scan range from m/z 150 to 2000 for Fr. 2. The capillary temperature was 350 °C. Nitrogen was used as the sheath gas and auxiliary gas, and the gas flow was set at 30 arb and 5 arb, respectively. The spray voltage was 4000 V for the positive mode and 3000 V for the negative mode. The collision energy was 35%, to adjust collision-induced dissociation for the best performance. The Xcalibur 2.1 software (Thermo Scientific) was used for data analysis.

The identification of compounds was determined on the basis of their retention times, UV spectra, and accurate mass data; a compound was positively identified when all the data matched those of the standard. Those with no available standards were tentatively identified by comparison with literature data. The mass errors for the quasi-molecular ions of all the identified compounds were within ±5 ppm.

3.9. UPLC-QqQ-MS/MS Analysis

The quantitation of compounds was performed on a UPLC-QqQ-MS/MS system, which consisted of a Waters ACQUITY H-CLASS UPLC instrument equipped with an autosampler (Waters, Milford, MA, USA), and a TSQ Quantum Ultra triple quadrupole tandem mass spectrometer (Thermo Scientific). The analytes were chromatographed by injecting 2 μL of sample into a Waters ACQUITY UPLC BEH C18 column (1.7 μm, 2.1 × 50 mm). The binary mobile phase consisted of 0.1% (v/v) acetic acid in acetonitrile (solvent A) and 0.1% (v/v) acetic acid in water (solvent B), and the solvent gradient was as follows: 0–5 min, 5–10% A; 5–7 min, 10–20% A; 7–8 min, 20–60% A; 8–9 min, 60–100% A; 9–10 min, 100–5% A. The flow rate was 0.3 mL/min.

An ESI source was used with negative ions in the MRM mode. The optimized ion spray voltage was 3000 V. The vaporizer and capillary temperature were 350 and 320 °C, respectively. Nitrogen was used as the sheath gas (30 arb) and auxiliary gas (5 arb), and argon was used as the collision gas (1.5 mTorr). The collision energy was optimized individually for each transition. Data acquisition and processing were performed using the Xcalibur 3.1 software (Thermo Scientific). The ion transitions, optimized MS parameters, and linear relationships of the 21 external standards are listed in Table S3 in the Supplementary Materials.

3.10. Statistical Analysis

All the assays were performed at least in triplicate and data were expressed as mean ± standard error. One-way analysis of variance (ANOVA) followed by Duncan's multiple range test were used to determine statistically different values at a significance level of $p < 0.05$. All the statistical analyses were performed using SPSS 19.0 for Windows (SPSS Inc., Chicago, IL, USA).

4. Conclusions

During this first investigation on the antioxidants from wild rice *Z. latifolia*, the ethanol extract of this species was demonstrated to be a potent source of natural antioxidants, that can be enriched in 10% (Fr. 1) and 20–30% ethanol-eluted fractions (Fr. 2) obtained by D101 macroporous resin column chromatography. The HPLC-LTQ-Orbitrap-MS^n analysis of the active fractions led to the identification of 34 phenolic acids and flavonoids, among which 14 compounds were firstly encountered in wild rice. We found that the active Frs. 1 and 2 mainly contained phenolic acids and flavonoids (including procyanidins and flavonoid glycosides), respectively. These first respective enrichments of phenolic acids and flavonoids provide references for the application of the two families of potential natural antioxidants from wild rice. Compared with phenolic acids, flavonoids may contribute more to the antioxidant activity of wild rice. This study offers new insights into the functional components of wild rice and may advance the understanding and development of the abundant but underutilized *Z. latifolia* resources in East Asia.

Supplementary Materials: Supplementary materials are available online. Table S1: Phenolic acids and flavonoids found in wild rice in previous reports; Table S2: Physical properties of six macroporous resins; Table S3: The ion transitions, optimized MS parameters, and linear relationships of the standards in UPLC-QqQ-MS/MS analysis; Figure S1: The radical scavenging activities of DPPH (A) and ABTS (B), reducing power (C), total flavonoid content (TFC) (D), and total phenolic content (TPC) (E) of different solvent extracts of wild rice collected from Jingzhou; Figure S2: Dynamic breakthrough curve of antioxidants on D101 resin column; Figure S3: Structures of phenolic compounds identified in wild rice; Figure S4: Base peak chromatograms of Frs. 1 (A) and 2 (B) in HPLC-LTQ-Orbitrap-MS^n analysis; Figure S5: HPLC fingerprint chromatograms at 360 nm (A) and 280 nm (B) of the four fractions (Frs. 1–4) eluted from D101 resin column. The gradient solvent system consisting of A (methanol) and B (water containing 0.1% acetic acid, v/v) was as follows: 0–10 min, 5–10% A; 10–30 min, 10–15% A; 30–40 min, 15–20% A; 40–50 min, 20–25% A; 50–60 min, 25–35% A; 60–70 min, 35–90% A; 70–80 min, 90–60% A.

Author Contributions: Z.-F.Z., Y.-M.D. and M.-J.C. conceived and designed the experiments. M.-J.C. and N.Y. performed the experiments. X.-M.L. and F.-Z.W. analyzed the data. M.-J.C. wrote the manuscript. All authors read and approved the final manuscript.

Funding: This research was funded by the Agricultural Science and Technology Innovation Program (ASTIP-TRIC05), the Postdoctoral Applied Research Project Fund of Qingdao, and the Science Foundation for Young Scholars of the Tobacco Research Institute of the Chinese Academy of Agricultural Sciences (2018A01).

Conflicts of Interest: The authors declare no conflict of interest.

References

1. Catling, P.M.; Small, E. Blossoming treasures of biodiversity: 2. North American wild rice (*Zizania species*)—A wild epicurean crop. *Biodiversity* **2001**, *2*, 24–25. [CrossRef]
2. Jiang, M.X.; Zhai, L.J.; Yang, H.; Zhai, S.M.; Zhai, C.K. Analysis of active components and proteomics of Chinese wild rice (*Zizania latifolia* (Griseb) Turcz) and *Indica* rice (*Nagina22*). *J. Med. Food* **2016**, *19*, 798–804. [CrossRef] [PubMed]
3. Han, S.F.; Zhang, H.; Zhai, C.K. Protective potentials of wild rice (*Zizania latifolia* (Griseb) Turcz) against obesity and lipotoxicity induced by a high-fat/cholesterol diet in rats. *Food Chem. Toxicol.* **2012**, *50*, 2263–2269. [CrossRef] [PubMed]
4. Yan, N.; Du, Y.M.; Liu, X.M.; Chu, C.; Shi, J.; Zhang, H.B.; Liu, Y.H.; Zhang, Z.F. Morphological characteristics, nutrients, and bioactive compounds of *Zizania latifolia*, and health benefits of its seeds. *Molecules* **2018**, *23*, 1561. [CrossRef] [PubMed]
5. Zhang, H.; Cao, P.; Agellon, L.B.; Zhai, C.K. Wild rice (*Zizania latifolia* (Griseb) Turcz) improves the serum lipid profile and antioxidant status of rats fed with a high fat/cholesterol diet. *Br. J. Nutr.* **2009**, *102*, 1723–1727. [CrossRef] [PubMed]
6. Lorenz, K.; Lund, D. Wild rice: The Indian's staple and the white man's delicacy. *Crit. Rev. Food Sci.* **1981**, *15*, 281–319. [CrossRef] [PubMed]

7. Qiu, Y.; Liu, Q.; Beta, T. Antioxidant properties of commercial wild rice and analysis of soluble and insoluble phenolic acids. *Food Chem.* **2010**, *121*, 140–147. [CrossRef]
8. Sumczynski, D.; Kotásková, E.; Orsavová, J.; Valášek, P. Contribution of individual phenolics to antioxidant activity and in vitro digestibility of wild rices (*Zizania aquatica* L.). *Food Chem.* **2017**, *218*, 107–115. [CrossRef] [PubMed]
9. Sumczynskia, D.; Koubová, E.; Šenkárová, L.; Orsavová, J. Rice flakes produced from commercial wild rice: Chemical compositions, vitamin B compounds, mineral and trace element contents and their dietary intake evaluation. *Food Chem.* **2018**, *264*, 386–392. [CrossRef] [PubMed]
10. Liu, R.H. Whole grain phytochemicals and health. *J. Cereal Sci.* **2007**, *46*, 207–219. [CrossRef]
11. Shao, Y.F.; Tang, F.F.; Huang, Y.; Xu, F.F.; Chen, Y.L.; Tong, C.; Chen, H.; Bao, J.S. Analysis of genotype × environment interactions for polyphenols and antioxidant capacity of rice by association mapping. *J. Agric. Food Chem.* **2014**, *62*, 5361–5368. [CrossRef] [PubMed]
12. Surendiran, G.; Alsaif, M.; Kapourchali, F.R.; Moghadasian, M.H. Nutritional constitutes and health benefits of wild rice (*Zizania* spp.). *Nutr. Rev.* **2014**, *72*, 227–236. [CrossRef] [PubMed]
13. Qiu, Y.; Liu, Q.; Beta, T. Antioxidant activity of commercial wild rice and identification of flavonoid compounds in active fractions. *J. Agric. Food Chem.* **2009**, *57*, 7543–7551. [CrossRef] [PubMed]
14. Zhai, C.K.; Jiang, X.L.; Xu, Y.S.; Lorenz, K.J. Protein and amino acid composition of Chinese and North American wild rice. *LWT—Food Sci. Technol.* **1994**, *27*, 380–383. [CrossRef]
15. Zhai, C.K.; Lu, C.M.; Zhang, X.Q.; Sun, G.J.; Lorenz, K.J. Comparative study on nutritional value of Chinese and North American wild rice. *J. Food Compos. Anal.* **2001**, *14*, 371–382. [CrossRef]
16. Han, S.F.; Zhang, H.; Qin, L.Q.; Zhai, C.K. Effects of dietary carbohydrate replaced with wild rice (*Zizania latifolia* (Griseb) Turcz) on insulin resistance in rats fed with a high-fat/cholesterol diet. *Nutrients* **2013**, *5*, 552–564. [CrossRef] [PubMed]
17. Zhuang, Y.L.; Ma, Q.Y.; Guo, Y.; Sun, L.P. Purification and identification of rambutan (*Nephelium lappaceum*) peel phenolics with evaluation of antioxidant and antiglycation activities in vitro. *Int. J. Food Sci. Technol.* **2017**, *52*, 1810–1819.
18. Wan, P.F.; Sheng, Z.L.; Han, Q.; Zhao, Y.L.; Cheng, G.D.; Li, Y.H. Enrichment and purification of total flavonoids from *Flos Populi* extracts with macroporous resins and evaluation of antioxidant activities in vitro. *J. Chromatogr. B* **2014**, *945–946*, 68–74. [CrossRef] [PubMed]
19. Arivalagan, M.; Roy, T.K.; Yasmeen, A.M.; Pavithra, K.C.; Jwala, P.N.; Shivasankara, K.S.; Manikantan, M.R.; Hebbar, K.B.; Kanade, S.R. Extraction of phenolic compounds with antioxidant potential from coconut (*Cocos nucifera* L.) testa and identification of phenolic acids and flavonoids using UPLC coupled with TQD-MS/MS. *LWT—Food Sci. Technol.* **2018**, *92*, 116–126. [CrossRef]
20. Fontes-Candia, C.; Ramos-Sanchez, V.; Chavez-Flores, D.; Salmeron, I.; Perez-Vega, S. Extraction of different phenolic groups from oats at a nonthermal pilot scale: Effect of solvent composition and cycles. *J. Food Process Eng.* **2018**, *41*, 12651. [CrossRef]
21. Bao, J.S.; Cai, Y.Z.; Sun, M.; Wang, G.Y.; Corke, H. Anthocyanins, flavonols, and free radical scavenging activity of Chinese bayberry (*Myrica rubra*) extracts and their color properties and stability. *J. Agric. Food Chem.* **2005**, *53*, 2327–2332. [CrossRef] [PubMed]
22. Gullón, B.; Eibes, G.; Moreira, M.T.; Herrera, R.; Labidi, J.; Gullón, P. Yerba mate waste: A sustainable resource of antioxidant compounds. *Ind. Crop. Prod.* **2018**, *113*, 398–405. [CrossRef]
23. Shao, Y.F.; Jin, L.; Zhang, G.; Lu, Y.; Shen, Y.; Bao, J.S. Association mapping of grain color, phenolic content, flavonoid content and antioxidant capacity in dehulled rice. *Theor. Appl. Genet.* **2011**, *122*, 1005–1016. [CrossRef] [PubMed]
24. Min, B.; McClung, A.M.; Chen, M.H. Phytochemicals and antioxidant capacities in rice brans of different color. *J. Food Sci.* **2011**, *76*, 117–126. [CrossRef] [PubMed]
25. Bao, Y.T.; Qu, Y.; Li, J.H.; Li, Y.F.; Ren, X.D.; Maffucci, K.G.; Li, R.P.; Wang, Z.G.; Zeng, R. In vitro and in vivo antioxidant activities of the flowers and leaves from *Paeonia rockii* and identification of their antioxidant constituents by UHPLC-ESI-HRMS^n via pre-column DPPH reaction. *Molecules* **2018**, *23*, 392. [CrossRef] [PubMed]
26. Xu, Z.Y.; Zhang, Q.X.; Chen, J.L.; Wang, L.S.; Anderson, G.K. Adsorption of naphthalene derivatives on hypercrosslinked polymeric adsorbents. *Chemosphere* **1999**, *38*, 2003–2011. [CrossRef]

27. Sandhu, A.K.; Gu, L. Adsorption/desorption characteristics and separation of anthocyanins from muscadine (*Vitis rotundifolia*) juice pomace by use of macroporous adsorbent resins. *J. Agric. Food Chem.* **2013**, *61*, 1441–1448. [CrossRef] [PubMed]
28. Gu, L.; Kelm, M.A.; Hammerstone, J.F.; Zhang, Z.; Beecher, G.; Holden, J.; Haytowitz, D.; Prior, R.L. Liquid chromatographic/electrospray ionization mass spectrometric studies of proanthocyanidins in foods. *J. Mass Spectrom.* **2003**, *38*, 1272–1280. [CrossRef] [PubMed]
29. Ambigaipalan, P.; de Camargo, A.C.; Shahidi, F. Phenolic compounds of pomegranate byproducts (outer skin, mesocarp, divider membrane) and their antioxidant activities. *J. Agric. Food Chem.* **2016**, *64*, 6584–6604. [CrossRef] [PubMed]
30. Li, S.Y.; Xiao, J.; Chen, L.; Hu, C.L.; Chen, P.; Xie, B.J.; Sun, Z.D. Identification of A-series oligomeric procyanidins from pericarp of *Litchi chinensis* by FT-ICR-MS and LC-MS. *Food Chem.* **2012**, *135*, 31–38. [CrossRef]
31. Figueroa, J.G.; Borrás-Linares, I.; Lozano-Sánchez, J.; Segura-Carretero, A. Comprehensive identification of bioactive compounds of avocado peel by liquid chromatography coupled to ultra-high-definition accurate-mass Q-TOF. *Food Chem.* **2018**, *245*, 707–716. [CrossRef] [PubMed]
32. Dudek, M.K.; Gliński, V.B.; Davey, M.H.; Sliva, D.; Kaźmierski, S.; Gliński, J.A. Trimeric and tetrameric A-type procyanidins from peanut skins. *J. Nat. Prod.* **2017**, *80*, 415–426. [CrossRef] [PubMed]
33. Álvarez-Fernández, M.A.; Cerezo, A.B.; Cañete-Rodríguez, A.M.; Troncoso, A.M.; García-Parrilla, M.C. Composition of nonanthocyanin polyphenols in alcoholic-fermented strawberry products using LC–MS (QTRAP), high-resolution MS (UHPLC-Orbitrap-MS), LC-DAD, and antioxidant activity. *J. Agric. Food Chem.* **2015**, *63*, 2041–2051. [CrossRef] [PubMed]
34. Lin, L.Z.; Chen, P.; Harnly, J.M. New phenolic components and chromatographic profiles of green and fermented teas. *J. Agric. Food Chem.* **2008**, *56*, 8130–8140. [CrossRef] [PubMed]
35. Farrell, T.; Poquet, L.; Dionisi, F.; Barron, D.; Williamson, G. Characterization of hydroxycinnamic acid glucuronide and sulfate conjugates by HPLC–DAD–MS^2: Enhancing chromatographic quantification and application in Caco-2 cell metabolism. *J. Pharm. Biomed. Anal.* **2011**, *55*, 1245–1254. [CrossRef] [PubMed]
36. Kargutkar, S.; Brijesh, S. Anti-inflammatory evaluation and characterization of leaf extract of *Ananas comosus*. *Inflammopharmacology* **2018**, *26*, 469–477. [CrossRef] [PubMed]
37. Santos, F.O.; de Lima, H.G.; de Souza Santos, N.S.; Serra, T.M.; Uzeda, R.S.; Alves Reis, I.M.; Botura, M.B.; Branco, A.; Moreira Batatinha, M.J. In vitro anthelmintic and cytotoxicity activities the *Digitaria insularis* (Poaceae). *Vet. Parasitol.* **2017**, *245*, 48–54. [CrossRef] [PubMed]
38. Yang, Q.Y.; Zhao, M.M.; Lin, L.Z. Adsorption and desorption characteristics of adlay bran free phenolics on macroporous resins. *Food Chem.* **2016**, *194*, 900–907. [CrossRef] [PubMed]
39. Yuan, Y.; Xu, X.; Jing, C.L.; Zou, P.; Zhang, C.S.; Li, Y.Q. Microwave assisted hydrothermal extraction of polysaccharides from *Ulva prolifera*: Functional properties and bioactivities. *Carbohydr. Polym.* **2018**, *181*, 902–910. [CrossRef] [PubMed]
40. Re, R.; Pellegrini, N.; Proteggente, A.; Pannala, A.; Yang, M.; Rice-Evans, C. Antioxidant activity applying an improved ABTS radical cation decolorization assay. *Free Radic. Biol. Med.* **1999**, *26*, 1231–1237. [CrossRef]
41. Tang, Y.; Li, X.H.; Zhang, B.; Chen, P.X.; Liu, R.H.; Tsao, R. Characterisation of phenolics, betanins and antioxidant activities in seeds of three *Chenopodium quinoa* Willd. genotypes. *Food Chem.* **2015**, *166*, 380–388. [CrossRef] [PubMed]

Sample Availability: Not available.

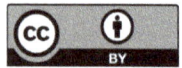

© 2018 by the authors. Licensee MDPI, Basel, Switzerland. This article is an open access article distributed under the terms and conditions of the Creative Commons Attribution (CC BY) license (http://creativecommons.org/licenses/by/4.0/).

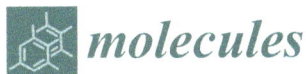

Article

An Accurate and Effective Method for Measuring Osimertinib by UPLC-TOF-MS and Its Pharmacokinetic Study in Rats

Song-Tao Dong [1,2], Ying Li [1], Hao-Tian Yang [1], Yin Wu [1], Ya-Jing Li [1], Cong-Yang Ding [1], Lu Meng [1], Zhan-Jun Dong [1,*] and Yuan Zhang [3,*]

1. National Clinical Drug Monitoring Center, Department of Pharmacy, Hebei Province General Center, Shijiazhuang 050051, China; dongsongtao8886@163.com (S.-T.D.); lyyaoda@126.com (Y.L.); yanghaotian0917@163.com (H.-T.Y.); Wuyin82@126.com (Y.W.); 15369305382@163.com (Y.-J.L.); dingcy1989@126.com (C.-Y.D.); M18203213683@163.com (L.M.); dzjhbgh@126.com (Z.-J.D.)
2. Department of Pharmaceutics, School of Pharmacy, China Medical University, Shenyang 110001, China
3. Department of Pharmacy, National Cancer Center/National Clinical Research Center for Cancer, Chinese Academy of Medical Sciences and Peking Union Medical College, Beijing 100021, China
* Correspondence: dzjhbgh@126.com (Z.-J.D.); 13840149878@163.com or zhangyuan@cicams.ac.cn (Y.Z.); Tel.: +86-0311-8598-8604 (Z.-J.D.); +86-010-8778-8040 (Y.Z.)

Academic Editor: In-Soo Yoon
Received: 15 October 2018; Accepted: 3 November 2018; Published: 6 November 2018

Abstract: Osimertinib, a new-generation inhibitor of the epidermal growth factor, has been used for the clinical treatment of advanced T790M mutation-positive tumors. In this research, an original analysis method was established for the quantification of osimertinib by ultra-performance liquid chromatography with time of flight mass spectrometry (UPLC-TOF-MS) in rat plasma. After protein precipitation with acetonitrile and sorafinib (internal standard, IS), they were chromatographed through a Waters XTerra MS C_{18} column. The mobile phase was acetonitrile and water (including 0.1% ammonia). The relative standard deviation (RSD) of the intra- and inter-day results ranged from 5.38 to 9.76% and from 6.02 to 9.46%, respectively, and the extraction recovery and matrix effects were calculated to range from 84.31 to 96.14% and from 91.46 to 97.18%, respectively. The results illustrated that the analysis method had sufficient specificity, accuracy and precision. Meanwhile, the UPLC-TOF-MS method for osimertinib was successfully applied into the pharmacokinetics of SD rats.

Keywords: osimertinib; UPLC-TOF-MS; rat; pharmacokinetics

1. Introduction

Osimertinib (AZD9291, Merelitinib, Tagriiso©), *N*-(2-{2dimethylaminoethyl-methylamino}-4-methoxy-5-{[4-(1-methylindol-3-yl)pyrimidin-2yl]amino}phenyl)prop-2-enamide (Figure 1), a third-generation, highly selective, irreversible covalent inhibitor has been created by AstraZeneca for the clinical therapy of advanced non-small cell lung cancer (NSCLC) [1–6]. NSCLC patients, who have epidermal growth factor receptor (EGFR) tyrosine kinase inhibitor (TKI) resistance, are mostly subject to a mutation of EGFR. Therefore, this has been the active target for the osimertinib [7–9]. In addition, the tablet formulation of osimertinib has been approved by the FDA (Food and Drug Administration of the USA) for NSCLC patients, who have progressed to or completed EGFR TKI therapy in 2015.

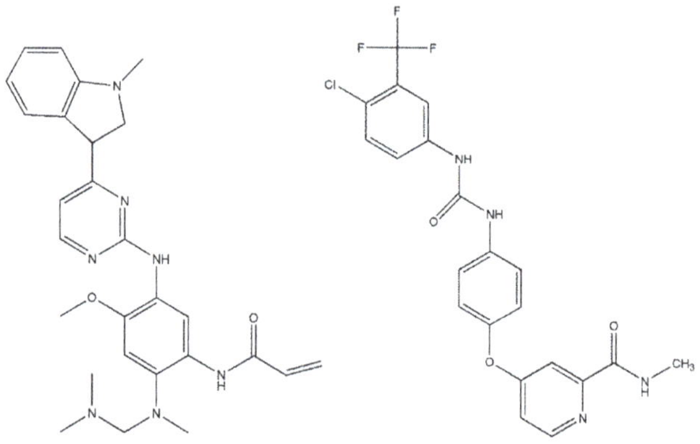

Figure 1. Structures of osimertinib (molecular weight = 499.619 Da) and sorafenib (molecular weight = 464.825 Da).

To the best of our knowledge, several papers have established the methods for the determination of osimertinib in biological samples, and the utilized apparatuses are all ultra-performance liquid chromatography coupled with tandem mass spectrometry (UPLC-MS/MS) [10–13]. There are some advantages of UPLC-MS/MS, including its high sensitivity, high stability, and short analytic time. Unlike UPLC-MS/MS, UPLC-TOF-MS has specific advantages such as its high working efficiency, wide measurable mass range, and high ratio of resolution [14–17]. In addition, the capability of simultaneous quantitative analysis and qualitative analysis greatly benefits the analysts, and it is very useful for the further study of agents, such as their metabolism, enzymology, transportation and so on [18]. However, to date, methods using UPLC-TOF-MS for the determination of osimertinib have not been reported. In the present study, we are the first to quantify osimertinib in rat plasma using UPLC-TOF-MS.

The objective of this study was to investigate a specific, sensitive, rapid and reliable UPLC-TOF-MS method for osimertinib quantification in rat plasma samples. Meanwhile, we have successfully investigated the pharmacokinetic study of osimertinib in rats using this UPLC-TOF-MS method.

2. Results and Discussion

2.1. UPLC-TOF-MS Method Development

By using the product scan mode, we could find the method of pyrolysis of osimertinib and ion of sorafenib (IS) in rat plasma under the UPLC-TOF-MS condition that we have optimized (see Section 2.3) (Figure 2). The parent ion m/z of osimertinib was 500.2768 and the characteristic product ion was 72.0810. In addition, the m/z of the parent ion and product ion of sorafenib (IS) were 465.0953 and 270.0882, respectively. All these results are consistent with previous studies [4–7,19].

However, the optimization of the UPLC condition became the key point in the process of investigating our UPLC-TOF-MS method. We used various proportions and gradients of water (containing 0.1% formic acid)–acetonitrile and water (containing 0.1% formic-ammonia formate)–acetonitrile to optimize the chromatographic conditions. However, the chromatographic peaks all displayed the trailing phenomenon (Figure S1). Since the pKa of osimertinib was 13.64, it needs a basic environment to keep its molecular state. Therefore, we decided to use 0.1% ammonia water–acetonitrile as the mobile phase, which enabled us to finally obtain the symmetrical chromatographic peak (Figure 3).

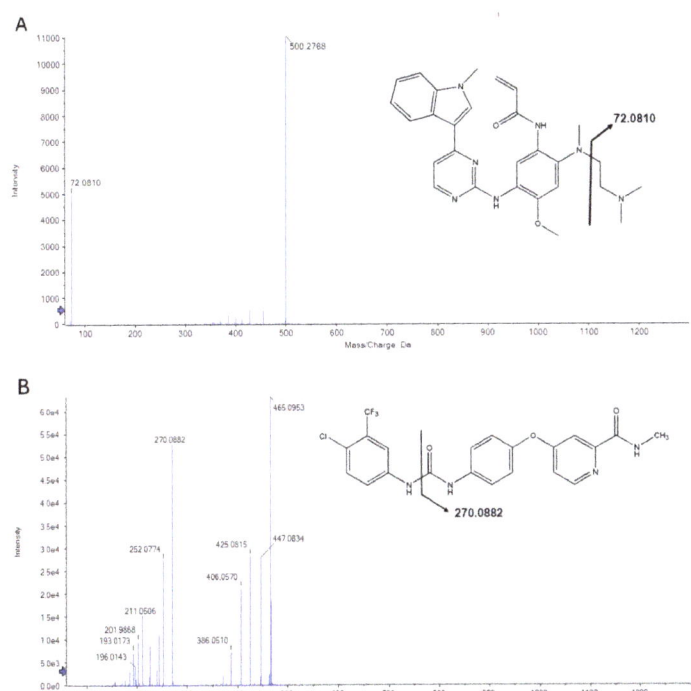

Figure 2. Product ion scan of osimertinib 500.2768 → 72.0810 (**A**), and IS 465.0953 → 270.0882 (**B**).

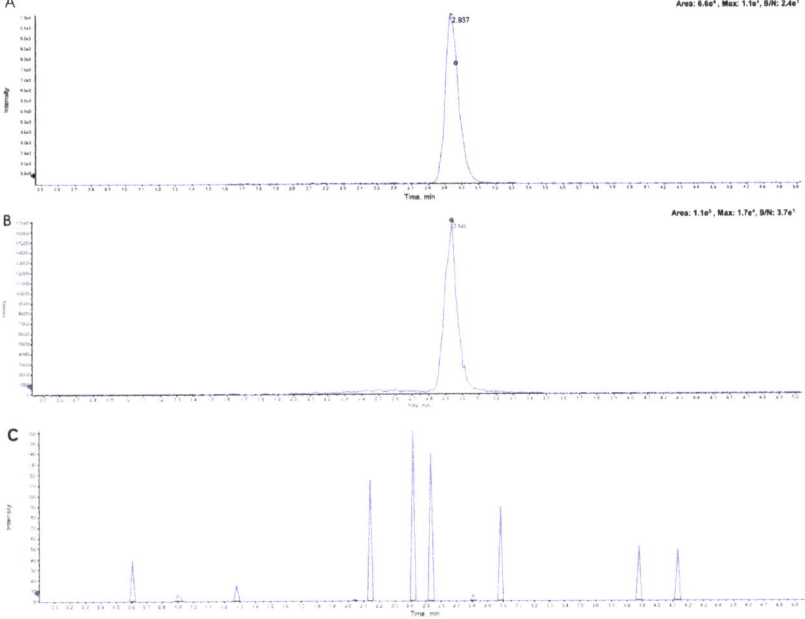

Figure 3. *Cont.*

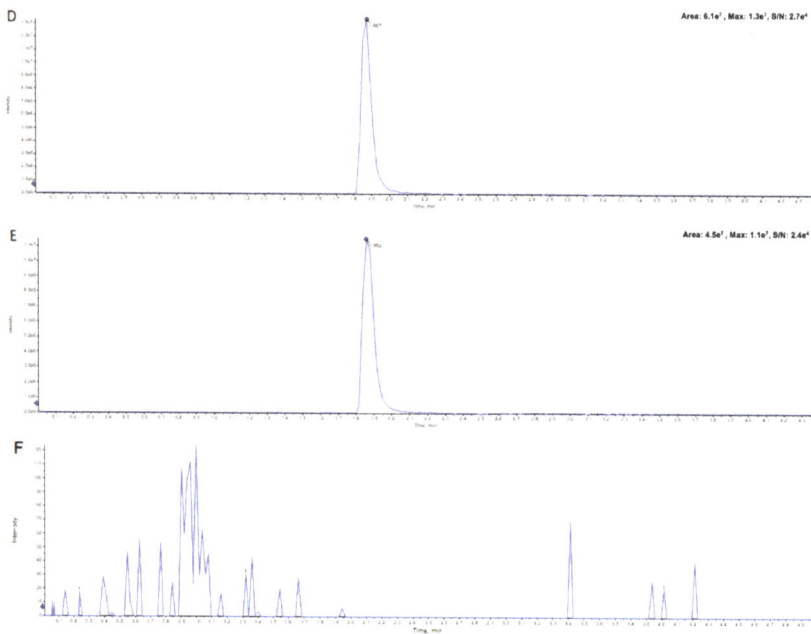

Figure 3. Typical chromatograms of (**A**) standard osimertinib (20 ng/mL) in rat plasma, (**B**) pharmacokinetic plasma sample, (**C**) blank plasma, (**D**) standard ion of sorafenib (IS) (500 ng/mL) in rat plasma, (**E**) pharmacokinetic plasma sample, and (**F**) blank plasma.

2.2. Method Validation

2.2.1. Specificity and Selectivity

The typical chromatograms of blank plasma, the plasma sample spiked with osimertinib and IS and rat plasma after treatment are shown in Figure 3. Figure 3A–C displays the characteristic peaks of standard osimertinib in rat plasma, the pharmacokinetic plasma sample and blank plasma, and the chromatograms showed a good specificity. In addition, Figure 3D–F exhibits the good specificity of standard sorafenib (IS). Moreover, these results also showed that there was no significant chromatographic interference with the osimertinib and IS in rat plasma.

2.2.2. Calibration and Lower Limit of Quantification (LLOQ)

To investigate the linearity of osimertinib and IS, nine calibration concentrations were analyzed in each validation batch, and the results showed the good linearity ($r^2 > 0.99$) of the calibration curve of osimertinib and IS over the range of 1 to 500 ng/mL. The lower limits of quantification (LLOQ) of osimertinib and IS were both 1 ng/mL, and the ratios of signal-to-noise were considerably higher than 5. In addition, the LLOQ of this UPLC-TOF-MS method was sufficient for the determination of the osimertinib pharmacokinetic study.

2.2.3. Precision and Accuracy

The intra- and inter-day precision and accuracy are shown in Table 1. In addition, the intra- and inter-day results of the HQC, MQC and LQC are investigated with the RSD ranging from 5.38–9.76% (intra-day) and 6.02–9.46% (inter-day), respectively. The results ranged within the standard acceptance limit of 15% and demonstrated the good accuracy and precision of osimertinib.

Table 1. Intra- and inter-day precision and accuracy of osimertinib in rat plasma. RSD: relative standard deviation.

Concentration (ng/mL)	Intra-Day (n = 7)			Inter-Day (n = 7)		
	Measured Conc. (ng/mL)	Precision, RSD (%)	Accuracy (%)	Measured Conc. (ng/mL)	Precision RSD (%)	Accuracy (%)
400	395.12 ± 21.27	5.38	98.78	401.13 ± 24.15	6.02	100.28
20	21.08 ± 1.42	6.74	105.40	19.34 ± 1.83	9.46	96.70
2	2.05 ± 0.20	9.76	102.50	1.98 ± 0.17	8.59	99.00

2.2.4. Extraction Recovery and Matrix Effect

Table 2 shows the extraction recovery of osimertinib and IS, and these results are sufficient for quantification. The matrix effects of osimertinib and IS range from 0.810 to 0.926 and from 0.798 to 0.934, respectively (Table 3). The calibration curves of the final concentrations of IS were the same as those of osimertinib. The results showed the high extraction recovery and lack of significant matrix effect of this method for osimertinib and IS in the rat plasma.

Table 2. Extraction recovery and matrix effect of osimertinib and IS in rat plasma.

Analyte	Concentration (ng/mL)	Extraction Recovery (%)	
		Mean ± SD	RSD
Osimertinib	400	95.24 ± 3.01	3.16
	20	96.14 ± 1.83	1.90
	2	84.31 ± 3.18	3.77
Sorafinib	500	87.22 ± 4.23	4.85

Table 3. The slope ratio of the solvent linear equation and the matrix linear equation.

Analyte	Calibration Curve	R^2	R_{slope}		
			Min	Max	ΔR
Osimertinib	Y = 0.085X + 0.1102	0.9997	0.810	0.926	0.116
Sorafinib	Y = 0.0781X + 0.2314	0.9996	0.798	0.934	0.136

R_{slope} = Slope of matrix standard calibration curve/slope of mobile phase standard calibration curve.

2.2.5. Stability

Table 4 shows the stability of HQC, MQC and LQC of osimertinib under four different storage conditions. According to the results, osimertinib was found to have good stability at room temperature (25 °C) and the autosampler temperature (4 °C) for 24 h and remained stable following three freeze (−80 °C) and thaw (0 °C) cycles. Moreover, the plasma samples of osimertinib were also stable at the storage temperature (−80 °C) for at least 30 days.

Table 4. Stability of osimertinib in rat plasma under various storage conditions.

Storage Condition	Concentration (ng/L)	Mean ± SD	RSD%
Autosampler (4 °C) temperature for 24 h	2	2.12 ± 0.23	10.85
	20	21.45 ± 1.81	8.44
	400	406.81 ± 5.64	1.39
Room temperature (25 °C) for 24 h	2	2.21 ± 0.26	3.66
	20	22.45 ± 2.18	9.71
	400	407.28 ± 5.12	1.26
Storage temperature (−80 °C) for 30 days	2	2.29 ± 0.25	10.92
	20	21.33 ± 1.74	8.16
	400	406.34 ± 7.51	1.85
Three freeze–thaw cycles (each at −80 °C for 24 h)	2	2.27 ± 0.19	8.37
	20	22.20 ± 1.92	8.65
	400	406.17 ± 6.19	1.52

2.3. Pharmacokinetic Application

After successfully establishing the analysis method of osimertinib by UPLC-TOF-MS, we applied this method into the pharmacokinetic study in SD rats. The dosage of the oral administration was 4.5 mg/kg and the mean plasma time-concentration of osimertinib in seven rats is shown in Figure 4. This showed that the osimertinib had the highest plasma concentration at 4.5 h after oral administration and the C_{max} was 28.49 ng/mL. In addition, Table 5 shows the following non-compartmental parameters of osimertinib in SD rats: a terminal half-life of (14.96 ± 3.44) h, a distribution volume of (233.82 ± 66.68) L/kg, and a clearance of about (10.84 ± 1.94) L/h/kg (Table 5). These pharmacokinetic data of osimertinib can provide more information regarding its application in clinical treatment.

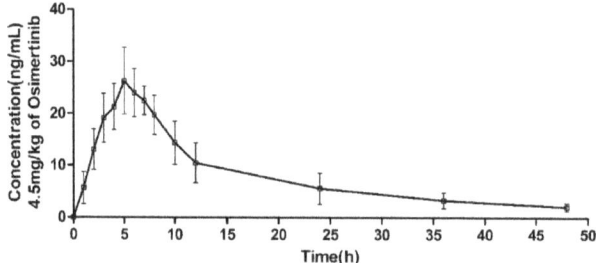

Figure 4. Plasma concentration-time profile after single oral administration of osimertinib (4.5 mg/kg) to rats. Data are expressed as the mean ± SD (n = 7).

Table 5. Pharmacokinetic parameters of osimertinib after oral administration of 4.5 mg/kg to rats.

Pharmacokinetic Parameter	Osimertinib
$AUC_{(0-t)}$, ng/mL·h	382.00 ± 69.00
$AUC_{(0-\infty)}$, ng/mL·h	426.01 ± 81.73
MRT, h	14.51 ± 1.91
$t_{1/2z}$, h	14.96 ± 3.44
t_{max}, h	4.80 ± 1.10
C_{max}, ng/mL	28.49 ± 3.97
V_z/F, L/kg	233.82 ± 66.68
CL_z/F, L/h/kg	10.84 ± 1.94

Data are expressed as the mean ± SD (n = 7).

3. Materials and Methods

3.1. Drugs and Materials

Osimertinib (purity >99%) and sorafenib (internal standard, IS) were purchased from Stanford Analytical Chemicals Inc. (Eugene, OR, USA). Dimethyl sulfoxide (DMSO) was purchased from Beijing Solarbio Science and Technology Co., Ltd. (Beijing, China). Ammonia and acetonitrile (HPLC grade) were provided by Tianjin Kemiou Chemical Reagent Co., Ltd. (Tianjin, China) and the Fisher Scientific Co., Ltd. (Pittsburgh, PA, USA), respectively. Ultrapure water was obtained from a milli-Q reagent water purification system (Millipore, Bedford, MA, USA).

3.2. Apparatus

The UPLC-TOF-MS/MS method was performed on a system that includes a Qtrap 5600-TOF mass spectrometer (AB Sciex, MA, USA) and an UPLC chromatographic analysis system (Shimadzu, Kyoto, Japan). An Xterra MS C_{18} column (100 × 2.1 mm, 3.5 μm) (Waters Corp., Milford, MA, USA) was used for the analytical separation at the temperature of 40 °C. A TGL-16M high speed centrifuge was purchased from Cence Co., Ltd. (Changsha, China).

3.3. Solution Preparation

DMSO was used to dissolve the accurately weighed standard of osimertinib and sorafenib (IS) to obtain the stock solutions of 1.0 mg/mL. Then, the working solutions of osimertinib were diluted serially with 50% acetonitrile in water to achieve 10, 20, 50, 100, 200, 500, 1000, 2000 and 5000 ng/mL. Next, 10 µL diluted solutions were diluted in 100 µL blank plasma to obtain the final calibration standard samples, and the range of the final concentrations of the calibration standards was from 1 to 500 ng/mL.

The working solution concentration of IS was 500 ng/mL, which was dissolved using 50% acetonitrile water (v/v). The quality controls (QCs) were diluted to achieve the lower limit of the quantification (10 ng/mL, LLOQ), low (20 ng/mL, LQC), medium (200 ng/mL, MQC), and high (4000 ng/mL, HQC) concentrations of osimertinib. After that step, 10 µL of the QC solutions were dissolved by 100 µL of blank plasma to get the final concentrations of LLOQ (1 ng/mL), LQC (2 ng/mL), MQC (20 ng/mL), HQC (400 ng/mL) and 50 ng/mL of IS. All samples and working solutions were kept at −20 °C before use.

3.4. UPLC-TOF-MS Condition

The chromatographic separation was performed using a C_{18} column, and its temperature was kept at 40 °C. The chromatographic separation consisted of a 0.1% ammonia (A) and acetonitrile (B) mixture and a 0.4 mL/min flow rate was maintained. The gradient ran linearly from 10% to 95% between 0 and 1.5 min, and then the mobile phase was kept at 95% for 5.0 min. 3.0 µL of samples was injected into the analysis system and the total analytical time of one sample was 5.1 min. The temperature of the autosampler was maintained at 4 °C.

The TOF-MS spectrometer was set up in the positive ion full scan electrospray and high sensitivity mode with an m/z range from 100 to 1000 Da, and the accumulation time was set as 0.25s. The parameters of TOF-MS were as follows: nebulizer gas (gas 1), 55 psi; heater gas (gas 2), 55 psi; curtain gas, 35 psi; ion spray voltage, 5500 V; turbo spray temperature, 550 °C; declustering potential (DP), 100 V; and collision energy (CE), 35 eV. The conditions of the information-dependent data acquisition (IDA) criteria were as follows. The eight most intense fragment ions of each analyte in 100 cps were chosen as the product ions, and the m/z of the product ions ranged from 600 to 1300 over a 0.08 s accumulation time. In addition, the CE and collision energy scope (CES) of the product ions scan were set at 35 eV and 15 eV, respectively.

3.5. Pharmacokinetic Application

The pharmacokinetic study of osimertinib was applied to seven male SD rats using oral administration by gavage and the dosage was 4.5 mg/kg. Osimertinib was diluted and suspended by 0.5% sodium carboxymethylcellulose. No less than 0.3 mL rat plasma was sampled at 0, 1, 2, 3, 4, 5, 6, 7, 8, 10, 12, 24, 36, and 48 h after oral administration through the oculi chorioideae vein under the condition of light ether anesthesia. After 10 min centrifuging of all analytes at 5000× g, the supernatant was collected and frozen at −40 °C until analysis. The use of animals in the presented study was permitted by the Ethics Committee of the Hebei Medical University, and all animal studies were carried out according to the Guidance for the Care and Use of Laboratory Animals of the US National Institute of Health.

3.6. Sample Preparation

Ten microliters of IS solution (500 ng/mL) was prepared in 100 µL rat plasma and vortex-mixed for 20 s. After that step, 500 µL of acetonitrile was added to precipitate the protein. Then, the mixture was vortexed for 1 min and centrifuged at 12,000 rpm for 10 min. The supernatant was transferred into a new Eppendorf tube and evaporated to dryness through nitrogen gas at 45 °C. After 100 µL of acetonitrile was added to reconstitute the residue and vortexed for 1 min, all samples were centrifuged at 12,000× *g* for 10 min. Finally, 80 µL of the supernatant was collected and injected into UPLC sample vials before use.

3.7. Method Validation

According to the US Food and Drug Administration (FDA) guidelines regarding the bioanalytical method's validation [20], the method validation was investigated and established, including the specificity and selectivity, the linearity and sensitivity, the recovery, the stability, and the precision, accuracy and matrix effect.

3.7.1. Selectivity and Specificity

The selectivity and specificity of the developed method was assessed by comparing the chromatography of the blank plasma and blank plasma spiked with the targets.

3.7.2. Linearity and Sensitivity

A series of calibration analytes from 1 to 500 ng/mL consisted of the calibration curve of osimertinib. In addition, the method to determine the linearity of calibration curve was the peak area ratios of osimertinib and IS, and these ratios were used to get a least-squares weighted regression (the weighting factor was 1/y, and y = peak area ratio of osimertinib/IS). The correlation coefficient (r^2) of all calibration curves, which were desirable for this method, were better than or equal to 0.99.

LLOQ was used to investigate the method sensitivity and follows these two criteria: (1) the comparison of the LLOQ and blank response should occur at least 5 times; and (2) the analyte peak of the LLOQ should be discrete, reproducible and identifiable, and its accuracy and precision should be at least 20%.

3.7.3. Precision, Accuracy and Matrix Effect

The intra-day accuracy and precision were investigated through the determination of six QC analytes of the high (HQC = 400 ng/mL), medium (MQC = 20 ng/mL), low (LQC = 2 ng/mL), and LLOQ (LLOQ = 1 ng/mL) concentrations. The inter-day accuracy and precision were conducted through the determination of the six replicates of the four levels of QCs using the same preparation on 3 separate days. The assay accuracy of the QC samples was compared to the corresponding standard calibration concentration. The precision of the replicates was evaluated by the RSD (relative standard deviation).

It can be accepted that the mean values of accuracy should not exceed 15% at the HQC and MQC, and LQC concentrations and LLOQ should not exceed 20%. Similarly, the relative standard deviation of the precision for HQC, MQC, and LQC concentration levels should not exceed 15% and the limitation of LLOQ was 20%.

The matrix effect was determined by dividing slopes of calibration curves of osimertinib in the rat blood matrix and mobile phase.

3.7.4. Recovery

The extraction recovery of osimertinib was evaluated by comparing the peak area ratios of standard solution samples and the same concentrations rat plasma samples through five replicates at HQC, MQC and LQC concentrations.

3.7.5. Stability

The stabilities of this method, which include the freeze–thaw stability, autosampler stability, short-term stability and long-term stability, were evaluated through three QC samples after the sample preparation method. The freeze (−80 °C)–thaw (room temperature) stability was conducted under the conditions of three free–thaw cycles. The autosampler stability of the plasma samples was investigated by the extracted QC samples that were kept in an autosampler (4 °C) for 12 h. In addition, the long-term stability was evaluated through the determination of three QC samples that were kept at −80 °C for 30 days. All samples were considered stable with RSDs < ±15%.

3.8. Data Analysis

Dynamic background subtraction is a novel technique performed using the Analyst software (AB Sciex, Foster City, CA, USA). In addition, the data of the pharmacokinetic study of osimertinib were collected and calculated by the DAS 2.1.1 software in the non-compartmental mode (Mathematical Pharmacology Professional Committee of China, Shanghai, China).

4. Conclusions

A sensitive UPLC-TOF-MS method for the determination of osimertinib has been established in this research. The method exhibited excellent precision, recovery and sensitivity. The results indicated that UPLC-TOF-MS could serve as a highly interesting analytical alternative for bioanalysis.

Supplementary Materials: The following are available online.

Author Contributions: Conceived and designed the experiments: Y.Z., Z.-J.D. and S.-T.D. Performed the experiments: S.-T.D., Y.L., H.-T.Y., Y.W., Y.-J.L., C.-Y.D., L.M. and Z.-J.D. Analyzed the data: S.-T.D. Wrote the paper: Y.Z. and S.-T.D. All authors read and approved the final manuscript.

Acknowledgments: This work was supported by the Liaoning Planning Program of Philosophy and Social Science (NO. L17BGL034), the Research Program on the Reform of Undergraduate Teaching in General Higher Schools in Liaoning (NO. 2016-346), the Key Program of the Natural Science Foundation of Liaoning Province of China (NO. 20170541027) and the Medical Education Scientific Research on the "12th Five-Year Plan" (Fifth Batch of Subjects) funded by China Medical University (NO. YDJK2015005).

Conflicts of Interest: The authors declared no conflict of interest.

References

1. Chen, Z.; Chen, Y.; Xu, M.; Chen, L.; Zhang, X.; To, K.K.; Zhao, H.; Wang, F.; Xia, Z.; Chen, X.; et al. Osimertinib (AZD9291) enhanced the efficacy of chemotherapeutic agents in ABCB1- and ABCG2-overexpressing cells in vitro, in vivo, and ex vivo. *Mol. Cancer Ther.* **2016**, *15*, 1845–1858. [CrossRef] [PubMed]
2. Cross, D.A.; Ashton, S.E.; Ghiorghiu, S.; Eberlein, C.; Nebhan, C.A.; Spitzler, P.J.; Orme, J.P.; Finlay, M.R.; Ward, R.A.; Mellor, M.J.; et al. AZD9291, an irreversible EGFR TKI, overcomes T790M-mediated resistance to EGFR inhibitors in lung cancer. *Cancer Discov.* **2014**, *4*, 1046–1061. [CrossRef] [PubMed]
3. Yang, M.; Tong, X.; Xu, X.; Zheng, E.; Ni, J.; Li, J.; Yan, J.; Shao, Y.W.; Zhao, G. Case Report: Osimertinib achieved remarkable and sustained disease control in an advanced non-small-cell lung cancer harboring EGFR H773L/V774M mutation complex. *Lung Cancer* **2018**, *121*, 1–4. [CrossRef] [PubMed]
4. Gao, X.; Le, X.; Costa, D.B. The safety and efficacy of osimertinib for the treatment of EGFR T790M mutation positive non-small-cell lung cancer. *Expert Rev. Anticancer Ther.* **2016**, *16*, 383–390. [CrossRef] [PubMed]
5. Ricciuti, B.; Chiari, R.; Chiarini, P.; Crino, L.; Maiettini, D.; Ludovini, V.; Metro, G. Osimertinib (AZD9291) and CNS response in two radiotherapy-naive patients with EGFR-Mutant and T790M-Positive advanced non-small cell lung cancer. *Clin. Drug Investig.* **2016**, *36*, 683–686. [CrossRef] [PubMed]
6. Uchino, J.; Nakao, A.; Tamiya, N.; Kaneko, Y.; Yamada, T.; Yoshimura, K.; Fujita, M.; Takayama, K. Treatment rationale and design of the SPIRAL study: A phase II trial of osimertinib in elderly epidermal growth factor receptor T790M-positive nonsmall-cell lung cancer patients who progressed during prior EGFR-TKI treatment. *Medicine* **2018**, *97*, e11081. [CrossRef] [PubMed]
7. Masuhiro, K.; Shiroyama, T.; Suzuki, H.; Takata, S.O.; Nasu, S.; Takada, H.; Morita, S.; Tanaka, A.; Morishita, N.; Okamoto, N.; et al. Impact of pleural effusion on outcomes of patients receiving Osimertinib for NSCLC harboring EGFR T790M. *Anticancer Res.* **2018**, *38*, 3567–3571. [CrossRef] [PubMed]
8. Mountzios, G. Making progress in epidermal growth factor receptor (EGFR)-mutant non-small cell lung cancer by surpassing resistance: Third-generation EGFR tyrosine kinase inhibitors (EGFR-TKIs). *Ann. Transl. Med.* **2018**, *6*, 140. [CrossRef] [PubMed]

9. Aguiar, P.N., Jr.; Haaland, B.; Park, W.; San Tan, P.; Del Giglio, A.; de Lima Lopes, G., Jr. Cost-effectiveness of Osimertinib in the First-Line treatment of patients with EGFR-Mutated advanced non-small cell lung cancer. *JAMA Oncol.* **2018**, *4*, 1080–1084. [CrossRef] [PubMed]
10. Rood, J.J.M.; van Bussel, M.T.J.; Schellens, J.H.M.; Beijnen, J.H.; Sparidans, R.W. Liquid chromatography-tandem mass spectrometric assay for the T790M mutant EGFR inhibitor osimertinib (AZD9291) in human plasma. *J. Chromatogr. B Analyt. Technol. Biomed. Life Sci.* **2016**, *1031*, 80–85. [CrossRef] [PubMed]
11. Xiong, S.; Deng, Z.; Sun, P.; Mu, Y.; Xue, M. Development and Validation of a Rapid and Sensitive LC-MS/MS Method for the Pharmacokinetic Study of Osimertinib in Rats. *J. AOAC Int.* **2017**, *100*, 1771–1775. [CrossRef] [PubMed]
12. Reis, R.; Labat, L.; Allard, M.; Boudou-Rouquette, P.; Chapron, J.; Bellesoeur, A.; Thomas-Schoemann, A.; Arrondeau, J.; Giraud, F.; Alexandre, J.; et al. Liquid chromatography-tandem mass spectrometric assay for therapeutic drug monitoring of the EGFR inhibitors afatinib, erlotinib and osimertinib, the ALK inhibitor crizotinib and the VEGFR inhibitor nintedanib in human plasma from non-small cell lung cancer patients. *J. Pharm. Biomed. Anal.* **2018**, *158*, 174–183. [CrossRef] [PubMed]
13. Zheng, X.; Wang, W.; Zhang, Y.; Ma, Y.; Zhao, H.; Hu, P.; Jiang, J. Development and validation of a UPLC-MS/MS method for quantification of osimertinib (AZD9291) and its metabolite AZ5104 in human plasma. *Biomed. Chromatogr.* **2018**, *17*, e4365. [CrossRef] [PubMed]
14. Lee, M.J.; Park, J.S.; Choi, D.S.; Jung, M.Y. Characterization and quantitation of anthocyanins in purple-fleshed sweet potatoes cultivated in Korea by HPLC-DAD and HPLC-ESI-QTOF-MS/MS. *J. Agric. Food Chem.* **2013**, *61*, 3148–3158. [CrossRef] [PubMed]
15. Park, J.S.; Jung, M.Y. Development of high-performance liquid chromatography-time-of-flight mass spectrometry for the simultaneous characterization and quantitative analysis of gingerol-related compounds in ginger products. *J. Agric. Food Chem.* **2012**, *60*, 10015–10026. [CrossRef] [PubMed]
16. Shintani-Ishida, K.; Kakiuchi, Y.; Ikegaya, H. Successful quantification of 4′-methyl-alpha-pyrrolidinohexanophenone (MPHP) in human urine using LC-TOF-MS in an autopsy case. *Forensic Toxicol.* **2016**, *34*, 398–402. [CrossRef] [PubMed]
17. Wille, K.; Kiebooms, J.A.; Claessens, M.; Rappe, K.; Vanden Bussche, J.; Noppe, H.; Van Praet, N.; De Wulf, E.; Van Caeter, P.; Janssen, C.R.; et al. Development of analytical strategies using U-HPLC-MS/MS and LC-ToF-MS for the quantification of micropollutants in marine organisms. *Anal. Bioanal. Chem.* **2011**, *400*, 1459–1472. [CrossRef] [PubMed]
18. Zhang, H.; Henion, J. Comparison between liquid chromatography-mass spectrometry for quantitative determination of idocifene in human plasma. *J. Chromatogr. B Biomed. Sci. Appl.* **2001**, *5*, 151–159. [CrossRef]
19. Abdelhameed, A.S.; Attwa, M.W.; Kadi, A.A. An LC-MS/MS method for ripad and sensitive high-throughput simultaneous determination of various protein kinase inhibitors in human plasma. *Biomed. Chromatogr.* **2017**, *31*. [CrossRef]
20. Smeraglia, J.; McDougall, S.; Elsby, K.; Companjen, A.; White, S.; Golob, M.; Brudny-Kloeppel, M.; Amsterdam, P.; Timmerman, P. Conference report: AAPS and US FDA Crystal City V meeting on Quantitative Bioanalytical Method Validation and Implementation: Feedback from the EBF. *Bioanalysis* **2014**, *6*, 729–732. [CrossRef] [PubMed]

Sample Availability: Samples of the compounds are available from the authors.

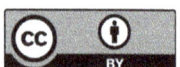

© 2018 by the authors. Licensee MDPI, Basel, Switzerland. This article is an open access article distributed under the terms and conditions of the Creative Commons Attribution (CC BY) license (http://creativecommons.org/licenses/by/4.0/).

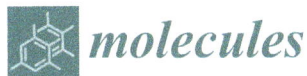

Article

Derivatization of Methylglyoxal for LC-ESI-MS Analysis—Stability and Relative Sensitivity of Different Derivatives

Stefan Fritzsche [1,2], Susan Billig [1], Robby Rynek [1], Ramarao Abburi [1,3], Elena Tarakhovskaya [1,4,5], Olga Leuner [1,6], Andrej Frolov [7] and Claudia Birkemeyer [1,*]

1. Institute of Analytical Chemistry, Faculty of Chemistry and Mineralogy, University of Leipzig, 04103 Leipzig, Germany; stefan.fritzsche@uni-leipzig.de (S.F.); billig@uni-leipzig.de (S.B.); r.rynek@live.de (R.R.); rams.abburi@gmail.com (R.A.); elena.tarakhovskaya@gmail.com (E.T.); leuner@ftz.czu.cz (O.L.)
2. Institute of Pharmacy, Faculty of Medicine, University of Leipzig, 04103 Leipzig, Germany
3. Department of Chemistry, Krishna University, Machilipatnam 521001, Andhra Pradesh, India
4. Department of Plant Physiology and Biochemistry, Faculty of Biology, Saint Petersburg State University, Saint Petersburg 199034, Russia
5. Library of the Russian Academy of Sciences, Saint Petersburg 199034, Russia
6. Faculty of Tropical AgriSciences, Czech University of Life Sciences Prague, 165 00 Prague-Suchdol, Czech Republic
7. Department of Bioorganic Chemistry, Leibniz Institute of Plant Biochemistry, 06120 Halle (Saale), Germany; andrej.frolov@ipb-halle.de
* Correspondence: birkemeyer@chemie.uni-leipzig.de; Tel.: +49-341-973-6092

Received: 12 October 2018; Accepted: 8 November 2018; Published: 16 November 2018

Abstract: The great research interest in the quantification of reactive carbonyl compounds (RCCs), such as methylglyoxal (MGO) in biological and environmental samples, is reflected by the fact that several publications have described specific strategies to perform this task. Thus, many reagents have also been reported for the derivatization of RCCs to effectively detect and quantify the resulting compounds using sensitive techniques such as liquid chromatography coupled with mass spectrometry (LC-MS). However, the choice of the derivatization protocol is not always clear, and a comparative evaluation is not feasible because detection limits from separate reports and determined with different instruments are hardly comparable. Consequently, for a systematic comparison, we tested 21 agents in one experimental setup for derivatization of RCCs prior to LC-MS analysis. This consisted of seven commonly employed reagents and 14 similar reagents, three of which were designed and synthesized by us. All reagents were probed for analytical responsiveness of the derivatives and stability of the reaction mixtures. The results showed that derivatives of 4-methoxyphenylenediamine and 3-methoxyphenylhydrazine—reported here for the first time for derivatization of RCCs—provided a particularly high responsiveness with ESI-MS detection. We applied the protocol to investigate MGO contamination of laboratory water and show successful quantification in a lipoxidation experiment. In summary, our results provide valuable information for scientists in establishing accurate analysis of RCCs.

Keywords: carbonyl derivatization; phenylhydrazine; phenylenediamine; hydroxylamine; water analysis; lipoxidation

1. Introduction

The research interest in the role of reactive carbonyl compounds (RCCs) for environmental and biomedical aspects has grown tremendously ever since their relevance for human metabolism was first discovered [1–3]. One of the biologically most important representatives of this compound group is methylglyoxal (MGO), which has been suggested to be involved in many lifestyle diseases, such as diabetes [4,5], cancer [6], aging [7,8] or even behavioral phenotypes, such as anxiety [9] and depression [10]. In biological samples, reactive carbonyl compounds are usually formed from carbohydrate and lipid metabolism [11,12], while in the environment, they may originate from degradation of volatile organic substances in the atmosphere, such as isoprene [13]. However, the analysis of RCCs is very challenging as most of them are UV-inactive and as they often feature only intermediate polarity. In addition, small RCCs are volatile, which complicates sample handling. Due to the transient, reactive nature of the analytes (e.g., MGO in the atmosphere has an average lifetime of 1.6 h [13]), trap reagents are often employed to avoid further reaction of the target compounds with other sample components. These trap reagents are usually selected to obtain derivatives with enhanced sensitivity compared to the parent compound with respect to the anticipated analytical detection technique.

Consequently, there are a few requirements for an optimal derivatization (or trap) agent: (i) solubility in or efficient miscibility with the sample or sample extract; (ii) a very fast reaction with the target compound (for efficient trapping of the analyte); (iii) modification of the original RCC to a derivative that can be very sensitively detected by the chosen analytical technique; and (iv) sufficient stability of the derivatives during analysis [14]. As RCCs are particularly reactive against amino groups, they are most often derivatized with reagents featuring a free amino group, such as hydroxylamines [15,16], amines [17,18], or hydrazines [14,19–21]. The reaction proceeds via the very well-known addition/elimination mechanism. This is depicted in Figure 1 with α,β-dicarbonyl compounds and phenylenediamines as an example.

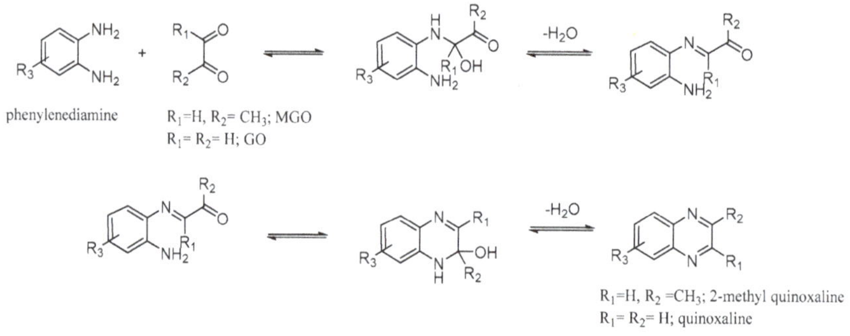

Figure 1. Reaction of dicarbonyl compounds (here methylglyoxal) with phenylenediamines (here o-phenylenediamine) as starting material. After addition of the two compounds, water is eliminated to form the mono-imine (**top**), which in a second addition-elimination cycle forms the quinoxaline (**bottom**).

For analysis of small RCCs, O-(2,3,4,5,6-pentafluorobenzyl)hydroxylamine (PFBHA, [16]) is one of the most frequently applied reagents for subsequent analysis with gas chromatography (GC) coupled with electron impact ionization mass spectrometry (EI-MS) [22,23]. Apart from stability, their derivatives feature a decreased volatility compared to the original compound and a lower polarity due to the shielding of the original molecule by the large nonpolar substituent. In addition, a very abundant, diagnostic fragment (m/z 181) enables very sensitive quantification of the derivatives in EI-MS. However, in aqueous samples, PFBHA derivatives first need to be extracted into a GC/MS-suitable organic solvent by liquid/liquid (l/l) partitioning to lengthen the sample preparation procedure and possibly decrease the recovery while increasing the analytical variance. Moreover, due to the required volatility of the analyte, the application of multitargeted analysis of RCCs by GC is limited to RCCs with small molecular weight, and two-step derivatization protocols need to be employed for hydroxylated representatives and carboxylates [24,25].

In contrast, liquid chromatography (LC) coupled with electrospray ionization (ESI) MS allows the direct analysis of aqueous samples, rendering l/l extraction of the derivatives from biological samples unnecessary. For LC-MS analysis of target analytes containing aldehyde and/or keto group, reaction with amines—such as o-phenylenediamine derivatives with RCCs resulting in imines or quinoxaline derivatives with α,β-dicarbonyl compounds and phenylenediamines (PD)—is frequently used (Figure 1). For hydrazines, the corresponding hydrazones are formed, while oximes are formed for hydroxylamines [16,20,24–27]. The introduction of small aromatic residues improves the required desorption of the target analyte ion during the ionization process. In addition, any other substituent of the reagent apart from the required amino group can be selected to further enhance the reactivity of the reagent (e.g., electron-donating substituents enhance nucleophilic attack during the addition) or improve ionization efficiency during electrospray. These are two very important requirements for successful analysis (electron-donating substituents also enhance the basicity of a compound for determining characteristic of a good ESI sensitivity [28]).

Many reagents and optimized protocols for derivatization of RCCs prior to analysis with LC-MS have already been reported. One of the most well-known reagents is 2,4-dinitrophenylhydrazine (DNPH), which was originally chosen for sensitive detection of RCCs with UV [20]. However, in the recent past, many alternatives to this reagent have been reported to provide a more sensitive and selective, and thereby more accurate, analysis. Moreover, new reagents have been tailored for use with mass spectrometric detection [24] to achieve a higher analytical sensitivity with this particular technique. In this report, we present a survey of 21 compounds for derivatization of MGO prior to LC-ESI-MS analysis with respect to analytical efficiency and robustness (stability). This consisted of 15 commercially available compounds (eight phenylenediamines, four hydrazines, two hydroxylamines and a coumarin hydrazide, Figure 2a) and six synthesized compounds (three hydrazines and their corresponding anilines featuring a permanent charge, Figure 2b).

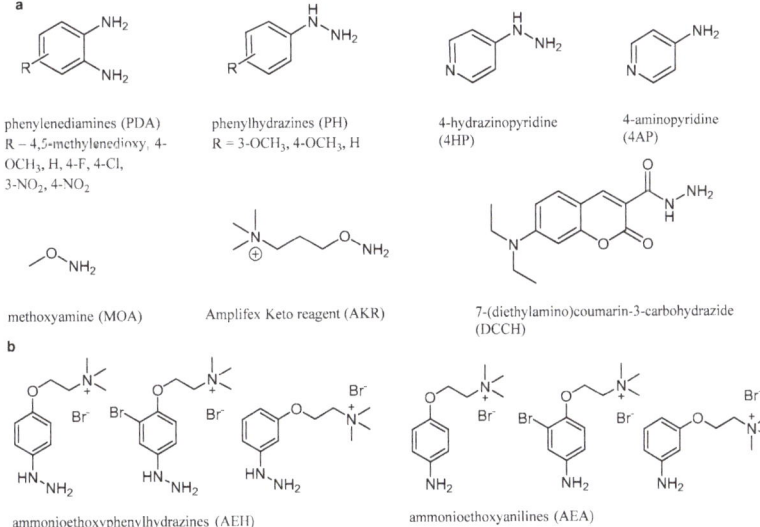

Figure 2. Chemical structure of the reagents tested for derivatization of methylglyoxal with subsequent ESI-MS detection: (**a**) commercially available compounds; (**b**) synthesized reagents for derivatization of carbonyl compounds, from left to right, 2-(4-hydrazineylphenoxy)-*N,N,N*-trimethylethan-1-aminium bromide (4-AEH), 2-(2-bromo-4-hydrazineylphenoxy)-*N,N,N*-trimethylethan-1-aminium bromide (3-BrAEH), 2-(3-hydrazineylphenoxy)-*N,N,N*-trimethylethan-1-aminium bromide (3-AEH), and the corresponding anilines including 2-(4-aminophenoxy)-*N,N,N*-trimethylethan-1-aminium bromide (4-AEA) according to Eggink et al. [24].

In this paper, we present a thorough comparison of the reagents to identify related problems and illustrate major obstacles in the accurate analysis of RCCs, which is still a challenge [29]. In conclusion, we discuss particularly efficient reagents and the requirements for further optimization and finally present the successful application of the best performing protocol for quantification of methylglyoxal in a lipoxidation experiment.

2. Results and Discussion

2.1. Relative Response of Methylglyoxal Derivatives in LC-MS Analysis

Although theoretically indicative, the ESI-MS responsiveness of carbonyl derivatives can be quite different from that of the original amine reagent; therefore, the responsiveness of the reagent is only a rough indicator for predicting the relative response of the corresponding derivative. For example, Figure 3a compares the change in response pattern of the protonated molecular ion of the phenylenediamines (left) and either their methylglyoxal (middle) or glyoxal (GO, right) quinoxaline derivatives depending on the phenylenediamine substituent R_3 (see Figure 2a). The corresponding m/z values of the MGO derivatization products that were used for quantification are given in Supplementary Table S1.

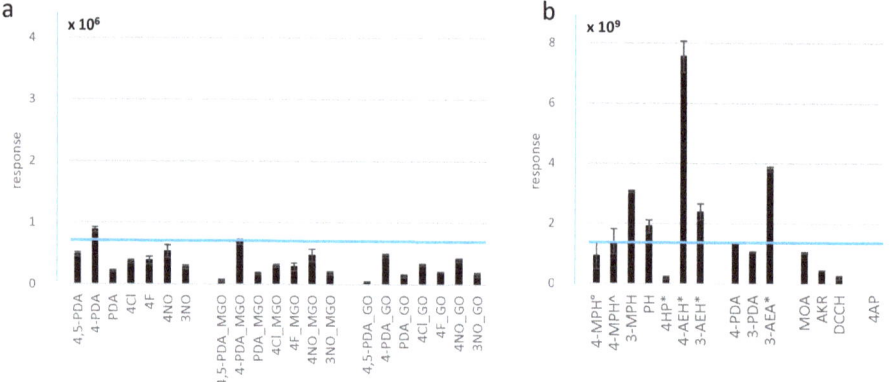

Figure 3. Relative abundances of the different reagents and their corresponding derivatives. Response is normalized to the peak of the two co-eluting products of MGO with 4-methoxyphenylenediamine within each experiment, the isomers 6- and 7-methoxy-2-methylquinoxaline (4-PDA_MGO in Figure 3a and 4-PDA in Figure 3b), illustrated by the blue horizontal line. (**a**) Relative response of the protonated molecular ions of phenylenediamine reagents (left) compared to the quinoxaline reaction products after incubation with MGO (middle) and GO (right). (**b**) Relative response of the most abundant reaction product of methylglyoxal with the corresponding reagent, including phenylhydrazines, methoxyphenylenediamines, and hydroxylamines. (° indole after two days incubation, ^ diimine after four days incubation, * monoderivative). The structure of all reagents is presented in Figure 2. All abbreviations are listed in Supplementary Table S2.

Among the phenylenediamines, signal intensity of the 4-methoxyphenylenediamine (4-PDA) product was consistently higher compared with those of other phenylenediamines, which was confirmed for different molar ratios of reagent and aldehyde (data not shown). As expected, the derivatives of reagents with strong mesomeric effect exhibited the highest signals with +M (e.g., methoxy) being better than -M (e.g., NO, nitro), and *para*-substituted (4-position) better than *meta*-substituted ones (3-position). According to these results, 4-PDA would be the best phenylenediamine reagent for detection of low amounts of methylglyoxal. Apart from ionization efficiency, the relative response of the reaction products may be caused by different reaction yields, e.g., due to insufficient incubation time. Thus, after 3 h incubation time, only 50% reaction yield was reported when using 2,4-dinitrophenylhydrazine (DNPH) for MGO derivatization [30], while reactions with 4-PDA and 4,5-methylenedioxyphenylenediamine (4,5-PDA) have been reported to be nearly complete after just 1 h [26,31]. These findings were in agreement with our results. Consequently, the characteristics supporting ionization efficiency, e.g., electron-donating substituents enhancing the basicity of compounds as the most important criterion for ESI-MS responsiveness of nitrogen bases [28], often foster the reactivity of the compound as well, resulting in faster reaction times. (Note that DNPH, which is the most commonly employed phenylhydrazine, was not included because with mass spectrometry the derivatives are usually detected in ESI negative ion mode, meaning the response cannot be easily compared to the other reagents. Moreover, the slow reaction times contradict the purpose of our study, which was to find a reagent candidate with a fast reaction time). However, we did not notice a significant time-dependent response effect between 2 and 4 h incubation time for all of the commercially available reagents and no response enhancement for the derivatives after that time, which also generally resulted in a satisfactory standard deviation of the replicates. As a general rule, signal response of the derivatives from reagents with electron-donating substituents slowly decreased up to 50% during the course of a day, so we prepared all samples for response comparison in situ.

4-PDA has only recently been introduced as a derivatization agent for methylglyoxal [26]. Among the tested, commercially available phenylenediamines, this reagent seems to produce the most sensitive signal response. Thus, we compared this particular reagent to phenylhydrazines, another group of commonly employed reagents for analysis of carbonyls that also promises to provide excellent performance for derivatization. The results are illustrated in Figure 3b.

It is clear that 3-methoxyphenylhydrazine (3-MPH)—which to our knowledge has not been suggested yet for derivatization of methylglyoxal—outperformed all other commercially available reagents we tested in our experiments. Only our synthesized phenylhydrazine carrying a permanent charge in *para* position (4-AEH) provided a higher intensity, although it mostly reacted with just the aldehyde function and we observed mainly monomers. For comparison, Table 1 lists the corresponding estimated limits of detection (LOD) for selected protocols, i.e., using the reagents 4-PDA, 3-MPH, 3-ammonioethoxyphenylhydrazine (3-AEH), 3-ammonioethoxyaniline (3-AEA), coumarin carbohydrazide (DCCH), Amplifex™ Keto Reagent (AKR, ABSciex, Framingham, MA, USA), and 4-MPH.

Table 1. Limit of detection (LOD, S/N > 3) for MGO derivatives of seven different reagents with LC-ESI-MS, estimated from factorial dilution series factor 3 involving concentrations below detection.

	LOD pmol/Injected	Literature Reference Value LOD pmol/Injected
4-PDA	0.01	0.1 with HPLC-FD [26]
3-MPH	0.05	n.a.
3-AEH	0.7	n.a.
3-AEA	1	n.a. [a]
DCCH	1.5	n.a. [b]
AKR	2	n.a. [c]
4-MPH	>50	n.a.

[a] 0.03 pmol/injected for malondialdehyde derivatized with 4-AEA analyzed with LC-ESI-MS/MS [24]; [b] 1 nmol/L 4-hydroxynonenal analyzed with continuous flow nanospray mass spectrometry [32]; [c] 0.035 fmol testosterone analyzed with LC-ESI-MS/MS [33].

The pattern of LODs did not exactly follow the relative response as obtained from signal intensities at 50 µM MGO (0.5 nmol injected). Thus, for 3-AEA, a surprisingly high value was found, while 4-PDA had a surprisingly low LOD in contrast. Our comparison confirms the notion that assessment of relative sensitivities based on peak areas far above the detection limit does not necessarily help to find the most sensitive protocol. According to these results, 4-PDA might be the preferred reagent by far for analysis of α-oxo-aldehydes, which quinoxaline derivative(s) of methylglyoxal (and glyoxal, not shown) were detected particularly sensitive. However, at higher concentrations of monocarbonyl compounds, multiple derivatives could be produced from phenylenediamines, which can be avoided when using the second-best candidate reagent, i.e., 3-MPH. Furthermore, the production of a diagnostic daughter ion from 3-MPH derivatives, m/z 122, provides a great advantage for identification of unknown carbonyl compounds by MS/MS analyses.

A drawback of using phenylhydrazines for quantification of nonsymmetric dicarbonyl compounds, such as methylglyoxal, compared to phenylenediamines is the formation of two mono- and two main bis-derivatives (for the latter, four isomers would be possible). For 3-MPH, the less abundant bis-derivative was present as a shoulder peak under our conditions, so we quantified the signal as the more robust sum of both peak areas. The same applied to the coumarin carbohydrazide DCCH, which was also the only reagent considerably retained beyond the dead volume of the LC column. Here, the two MGO monoderivatives eluting within the broad tailing of the reagent peak were nearly twice as abundant as the late eluting bis-derivatives, indicating insufficient reactivity against ketones. (Note that another reason for the observed low abundance of the bis-derivative might be the expected very poor solubility, with a logS of 6.78 in the ChemAxon's solubility predictor [34] corresponding to maximal 3 µM dissolved substance vs. 50 µM starting material used in this experiment.). Considering the use of the reagent for a generally applicable multimethod to analyze aldehydes and ketones beyond the analysis of α-oxo-aldehydes, 3-MPH would still be favorable due to its nonselective high reactivity. In return, the presence of two isomers also enables an easier identification of corresponding derivatives in an unknown mixture or for derivatization of unknown carbonyl compounds.

The most curious result, however, is the bad performance of 4-MPH as derivatizing reagent. With this reagent, the base peak chromatogram of the reaction mixture was dominated by multiple degradation products rather than by the expected MGO derivatives. Thus, the only intermediate response of the main derivative (m/z 296) and the corresponding high variance of this species may be the consequence of ion suppression by a very abundant coeluting reagent dimer (m/z 243, see Section 2.2.1 or Figure 4). Stability tests suggested that extensive oxidation processes within the reaction mixture hampered reproducibility of the results and led not only to the degradation of derivatives and reagent but also to precipitations in reaction mixtures with high concentration of GO.

2.2. Extent of Degradation, Solubility, and Practical Considerations

2.2.1. Multiple Reaction Products in the Chromatograms of 4-MPH and 4-PDA Reaction Mixtures

Particularly with the successful derivatization reagents, we noticed extensive, time-dependent reactive processes within the reaction mixtures, which were not inhibited by addition of antioxidants such as 2-mercaptoethanol or di-tert-butyl-hydroxytoluene (BHT) after incubation (not shown); these results were in agreement to the observations reported by Nemet et al. [31]. Indeed, the addition of mercaptoethanol, which has been described for the derivatization with 4-PDA [26], led to a slightly but consistently reduced response (90%) of the MGO derivative that was even more prominent for the phenylhydrazines. Therefore, we omitted this additive from our comparison. However, after the addition of mercaptoethanol, the response of the reagent dimer peaks, m/z 241 and 273, indeed decreased, indicating an inhibition of reagent polymerization. Moreover, a reduced form of the reagent (e.g., m/z 137 for 4-PDA) was observed in mercaptoethanol-containing preparations.

Figure 4 illustrates the appearance of typical LC-MS chromatograms obtained from the reaction mixtures of MGO, with 4-PDA, 4-MPH, and 3-MPH as an example to illustrate the formation of such by-products.

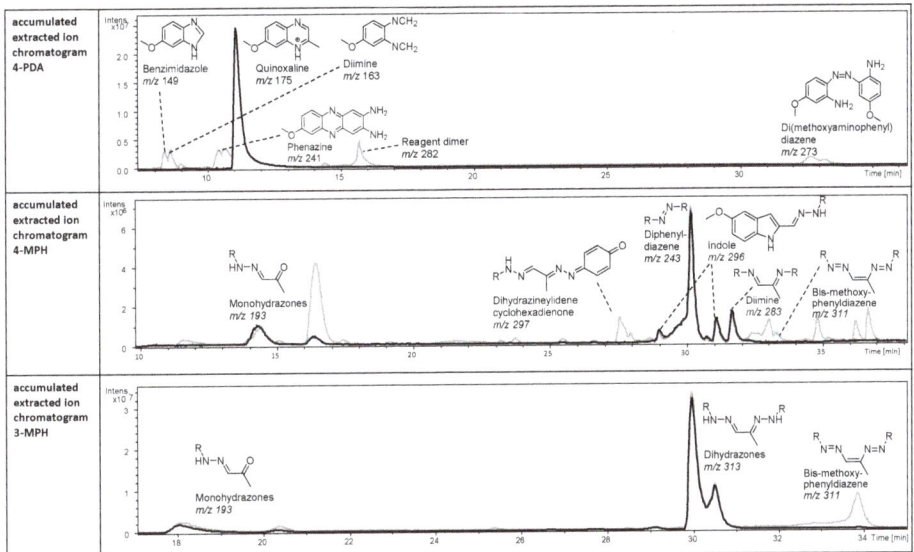

Figure 4. LC-ESI-MS analysis of reaction mixtures of methylglyoxal with phenylenediamines or phenylhydrazines. **Top**: reaction mixture with 4-PDA. **Middle**: reaction mixture with 4-MPH. **Bottom**: reaction mixture with 3-MPH. Black: ion current of selective mass traces, m/z 175 (extracted ion chromatogram for the reaction mixture with 4-PDA) or m/z 193, 243, 283, 296, 313 (reconstructed ion current for the reaction mixtures with 4-MPH and 3-MPH). Grey: base peak chromatogram, BPC (intensity of the base peak at a given retention time).

In the 4-PDA reaction mixture, m/z 175 from the protonated reaction product methoxy-2-methylquinoxaline exhibited the most abundant signal. Other abundant peaks with m/z such as 149, 163, 241, 282, and 273 have been earlier shown to appear after electrolytic oxidation of the reagent during the electrospray ionization process [35]. As we found the compounds corresponding to these peaks also separated in LC-MS analysis of the reaction mixture, we concluded them to have been formed spontaneously here by reagent oxidation in solution. In addition, after multiple measurements, we observed a very abundant compound with m/z 124 eluting at higher acetonitrile (ACN) phase. This m/z corresponds to another potential degradation product of 4-PDA—4-methoxyaniline; the signal hardly decreased even after long flushing times of the column. In contrast, the signal intensity of the MGO derivative methoxy-2-methylquinoxaline itself was reduced to 75% after 12 h.

The different hydrazines are known to produce many analytical artifacts in solution, such as by degradation to the corresponding aniline, aryldiazene, or diarylamine [36,37]. Nevertheless, they have long been used as derivatization agents of carbonyls for analytical purposes [20]. This is most likely due to the good sensitivity that can be achieved, the sufficient stability of the target derivatives, and reproducibility [38]. The stability of hydrazines and their derivatives from the reaction with carbonyl compounds, i.e., the hydrazones, is related to the type of substituent and the extent of protonation of the hydrazine/hydrazone group. Thus, phenylhydrazines with electron-donating substituents, such as the alkoxy phenylhydrazines used in this study, are less stable but are much more reactive at the same time due to the higher electron density in the aromatic ring and at the hydrazine group itself. Last but not least, electron-donating substituents make their carrier molecules particularly responsive to ESI-MS in positive mode [28] and promise to introduce high sensitivity to the analysis of the derivatives, a point that is particularly relevant for our investigation.

At low pH, these electron-rich phenylhydrazines exist as the more stable ions; however, degradation to the corresponding aniline already starts in these conditions [39]. Thus, we tentatively identified the diimine with 4-MPH (*m/z* 283, Figure 3) and mixed aniline/hydrazine derivatives with our synthesized, permanently charged phenylhydrazines (data not shown). Moreover, fast reagent polymerization was indicated by the presence of dimethoxyphenyldiazenes from 4-MPH and, to a lesser extent, 3-MPH (*m/z* 243) (Note that reagent dimers were also immediately observed for the phenylenediamines, e.g., *m/z* 241 and 273 for 4-PDA in Figure 4). In agreement, in the reaction mixture of 4-MPH with high concentrations of GO in 20% ACN, a precipitation already occurred after 2 h (Note that no precipitates were observed for MGO at used concentrations).

In the analysis of the reaction mixture from the derivatization with 4-MPH, only a small signal of a tentative oxidation product of the expected derivative—the dehydro-dihydrazone, i.e., the propenediyl-bis(methoxyphenyl)diazene (*m/z* 311)—was detected instead of the dihydrazone, while the main peak appeared to be the di(methoxyphenyl)diazene (*m/z* 243), a chemically formed reagent dimer whose formation should be particularly favored with the methoxy group in *para* position to the hydrazino group. The two main products with MGO were the tentatively identified diimine (*m/z* 283) and an indole (*m/z* 296) related to the MGO–dihydrazone intermediate, which formally cleaves ammonia in a [3,3]-sigmatropic rearrangement known as Fischer indole synthesis. In summary, a minimum of eight abundant, reagent-borne species and six derivatives of MGO were detected in the reaction mixture. The reaction speed of all these products was found to be inversely related to the organic content in the solvent composition of the reaction mixture (data not shown). Consequently, 4-MPH was deemed not suitable for derivatization in LC-MS profiling of reactive carbonyl compounds, and the protocol would require further method development before efficient application. However, we refrained from further optimization given the only-moderate responsiveness for MGO with this protocol.

2.2.2. 3-MPH, Anilines, and Hydroxylamines Exhibit Higher Stability Compared to 4-MPH

In comparison to 4-MPH, 3-MPH produced considerably less by-products (Figure 4); not only were the tentative diphenyldiazene, diimine, and demethylated dihydrazone absent from the reagent mixture, but the monohydrazones also had a very low relative intensity. Thus, 3-MPH produced the expected dihydrazone derivative as base peak in the corresponding chromatogram (*m/z* 313). However, the bis-diazene was also observed due to oxidation in the reaction mixture. In agreement, the derivative of our 3-substituted aniline also gave higher signals compared to the 4-subsituted analogue (data not shown). However, the stability of the 3-MPH derivative was still not satisfactory; after 2–3 hours, signal intensity decreased constantly to 50% at 12 h. However, as response with this reagent was favorable compared to other reagents, we tested the influence of other parameters such as reaction buffers at different pH, the addition of antioxidants or the reducing agent $NaCNBH_3$, and storage at lower temperature. Finally, we observed that in higher organic phase, the stability of the derivatives was crucially enhanced, which led to the development of an optimized protocol; shortly after mixing (after ~30 min) the reagent and target analyte, the aqueous sample was almost completely dried and needed to be re-dissolved in methanol before analysis. These samples did not produce any signal decline over the tested period of 24 h, providing satisfactory stability for proper handling in the lab. Moreover, the procedure offers the possibility of sample concentration with respect to a reasonable evaporation time below 2 h in the vacuum centrifuge (otherwise lyophilization might be recommended). The estimated LOD did not change in comparison to immediate analysis in the aqueous sample.

For 3- and 4-PDA using the intensity of the reagent dimer as an indicator, polymerization [35] was observed with both reagents from the very beginning, i.e., after 2 h incubation. The intensity of the signal corresponding to 5-methoxy-3-methylquinoxaline, the product with 3-PDA, was only 75% of the corresponding product from 4-PDA (Figure 3b). However, in agreement with the extent of degradation of the *meta*- compared to the *para*-substituted phenylhydrazine, the intensity of the corresponding reagent dimer peak was 10 times higher in 4-PDA compared to 3-PDA.

Unlike the phenylenediamines and phenylhydrazines, the anilines synthesized according to Eggink et al. [24] appeared to be rather stable. In addition, the MGO derivatives of the anilines provided an excellent stability within one week storage. Given their competitive signal response (Figure 3b), reagents of this type would have been the most promising approach for derivatization of aldehydes to achieve a very sensitive ESI-MS detection within our comparison. Unfortunately though, the reactivity against the keto group was negligible.

Finally, after multiple injections, we experienced undesirable precipitations for most reagents in the ESI source on the spray shield. As a general rule, the more pronounced the precipitation, the more the reagent tended to polymerize, degrade, and form late eluting products not directed to waste during the first minutes of LC separation. In this context, DCCH, which was hardly soluble in water or organic phase other than dimethylformamide, was the reagent that was most prone to precipitation. Its derivatives were indeed expected to exhibit a very low solubility in aqueous solvents, and we experienced particularly serious, hardly removable source contamination during these experiments. Moreover, we observed a fast deterioration of the LC column signal background and performance using this derivatization agent as well as abundant, long-tailing memory peaks. The solutions of this reagent would have to be strongly diluted or the reagent would have to be removed before analysis to avoid any precipitation in the ESI source or accumulation on the column due to precipitation, which might compromise the limit of detection for the method. In the literature, this reagent is instead used for analysis of lipoxidation products from polyunsaturated fatty acids of higher molecular weight compared to MGO [40], where the chromatographic separation of the reagent by elution within the dead volume is easier to achieve with other chromatographic systems than that used for the small RCC investigated here. In addition, reagent removal by liquid extraction of derivatives from the aqueous sample to nonpolar solvents after incubation time might be a useful approach to improve the situation; however, this would lengthen the sample preparation procedure and manual effort.

2.2.3. Reaction Products of Phenylhydrazines Featuring a Permanent Charge Provide Excellent Solubility but Insufficient Stability

When it comes to reversed phase (RP) LC analysis of aqueous samples, a particular problematic aspect of the hydrazines and their reaction products is the poor solubility in water, which leads to precipitation in the samples, possibly disturbing the injection process or, worse, to precipitation in the separating column. Therefore, we investigated the suitability of permanently charged reagents in analogy to the aniline 4-AEA [24] to improve the solubility of the reagent and any obtained products. Given the results we obtained with our test candidates, including 3-MPH, we also developed synthesis routes leading to the corresponding permanently charged phenylhydrazine (4-AEH), the corresponding 3-substituted phenylhydrazine, and a third hydrazine by additionally introducing bromine as inductive electron-withdrawing substituent in *ortho* position to improve the stability of the molecule (Figure 2b, protocols described in the supplement). These reagents were tested with methylglyoxal.

As expected, precipitate formation did not appear in the reaction mixtures with these reagents featuring a permanent charge. However, unfortunately, the synthesized hydrazines were still very unstable in aqueous solution and produced several oxidation products at later retention times. Thus, the signal response of all synthesized hydrazines was significantly decreased after just a few hours (data not shown), indicating a particularly bad stability of the reagents in aqueous solution. The reaction with MGO appeared to be very fast as the maximum response was observed as early as after 30–45 min incubation, while the derivative with bromine as substituent provided the worst response (data not shown), possibly due to a lower reactivity of the starting material from the inductive electron-withdrawing effect or a worse ionization efficiency of the derivative. Figure 5 illustrates the appearance of the chromatogram of the reagent mixtures with 3-AEH after 1 h incubation time.

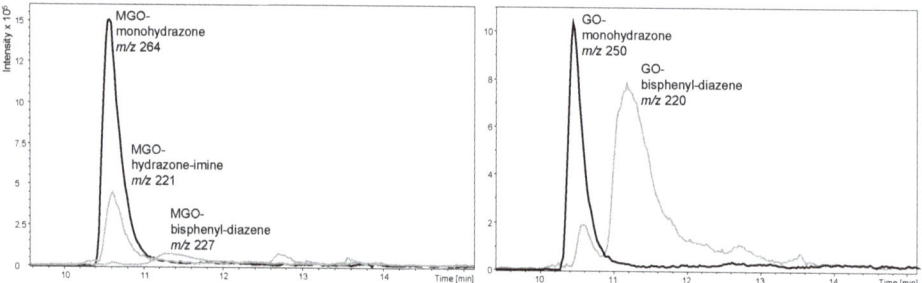

Figure 5. LC-ESI-MS analysis of the reaction mixtures from the derivatization of MGO (**left**) and GO (**right**) with 3-AEH after 1 h incubation time in aqueous ACN. Black: ion current of selective mass traces (extracted ion chromatogram) for the monohydrazone derivatives of MGO, *m/z* 264, and GO, *m/z* 250. Grey: ion current of selective mass traces of the MGO hydrazone-imine and bisphenyldiazene (*m/z* 221 and 227) and GO bisphenyldiazene (*m/z* 220) derivatives.

Unfortunately, in addition to the insufficient stability of the reagents, a clear discrimination in reactivity against the keto (MGO) and even the second aldehyde group (GO) obviously led to abundant multiple derivatives, exhibiting a disadvantage of the use of these reagents in the development of multiselective methods, including ketones as target compounds. Finally, though the permanently charged hydrazines produced derivatives with satisfactory responsiveness (e.g., factor 2.5 for the MGO monoderivative of 4-AEH compared to 3-MPH), in agreement with the behavior of the reagents, the stability of these derivatives was also less satisfactory. Thus, the response of the derivatives obtained with 4-AEH continuously decreased to 50% of the original value during 7 h incubation time (for the 3-AEH derivative, the half-life was as short as ~30 min). The highest response of the derivative was always observed with the shortest possible incubation time.

The corresponding anilines featuring a permanent charge [24] were expected to be more stable than the hydrazines. However, we did not obtain any products in the course of 10 h without adding sodium cyanoborohydride as reduction agent for the formed imines to the corresponding amines, which could only then be detected with high sensitivity. As reported, the keto group of MGO hardly reacted, meaning these reagents would only be suitable for reactive carbonyls carrying an aldehyde function.

In conclusion, among the reagents whose derivatives exhibited a high signal response after reaction with MGO, we found 3-MPH and 4-PDA produced the least number and intensity of by-products, which is an important advantage when it comes to the establishment of multitargeted methods. While MGO derivatives were successfully separated from the most abundant by-products of all investigated reagents, derivatives of other carbonyl compounds might coelute and therefore be prone to be suppressed by these abundant signals as was found for the derivative of 3-deoxyglucosone and the 4-PDA dimer at *m/z* 241 (data not shown). In such situations, further method optimization, such as improvement of chromatographic separation or the addition of 2-mercaptoethanol to reduce the reagent dimer formation, may be recommended.

2.3. Application of 3-MPH as Derivatizing Agent to Explore the Contamination of Laboratory Water with Methylglyoxal

Another well known, serious problem in the quantitative analysis of methylglyoxal is the fact that it is hard to produce a clean solvent blank as required, for instance, for LOD determination [41]. As illustrated below using 3-MPH as reagent, even high-quality equipment and several tested cleaning procedures were not able to completely remove methylglyoxal from the blank (Figure 6).

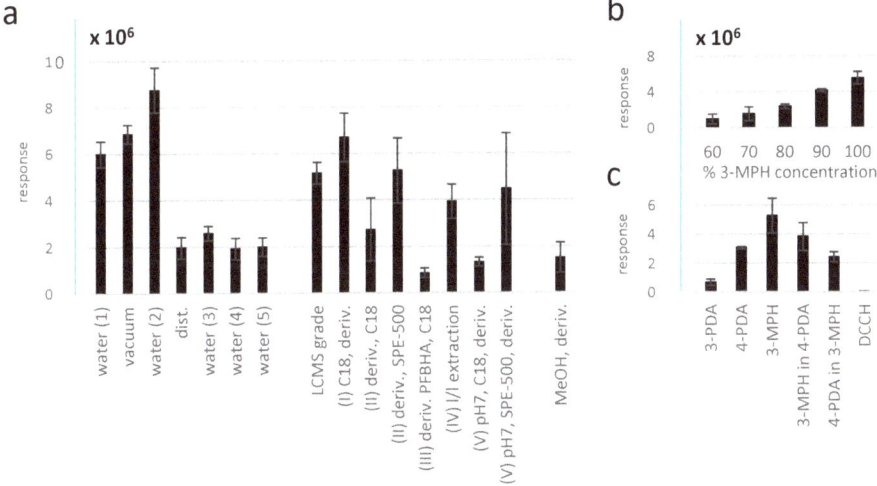

Figure 6. (a) Water contamination with MGO analyzed as MGO–dihydrazone after incubation with 3-MPH. Different quality laboratory water and different procedures for purification of water were tested, refer to Section 2.3. (b) Response of the MGO–dihydrazone in preparations containing different concentrations of 3-MPH in relation to the original 5 mM solution. (c) Response of the corresponding MGO derivatives in blank solutions of four different reagents and response of the dihydrazone after incubation of a 3-MPH solution with 4-PDA and the quinoxaline in a 4-PDA solution with 3-MPH.

MGO response in methanol equaled the one from distilled water and water purification systems 3, 4, and 5, suggesting that these purification protocols indeed performed the best. However, successful purification by SPE procedures appeared to be much more cumbersome, expensive, and laborious and required a very careful optimization in advance. Thus, we believe the favorable value achieved with the PFBHA (III) protocol could at least partially be a consequence of signal suppression by bulk unreacted PFBHA, which was not satisfactorily removed by SPE. Excess PFBHA is usually removed by l/l extraction after selective protonation of the reagent [16], after which a higher response of blank contamination can be obtained (protocol IV). Moreover, complete elimination of the reagent employed for MGO removal from the solvent used for analysis is indispensable to avoid subsequent competitive reaction with the reagent of choice for determination of MGO in the sample. Using the same reagent for purification of water and analytical derivatization itself [26], on the other hand, may still lead to an overestimation of MGO in the sample in case the residue is not completely removed.

Curiously, we still obtained a response for MGO when injecting 3-MPH in methanol only. This finding prompted us to further test the potential origins of the contamination. Considering that excess reagent is used for derivatization, MGO response in the water blank was expected to stay constant with decreasing reagent concentration until a certain threshold. Instead, we observed an immediate decrease in response with decreasing concentrations of the reagent at all levels (Figure 6b), indicating reagent contamination with the derivative. Reagent contamination was further confirmed by dissolving one reagent in a solution of another after 2 h incubation, i.e., 3-MPH in 4-PDA and 4-PDA in 3-MPH solutions without adding MGO, where derivatives of MGO with both reagents were found (Figure 6c). We conclude that the reagents themselves are a source of blank contamination and require thorough purification and subsequent storage under appropriate conditions, particularly if quantification near or below the concentration of the corresponding contamination is anticipated (5 nM for 3-MPH in our case). In addition, appropriate blank replication is required for quantification above the blank level for which, theoretically, the reagents can be used without prior purification employing blank subtraction. Thus, 3-PDA, 4-PDA, and 3-MPH were all suitable to determine concentrations down to 10 nM MGO (0.1 pmol injected) before blank contamination prevented quantification of lower concentrations. For comparison, typical concentrations of MGO in biological samples are, for example, ~250 nM in whole blood and 170 nM in human plasma [17], 1 nmol/g in U87 cancer cells [22], ~15 µM in wine [42], and >200 nM in urine [26].

2.4. Analysis of Carbonyl Reaction Products of Linoleic and Linolenic Acids Oxidation by Cu(II) and Hydrogen Peroxide After Derivatization with 3-MPH

As a proof of concept and to show the applicability of our derivatization agent, we analyzed reaction mixtures after oxidation of linoleic and linolenic acids—two very important native fatty acids that are present, for instance, in human epidermis. Oxidation of these acids is known to produce mainly hydroxylated acids, such as 8,13-dihydroxy-9,11-octadecadienoic and 9,14-dihydroxy-10,12-octadecadienoic acids [43], but oxo-octadecadienoic acids were also observed [44]. Recently, the formation of several carbonyl compounds, such as acrolein and crotonaldehyde as well as glyoxal and methylglyoxal after oxidation of linoleic and linolenic acids, has been reported [45] but no quantitative information has been added. Because lipoxidation mechanisms are a highly interesting topic in biomedical research and because there is already information available to rate the validity of our own results, we selected this model system to show the performance of our method. Firstly, we detected signals that could be produced by approximately 60 possible RCC candidates (although this tentative identification would have to be subjected to future confirmation). Moreover, we were able to quantify methylglyoxal in the reaction mixture (4.6 µM in the linoleic acid and 1.1 µM in the linolenic acid mixtures) and used the average comparison for other test candidates. As an example, we present a small table with ratios and average comparisons of selected potential target compounds (Table 2).

Table 2. Average comparison of selected, tentatively identified carbonyl compounds between the reaction mixtures of linoleic and linolenic acids. Values below one represent candidates that were more abundant in linolenic acid mixtures, and those above one represent candidates preferentially formed from linoleic acid.

Tentative Identification	Ratio C18:2/C18:3	p-Value t-Test
oxobutanal *	11	0.005
oxopentanal *	10	0.056
oxononanoic acid *	1.9	0.035
methylglyoxal	1.7	0.013
glyoxal	0.7	0.031
acrolein *	0.7	0.056
pentenal *	0.6	0.071
malondialdehyde *	0.4	0.015
hexenedial *	0.1	0.005

* tentative assignment by m/z.

Although an exhaustive evaluation of such an experiment would require prior establishment of a proper multimethod, in particular the assessment of appropriate retention times and MS-MS data for differentiation of derivatives with the same mass but different structure (e.g., methylglyoxal and malondialdehyde), this experiment already shows the capability of the reagent for application in such multitargeted methods to assess the presence and concentration of many carbonyl compounds in a sample in one analytical run. However, compared to our standard samples, we observed not only a significantly enhanced background in the hydrogen peroxide and metal ion (Cu II)-containing solutions of this experiment but also an enhanced formation of the reagent dimer (m/z 243) as indicator of oxidative degradation of the reagent. (Note that similar effects were observed for 4-PDA as derivatization agent in a glycation mixture from a glucose solution with Fe II/III; data is not shown). Copper and iron salts are additives with the particular purpose of enhancing the reactivity of lipids and carbohydrates toward oxidative degradation; therefore, not surprisingly, we found that the presence of these Lewis acids may become very problematic in investigations such as ours. Their interaction with the lone electron pairs of the heteroatoms could enhance the reactivity of the reagents and the carbonyls. Thus, in such experiments, the immediate analysis of the derivatized sample would be of particular importance. Our advanced protocol, which changed the solvent directly after derivatization, is expected to decrease the concentration of these metal ions in the reaction mixture and would therefore provide a significant advantage to improve experimental variance.

3. Materials and Methods

3.1. Materials and Chemicals

Acetonitrile (ACN; ROTISOLV®, ≥99.95%, LC-MS Grade), cyclohexane, and formic acid (>98%, p.s.) were purchased from Carl Roth, Karlsruhe, Germany. Bakerbond SPE-500, C18 and empty cartridges (all J.T.Baker, Philipsburg, MT, USA), LiChrosorb C18 bulk material (Merck, Darmstadt, Germany), and water (HiPerSolv® CHROMANORM®, LC-MS Grade) were purchased from VWR Chemicals, Darmstadt, Germany. Sodium cyanoborohydride (95%) was purchased from Alfa Aesar, Karlsruhe, Germany. All other chemicals were purchased from Sigma-Aldrich, Taufkirchen, Germany. The experimental details for synthesis and analytical confirmation of the permanently charged anilines and hydrazines, i.e., 2-(4-hydrazineylphenoxy)-*N,N,N*-trimethylethan-1-aminium (4-AEH), 2-(2-bromo-4-hydrazineylphenoxy)-*N,N,N*-trimethylethan-1-aminium (3-BrAEH), and 2-(3-hydrazineylphenoxy)-*N,N,N*-trimethylethan-1-aminium (3-AEH) bromides and the corresponding aminoethoxyanilines (AEA), are given in the supplementary.

All solvents were degassed with Argon 4.6 (Air Liquide, Düsseldorf, Germany). All reagent solutions were prepared in situ, sonicated, and handled under argon in the dark. The pH was adjusted using the pH meter Level 1 (WTW, Weilhcim, Germany) with the pH electrode BlueLine 24 pH (Schott Instruments, Mainz, Germany).

MGO contamination was analyzed in water from the following water purification systems: BWT Permaq Pico 10-90 (1, BWT Wassertechnik GmbH, Schriesheim, Germany), Veolia Berkesoft Midi with Berkefeld miniRO 5 (2, Veolia Water Technologies, Celle, Germany), Millipore Milli-Q Integral 5 (3), Millipore Elix 3 with Element A10 (4), and Millipore Direct-Q 3UV (5); the latter three were from Merck, Darmstadt, Germany.

3.2. Response and Stability of Methylglyoxal Derivatives

A total of 21 reagents were used for analytical derivatization of methylglyoxal with subsequent LC-MS analysis of the derivatives. The detailed structures of all reagents are illustrated in Figure 2, and all used abbreviations are summarized in Table S2. The selection of the reagents was guided by reported frequent use for carbonyl derivatization and mainly comprised two groups of chemical substances: aromatic amines [41,46] and hydrazines [47]. In our experiments, we included further reagents from these two groups with substituents, allowing a more systematic comparison of signal response featuring electron-withdrawing and electron-donating substituents in different positions to the reacting amino group.

Below, we describe the protocols used for derivatization as adopted from the literature and optimized if required. Stability of the reagents and the reaction mixtures was assessed over the course of one week.

3.2.1. Reaction with Anilines

Anilines were dissolved in 50 mM ammonium acetate pH 5.7 to prepare mixtures of 2.5 mM reagent and 25 µM MGO [24]. Alternatively, these samples contained 2.5 mM sodium cyanoborohydride as reduction agent. Reagent blanks and reagent mixtures without sodium cyanoborohydride were analyzed by LC-MS after 1, 3, and 10 h incubation time; reagent mixtures with sodium cyanoborohydride were analyzed after 3 h incubation time [24]. Five millimolar 4-aminopyridine and 250 µM MGO in 20% ACN (v/v) were incubated for 2 h and analyzed in triplicate by LC-MS after appropriate dilution.

3.2.2. Comparison of Phenylenediamines (PDA)

Responsiveness of formed quinoxalines was studied after mixing equal volumes of 16 mM reagent stock solutions in methanol (pH 4) with 3 mM MGO or GO for incubation at 37 °C for 70 minutes in the dark at 550 rpm shaking. Reaction mixtures were diluted and analyzed with flow injection analysis in ESI positive mode.

3.2.3. Reaction with Phenylhydrazines, 4-Hydrazinopyridine, and Methoxyphenylenediamines

Ten millimolar 4-methoxyphenylhydrazine (4-MPH), 3-methoxyphenylhydrazine (3-MPH), phenylhydrazine (PH), 4-hydrazinopyridine (4-HP), 3-methoxyphenylenediamine (3-PDA), and 4-methoxyphenylenediamine (4-PDA), were used to prepare reaction mixtures containing 50 µM MGO in 20% ACN (v/v) at pH ~4. For the synthesized hydrazines, 50 mM ammonium acetate pH 5.7 was used instead (n = 3) [24]. Reaction vessels were closed firmly and incubated for 2 h shaking in the dark before analysis by LC-MS.

3.2.4. Reaction with the Amplifex™ Keto Reagent, Methoxyamine, and 7-(Diethylamino)coumarin-3-carbohydrazide

The derivatization with the Amplifex™ Keto Reagent Kit (AKR) [33] was carried out according to the manufacturer's instructions (ABSciex, Framingham, MA, USA). Briefly, 50 µM MGO was incubated with the reagent working solution for 1 h at room temperature.

Ten millimolar aqueous methoxyamine (MOA) and 100 µM MGO were incubated for 2 h at room temperature, diluted, and analyzed in triplicate.

Derivatization with 7-(diethylamino)coumarin-3-carbohydrazide (DCCH) was accomplished in triplicates as described in Reference [40]: 5 µL of a 100 mM stock solution in DMF was mixed with 40 µL 50% ACN and added with 5 µL of a 10 mM MGO solution. The mixture was incubated for 1 h at 37 °C and diluted with 20% ACN (1:20) prior to LC-MS analysis.

3.2.5. Relative Response for Different Types of Reagents

Prior to comparison of responsiveness, we confirmed the dynamic behavior from 10 to 300 µM MGO (n ≥ 3). Based on this investigation, we selected a concentration of 50 µM (0.5 nmol on column) in the final sample as the basis for our comparison (n ≥ 3). This concentration is in the lower dynamic range and not hampered by any blank contamination. We refrained from comparison of responsiveness at high concentrations because the concentration of RCCs in biological and environmental samples is usually rather low.

However, for particularly successful protocols, we additionally estimated the limit of detection (S/N ≥ 3). A factorial dilution series (factor 3) of the derivatization products of MGO with 3-PDA, 4-PDA, 4-MPH, 3-MPH, DCCH, AKR, 3-trimethylammonioethoxyphenylhydrazine (3-AEH), and 3-trimethylammonioethoxyaniline (3-AEA) was used to assess the agreement with the relative response at 50 µM.

3.2.6. Optimized Derivatization Protocol with 3-MPH

Ten millimolar 3-MPH in methanol was mixed with an equal volume of the sample in 50 mM ammonium acetate buffer of pH 4 and incubated for 30 min in the dark. Subsequently, the sample was completely evaporated in a vacuum centrifuge. The sample was dissolved in methanol before LC-ESI-MS analysis. If diluted in an aqueous solvent, dilution was made very shortly before analysis of the sample.

3.3. Application of 3-MPH as Derivatization Agent to Explore the Contamination of Laboratory Water with Methylglyoxal

We determined MGO blank contamination in water from five different water purification systems as outlined under 3.1. In addition, several protocols were assessed for their ability to completely remove methylglyoxal from blank water (HiPerSolv® CHROMANORM®, LC-MS Grade from VWR Chemicals, Darmstadt, Germany).

Thus, apart from heating for 20 min at 100 °C under the fume, distillation, and vacuum centrifugation without heating to reduce the solvent volume by ~25% before LC-MS analysis, we also applied several solid phase extraction protocols. For solid phase extractions, cartridges were conditioned with methanol before application: (1) Water was applied to a Bakerbond C18 cartridge and the eluate was subjected to derivatization with 3-MPH. (2) Water was derivatized with 3-MPH and applied to SPE extraction with Bakerbond C18, LiChrosorb C18 and SPE-500. (3) 25 mg O-(2,3,4,5,6-pentafluorobenzyl) hydroxylamine (PFBHA) was dissolved in 20 mL water, incubated 1 h at 40 °C, applied to SPE extraction with Bakerbond C18, and subsequently derivatized with 3-MPH. (4) 2.5 mg/mL PFBHA in water was subjected to l/l extraction against equal volumes of cyclohexane. The aqueous phase was subjected to derivatization with 3-MPH. (5) Water was adjusted to pH 7 by ammonia, extracted with Bakerbond C18 and SPE-500 and subsequently derivatized with 3-MPH.

All purified extracts were subjected to LC-MS analysis (n $\geq$ 3).

3.4. Analysis of Carbonyl Reaction Products of Linoleic and Linolenic Acids Oxidation by Hydrogen Peroxide After Derivatization with 3-MPH

Three replicates of the following samples were prepared in 100 µL water: 500 nmol linoleic or linolenic acids (5 mM, 1.4 mg/mL) and 300 nmol $Cu(NO_3)_2$ (3 mM) were added with 10 µmol hydrogen peroxide (100 mM) and incubated overnight at 37 °C while shaking. Afterwards, samples were derivatized with 3-MPH as described under 3.2.6 and analyzed by LC-ESI-MS as described below.

3.5. Instrumental Parameters of LC-ESI-MS

LC-MS analysis was carried out using an HPLC system 1100 series (Agilent, Waldbronn, Germany) equipped with a Gemini C18 reversed-phase column 5 µm, 110 Å, 150 mm × 2 mm (Phenomenex, Aschaffenburg, Germany). For separation of the derivatives obtained with the permanently charged Amplifex™ Keto Reagent (Figure 2a), 3-AEH and 3-AEA, an Accucore aQ LC column (100 × 2.1 mm, 2.6 µm, Thermo Fisher Scientific GmbH) was used. The columns were kept at 40 °C, and 10 µL sample was injected.

The gradients were established with 0.1% formic acid in ACN as Eluent A and in water as Eluent B according to the required performance (Table 3).

Table 3. Gradients used for HPLC separation of the carbonyl derivatives.

Experiment	Gradient [min]/[%B]	Flow mL/min
3- and 4-MPH, PDAs and MOA	0/80, 5/80, 20/70, 30/30, 35/0, 42/0, 47/80, 54/80	0.6
DCCH, 4-AEH	0/90, 5/90, 15/0, 30/0, 40/90, 45/90	0.5
Amplifex™ (AKR)	0/0, 10/0, 30/50, 40/98, 45/98, 46/0, 56/0	0.3
3-AEH, 3-AEA	0/98, 5/98, 15/0, 20/0, 20.1/98, 25/98	0.3

The LC system was coupled with a Bruker ESI ion trap mass spectrometer Esquire 3000+ (Bruker Daltonik GmbH, Bremen, Germany) operated in positive ion mode. The source parameters were as follows: nitrogen as nebulizer (55 psi) and dry gas (12 L/min) with a temperature of 365 °C; ICC 20,000, target mass m/z 250, scan range m/z 50–700.

Flow injection analysis by full scan MS was carried out on the Esquire 3000 Plus using a syringe pump (KD Scientific, Hollisten MA, USA) at a flow rate of 4 µL/min. For this, the nebulizer was set to

11 psi, and the dry gas was set to 5 L/min at 280 °C. Target mass was set to the anticipated m/z value and a scan range from m/z 50–500.

Bruker Data analysis 4.2 (Bruker Daltonik GmbH, Bremen, Germany), was used for raw data assessment based on peak areas (LC-MS analyses) or peak height (flow injection analysis) of selected mass traces for the derivatives listed in Table S1.

Student's t-test for average comparisons was performed with MS Excel 2013 (Microsoft, Redmond, WA, USA).

4. Conclusions

In our survey, the commercially available substances 4-methoxyphenylenediamine followed by 3-methoxyphenylhydrazine were the best performing reagents for derivatization of methylglyoxal in LC-ESI-MS analysis considering handling, analysis time, sensitivity of the derivatives, and stability of the reagent mixture at room temperature. With respect to reactive carbonyl compounds in general, permanently charged anilines might still be a better choice for derivatization of aldehydes with subsequent LC-MS analysis due to the high response and stability of the corresponding N-substituted anilines obtained after reductive amination of the formed imines; however, they cannot be employed for ketones. Moreover, the very quick reaction time achieved with 4-PDA and 3-MPH exhibits a great advantage over reagents requiring longer incubation times, especially because MGO can be released or produced de novo from certain sample matrix components during procedural steps and because the remaining metabolic activity in biological samples may result in an overestimation of its concentration in the sample [41]. Finally, apart from stability, sensitivity can also be greatly enhanced when drying the samples and dissolving in a smaller volume of a nonaqueous solvent. Using this improved protocol, we showed the capability of employing 3-MPH for quantification of methylglyoxal during a lipoxidation experiment and demonstrated the potential of this method to analyze different carbonyl compounds simultaneously.

A particularly bothersome fact, however, appeared to be the solvent and reagent contamination with methylglyoxal at very low concentration levels. While contamination of water used as sample solvent could be removed by repeated distillation or high-quality water purification systems, the development of a protocol for satisfactory reagent purification is tedious and requires very careful optimization.

In addition, the stability of the derivatives with trapping reagents still needs very careful consideration, particularly when applying lengthy deproteinization procedures as often required for biological samples or extended trapping times of MGO from environmental samples. Here, an insufficient stability of the derivatives may lead to an underestimation of MGO concentration in the samples. With only intermediate stability of the derivatives, nested online sampling and derivatization [48,49] might be considered when analyzing large sample batches.

Supplementary Materials: The following are available online at http://www.mdpi.com/1420-3049/23/11/2994/s1, Materials and Methods for the synthesis of the permanently charged hydrazines and anilines; Table S1: Selective m/z for quantification of the MGO derivatives, Table S2: Abbreviations of the used reagents.

Author Contributions: S.F., S.B., R.R. and R.A. equally contributed. S.F. carried out synthesis of permanently charged anilines and phenylhydrazines; S.B. carried out most LC-MS analyses and the lipoxidation experiment, LODs; R.R. carried out blank experiments, sensitivity, and LOD analyses of 3- and 4-MPH and 3- and 4-PDA; R.A. carried out phenylenediamine comparison; E.T. carried out LOD analysis of 4-MPH and DCCH; O.L. did data evaluation of stability tests with DCCH, AKR, and synthesized reagents; A.F. contributed to project design and protocol applications; C.B. contributed with the project idea, experimental design, and manuscript writing.

Funding: E.T. and C.B. thank the German Academic Exchange Service (DAAD, Deutscher Akademischer Austauschdienst) for funding within the Dmitrij Mendeleev Programme. E.T. further thanks the Russian Foundation for Basic Research (project No. 17-04-01331). O.L. and C.B. thank the German Research Foundation (Deutsche Forschungsgemeinschaft, DFG) for funding of international collaborations (project No. 408121020) and the European Commission for funding within the Erasmus+ Training Mobility Programme. The University of Leipzig funded all other work. We acknowledge the support of the German Research Foundation (DFG) and Universität Leipzig within the program of Open Access Publishing.

Acknowledgments: The authors would like to sincerely thank the Stefan Berger, Jörg Matysik, Detlef Briel—all from University of Leipzig—and Thorsten Reemtsma (University of Leipzig and UFZ Leipzig, Germany) for their continuing, kind support. Alice Grün, Alex Kowar, Alena Soboleva, Ahyong Kim, Mareike Lochas, Natasha Frolova, Ramona Oehme (MS), Lothar Hennig, and Matthias Findeisen (NMR), and Manuela Roßberg (elemental analyses)—all from University of Leipzig—performed analyses in preparation and periphery of the presented experiments. Andreas Kiontke (University of Leipzig) kindly provided general technical support and daily advice to the students involved in the experiments. Professor Dieter Sicker (University of Leipzig) helped with purification of solvents during blank contamination assessment.

Conflicts of Interest: The authors declare no conflict of interest. The funders had no role in the design of the study; in the collection, analyses, or interpretation of data; in the writing of the manuscript, or in the decision to publish the results.

References

1. Dakin, H.D.; Dudley, H.W. An enzyme concerned with the formation of hydroxy acids from ketonic aldehydes. *J. Biol. Chem.* **1913**, *14*, 155–157.
2. Dakin, H.D.; Dudley, H.W. The interconversion of alpha-amino acids, alpha-hydroxy acids and alpha-ketonic aldehydes. Part II. *J. Biol. Chem.* **1913**, *15*, 127–143.
3. Neuberg, C. Über die Zerstörung von Milchsäurealdehyd und Methylglyoxal durch tierische Organe. *Biochem. Z.* **1913**, *49*, 502–506.
4. Beisswenger, P.J. Methylglyoxal in diabetes: Link to treatment, glycemic control and biomarkers of complications. *Biochem. Soc. Trans.* **2014**, *42*, 450–456. [CrossRef] [PubMed]
5. Brownlee, M. Biochemistry and molecular cell biology of diabetic complications. *Nature* **2001**, *414*, 813–820. [CrossRef] [PubMed]
6. Szent-Györgyi, A. The living state and cancer. *Proc. Natl. Acad. Sci. USA* **1977**, *74*, 2844–2847. [CrossRef] [PubMed]
7. Baynes, J.W.; Thorpe, S.R. Glycoxidation and lipoxidation in atherogenesis. *Free Radic. Biol. Med.* **2000**, *28*, 1708–1716. [CrossRef]
8. Thornalley, P.J. Protein and nucleotide damage by glyoxal and methylglyoxal in physiological systems - role in ageing and disease. *Drug Metabol. Drug Interact.* **2008**, *23*, 125–150. [CrossRef] [PubMed]
9. Hovatta, I.; Tennant, R.S.; Helton, R.; Marr, R.A.; Singer, O.; Redwine, J.M.; Ellison, J.A.; Schadt, E.E.; Verma, I.M.; Lockhart, D.J.; et al. Glyoxalase 1 and glutathione reductase 1 regulate anxiety in mice. *Nature* **2005**, *438*, 662–666. [CrossRef] [PubMed]
10. Benton, C.S.; Miller, B.H.; Skwerer, S.; Suzuki, O.; Schultz, L.E.; Cameron, M.D.; Marron, J.S.; Pletcher, M.T.; Wiltshire, T. Evaluating genetic markers and neurobiochemical analytes for fluoxetine response using a panel of mouse inbred strains. *Psychopharmacology* **2012**, *221*, 297–315. [CrossRef] [PubMed]
11. Allaman, I.; Bélanger, M.; Magistretti, P.J. Methylglyoxal, the dark side of glycolysis. *Front. Neurosci.* **2015**, *9*, 23. [CrossRef] [PubMed]
12. Semchyshyn, H.M. Reactive carbonyl species in vivo: Generation and dual biological effects. *Sci. World J.* **2014**, *2014*. [CrossRef] [PubMed]
13. Fu, T.-M.; Jacob, D.J.; Wittrock, F.; Burrows, J.P.; Vrekoussis, M.; Henze, D.K. Global budgets of atmospheric glyoxal and methylglyoxal, and implications for formation of secondary organic aerosols. *J. Geophys. Res.* **2008**, *113*. [CrossRef]
14. Vogel, M.; Büldt, A.; Karst, U. Hydrazine reagents as derivatizing agents in environmental analysis—A critical review. *Fresenius J. Anal. Chem.* **2000**, *366*, 781–791. [CrossRef] [PubMed]
15. Chalmers, R.A.; Watts, R.W.E. Derivatives for the identification and quantitative determination of some keto- and aldo-carboxylic acids by gas-liquid chromatography. *Analyst* **1972**, *97*, 951–957. [CrossRef] [PubMed]
16. Kobayashi, K.; Tanaka, M.; Kawai, S. Gas chromatographic determination of low-molecular-weight carbonyl compounds in aqueous solution as their O-(2,3,4,5,6-pentafluorobenzyl) oximes. *J. Chromatogr. A* **1980**, *187*, 413–417. [CrossRef]
17. McLellan, A.C.; Phillips, S.A.; Thornalley, P.J. The assay of methylglyoxal in biological systems by derivatization with 1,2-diamino-4,5-dimethoxybenzene. *Anal. Biochem.* **1992**, *206*, 17–23. [CrossRef]
18. Rotondo, A.; Bruno, G.; Brancatelli, G.; Nicolò, F.; Armentano, D. A phenyl-salicyliden-imine as a suitable ligand to build functional materials. *Inorganica Chim. Acta* **2009**, *362*, 247–252. [CrossRef]

19. Pal, R.; Kim, K.-H. Experimental choices for the determination of carbonyl compounds in air. *J. Sep. Sci.* **2007**, *30*, 2708–2718. [CrossRef] [PubMed]
20. Brady, O.L.; Elsmie, G.V. The use of 2,4-dinitrophenylhydrazine as a reagent for aldehydes and ketones. *Analyst* **1926**, *51*, 77–78. [CrossRef]
21. Fischer, E. Über einige Osazone und Hydrazone der Zuckergruppe. *Ber. Dtsch. Chem. Ges.* **1894**, *27*, 2486–2492. [CrossRef]
22. Oppermann, H.; Ding, Y.; Sharma, J.; Berndt Paetz, M.; Meixensberger, J.; Gaunitz, F.; Birkemeyer, C. Metabolic response of glioblastoma cells associated with glucose withdrawal and pyruvate substitution as revealed by GC-MS. *Nutr. Metab.* **2016**, *13*. [CrossRef] [PubMed]
23. Bilova, T.; Lukasheva, E.; Brauch, D.; Greifenhagen, U.; Paudel, G.; Tarakhovskaya, E.; Frolova, N.; Mittasch, J.; Balcke, G.U.; Tissier, A.; et al. A snapshot of the plant glycated proteome-structural, functional, and mechanistic aspects. *J. Biol. Chem.* **2016**, *291*, 7621–7636. [CrossRef] [PubMed]
24. Eggink, M.; Wijtmans, M.; Ekkebus, R.; Lingeman, H.; de Esch, I.J.P.; Kool, J.; Niessen, W.M.A.; Irth, H. Development of a selective ESI-MS derivatization reagent: Synthesis and optimization for the analysis of aldehydes in biological mixtures. *Anal. Chem.* **2008**, *80*, 9042–9051. [CrossRef] [PubMed]
25. Milkovska-Stamenova, S.; Schmidt, R.; Frolov, A.; Birkemeyer, C. GC-MS Method for the Quantitation of Carbohydrate Intermediates in Glycation Systems. *J. Agric. Food Chem.* **2015**, *63*, 5911–5919. [CrossRef] [PubMed]
26. Ojeda, A.G.; Wrobel, K.; Escobosa, A.R.C.; Garay-Sevilla, M.E.; Wrobel, K. High-performance liquid chromatography determination of glyoxal. methylglyoxal, and diacetyl in urine using 4-methoxy-*o*-phenylenediamine as derivatizing reagent. *Anal. Biochem.* **2014**, *449*, 52–58. [CrossRef] [PubMed]
27. Thornalley, P.J.; Yurek-George, A.; Argirov, O.K. Kinetics and mechanism of the reaction of aminoguanidine with the α-oxoaldehydes glyoxal, methylglyoxal, and 3-deoxyglucosone under physiological conditions. *Biochem. Pharmacol.* **2000**, *60*, 55–65. [CrossRef]
28. Kiontke, A.; Oliveira-Birkmeier, A.; Opitz, A.; Birkemeyer, C. Electrospray ionization efficiency is dependent on different molecular descriptors with respect to solvent pH and instrumental configuration. *PLoS ONE* **2016**, *11*. [CrossRef] [PubMed]
29. Hoyen, H.; Vogel, M.; Karst, U. Recent developments in the determination of formaldehyde in air samples using derivatizing agents. *Air Qual. Control* **2003**, *63*, 295–298.
30. Zwiener, C.; Glauner, T.; Frimmel, F.H. Method optimization for the determination of carbonyl compounds in disinfected water by DNPH derivatization and LC-ESI-MS-MS. *Anal. Bioanal. Chem.* **2002**, *372*, 615–621. [CrossRef] [PubMed]
31. Nemet, I.; Varga-Defterdarović, L.; Turk, Z. Preparation and quantification of methylglyoxal in human plasma using reverse-phase high-performance liquid chromatography. *Clin. Biochem.* **2004**, *37*, 875–881. [CrossRef] [PubMed]
32. Milic, I.; Hoffmann, R.; Fedorova, M. Simultaneous detection of low and high molecular weight carbonylated compounds derived from lipid peroxidation by electrospray ionization-tandem mass spectrometry. *Anal. Chem.* **2013**, *85*, 156–162. [CrossRef] [PubMed]
33. Star-Weinstock, M.; Williamson, B.L.; Dey, S.; Pillai, S.; Purkayastha, S. LC-ESI-MS/MS analysis of testosterone at sub-picogram levels using a novel derivatization reagent. *Anal. Chem.* **2012**, *84*, 9310–9317. [CrossRef] [PubMed]
34. ChemAxon's Solubility Predictor. Available online: https://docs.chemaxon.com/display/docs/Solubility+Predictor (accessed on 7 May 2018).
35. Abburi, R.; Kalkhof, S.; Oehme, R.; Kiontke, A.; Birkemeyer, C. Artifacts in amine analysis from anodic oxidation of organic solvents upon electrospray ionization for mass spectrometry. *Eur. J. Mass Spectrom.* **2012**, *18*, 301–312. [CrossRef] [PubMed]
36. Hardie, R.L.; Thomson, R.H. 488. The oxidation of phenylhydrazine. *J. Chem. Soc.* **1957**, *0*, 2512–2518. [CrossRef]
37. Huang, P.-K.C.; Kosower, E.M. Diazenes. III. Properties of phenyldiazene. *J. Am. Chem. Soc.* **1968**, *90*, 2367–2376. [CrossRef]
38. Henning, C.; Liehr, K.; Girndt, M.; Ulrich, C.; Glomb, M.A. Extending the spectrum of α-dicarbonyl compounds in vivo. *J. Biol. Chem.* **2014**, *289*, 28676–28688. [CrossRef] [PubMed]

39. Enders, E.; Kolbah, D.; Korunčev, D.; Müller, E. Hydrazines, Azines; Azo-, Azoxy-Compounds I; Diazenes I. In *Methoden der Organischen Chemie*, 4th ed.; Thieme: Stuttgart, Germany, 1967; ISBN 9783131959249.
40. Milic, I.; Fedorova, M. Derivatization and detection of small aliphatic and lipid-bound carbonylated lipid peroxidation products by ESI-MS. *Methods Mol. Biol.* **2015**, *1208*, 3–20. [CrossRef] [PubMed]
41. Nemet, I.; Varga-Defterdarović, L.; Turk, Z. Methylglyoxal in food and living organisms. *Mol. Nutr. Food Res.* **2006**, *50*, 1105–1117. [CrossRef] [PubMed]
42. Rodríguez-Cáceres, M.I.; Palomino-Vasco, M.; Mora-Diez, N.; Acedo-Valenzuela, M.I. Novel HPLC—fluorescence methodology for the determination of methylglyoxal and glyoxal. Application to the analysis of monovarietal wines "Ribera del Guadiana". *Food Chem.* **2015**, *187*, 159–165. [CrossRef] [PubMed]
43. Hamberg, M. Autoxidation of linoleic acid: Isolation and structure of four dihydroxyoctadecadienoic acids. *Biochim. Biophys. Acta Lipids Lipid Metab.* **1983**, *752*, 353–356. [CrossRef]
44. Banni, S.; Contini, M.S.; Angioni, E.; Deiana, M.; Dessì, M.A.; Melis, M.P.; Carta, G.; Corongiu, F.P. A novel approach to study linoleic acid autoxidation: Importance of simultaneous detection of the substrate and its derivative oxidation products. *Free Radic. Res.* **1996**, *25*, 43–53. [CrossRef] [PubMed]
45. Wang, Y.; Cui, P. Reactive carbonyl species derived from Omega-3 and Omega-6 fatty acids. *J. Agric. Food Chem.* **2015**, *63*, 6293–6296. [CrossRef] [PubMed]
46. Shibamoto, T. Analytical methods for trace levels of reactive carbonyl compounds formed in lipid peroxidation systems. *J. Pharmaceut. Biomed. Anal.* **2006**, *41*, 12–25. [CrossRef] [PubMed]
47. Qi, B.-L.; Liu, P.; Wang, Q.-Y.; Cai, W.-J.; Yuan, B.-F.; Feng, Y.-Q. Derivatization for liquid chromatography-mass spectrometry. *Trends Anal. Chem. TrAC* **2014**, *59*, 121–132. [CrossRef]
48. El-Maghrabey, M.H.; Kishikawa, N.; Ohyama, K.; Imazato, T.; Ueki, Y.; Kuroda, N. Determination of human serum semicarbazide-sensitive amine oxidase activity via flow injection analysis with fluorescence detection after online derivatization of the enzymatically produced benzaldehyde with 1,2-diaminoanthraquinone. *Anal. Chim. Acta* **2015**, *881*, 139–147. [CrossRef] [PubMed]
49. Grosjean, D.; Fung, K. Collection efficiencies of cartridges and microimpingers for sampling of aldehydes in air as 2,4-dinitrophenylhydrazones. *Anal. Chem.* **2002**, *54*, 1221–1224. [CrossRef]

Sample Availability: Samples of methylglyoxal, 4-PDA and 3-MPH and most of the synthesized compounds and intermediates are available from the authors at the date of publication.

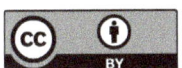

© 2018 by the authors. Licensee MDPI, Basel, Switzerland. This article is an open access article distributed under the terms and conditions of the Creative Commons Attribution (CC BY) license (http://creativecommons.org/licenses/by/4.0/).

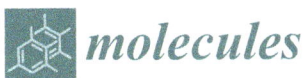

Article

Identification, Characterization and Quantification of Process-Related and Degradation Impurities in Lisdexamfetamine Dimesylate: Identifiction of Two New Compounds

Shenghua Gao [1], Lili Meng [1], Chunjie Zhao [2], Tao Zhang [1], Pengcheng Qiu [1,*] and Fuli Zhang [1,*]

1. Shanghai Institute of Pharmaceutical Industry, China State Institute of Pharmaceutical Industry, No. 285 Gebaini Road, Shanghai 201203, China; shh_gao@163.com (S.G.); 18221816872@163.com (L.M.); zt0414@126.com (T.Z.)
2. College of Pharmacy, Shenyang Pharmaceutical University, Shenyang 110016, China; zcjjlj@sina.com
* Correspondence: pcqiu@aliyun.com (P.Q.); zhangfuli1@sinopharm.com (F.Z.);
  Tel.: +86-21-2057-2000 (ext. 5077) (P.Q.); +86-21-2057-2000 (ext. 5036) (F.Z.)

Academic Editor: In-Soo Yoon
Received: 4 November 2018; Accepted: 27 November 2018; Published: 29 November 2018

Abstract: Twelve impurities (process-related and degradation) in lisdexamfetamine dimesylate (LDX), a central nervous system (CNS) stimulant drug, were first separated and quantified by high-performance liquid chromatography (HPLC) and then identified by liquid chromatography mass spectrometry (LC-MS). The structures of the twelve impurities were further confirmed and characterized by IR, HRMS and NMR analyses. Based on the characterization data, two previously unknown impurities formed during the process development and forced degradation were proposed to be (2S)-2,6-di-(lysyl)-amino-N-[(1S)-1-methyl-2-phenyl ethyl]hexanamide (Imp-II) and (2S)-2,6-diamino-N-[(1S)-1-methyl-2-(2-hydroxyphenyl)ethyl] hexanamide (Imp-M). Furthermore, these two compounds are new. Probable mechanisms for the formation of the twelve impurities were discussed based on the synthesis route of LDX. Superior separation was achieved on a YMC-Pack ODS-AQ S5 120A silica column (250 × 4.6 mm × 5 μm) using a gradient of a mixture of acetonitrile and 0.1% aqueous methanesulfonic acid solution. The HPLC method was optimized in order to separate, selectively detect, and quantify all the impurities. The full identification and characterization of these impurities should prove useful for quality control in the manufacture of lisdexamfetamine dimesylate.

Keywords: lisdexamfetamine dimesylate; impurities; structural elucidation; forced degradation; HPLC validation

1. Introduction

Lisdexamfetamine dimesylate (LDX; formerly NRP-104), (2S)-2,6-diamino-N-[(1S)-1-methyl-2-phenylethyl]hexanamide dimethanesulfonate) is a novel, long-acting, central nervous system (CNS) stimulating drug with low toxicity used as an abuse-resistant treatment of attention-deficit/hyperactivity disorder (ADHD). LDX is a therapeutically inactive amphetamine prodrug, and the pharmacologically active D-amphetamine is gradually released by rate-limited hydrolysis following ingestion [1]. The drug, originally developed by Shire Development Inc. (London, UK) and New River Pharmaceutical Inc. (Washington, DC, US) is currently marketed under the trade name of Vyvanse since its launch in February 2007 [2,3].

The industrial manufacturing process of LDX was developed by New River Pharmaceutical Inc. (Figure 1) [2]. Impurities in drugs are closely related to their adverse reactions and pharmacological activity. For example, degradation products, precursors, and byproducts in drugs can produce fatal immune responses, which may be responsible for some clinical allergic reactions [4,5]. After a comprehensive literature survey, we found that only one patent cursorily referred to six impurities of LDX [3]. Unfortunately, there was no information about the synthesis and spectroscopic data of LDX process-related and degradation impurities. There was only one analytical method available for quantitative analysis of LDX in the literature [6]. However, the paper only focused on comparison of CAD and UV detectors, but did not include information on process-related impurities of LDX. Furthermore, we did not get good separation resolution between LDX and process-related impurities according to the literature. According to the guidelines recommended by the International Conference on Harmonization (ICH), impurities present in drug substances exceeding the accepted level of 0.1% should be identified and characterized [7]. Hence, a thorough study was conducted to develop an effective and sensitive method for separation and identification of impurities in LDX.

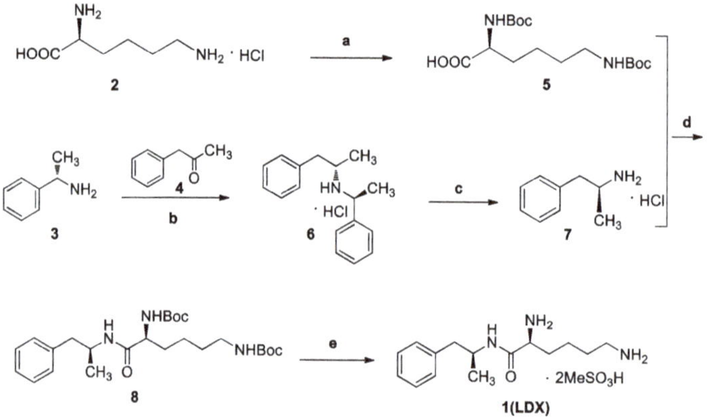

Figure 1. The synthesis route of LDX. *Reagents and conditions*: (**a**) Boc$_2$O, acetone/2N NaOH, 25 °C, 4 h, 94%–98%; (**b**) (*i*) NaBH(AcO)$_3$, DCM, rt., 9h; (*ii*) THF, 36% hydrochloric acid, 73%–78%; (**c**) ammonium formate, MeOH, 65 °C, 3 h, 92%–96%; (**d**) (*i*) EDCI, HOBt, NMM, DMF, rt., 20 h, 92–95%; (*ii*) recrystallization (acetone:*n*-heptane = 1:10, *v*/*v*); (**e**) MeSO$_3$H, THF, 50 °C, 6 h, 95%–96%.

This study aimed to: (1) identify impurities formed during the preparation of LDX and its forced degradation study; (2) characterize and confirm structures of process-related and degradation impurities by IR, HRMS and NMR. The impurities were proposed based on the molecular weight revealed by LC-MS, and confirmed by their synthesis followed by spectroscopic analysis; (3) develop an effective and sensitive HPLC method to separate and quantify all the related substances of LDX. To our knowledge, this is the first comprehensive study on process-related and degradation impurities in LDX including their characterization and probable mechanisms of formation, and on development of an effective HPLC method to separate and quantify them.

2. Results and Discussion

2.1. Detection of Process-Related Impurities and Forced Degradation of LDX

After analysis of different laboratory batches of LDX, process-related impurities were detected in the range of 0.05–1.61%. The HPLC method described in Section 3.2 was used to obtain a typical LC-UV chromatogram of a bulk drug sample of LDX, presenting eleven peaks (the retention time of Imp-B and Imp-C was the same due to their being enantiomers), Imp-H (RT = 8.667, relative retention time (RRT) = 0.725); Imp-L (RT = 9.908, RRT = 0.828); Imp-M (RT = 10.305, RRT = 0.862); Imp-E (RT = 10.728, RRT = 0.897); Imp-D (RT = 11.145, RRT = 0.932); Imp-B and Imp-C (RT = 13.467, RRT = 1.126); Imp-A (RT = 14.025, RRT = 1.173); Imp-K (RT = 25.740, RRT = 2.153); Imp-G (RT = 26.907, RRT = 2.251), Imp-F

(RT = 28.440, RRT = 2.379); Imp-J (RT = 36.838, RRT = 3.082), which were shown in Figure 2. Moreover, the LDX samples were analyzed by LC-MS and the molecular weights were 135.1 (Imp-A), 263.2 (Imp-B and Imp-C), 391.2 (Imp-D), 391.2 (Imp-E), 363.2 (Imp-F), 363.2 (Imp-G), 519.3 (Imp-H), 463.3 (Imp-J), 163.1 (Imp-K), 249.2 (Imp-L) and 279.2 (Imp-M), respectively (Figure S5).

During the course of degradation studies (under acidic, thermal and photolytic conditions), no significant change in the sample purity was observed. However, three degraded products (Imp-A, -B and -C) under alkaline and one degradation product (Imp-M) under oxidative conditions were detected.

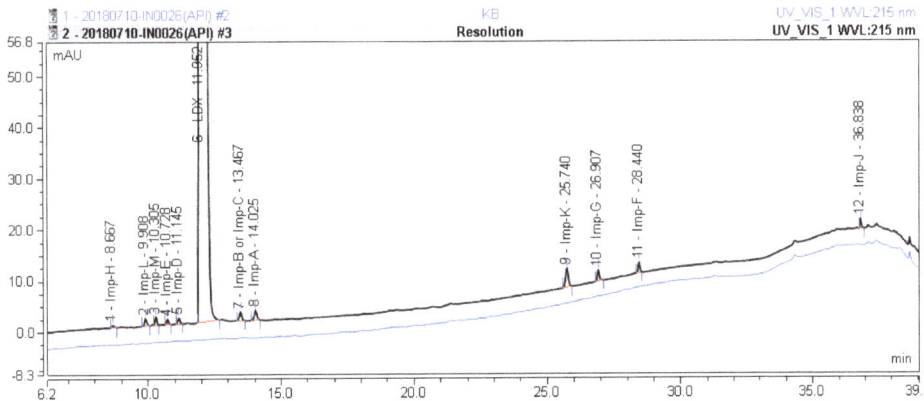

Figure 2. Typical HPLC chromatogram of LDX spiked with its impurities.

2.2. Impurity Preparation and Structural Confirmation

All twelve LDX impurities were synthesized in our laboratory and further confirmed by IR, HRMS, NMR, and MS/MS spectroscopy. The HRMS data and carbon atom numbering scheme were shown in Table 1 and the ^{1}H-NMR and ^{13}C-NMR spectral data of the impurities were shown in Tables 2 and 3, respectively. There were detailed descriptions on the structural characterization of (1S)-1-phenyl propan-2-amine (Imp-A) [8,9], (2S)-2,6-di-((tert-butoxycarbonyl)amino)-N-[(1S)-1-methyl-2-phenyl ethyl]hexanamide (Imp-J) [10] and N-[(1S)-1-methyl-2-phenylethyl]formamide (Imp-K) [11] in the literature. Accordingly, the structures of Imp-A, Imp-J and Imp-K were confirmed by comparison with published spectral data. All the relevant spectral data for structural confirmation are shown in the Supporting Information.

2.2.1. Structural Elucidation and Control Strategy of Imp-B and Imp-C

Imp-B and Imp-C originated from the enantiomers of two different starting materials **2**, **3**. The synthetic route of Imp-B and Imp-C were consistent with LDX (Figure 3), except that L-lysine (**2**) was replaced by D-lysine (**2a**) or (S)-1-phenylethanamine (**3**) was replaced by (R)-1-phenylethanamine (**3a**). Imp-B and Imp-C, were obtained as white solids and their HPLC purities were 98.63% and 96.71%, respectively. The HRMS of Imp-B and Imp-C showed an [M + H]$^+$ at m/z 264.2071 and 264.2069, respectively, suggesting the same elemental composition of $C_{15}H_{26}N_3O$ (Table 1) as LDX. Imp-B and Imp-C were at the same position in reversed-phase liquid chromatography but were displayed as two different peaks (RT = 12.740 min and 14.288 min) in normal-phase chromatography (in Supporting Information Figure S6), which indicated that they were isomers instead of an identical compound. Specific rotations of Imp-B and Imp-C were +6.512 and −6.847, respectively, further supporting that Imp-B and Imp-C, with identical molecular formulae, were diastereoisomers of LDX. Detailed ^{1}H-NMR spectral data were given in Table 2. The control strategy of Imp-B and Imp-C was to minimize the isomers of intermediate **8** by recrystallization (acetone:n-heptane = 1:10, v/v). Furthermore, by means of recrystallization of LDX, Imp-B and Imp-C were easily removed leaving less than 0.1% content in the bulk drug.

Table 1. Retention time, HRMS and structures of LDX and its impurities.

Compound	RRT	HRMS		Structure	Source
		[M + H]$^+$	Chemical Formula		
LDX	1.00	264.2076	$C_{15}H_{26}N_3O$		Target compound
Imp-A	1.17	136.1121	$C_9H_{13}N$		Process and alkaline degradation
Imp-B	1.12	264.2071	$C_{15}H_{26}N_3O$		Process and alkaline degradation
Imp-C	1.12	264.2069	$C_{15}H_{26}N_3O$		Process and alkaline degradation
Imp-D	0.93	392.3205	$C_{21}H_{38}N_5O_2$		Process
Imp-E	0.89	392.3207	$C_{21}H_{38}N_5O_2$		Process
Imp-F	2.38	364.2595	$C_{20}H_{34}N_3O_3$		Process
Imp-G	2.25	364.2590	$C_{20}H_{34}N_3O_3$		Process
Imp-H	0.72	520.3975	$C_{27}H_{50}N_7O_3$		Process
Imp-J	3.08	464.3118	$C_{25}H_{41}N_3O_5$		Process
Imp-K	2.15	186.0889 (M + Na$^+$)	$C_{10}H_{13}NO$		Process
Imp-L	0.82	250.1908	$C_{14}H_{24}N_3O$		Process
Imp-M	0.86	280.2020	$C_{15}H_{26}N_3O_2$		Oxidative degradation

Table 2. ^{1}H-NMR assignment for LDX and its impurities.

Position	LDX	Imp-B	Imp-C	Imp-D	Imp-E	Imp-F	Imp-G	Imp-H	Imp-L	Imp-M
2	3.66–3.63 (t,1H)	3.67–3.63 (t,1H)	3.67–3.63 (t,1H)	4.22–4.18 (t,1H)	3.63–3.61 (t,1H)	3.10–3.07 (t,1H)	3.99–3.95 (t,1H)	4.20–4.12 (dt,1H)	4.93–4.88 (m,1H)	3.65–3.63 (t,1H)
3	1.48–1.40 (m $^{(c)}$,4H)	1.76–1.67 (dd $^{(d)}$,2H)	1.76–1.68 (dd,2H)	1.79–1.69 (m,2H)	1.75–1.68 (m,2H)	1.47,1.30 (m,2H)	1.54–1.46 (m,2H)	1.49–1.43 (m,2H)	1.53–1.46 (m,2H)	1.54–1.46 (dd,2H)
4	1.03–0.92 (m,2H)	1.35–1.26 (m,2H)	1.35–1.26 (m,2H)	1.39–1.31 (m,2H)	1.38–1.27 (m,4H)	1.24–1.17 (m,2H)	1.28–1.23 (dd,2H)	1.13–1.11 (d,2H)	1.25–1.14 (m,2H)	1.08–0.86 (m,2H).
5	1.48–1.44 (m,4H)	1.59–1.47 (m,2H)	1.59–1.47 (m,2H)	1.63–1.48 (m,6H)	1.49–1.45 (m,2H)	1.34–1.26 (m,2H)	1.43–1.34 (m,2H)	1.38–1.34 (m,6H)	1.69–1.66 (m,2H)	1.44–1.39 (m,2H),
6	2.78–2.73 (m,2H)	2.78–2.71 (m,2H)	2.78–2.70 (m,2H)	2.82–2.76 (m,4H)	3.03–2.98 (m,2H)	2.89–2.84 (dd,2H)	2.69–2.61 (m,2H)	3.06–3.01 (m,2H)	2.67–2.61 (dd,2H)	2.68–2.61 (m,2H),
7	4.16–4.04 (m,1H)	3.97–3.93 (m,1H)	3.97–3.93 (m,1H)	3.97–3.92 (m,1H)	4.15–4.07 (m,1H)	3.93–4.03 (m,1H)	4.32–4.32 (m,1H)	4.02–3.95 (m,1H)	–	4.20–4.09 (m,1H),
8	1.13 (d $^{(b)}$,3H)	1.03 (d,3H)	1.02 (d,3H)	1.01 (d,3H)	1.14 (d,3H)	1.03 (d,3H)	1.15 (d,3H)	1.07 (d,3H)	1.38 (d,3H)	1.11–1.10 (d,3H),
9	2.65,2.75 (dd,2H)	2.62,2.82 (dd,2H)	2.62,2.82 (dd,2H)	2.62,2.79 (dd,2H)	2.68,2.76 (dd,2H)	2.77,2.63 (dd,2H)	2.84–2.71 (dd,2H)	2.69–2.67 (d,2H)	3.79 (t,1H)	2.72.2.56 (dd,2H)
11,13	7.24–7.18 (m,3H)	7.23–7.17 (m,3H)	7.23–7.16 (m,3H)	7.23–7.17 (m,3H)	7.23–7.18 (m,3H)	7.20–7.17 (m,3H)	7.24–7.18 (m,3H)	7.20–7.19 (m,3H)	7.34–7.28 (m,4H)	7.04(d,1H), 7.01(t,H)
12,14	7.31–7.26 (m,2H)	7.32–7.26 (m,2H)	7.32–7.25 (m,2H)	7.31–7.26 (m,2H)	7.30–7.26 (m,2H)	7.29–7.26 (m,2H)	7.31–7.28 (m,2H)	7.30–7.23 (m,2H)	7.34–7.28 (m,4H)	6.69(d,1H), 6.78(t,H)
15	7.24–7.18 (m,3H)	7.23–7.17 (m,3H)	7.23–7.16 (m,3H)	7.23–7.17 (m,3H)	7.23–7.18 (m,3H)	7.20–7.17 (m,3H)	7.24–7.18 (m,3H)	7.20–7.19 (m,3H)	7.34–7.28 (m,4H)	–
16	8.38–8.32 (d,1H)	8.43–8.37 (d,1H)	8.43–8.37 (d,1H)	8.01–7.99 (d,1H)	8.43–8.40 (t,1H)	7.80–7.77 (d,1H)	5.15 (d,1H)	7.99–7.97 (d,1H)	8.95–8.93 (d,1H)	8.27 (d,1H)
17	8.15–7.56 (s,6H)	8.20–8.10 (s,3H)	8.20–8.10 (s,3H)	8.65–8.63 (d,1H)	8.10–8.09 (d,3H)	–	6.16 (s,1H)	8.43–8.42 (d,2H)	8.18–8.13 (m,3H)	8.08 (s,2H)
18	8.15–7.56 (s $^{(a)}$,6H)	7.82–7.72 (s,3H)	7.82–7.72 (s,3H)	7.78 (s,3H)	8.33–8.30 (d,1H)	6.75–6.73 (t,1H)	–	8.43–8.42 (d,2H)	7.78 (s,3H)	7.86 (s,2H)
19	2.39 (s,6H)	2.42 (s,6H)	2.42 (s,6H)	2.39 (s,9H)	2.38 (s,9H)	–	–	2.45 (s,12H)	2.45 (s,6H)	9.43 (s,1H)
21,29				3.88–3.83 (t,1H)	3.72–3.69 (t,1H)	1.37 (s,9H)	1.45 (s,9H)	3.82–3.73 (t,1H)		
22,31				1.63–1.48 (m,6H)	1.60–1.52 (dd,2H)	1.37 (s,9H)	1.45 (s,9H)	1.72–1.70 (d,4H)		
23,32				1.25 (d,2H)	1.04,0.93 (m,2H).	1.37 (s,9H)	1.45 (s,9H)	1.38–1.34 (m,6H)		
24,33				1.63–1.48 (m,6H)	1.38–1.27 (m,4H)			1.62–1.53 (dd,4H)		
25,34				2.82–2.76 (m,4H)	2.79–2.74 (dd,2H)			2.84–2.71 (dd,4H)		
26,(35)				7.78 (s,3H)	7.70 (s,3H)			7.75 (s,6H)		
27,(30)				8.14 (s,3H)	7.99 (d,3H)			8.09 (s,6H)		

$^{(a)}$ Single; $^{(b)}$ Double; $^{(c)}$ Multiple; $^{(d)}$ Doublet doublet.

Table 3. ^{13}C-NMR assignment for LDX and its impurities.

Position	LDX δC DEPT	Imp-D δC DEPT	Imp-E δC DEPT	Imp-F δC DEPT	Imp-G δC DEPT	Imp-H δC DEPT	Imp-L δC DEPT	Imp-M δC DEPT
1	167.41–	168.88–	167.87–	174.25–	174.17–	170.61–	167.96–	167.69–
2	52.02 CH	53.35 CH	52.61 CH	54.98 CH	54.97 CH	53.34 CH	52.33 CH	52.47 CH
3	30.38 CH$_2$	30.89 CH$_2$	30.88 CH$_2$	35.00 CH$_2$	34.55 CH$_2$	28.97 CH$_2$	30.78 CH	30.88 CH$_2$
4	20.73 CH$_2$	21.58 CH$_2$	21.57 CH$_2$	22.88 CH$_2$	22.72 CH$_2$	22.96 CH$_2$	22.74 CH$_2$	21.27 CH$_2$
5	26.38 CH$_2$	26.72 CH$_2$	26.78 CH$_2$	29.89 CH$_2$	29.83 CH$_2$	26.72 CH$_2$	26.66 CH$_2$	27.01 CH$_2$
6	38.53 CH$_2$	38.98 CH$_2$	38.90 CH$_2$	40.25 CH$_2$	40.09 CH$_2$	32.14 CH$_2$	38.95 CH$_2$	38.93 CH$_2$
7	46.45 CH	46.66 CH	46.84 CH	46.00 CH	45.83 CH	46.54 CH	–	45.31 CH
8	20.83 CH$_3$	20.17 CH$_3$	21.22 CH$_3$	20.54 CH$_3$	20.23 CH$_3$	21.02 CH$_3$	21.46 CH$_3$	21.47 CH$_3$
9	41.77 CH$_2$	41.99 CH$_2$	42.17 CH$_2$	42.29 CH$_2$	42.62 CH$_2$	42.19 CH$_2$	48.91 CH	36.97 CH$_2$
10	138.99 C	139.34 C	139.34 C	139.43 C	138.55 C	139.51 C	144.61 C	125.37 C
11	128.13 CH	128.62 CH	128.50 CH	128.55 CH	128.30 CH	128.46 CH	127.32 CH	131.29 CH
12	129.20 CH	129.61 CH	129.57 CH	129.62 CH	129.38 CH	129.59 CH	128.78 CH	118.94 CH
13	126.18 CH	128.62 CH	126.56 CH	126.45 CH	126.37 CH	126.47 CH	126.37 CH	127.73 CH
14	129.20 CH	129.61 CH	129.57 CH	129.62 CH	129.38 CH	129.55 CH	128.78 CH	115.28 CH
15	128.13 CH	128.62 CH	128.50 CH	128.55 CH	128.30 CH	128.49 CH	127.32 CH	155.85 C
19	39.80 CH$_3$	40.07 CH$_3$	40.13 CH$_3$	156.03–	156.10–	40.16 CH$_3$	40.11 CH$_3$	–
20		170.61–	168.67–	77.73 C	79.07 C	168.63–		
21		52.47 CH	52.53 CH	28.74 CH$_3$	28.42 CH$_3$	52.53 CH		
22		31.98 CH$_2$	31.07 CH$_2$	28.74 CH$_3$	28.42 CH$_3$	30.90 CH$_2$		
23		22.63 CH$_2$	21.64 CH$_2$	28.74 CH$_3$	28.42 CH$_3$	21.65 CH$_2$		
24,33		26.86 CH$_2$	28.83 CH$_2$			26.78 CH$_2$		
25,34		39.10 CH$_2$	38.96 CH$_2$			38.97 CH$_2$		
28						168.69–		
29						52.25 CH		
31						30.84 CH$_2$		
32						21.33 CH$_2$		

Note: ^{13}C-NMR assignment for Imp-B and Imp-C was identical to LDX.

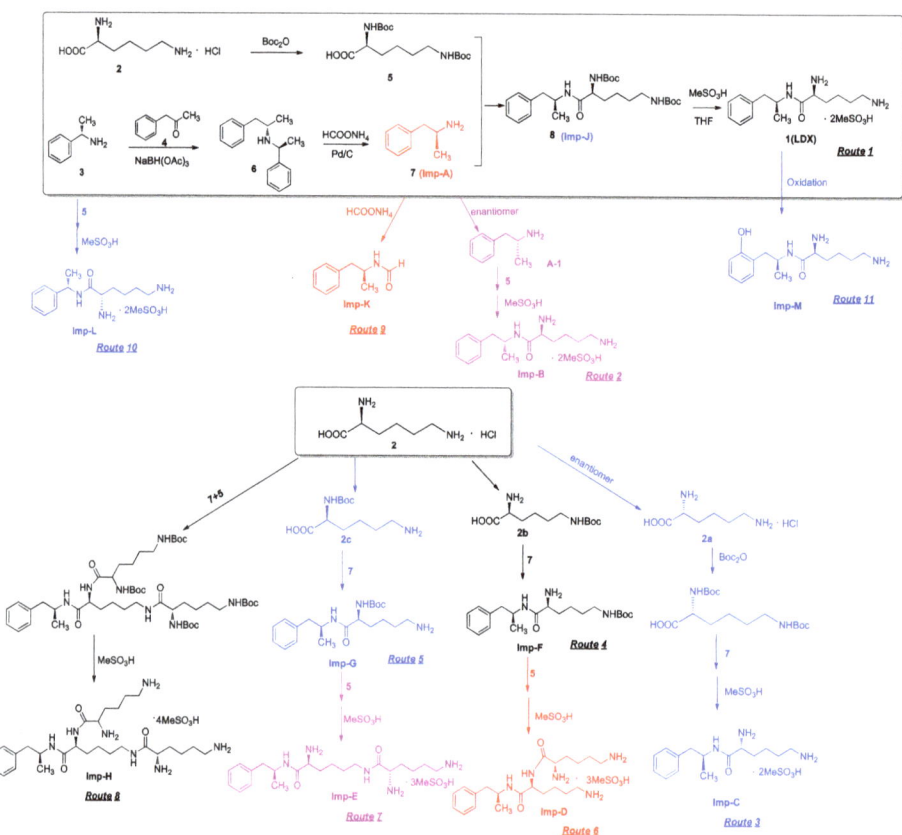

Figure 3. Eleven routes for the formation of LDX and its impurities.

2.2.2. Structural Elucidation and Control Strategy of Imp-F and Imp-G

Both of the protonated molecular ions for Imp-F and Imp-G, were obtained at an [M + H]⁺ of m/z 364.2 (Figure S5), which was 100 a.m.u. more than that of LDX. The 100 may correspond to one t-butyloxy carbonyl (Boc) moiety and thus we speculated that the two impurities were possibly (2S)-2-amino-6-((tert-butoxycarbonyl)amino)-N-[(1S)-1-methyl-2-phenylethyl]hexan-amide (Imp-F) and (2S)-2-((tert-butoxycarbonyl)amino)-6-amino-N-[(1S)-1-methyl-2-phenyl-ethyl]hexanamide (Imp-G), respectively. According to the synthetic route (Figure 3), Imp-F was obtained as a colorless oil with 97.63% HPLC purity while Imp-G was obtained as a white solid with 98.63% HPLC purity.

The HRMS of impurities F and G showed an [M + H]⁺ at m/z 364.2595 and 364.2590, respectively, suggesting an identical elemental composition of $C_{20}H_{34}N_3O_3$ (Table 1). The structures were further confirmed by the IR, ¹H-NMR, ¹³C-NMR, and DEPT spectra. Both of these impurities had one additional t-butyloxycarbonyl compared with LDX. In the ¹³C-NMR of Imp-F, the additional Boc group was deshielded to δ_{C20} = 77.73 ppm and δ_{C21} = 28.74 ppm. In the ¹H-NMR, the chemical shift of the additional Boc was deshielded to δ_{H21} = 1.37 ppm. The NMR spectrum of Imp-G was similar to that of Imp-F, except that H-2 was appeared at a lower field of the ¹H-NMR spectrum (chemical shift of δ_H = 3.98 ppm) that impurity G, which was affected by the acyl-amino groups at C1 and C19. This phenomenon also ocurrs between **2b** and **2c** (Supporting Information Figure S7). Detailed information about the ¹H-NMR and ¹³C-NMR spectra can be seen in Tables 2 and 3. To the best of our knowledge, this is the first report of all the spectroscopic data of Imp-F and Imp-G.

There were two ways whereby Imp-F and Imp-G can be formed in the bulk drug. First, intermediate **5** may contain **2b** and **2c** if the amino protection was not complete during its synthesis, affording, respectively, Imp-F and Imp-G. Second, the presence of Imp-J in LDX drug substance indicated that Imp-F and Imp-G were also likely formed due to the incomplete de-Boc in the final step of LDX. Accordingly, the control strategy of Imp-F and Imp-G was to increase the equivalents of (Boc)$_2$O to 2.2 during the amino protection, so that L-lysine reacted completely as far as possible, thereby reducing the content of **2b** and **2c**. Moreover, the amount of methanesulfonic acid was increased to 5 equivalents in the last step to ensure he complete deprotection. The content of Imp-F, Imp-G and Imp-J can thus be reduced to below 0.1% after recrystallization.

2.2.3. Structural Elucidation and Control Strategy of Imp-D and Imp-E

On-line LC-MS spectra of Imp-D and Imp-E in LDX suggested that they were likely (2S)-2-lysyl-6-amino-N-[(1S)-1-methyl-2-phenylethyl]hexanamide (Imp-D), and (2S)-2-amino-6-lysyl-N-[(1S)-1-methyl-2-phenylethyl]hexanamide (Imp-E), both of which were colorless oils with ≥96% HPLC purity. The HRMS of impurity D and E revealed their [M + H]$^+$ at m/z 392.3205 and 392.3207, respectively, suggesting that they share the same elemental composition of C$_{21}$H$_{38}$N$_5$O$_2$ (Table 1). Their structures were further confirmed by IR, ^{1}H-NMR, ^{13}C-NMR, DEPT, HSQC and HMBC spectral data. The ^{1}H-NMR spectra of Imp-D and Imp-E showed 17 signals, corresponding to 49 protons, which were consistent with the molecular structures of Imp-D and Imp-E. Both of them had an additional L-lysine on different amino groups (H17 and H18) compared with LDX. In the ^{13}C-NMR spectrum of Imp-E, the chemical shift of the additional L-lysine (C20, C21, C22, C23, C24, C25) was deshielded to δ_C = 168.64, 52.53, 31.07, 21.64, 28.83, 38.96 ppm, respectively. The ^{13}C-NMR spectrum of Imp-D was similar to that of Imp-E. In the ^{1}H-NMR spectrum of Imp-D (Supporting Information Figure S7, D-1), affected by the two carbonyl groups (C1 and C20), the H-2 proton appeared at a lower field (chemical shift of δ_{H2} = 4.20 ppm) while its chemical shift is 3.60 ppm in the ^{1}H-NMR spectrum of Imp-E (Figure S7, E-1). Besides, compared with the H-6 of Imp-D (δ_{H6} = 2.80 ppm), the H-6 of Imp-E, affected by the acyl-amino group (C20), shifted to a lower field (δ_{H6} = 3.02 ppm). The HSQC spectrum provided further evidence for the difference on the structures of Imp-D and Imp-E (Figures S7, D-5, E-5). In the HMBC spectrum of Imp-D (Figure S7, D-6), H-2 was correlated with C1 and C20, but the key long-range correlation between H-2 and C20 in Imp-E was not existed (Figure S7, E-6). In the meantime, there was no correlation between H-6 and C20 in Imp-D (Figure S7, D-6), while the H-6 was correlated with C20 in Imp-E (Figure S7, E-6). The correlation peaks of two-dimensional NMR spectra indicated that Imp-D and Imp-E were not the same compound, but rather positional isomers. The detailed ^{1}H-NMR and ^{13}C-NMR spectra information can be seen in Tables 2 and 3. The HRMS and NMR spectra of the two impurities have never been reported in the literature.

In order to control the amount of Imp-D and Imp-E, we decreased the content of **2b** and **2c** by optimizing the process parameters in the amino protection step. In addition, intermediate **8** was recrystallized (acetone:n-heptane = 1:10, v/v) to reduce the precursors of Imp-D and Imp-E. As a result, the content of the two impurities in LDX were eliminated to below 0.05%.

2.2.4. Structural Elucidation and Control Strategy of Imp-H

Inspired by the formation of Imp-D and Imp-E and a [M + H]$^+$ m/z 520.3 peak for Imp-H (Figure S5), we speculated that Imp-H was (2S)-2,6-di-(lysyl)-amino-N-[(1S)-1-methyl-2-phenylethyl] hexanamide. Imp-H was obtained as a white solid and its HPLC purity was found to be 99.61%. By comparison of retention times in HPLC, we found that the quantity of Imp-H was about 0.05% in the bulk drug (Figure 2). The HRMS of impurity H revealed an [M+H]$^+$ at m/z 520.3975, suggesting an elemental composition of C$_{27}$H$_{50}$N$_7$O$_3$ (Table 1). Besides, the fragments 503.4, 392.3, 385.3, 264.2, 257.2, 129.1 appeared in the MS/MS spectrum of Imp-H, which supported the proposed molecular structure (Figure 4). The structure was further confirmed by IR, 1D NMR (^{1}H, ^{13}C, DEPT) and 2D NMR (COSY, HSQC, HMBC) spectral data. The IR spectrum displayed characteristic absorptions at 3431.0, 1671.4,

1555.5 and 1192.9/cm which were indicatives of an amino (N-H) stretching vibration, a C=O stretching vibration, an N-H bending vibration, and a C-N stretching vibration, respectively. Imp-H had two additional acyl-amino groups (-CONH) and two additional amino-groups (-NH$_2$) compared with LDX. The chemical shift of the additional active hydrogens (H17, H18) were deshielded to δ_H = 7.8–8.5 ppm compared with the ^{1}H-NMR spectrum of LDX. The additional amino groups were assigned to be H-27, H-30, H-26, H-35 on the basis of the HMBC spectrum in the Supporting Information (Figure S7) showing correlations of H-27, H-30 (δ_H =8.08 ppm) with C-20, C-28 (δ_C = 168.69, 168.63 ppm) and correlations of C-20, C-28 (δ_C = 168.69, 168.63 ppm) with H-17, H-18 (δ_H =8.43–8.42 ppm) (Figure S7, H-5). The above results indicated that Imp-H had two additional L-lysines compared with LDX. Furthermore, the H-2 and H-6 signals appeared at a lower field in the ^{1}H-NMR spectrum (chemical shift of δ_{H2} = 4.18 ppm and δ_{H2} = 3.04 ppm, respectively) of impurity H (Figure S7), which indicated that the amino-group (-NH$_2$) was transformed to an acylmino (-CONH). The COSY spectrum showed correlation of H-17 (δ_H = 8.42 ppm) with H-2 (δ_H = 4.18 ppm) and correlation of H-18 (δ_H = 8.43 ppm) with the methylene H-6 (δ_H = 3.04 ppm). In the meantime, there were twelve more carbon atoms in Imp-H than in LDX, and the chemical shifts of δ_{C28} = 168.69 ppm, δ_{C20} = 168.63 ppm and δ_{C1} = 170.61 ppm in the ^{13}C-NMR spectrum provided further evidence for the existence of amides. The assignment of ^{1}H- and ^{13}C-NMR signals was performed for Imp-H on the basis of the ^{1}H-, ^{13}C- and 2D NMR data in Tables 2 and 3. Further detailed information of the HSQC, HMBC and COSY spectra of Imp-H can be seen in Figure S7. To our knowledge, this compound is reported for the first time. The control strategy of Imp-H is identical to that of Imp-D and Imp-E.

2.2.5. Structural Elucidation and Control Strategy of Imp-L

The synthetic route of (2S)-2,6-di-amino-N-((1S)-phenylethyl) hexanamide (Imp-L) was similar to that of LDX (Figure1), except that Imp-A was replaced by (S)-1-phenylethylamine (3) in the amide condensation step. Imp-L was obtained as a white solid and its HPLC purity was found to be 98.63%. The HRMS of Imp-L revealed an [M + H]$^+$ at m/z 250.1908, which suggested an elemental composition of C$_{14}$H$_{24}$N$_3$O (Table 1). Compared with LDX, Imp-L was missing a -CH$_2$ group. In the ^{1}H-NMR spectrum, no benzyl (H7) was found at δ_H = 2.6–2.9 ppm and the chemical shift of H$_8$ was deshielded from 1.14–1.15 ppm to 1.37–1.39 ppm. Detailed information about the ^{1}H-NMR and ^{13}C-NMR spectra is given in Tables 2 and 3. The IR spectrum of Imp-L displayed characteristic absorptions at 3449.5, 1597.1 and 1198.5/cm which were indicative of an amino (N-H) stretching vibration, a C=O stretching vibration and a C-N stretching vibration, respectively.

The residue of (S)-1-phenylethanamine (3) in intermediate 7 led to Imp-L. Hence, the control strategy of Imp-L was to make 3 react as completely as possible in the reductive amination reaction. Thus, the equivalent ratio of (S)-1-phenylethanamine (3) and phenylacetone (4) was set to 1:1.1. On the other hand, the chemical and optical purity of intermediate 6 were improved by salt formation with hydrochloric acid, thereby reducing the production of Imp-L from the source.

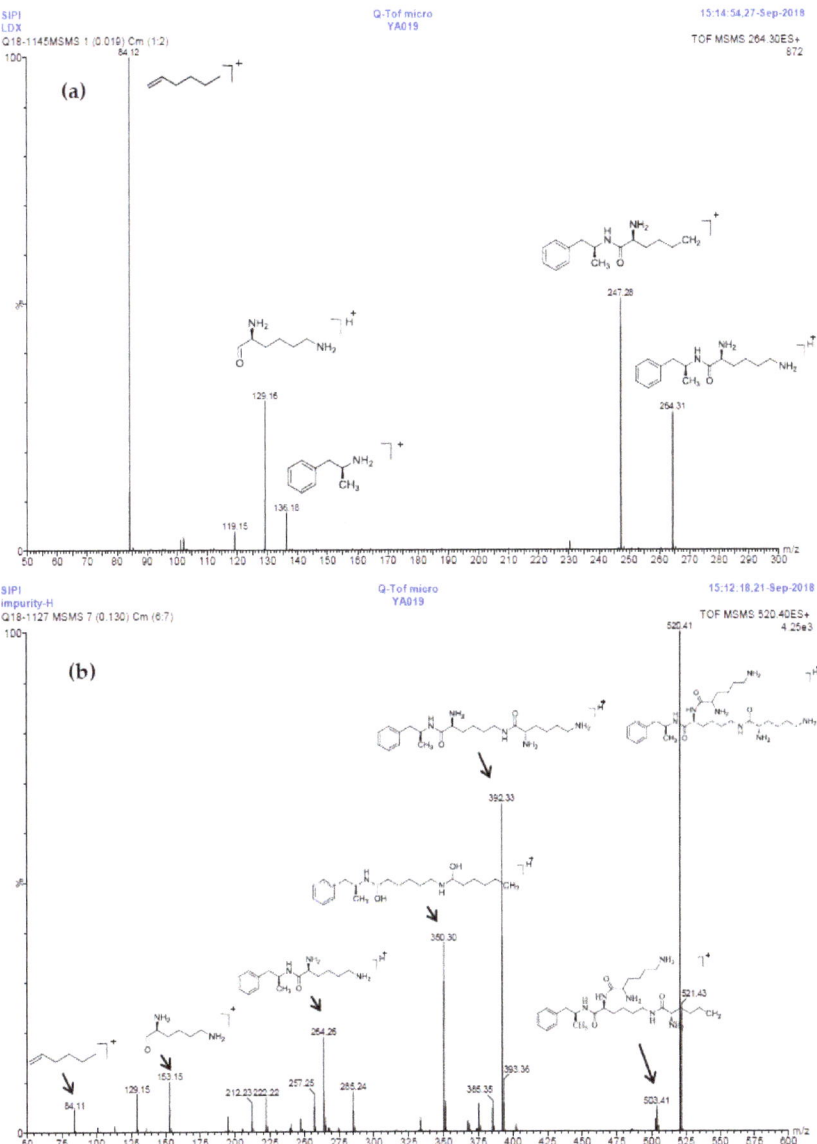

Figure 4. *Cont.*

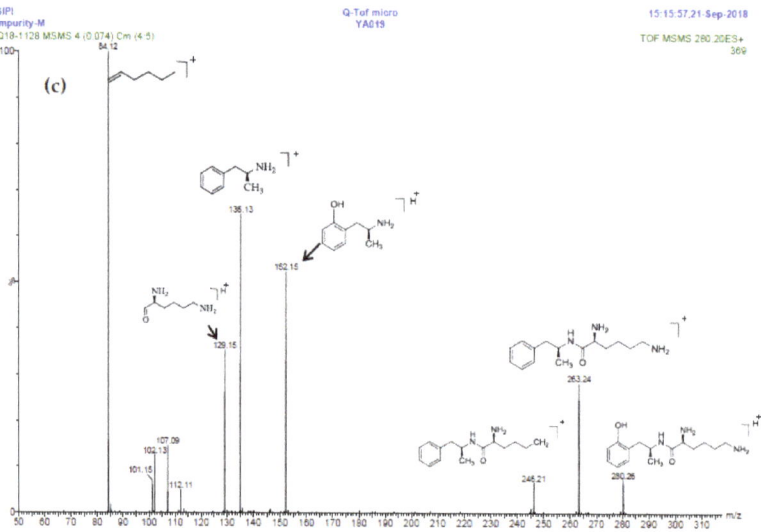

Figure 4. MS/MS spectra and plausible fragments of LDX (**a**), Imp-H (**b**) and Imp-M (**c**).

2.2.6. Structural Elucidation and Control Strategy of Imp-M

Oxidative degradation was performed in 5% H_2O_2 at room temperature in the dark for 4h. Considering that the purpose of the degradation experiment is to provide recommendations for transport and storage of drugs, we focused on the impurity with the maximum content under this oxidative condition. The on-line LC-MS spectrum indicated that the molecular weight of the major degradation product was 279.2 (Figure S5), 16 more than LDX. The HRMS of impurity M showed an $[M + H]^+$ at m/z 280.2020, suggesting an elemental composition of $C_{15}H_{26}N_3O_2$ (Table 1). Furthermore, there was only four hydrogen atoms on the benzene ring accorded with the ^{1}H-NMR spectrum. In other words, impurity M had more than one substituent group on the benzene ring and not the two primary amines of LDX. It was supposed that the two primary amines had formed salts with methanesulfonic acid, making them more stable in hydrogen peroxide. Furthermore, the identical oxidative experiment had been conducted with the free base of LDX, but the degraded products showed different retention time with Imp-M in HPLC. Moreover, it was reported that hydrogen peroxide with strong acid or Lewis acid converted benzene and alkylbenzenes into their hydroxylated products [12]. On the basis of molecular weight (279.2), we speculated that the additional group was a hydroxyl group. In addition, the ^{1}H-NMR spectrum showed that there were four different kinds of hydrogen on the benzene ring in the low field. Thus, we excluded the para-hydroxyl degradant. Moreover, the splitting of these four kinds of hydrogen are double and triple peaks, but not single, which indicated the hydroxyl group was not located in the *meta*-position. The HMBC spectrum of Imp-M in Supporting Information Figure S7 showed correlations of the additional hydroxyl group (H-19) (δ_H =9.43 ppm) with C-10, C-14 and C-15 (δ_C = 125.30, 115.25, 155.85 ppm) and correlations of H-9 (δ_H = 2.73, 2.56 ppm, dd) with C-10, C-11 and C-15 (δ_C = 125.30, 131.29, 155.85 ppm). The above results supported that the additional OH was located in the *ortho*-position. The structure was further confirmed by ^{13}C-NMR and DEPT. In the ^{13}C-NMR, the carbon atom connecting to the additional OH shifted to the low field (δ_{C15} = 155.85 ppm) compared to that of LDX. In the meantime, the DEPT spectrum showed that only four carbons appeared in the aromatic region (110–160 ppm), and the C-15 (δ_{C15} = 155.85 ppm) disappeared, which confirmed again that the OH was on the benzene ring. The HSQC spectrum of Imp-M (Figure S7, M-5) showed that there was no hydrogen atom correlated with C-10 and C-15 (δC-10 = 1125.30 ppm, δC-15 = 155.85 ppm), which provided further evidence for the above conclusion. Based on the abovementioned spectral data, the new compound was identified as (2*S*)-2,6-diamino-*N*-[(1*S*)-1-methyl-2-(2-hydroxyphenyl) ethyl] hexanamide. Fragments 263.2, 246.2, 152.1, 135.1, 129.1, 84.1 were visible in the MS/MS spectrum of Imp-M, which further supports the proposed molecular structure (Figure 4). The assignment of ^{1}H- and ^{13}C-NMR signals was completed by means of COSY, HSQC and HMBC spectroscopic data sets (Figure S7). The detailed information about the ^{1}H-NMR, ^{13}C-NMR and DEPT spectra can be seen in Tables 2 and 3. This novel degradation product has not yet been disclosed in any other published work.

2.3. Possible Mechanisms for Formation of the Impurities

Taking into account the synthetic process of LDX in combination with some published research, we proposed eleven possible routes for the formation of the twelve impurities (process-related and degradation) (Figure 3). Imp-A and Imp-J were the residues of intermediate **7** and intermediate **8** in the synthetic process of LDX in route 1. In routes 2 and 3, both intermediate **7** and L-lysine (**2**) contained trace amounts of enantiomers **A-1** and **2a**. The synthetic routes of Imp-B and Imp-C were consistent with that of LDX (Figure 1), except that L-lysine (**2**) was replaced by D-lysine (**2a**) while intermediate **7** was replaced by (R)-1-phenylpropan-2-amine (**A-1**). On the other hand, LDX can produce Imp-B or Imp-C in alkaline condition. In routes 4 and 5, intermediate **5** may contain (2S)-2-amino-6-((tert-butoxycarbonyl)amino)hexanoic acid (**2b**) and (2S)-6-amino-2-((tert-butoxycarbonyl)-amino)hexanoic acid (**2c**) as impurities when the amino protection was not completed during its synthesis, affording, respectively, Imp-F and Imp-G which, generated Imp-D (route 6) and Imp-E (route 7) after sequentially reacting with intermediate **5**, and both underwent the same reaction that gave LDX. In route 8, intermediate **5** may contain the residue of L-lysine (**2**) in its synthesis process, affording Imp-H with the same reaction that gave LDX in the last step. In route 9, during the debenzyl reaction, excessive amounts of ammonium formate may continuously react with intermediate **7**, affording Imp-K as a residue in LDX. In route 10, as an impurity, **3** might exist in intermediate **7**, and Imp-L was obtained by the same reaction for LDX. In route 11, Imp-M was produced under oxidative condition.

2.4. Optimization of the HPLC-UV Method

According to the foregoing analysis, twelve impurities were detected and successfully identified by LC-MS, HRMS, NMR and IR spectroscopy. Initially, different types of HPLC columns, such as Thermo Accucore XL C8 (150 × 4.6 mm, 4 μm) column, Thermo Syncronis C18 (250 × 4.6 mm × 5 μm) column and YMC-Pack ODS-AQ (250 × 4.6 mm × 5 μm) were tested to analyze LDX. The capability of separating LDX and its impurities was evaluated mainly through the performance characteristics of the columns. The best resolution was obtained on the discovery YMC-Pack ODS-AQ column which was thereafter used for further optimization of the method.

Different mobile phase conditions and gradient progress were tested together to develop a selective separation method. We used a variety of organic acids and the tailing peak was found to appear when trifluoroacetic acid was used as the mobile phase. Fortunately, better shape symmetrical peaks were obtained with methanesulfonic acid. In the meantime, the addition of 0.1% methanesulfonic acid to acetonitrile improved the baseline fluctuation. The separation of these impurities was not satisfactory by a continuous gradient elution program. The initial gradient elution condition was as follows: 0–10 min, linear from 5% to 20% B, however, the polar impurities (D, E, L, M) cannot be well separated under this condition. For the separation of Imp-D, Imp-E, Imp-L and Imp-M, the gradient profile was optimized. On the one hand, we reduced the slope of B increase (0–15 min, linear from 3% to 20% B). Alternatively, the separation can be improved by reducing the initial proportion of the organic phase to 3%. The method was initially optimized by comparing the separation of related substance, shape symmetrical peaks of LDX and its impurities, and then by optimizing the effect of column types, mobile phase and gradient elution mode afterwards shown in Section 2.2.

2.5. Validation of the HPLC-UV Method

The HPLC method, used to identify the related substances in LDX bulk drug, was validated in terms of the linearity, accuracy, precision, limit of quantitation (LOQ), limit of detection (LOD), robustness and system suitability. The validation was in accordance with ICH Q2 guideline [13] and the details are shown in Tables 4 and 5.

Table 4. Summary of method validation.

Compound	System Suitability				Linearity					Sensitivity	
	RRT [a]	PC [b]	SF [c]	R [d]	Range (µg/mL)	R [e]	Slope	Intercept	CF [f]	LOD [g] (µg/mL)	LOQ [h] (µg/mL)
LDX	-	19755	1.28	6.09	0.5100–20.4000	0.9999	0.1461	−0.0055	-	0.3060	0.5100
Imp-A	1.17	105353	1.15	66.28	0.5025–20.1000	1.0000	0.2271	−0.0276	0.61	0.3028	0.5025
Imp-B	1.12	121354	1.02	3.50	0.5110–20.4400	1.0000	0.1262	−0.0141	1.10	0.3010	0.5105
Imp-C	1.12	125659	1.03	3.50	0.5047–20.1900	1.0000	0.1119	−0.0010	1.31	0.3026	0.5105
−Imp-D	0.93	98972	1.09	3.33	0.5160–20.6400	1.0000	0.1112	−0.0079	1.04	0.3035	0.5070
Imp-E	0.89	118365	1.14	3.19	0.5135–20.5400	1.0000	0.0836	−0.0013	1.66	0.3041	0.5051
Imp-F	2.38	749255	1.63	12.44	0.5022–20.0900	1.0000	0.1700	−0.0061	0.86	0.3013	0.5023
Imp-G	2.25	864920	1.16	80.95	0.5070–20.2800	1.0000	0.1641	−0.0119	0.89	0.3042	0.5070
Imp-H	0.725	46840	1.28	8.53	0.5028–20.1900	1.0000	0.1524	−0.0085	0.92	0.3028	0.5062
Imp-J	3.08	28465	1.14	-	0.5080–20.3200	0.9998	0.1269	0.0110	1.15	0.3028	0.5041
Imp-K	2.15	322224	1.12	7.00	0.5105–20.256	0.9999	0.1389	0.0105	1.32	0.3036	0.5075
Imp-L	0.83	90222	1.02	8.53	0.5180–20.7200	1.0000	0.1159	−0.0056	1.19	0.3041	0.5180
Imp-M	0.86	114119	1.17	3.40	0.5240–20.9592	1.0000	0.1614	−0.0011	0.91	0.3060	0.5140

[a] Relative retention time; [b] (USP) plate count; [c] Symmetry factor; [d] (USP) resolution; [e] Correlation factor. [f] Calibration response factor. [g] (S/N ≥ 3). [h] (S/N ≥10).

Table 5. Summary of accuracy.

Impurity	0.05%–1%	0.05%–2%	0.05%–3%	0.10%–1%	0.10%–2%	0.10%–3%	0.15%–1%	0.15%–2%	0.15%–3%	Mean	RSD (n = 9)
Imp-A	91.8	90.2	92.6	89.6	92.7	94.1	92.0	92.5	94.1	92.0	1.83
Imp-B	102.6	105.1	100.2	100.9	91.3	97.3	92.6	90.8	90.5	96.8	5.82
Imp-C	92.8	90.4	91.2	100.6	98.7	99.5	97.4	102.4	98.5	96.8	4.44
Imp-D	99.7	96.3	95.8	97.7	96.3	97.6	94.1	97.0	93.1	96.4	2.04
Imp-E	99.1	101.0	102.7	101.6	96.5	95.7	103.5	103.4	102.6	100.6	2.91
Imp-F	103.9	96.6	97.1	103.3	105.6	99.3	98.8	100.3	98.1	100.3	3.19
Imp-G	101.5	102.4	100.3	103.3	96.6	102.6	95.8	100.9	100.5	100.4	2.59
Imp-H	99.5	98.7	102.5	101.8	98.9	103.5	96.9	99.5	102.1	100.3	2.16
Imp-J	92.7	95.4	93.9	95.0	96.2	93.5	91.0	99.4	94.0	94.5	2.50
Imp-K	99.7	103.5	101.6	98.7	99.5	96.4	105.1	103.6	104.2	101.3	2.90
Imp-L	91.4	90.6	101.2	95.7	95.5	94.8	96.7	90.0	94.9	94.5	3.69
Imp-M	97.8	98.5	93.2	95.1	94.4	97.6	91.3	95.5	92.7	95.1	2.62

2.5.1. System Suitability

In order to obtain a satisfactory performance using the analytical method, a system suitability test was carried out before each run. The results showed that the United States Pharmacopoeia (USP) theoretical plates of LDX and its impurities were greater than 19755, the USP resolution between any two compounds was greater than 3.19, and the peak asymmetry for all the analytes was between 1.02 and 1.28 (Table 4). The HPLC chromatogram of the separation of LDX and its impurities can be seen in Figure 2.

2.5.2. Linearity, LOD, and LOQ

Using the least squares method, linear regression analysis of the response values of sample solutions with different concentrations and the corresponding concentration was carried out to calculate the slope and intercept. The measurements indicated that the response value and concentration had a positive linear relationship over the concentration range of 0.50–20.00 µg/mL. The LOQ solution (0.50 µg/mL), equivalent to 0.05% of the LDX sample solution, was prepared and used to calculate the (S/N) of LDX and its twelve impurities. S/N of LDX and its impurities was greater than 10, and the LOQ of the method was 0.05% while the minimum quantitative concentration was 0.50 µg/mL. Using the same injection, the calculated LOD of the method was 0.02% and the S/N of LDX and its impurities was 3:1. The LOQ level by injecting six individual preparations and calculating the percentage RSD of the areas. The results were shown in Table 4.

2.5.3. Accuracy, Precision, and Robustness

Recovery and RSD values of sample solution at concentration levels of 0.05%, 0.10%, and 0.15% were measured in triplicate after the addition of a certain amount of the twelve impurities to LDX test solutions (1.0 mg/mL) and then the accuracy was calculated. The recovery of all the impurities was 80%–120%, confirming the acceptable good accuracy of the method (Table 5). The precision of the method was evaluated through parallel preparation of six individual 1.0 mg/mL LDX sample solution for injection and calculating the RSD for each peak. The RSD of all individual impurities was not more than 5%, indicating good precision of the method (Table 6). The robustness of the developed method was studied by changing the column temperature (30 ± 3 °C) flow rate (1.0 ± 0.1 mL/min), detection wavelength (215 ± 2 nm) of the original HPLC conditions. Under different conditions, excluding the isomer of impurities B and C, resolution between any two compounds was >1.5. Compared with the original HPLC method, difference measured values of the individual impurities in the sample solution was not more than 0.02%, suggesting excellent robustness of the method (Table 7).

Table 6. Summary of precision.

Compound	1	2	3	4	5	6	RSD (n = 6)
	\multicolumn{6}{c}{C (mg/mL)}	
	1.0080	1.0225	1.0180	1.0290	1.0130	1.0095	
Imp-A	0.10	0.10	0.09	0.10	0.10	0.10	4.22
Imp-B	0.10	0.11	0.11	0.11	0.11	0.11	2.19
Imp-C	0.12	0.12	0.12	0.12	0.12	0.13	3.24
Imp-D	0.09	0.09	0.09	0.09	0.09	0.08	1.67
Imp-E	0.10	0.10	0.10	0.11	0.10	0.10	1.83
Imp-F	0.12	0.12	0.12	0.12	0.11	0.11	1.20
Imp-G	0.10	0.10	0.10	0.10	0.10	0.10	1.30
Imp-H	0.10	0.11	0.11	0.10	0.10	0.10	1.51
Imp-J	0.11	0.11	0.10	0.10	0.10	0.10	2.14
Imp-K	0.11	0.11	0.11	0.10	0.10	0.11	1.63
Imp-L	0.11	0.11	0.11	0.11	0.11	0.11	1.32
Imp-M	0.12	0.11	0.11	0.11	0.11	0.11	1.87
RRT = 1.32	0.01	0.01	0.01	0.02	0.02	0.01	2.85

Table 7. Summary of robustness.

Compound	Column Temperature			Flow Rate			UV		
	27 °C	30 °C	33 °C	0.9 mL/min	1.0 mL/min	1.1 mL/min	213 nm	215 nm	217 nm
Imp-A	0.10	0.10	0.09	0.10	0.10	0.09	0.11	0.10	0.10
Imp-B	0.13	0.12	0.13	0.12	0.13	0.12	0.12	0.13	0.13
Imp-C	0.10	0.11	0.10	0.13	0.12	0.13	0.11	0.10	0.12
Imp-D	0.09	0.09	0.08	0.09	0.09	0.10	0.09	0.09	0.08
Imp-E	0.11	0.10	0.11	0.11	0.10	0.10	0.10	0.10	0.10
Imp-F	0.10	0.09	0.09	0.09	0.10	0.10	0.09	0.10	0.09
Imp-G	0.09	0.09	0.09	0.10	0.09	0.10	0.09	0.09	0.10
Imp-H	0.09	0.09	0.08	0.09	0.09	0.08	0.09	0.09	0.09
Imp-J	0.08	0.09	0.08	0.07	0.08	0.07	0.07	0.07	0.07
Imp-K	0.10	0.10	0.11	0.10	0.10	0.11	0.11	0.10	0.10
Imp-L	0.11	0.12	0.12	0.11	0.11	0.12	0.12	0.12	0.12
Imp-M	0.08	0.08	0.09	0.08	0.09	0.08	0.09	0.09	0.09

3. Materials and Methods

3.1. Chemicals and Reagents

Crude LDX and its impurities were synthesized in our laboratory. L-Lysine hydrochloride (**2**), (*S*)-1-phenylethanamine (**3**) and methanesulfonic acid were purchased from Energy Chemical Corporation (Shanghai, China). The purity of all substances was >98%. HPLC-grade methanesulfonic acid were purchased from Fisher Scientific (Waltham, MA, USA). HPLC-grade acetonitrile (ACN) was purchased from Honeywell (Newark, NJ, USA). Deionized water for preparing the aqueous phase was obtained using a water purification system and all other chemicals were of analytical grade.

3.2. Analytical HPLC Conditions

Studies were conducted on a Dionex Ultimate 3000 HPLC instrument (Waltham, MA, USA) equipped with a quaternary pump and a DAD detector. An analytical silica column YMC-Pack ODS-AQ S5 120A (250 × 4.6 mm × 5 μm, YMC, Nagoya, Japan) maintained at 30 °C was used for separation. Mobile phase A was 0.1% methanesulfonic acid (v/v) in water, while B was 0.1% methanesulfonic acid in acetonitrile. The HPLC gradient program was set as follows: Time (min)/% of solvent B: 0/3, 15/20, 30/50, 35/95, 37/95, 37.1/3, 45/3. The flow rate was 1.0 mL/min for a total run time of 45 min, and the detection wavelength was 215 nm. The crude LDX was accurately weighed and dissolved in the mixture of water and ACN (70:30, v/v) to obtain a test solution of 1.0 mg/mL. Samples (10 μL) were injected into the HPLC system for analysis.

3.3. LC-MS Conditions

LC-MS was performed on an Agilent LC/MS system consisting of an Agilent 1260-LC system equipped with a single quadruple mass detector and electrospray ionization (ESI) interface (Agilent Technologies, Santa Clara, CA, USA). The column and mobile phase composition are the same as in the HPLC analysis, except that formic acid was used instead of methanesulfonic acid. The LC gradient program was set as follows: Time (min)/% of solvent B: 0/5, 40/15, 50/50, 55/95, 60/95, 60.1/5, 65/5. The flow rate was 1.0 mL/min for a total run time of 65 min. The mass instrument was operated in positive-ion ESI mode. Optimized mass conditions are as follows: drying gas (N_2) flow rate of 12.0 L/min, drying gas temperature 300 °C, nebulizer pressure 50 psig, capillary voltage 3.0 kV. Scans were acquired from 50 to 800 amu with a 0.1 s/scan. The high-resolution mass spectra and MS/MS were recorded on a Q-TOF micro YA019 instrument (Waters, Milford, MA, USA).

3.4. NMR Spectroscopy

^{1}H-NMR, ^{13}C-NMR, distortionless enhancement by polarization transfer (DEPT), correlation spectroscopy (COSY), heteronuclear multiple bond correlation (HMBC), and heteronuclear singular quantum correlation (HSQC) NMR spectra were recorded on an Avance III 400 MHz spectrometer (Bruker, Karlsruhe, Germany). Solvents used were DMSO-d_6 or CDCl$_3$.

3.5. FT-IR Spectroscopy

IR spectra were recorded in the solid state as KBr dispersions using a 670 FT-IR spectrophotometer (NICOLET Waltham, MA, USA). Data were collected between 400 and 4000/cm, at a resolution of 4.0/cm.

3.6. Preparation of Standard and Sample Solutions

Samples was prepared using a water and acetonitrile mixture (70:30, v/v) as the diluent. In each trial, the HPLC conditions were investigated by injecting test solution added with the twelve impurities into the HPLC system. The concentration of LDX sample was 1.0 mg/mL, prepared by spiking the twelve impurities (Imp-A, Imp-B, Imp-C, Imp-D, Imp-E, Imp-F, Imp-G, Imp-H, Imp-J, Imp-K, Imp-L and Imp-M) into LDX at a concentration of 1.0 μg/mL and used to investigate the system suitability.

3.7. Forced Degradation Study

For forced degradation solutions, LDX was subjected to stress conditions according to ICH guidelines [14]. The forced degradation of LDX was performed under hydrolytic (acidic and alkaline), oxidative, thermal and photolytic conditions. The hydrolytic degradation was carried out separately in 1.0 M HCl (2.0 mL) as well as 5.0 M NaOH (2.0 mL) and kept in water bath at 90 °C for 3 h. The oxidative degradation was performed in 5% H_2O_2 (5.0 mL) at room temperature in the dark for 4 h. LDX was also subjected to thermolytic (90 °C, 48 h) and photolytic (UV light, 4500 lx, 24 h) degradation. After completion of the experiment, the samples were cooled to ambient temperature, neutralized with a base or an acid, respectively. All of the stressed samples were kept at a concentration of 1.0 mg/mL for assay determination.

4. Conclusions

An effective and selective HPLC method, used for the separation and determination of the twelve impurities (process-related and degradation) in LDX bulk drug, was developed and optimized. Structures of the two new compounds, Imp-H and Imp-M, were proposed by the synthesis route of LDX and LC-MS analyses, and then confirmed and characterized using HRMS, ESI-MS/MS, 1D NMR (^{1}H-, ^{13}C-, DEPT 135) and 2D NMR (COSY, HSQC, HMBC). Furthermore, probable mechanisms for the formation of the process-related and degradation impurities were proposed based on the synthesis route of LDX. The HPLC method was validated in terms of its linearity, accuracy, robustness, limits of detection, and quantification. Full identification and characterization of these impurities is useful in quality control in the manufacture of LDX.

Supplementary Materials: The following are available online, Table of contents; Figure S5 the LC-MS spectrum of LDX and its impurities; Figure S6 The spectrum of Imp-B and Imp-C in normal-phase chromatography; Figure S7 NMR, HRMS and IR spectrogram of LDX and its impurities.

Author Contributions: S.G. designed and carried out the synthetic experiments, analyzed the data and wrote the paper. L.M. performed HPLC analysis and other analysis work. C.Z. and F.Z. reviewed and edited the manuscript. All authors read and approved the manuscript.

Acknowledgments: The authors are thankful to the teachers of the China State Institute of Pharmaceutical Industry for supporting this study and the cooperation from other colleagues is also highly appreciated.

Conflicts of Interest: The authors declare no conflict of interest.

References

1. Biederman, J.; Krishnan, S.; Zhang, Y.X.; McGough, J.; Findling, R. Efficacy and tolerability of lisdexamfetamine dimesylate(NRP-104) in children with attention-deficit/hyperactivity disorder: A phase III, multicenter, randomized, double-blind, forced dose, parallel-group study. *Clin. Ther.* **2007**, *29*, 450–463. [CrossRef]
2. Michel, T.; Krishnan, S.; Bishop, B.; Lauderback, C.; Moncrief, J.; Oberlender, R.; Piccariello, T. Abuse-resistant Amphetamine Compounds. U.S. Patent 20050054561A1, 10 March 2005.
3. Michel, T.; Krishnan, S.; Bishop, B.; Lauderback, C.; Moncrief, J.; Oberlender, R.; Piccariello, T. Abuse-resistant Amphetamine Prodrugs. U.S. Patent 20070042955A1, 22 January 2007.
4. Lu, C.Y.; Feng, C.H. Identification of dimer impurities in ampicillin and amoxicillin by capillary LC and tandem mass spectrometry. *J. Sep. Sci.* **2007**, *30*, 329–332. [CrossRef] [PubMed]
5. Sun, Q.S.; Li, Y.; Qin, L. Isolation and identification of two unknown impurities from the raw material of clindamycin hydrochloride. *J. Sep. Sci.* **2014**, *37*, 2682–2687. [CrossRef] [PubMed]
6. Carlos, G.; Comiran, E.; Herbstrith, M.; Limberger, R.; Bergold, A.; Froehlich, P. Development, validation and comparison of two stability-indicating RP-LC methods using charged aerosol and UV detectors for analysis of lisdexamfetamine dimesylate in capsules. *Arab. J. Chem.* **2016**, *9*, S1905–S1914. [CrossRef]
7. Guideline, I.H.T. ICH Harmonised Tripartite Guideline: Impurities in new drug substances Q3A(R2). In Proceedings of the International Conference on Harmonization of Technical Requirements for Registration of Pharmaceuticals for Human Use, Geneva, Switzerland, 25 October 2006.
8. Yang, B.; Zhang, Y.J.; Zhang, S.S. Amidation of amines with eaters catalyzed by candida Antarctica lipase (CAL). *Cheminform* **2010**, *36*, 1312–1316.
9. Routaboul, L.; Vanthuyne, N.; Gastaldi, S.; Gil, G.; Bertrand, M. Highly efficient photochemically induced thiyl radical-mediated racemization of aliphatic amines at 30 °C. *J. Org. Chem.* **2008**, *73*, 364–368. [CrossRef] [PubMed]

10. Goudriaan, P.E.; Kaiser, J.; Ibrahim, H.; Verspui, G.A.; Cox, D.P. Process for the preparation of lisdexamfetamine and related derivatives. U.S. Patent 20160376618A1, 29 December 2016.
11. Enders, D.; Haertwig, A.; Raabe, G.; Runsink, J. Diastereo- and enantio-selective synthesis of vicinal amino alcohols by oxa-michael addition of *N*-formylnorephedrine to nitro alkenes. *Eur. J. Org. Chem.* **1998**, 1771–1792. [CrossRef]
12. Olah, G.A.; Fung, A.P.; Keumi, T. Oxyfunctionalization of hydrocarbons, hydroxylation of benzene and alkylbenzenes with hydrogen peroxide in hydrogen fluoride/boron trifluoride. *J. Org. Chem.* **1981**, *46*, 4305–4306. [CrossRef]
13. Guideline, I.H.T. Validation of analytical procedures: text and methodology. In Proceedings of the International Conference on Harmonization, Geneva, Switzerland, November 2005; pp. 11–12.
14. Guideline, I.H.T. Stability testing of new drug substances and products. *Curr. Step* **2003**, *4*, 1–24.

Sample Availability: Samples of the impurities A–M are available from the authors.

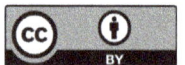

© 2018 by the authors. Licensee MDPI, Basel, Switzerland. This article is an open access article distributed under the terms and conditions of the Creative Commons Attribution (CC BY) license (http://creativecommons.org/licenses/by/4.0/).

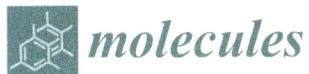

Article

Identification and Analysis of Compound Profiles of Sinisan Based on 'Individual Herb, Herb-Pair, Herbal Formula' before and after Processing Using UHPLC-Q-TOF/MS Coupled with Multiple Statistical Strategy

Jia Zhou [1,2,†], Hao Cai [1,2,*,†], Sicong Tu [3,4,†], Yu Duan [1,2,†], Ke Pei [5], Yangyang Xu [1,2], Jing Liu [1,2], Minjie Niu [1,2], Yating Zhang [1,2], Lin Shen [1,2] and Qigang Zhou [6]

1. School of Pharmacy, Nanjing University of Chinese Medicine, Nanjing 210023, China; zhoujia19931005@126.com (J.Z.); duanyu1681@sina.com (Y.D.); yangyangxu92@126.com (Y.X.); 15951921665@163.com (J.L.); someonearis@163.com (M.N.); zhangyatingzyt@126.com (Y.Z.); sonesunfany@sina.cn (L.S.)
2. Engineering Center of State Ministry of Education for Standardization of Chinese Medicine Processing, Nanjing University of Chinese Medicine, Nanjing 210023, China
3. Medical Sciences Division, University of Oxford, Oxford OX3 7BN, UK; Sicong.tu@sydney.edu.au
4. Sydney Medical School, The University of Sydney, Sydney, NSW 2006, Australia
5. Institute of Pharmaceutical and Food Engineering, Shanxi University of Traditional Chinese Medicine, Taiyuan 030024, China; peike_pk@126.com
6. School of Pharmacy, Nanjing Medical University, Nanjing 210026, China; qigangzhou@njmu.edu.cn
* Correspondence: haocai_98@126.com; Tel./Fax: +86-025-86798281
† These authors contributed equally to this work.

Academic Editors: In-Soo Yoon and Hyun-Jong Cho
Received: 1 November 2018; Accepted: 26 November 2018; Published: 29 November 2018

Abstract: Sinisan has been widely used to treat depression. However, its pharmacologically-effective constituents are largely unknown, and the pharmacological effects and clinical efficacies of Sinisan-containing processed medicinal herbs may change. To address these important issues, we developed an ultra-high performance liquid chromatography coupled with electrospray ionization tandem quadrupole-time-of-flight mass spectrometry (UHPLC-Q-TOF/MS) method coupled with multiple statistical strategies to analyze the compound profiles of Sinisan, including individual herb, herb-pair, and complicated Chinese medicinal formula. As a result, 122 different constituents from individual herb, herb-pair, and complicated Chinese medicinal formula were identified totally. Through the comparison of three progressive levels, it suggests that processing herbal medicine and/or altering medicinal formula compatibility could change herbal chemical constituents, resulting in different pharmacological effects. This is also the first report that saikosaponin h/i and saikosaponin g have been identified in Sinisan.

Keywords: chemical constituent profiles of Sinisan; chinese medicine processing; chinese medicinal formula compatibility

1. Introduction

Chinese medicine processing and Chinese medicinal formula compatibility are two outstanding characteristics in the clinical applications of Chinese medicine. However, current studies often focus on the compatibility mechanism or processing mechanism alone without combining them together organically, and reports discussing Chinese medicine processing mechanisms in Chinese medicinal formulae have been rarely involved. Therefore, the selection of the processed products of Chinese herbal medicines contained in Chinese medicinal formulae has only to rely on the experiences of clinicians without sufficient basis of scientific theories.

Sinisan (SNS), an ancient well-known Chinese medicinal formula consisting of four Chinese herbal medicines—Bupleuri Radix (BR), Paeoniae Radix Alba (PRA), Aurantii Fructus Immaturus (AFI), and Glycyrrhizae Radix et Rhizoma Praeparata Cum Melle (GRM), has been regarded as an effective anti-depression prescription according to the traditional Chinese medicine (TCM) theories of six channels and depression. SNS was initially described by Zhongjing Zhang in 'Treatise on Febrile Diseases' as a traditional Chinese herbal formula to cure mental disorders. It has been widely used for thousands of years, and even today it is still the fundamental and essential prescription for the treatment of depression [1,2]. However, the application of processed BR and processed PRA contained in SNS is quite controversial, which is necessary to improve our understanding whether the processing procedures has changed any chemical constituents of the herbal medicine.

At present, ultra-high performance liquid chromatography coupled with electrospray ionization tandem quadrupole/time of flight mass spectrometry (UHPLC-Q-TOF/MS) is a powerful tool for the analysis of complex samples in TCM and possesses high resolution, efficiency, and sensitivity to obtain accurate mass information [3–6]. Multivariate statistical analysis based on all the available chemical information has made the identification of potential chemical markers possible. In this report, we successfully developed an UHPLC-Q-TOF/MS method coupled with multiple statistical strategy to analyze the compound profiles of SNS.

Based on the theory of TCM, processing with vinegar can enhance the effects of coursing liver and resolving depression [7]. A previous report has suggested that vinegar-processed BR (VPBR) is more effective in the treatment of liver disorders, including hepatitis, cirrhosis, and liver cancer [8]. In this study, we creatively analyzed the compound profiles of individual herb, herb-pair, and complicated Chinese herbal formula according to their representative herbal medicine: BR, PRA, BR-PRA herb-pair, and SNS, respectively, and also systematically compared the changes of chemical constituents of BR, PRA, BR-PRA herb-pair, and SNS before and after processing to reveal the scientific connotation of processing and formula compatibility. We are looking forward to seeking out the common mechanism of processing and formula compatibility of Chinese herbal medicine in order to provide scientific theory for safe clinical applications of Chinese medicine and rational herbal medicine processing in Chinese medicinal formula.

2. Results and Discussion

2.1. Identification of Compounds

According to the previous reports [9–12], saponins, terpenoids, and flavones are the main chemical components in BR (VPBR), PRA (VPPRA), AFI, and GRM. These components easily lose a proton under mass spectrum detection, resulting in a better mass response in negative ion mode than in positive one. As shown in Table 1, 101 compounds were identified in negative ion mode and 21 compounds were identified in positive ion mode [13–15]. The typical total ion chromatograms (TICs) of BR, VPBR, PRA, vinegar-processed PRA (VPPRA), BR-PRA herb-pair, VPBR-VPPRA herb-pair, SNS, and SNS-containing VPBR and VPPRA in both ion modes are shown in Figure 1.

Table 1. Identification of chemical compounds by ultrahigh performance liquid chromatography coupled with electrospray ionization tandem quadrupole-time-of-flight mass spectrometry (UHPLC-Q-TOF-MS/MS).

No.	Compound	T$_R$ (min)	Molecular Formula	Detected Mass (m/z) Ion Type	Mass Error (ppm)	MS/MS (m/z)	Purity Score	Source
1	Adonitol	0.82	C$_5$H$_{12}$O$_5$	151.0612 [M − H]$^−$	4.0	101.0283,83.0141,71.0171	88.30%	BR
2	Sucrose	0.83	C$_{12}$H$_{22}$O$_{11}$	387.1133 [M + HCOOH-H]$^−$	1.0	341.1099,161.0458,89.0264	100.00%	PRA
3	Synephrine	1.22	C$_9$H$_{13}$NO$_2$	168.1019 [M + H]$^+$	−2.4	150.0912,121.0653,91.0553	76.20%	AFI
4	Gallic acid	1.97	C$_7$H$_6$O$_5$	169.0142 [M − H]$^−$	2.4	125.0246,79.0210,51.0283	79.40%	PRA
5	1-O-β-D-glucopyranosyl-paeonisuffrone	2.39	C$_{15}$H$_{24}$O$_9$	405.1391 [M + HCOOH-H]$^−$	1.3	197.0814,137.0603,85.0304	83.90%	PRA
6	6-O-β-D-glucopyranosyl lactinolide	3.16	C$_{15}$H$_{26}$O$_9$	407.1547 [M + HCOOH-H]$^−$	1.4	361.1514,199.0974,101.0250	100.00%	PRA
7	Mudanpioside f	3.31	C$_{15}$H$_{24}$O$_8$	389.1442 [M + HCOOH-H]$^−$	0.9	181.0835,151.0767,109.0646	88.10%	PRA
8	Neochlorogenic acid	3.48	C$_{16}$H$_{18}$O$_9$	353.0884 [M − H]$^−$	1.6	191.0555, 135.0449, 85.0305	93.90%	BR
9	Oxypaeoniflora	3.83	C$_{23}$H$_{28}$O$_{12}$	495.1508 [M − H]$^−$	−0.9	495.1560,137.0238	100.00%	PRA
10	4″-Hydroxy-3″-methoxyalbiflorin	4.16	C$_{24}$H$_{30}$O$_{13}$	571.1658 [M + HCOOH-H]$^−$	−2.0	525.1653,363.1080,167.0345	100.00%	PRA
11	Chlorogenic acid	4.18	C$_{16}$H$_{18}$O$_9$	353.0878 [M − H]$^−$	0.9	191.0558,85.0300	100.00%	BR
12	Cryptochlorogenic acid	4.35	C$_{16}$H$_{18}$O$_9$	353.0888 [M − H]$^−$	2.7	191.0554, 155.0330, 93.0353	93.50%	BR
13	Cianidanol	4.40	C$_{15}$H$_{14}$O$_6$	289.0718 [M − H]$^−$	2.0	245.0824,137.0238,109.0294	81.10%	PRA
14	Fabiatrin	4.52	C$_{21}$H$_{26}$O$_{13}$	531.1345 [M + HCOOH-H]$^−$	2.3	177.0189	100.00%	AFI
15	6′-O-β-D-glucopyranosylalbiflorin	4.76	C$_{29}$H$_{36}$O$_{16}$	687.2131 [M + HCOOH-H]$^−$	−8.7	641.2078,489.1612,183.0668	100.00%	PRA
16	5,7-dihydroxycoumarin	4.99	C$_9$H$_6$O$_4$	177.0193 [M − H]$^−$	6.3	177.0205,69.0003	72.80%	AFI
17	Lonicerin	5.03	C$_{27}$H$_{30}$O$_{15}$	593.-512 [M − H]$^−$	−0.7	593.1543,353.0670,297.0776	100.00%	AFI
18	Isomaltopaeoniflorin	5.13	C$_{29}$H$_{38}$O$_{16}$	687.2131 [M + H]$^+$	0.2	611.2036,323.0995,165.0563	100.00%	PRA
19	Albiflorin	5.49	C$_{23}$H$_{28}$O$_{11}$	481.1704 [M + H]$^+$	1.0	319.1183,133.0645,105.0334	100.00%	PRA
20	Paeoniflorigenone	5.58	C$_{17}$H$_{18}$O$_6$	319.1176 [M + H]$^+$	2.5	151.0757,105.0349,77.0406	100.00%	PRA
21	Isomaltoalbiflorin	5.61	C$_{29}$H$_{38}$O$_{16}$	687.2131 [M + HCOOH-H]$^−$	−9.1	641.2088,491.1763	100.00%	GRM
22	Schaftoside	5.91	C$_{26}$H$_{28}$O$_{14}$	563.1406 [M − H]$^−$	1.0	563.1478,443.1016,365.0682	100.00%	PRA
23	Paeoniflorin	5.98	C$_{23}$H$_{28}$O$_{11}$	525.1603 [M + HCOOH-H]$^−$	5.3	449.1492,165.0558,121.0301	100.00%	PRA
24	Paeonol	6.70	C$_9$H$_{10}$O$_3$	165.0557 [M − H]$^−$	1.8	119.0507,96.9579	100.00%	PRA
25	Ethyl gallate	6.90	C$_9$H$_{10}$O$_5$	197.0456 [M − H]$^−$	2.5	162.8362,89.0271,59.0154	100.00%	PRA
26	SSq	7.32	C$_{54}$H$_{88}$O$_{24}$	1165.5639 [M + HCOOH-H]$^−$	0.2	1119.5784, 1089.5630	91.00%	BR
27	Rutin	7.57	C$_{27}$H$_{30}$O$_{16}$	611.1607 [M + H]$^+$	−1.4	303.0506	100.00%	BR
28	liquiritin apioside	7.75	C$_{26}$H$_{30}$O$_{13}$	549.1614 [M − H]$^−$	1.2	549.1659,255.0666,135.0088	100.00%	GRM
29	Liquiritin	7.93	C$_{21}$H$_{22}$O$_9$	417.1191 [M − H]$^−$	0.5	255.0667,135.0090	100.00%	GRM
30	Neoeriocitrin	8.18	C$_{27}$H$_{32}$O$_{15}$	595.1568 [M − H]$^−$	0.8	595.1719,287.0566,135.0449	100.00%	AFI
31	Scopoletin	9.04	C$_{10}$H$_8$O$_4$	237.0394 [M + HCOOH-H]$^−$	6.7	121.0295,93.0328,71.0160	100.00%	AFI
32	Kaempferol	9.19	C$_{15}$H$_{10}$O$_6$	287.0550 [M + H]$^+$	−0.7	287.0533,93.0374	100.00%	BR
33	SSv	9.47	C$_{53}$H$_{86}$O$_{24}$	1151.5480 [M + HCOOH-H]$^−$	−3.1	1105.5579,791.4285,313.1119	95.90%	BR
34	Narirutin	9.50	C$_{27}$H$_{32}$O$_{14}$	579.1719 [M − H]$^−$	2.9	271.0622,151.0033	100.00%	AFI
35	Isorhamnetin	9.56	C$_{16}$H$_{12}$O$_7$	317.0656 [M − H]$^−$	0.2	317.0648,257.0430	73.60%	BR
36	Isorhamnetin-3-rutinoside	9.65	C$_{28}$H$_{32}$O$_{16}$	623.1618 [M − H]$^−$	−0.1	623.1665,315.0513,299.0196	75.50%	BR
37	Isochlorogenic acid b	9.68	C$_{25}$H$_{24}$O$_{12}$	561.1239 [M + HCOOH-H]$^−$	0.3	385.0916,193.0504,147.0257	83.60%	BR
38	Naringin	10.07	C$_{27}$H$_{32}$O$_{14}$	579.1719 [M − H]$^−$	0.9	579.1771,271.0614,151.0032	100.00%	AFI
39	Benzoic acid	10.08	C$_7$H$_6$O$_2$	123.0441 [M + H]$^+$	−5.6	105.0358,77.0394	90.50%	PRA
40	Isorhamnetin-3-glucoside	10.11	C$_{22}$H$_{22}$O$_{12}$	479.1184 [M + H]$^+$	−2.0	317.0667	89.10%	BR
41	Mudanpioside i	10.18	C$_{23}$H$_{28}$O$_{11}$	479.1559 [M − H]$^−$	−1.5	121.0302,77.0416	100.00%	PRA

Table 1. Cont.

No.	Compound	T_R (min)	Molecular Formula	Detected Mass (m/z) Ion Type	Mass Error (ppm)	MS/MS (m/z)	Purity Score	Source
42	Galloylpaeoniflorin	10.19	$C_{23}H_{28}O_{14}$	509.1654 [M + HCOOH-H]$^-$	1.1	121.0302,77.0415	100.00%	PRA
43	Neohesperidin	10.23	$C_{28}H_{34}O_{15}$	609.1825 [M − H]$^-$	1.4	325.0730,301.0726	70.40%	AFI
44	Hesperetin	10.39	$C_{16}H_{14}O_6$	303.0863 [M + H]$^+$	1.4	303.0872,153.0181,67.0204	100.00%	AFI
45	Hesperidin	10.40	$C_{28}H_{34}O_{15}$	609.1825 [M − H]$^-$	0.8	609.1887,301.0725,283.0621	72.60%	AFI
46	Isoliquiritin apioside	10.56	$C_{26}H_{30}O_{13}$	549.1614 [M − H]$^-$	2.3	549.1667,255.0663,135.0082	100.00%	GRM
47	Isochlorogenic acid a	10.61	$C_{25}H_{24}O_{12}$	561.1239 [M + HCOOH-H]$^-$	−0.9	323.0849,193.0482,147.0296	82.60%	BR
48	Lactiflorin	10.68	$C_{23}H_{26}O_{10}$	480.1864 [M + NH$_4$]$^+$	0.5	301.1076,151.0752,105.0343	100.00%	PRA
49	Ononin	10.83	$C_{22}H_{22}O_9$	431.1337 [M + H]$^+$	1.1	269.0807	100.00%	GRM
50	Rhoifolin	10.94	$C_{27}H_{30}O_{14}$	577.1563 [M − H]$^-$	−0.9	271.0613,151.0030	100.00%	AFI
51	Isochlorogenic acid c	11.06	$C_{25}H_{24}O_{12}$	561.1239 [M + HCOOH-H]$^-$	0.2	323.0766,193.0494,147.0452	75.70%	BR
52	Clinoposaponin XII	11.19	$C_{42}H_{68}O_{14}$	795.4536 [M − H]$^-$	−0.4	795.4661,633.4072,471.3084	100.00%	BR
53	epinortrachelogenin	11.86	$C_{20}H_{22}O_7$	373.1293 [M − H]$^-$	0.3	179.0711,99.0091	70.90%	BR
54	Heraclenin	11.93	$C_{16}H_{14}O_5$	287.0914 [M + H]$^+$	0.9	287.0906,153.0176,133.0640	100.00%	AFI
55	Liquiritigenin	11.98	$C_{15}H_{12}O_4$	255.0663 [M − H]$^-$	2.6	135.0082,119.0505,91.0195	100.00%	GRM
56	HOSSa	12.17	$C_{42}H_{70}O_{14}$	797.4693 [M − H]$^-$	−1.9	635.4196	100.00%	BR
57	Puerarin	12.29	$C_{21}H_{20}O_9$	417.1180 [M + H]$^+$	−0.2	417.1094,367.0811,131.0498	77.70%	BR
58	5,4′′-dihydroxy-3,7-dimethoxyflavone	12.65	$C_{17}H_{14}O_6$	315.0863 [M + H]$^+$	1.4	315.0856,243.0647,175.0386	72.50%	GRM
59	HOSSd	12.79	$C_{42}H_{70}O_{14}$	797.4693 [M − H]$^-$	−0.9	635.4235	100.00%	BR
60	Buddlejasaponin IV	13.24	$C_{48}H_{78}O_{18}$	987.5159 [M + HCOOH-H]$^-$	0.3	941.5229,795.4616	100.00%	BR
61	Clinoposaponin XIV	13.45	$C_{42}H_{68}O_{14}$	795.4536 [M − H]$^-$	0.0	795.4627,633.3986,457.3314	100.00%	BR
62	Benzoylpaeoniflorin	13.96	$C_{30}H_{32}O_{12}$	629.1864 [M + HCOOH-H]$^-$	1.0	165.0562,121.0307	100.00%	PRA
63	Benzoylalbiflorin	14.09	$C_{30}H_{32}O_{12}$	585.1967 [M + H]$^+$	−1.0	319.1172,197.0798,133.0643	100.00%	PRA
64	Licoricesaponin A$_3$	14.83	$C_{48}H_{72}O_{21}$	983.4493 [M − H]$^-$	0.2	983.4633,497.1162	100.00%	GRM
65	(+/−)-Naringenin	14.85	$C_{15}H_{12}O_5$	271.0612 [M − H]$^-$	2.7	187.0396,119.0511	100.00%	AFI
66	4,4′-dihydroxy-2-methoxychalcone	15.30	$C_{16}H_{14}O_4$	269.0819 [M − H]$^-$	4.4	269.0707,133.0297,117.0337	73.50%	GRM
67	SSc	15.79	$C_{48}H_{78}O_{17}$	971.5210 [M + HCOOH-H]$^-$	−0.7	925.5193,779.4675	100.00%	BR
68	SSi/h	15.90	$C_{48}H_{78}O_{17}$	971.5209 [M + HCOOH-H]$^-$	−0.1	925.5296, 779.4640	100.00%	BR
69	Salicifoline	16.13	$C_{20}H_{20}O_6$	355.1187 [M − H]$^-$	−2.7	184.9549,129.0726	85.90%	BR
70	Licoricesaponin G$_2$	16.42	$C_{42}H_{62}O_{17}$	837.3914 [M − H]$^-$	−0.5	837.4008,351.0573,193.0347	96.60%	GRM
71	Deacetylnomilinic acid	16.50	$C_{26}H_{34}O_9$	489.2130 [M − H]$^-$	−1.6	489.2174,333.1706,203.0687	93.20%	AFI
72	Licoricesaponin E$_2$	16.55	$C_{42}H_{60}O_{16}$	819.3809 [M − H]$^-$	−0.9	819.3925,351.0577,193.0343	100.00%	GRM
73	Enoxolone	16.61	$C_{30}H_{46}O_4$	471.3469 [M + H]$^+$	0.5	471.3489,219.1769,177.1636	81.70%	GRM
74	SSh/i	16.62	$C_{48}H_{78}O_{17}$	971.5210 [M + HCOOH-H]$^-$	0.9	925.5193	100.00%	GRM
75	Licoricesaponin D$_3$	16.64	$C_{50}H_{76}O_{21}$	1011.4886 [M − H]$^-$	−0.9	1011.4976,497.1175	100.00%	GRM
76	SSb$_3$/b$_4$	16.96	$C_{43}H_{72}O_{14}$	857.4893 [M + HCOOH-H]$^-$	−4.1	811.4911,649.4320,161.0409	92.40%	BR
77	Glycyrrhizic acid	17.00	$C_{42}H_{62}O_{16}$	823.4111 [M + H]$^+$	0.9	647.3782,471.3467,453.3356	100.00%	GRM
78	Isoliquiritigenin	17.09	$C_{15}H_{12}O_4$	255.0663 [M − H]$^-$	0.4	135.0074,119.0495,91.0186	100.00%	GRM
79	Formononetin	17.31	$C_{16}H_{12}O_4$	269.0808 [M + H]$^+$	1.0	269.0811,197.0600	100.00%	GRM
80	Acetyl-SSc	17.32	$C_{50}H_{80}O_{18}$	1013.5316 [M + HCOOH-H]$^-$	−2.8	967.5370,779.4628	81.80%	BR
81	Betulonicacid	17.68	$C_{30}H_{46}O_3$	455.3520 [M − H]$^-$	0.0	453.3525,285.2216,133.1008	96.60%	GRM
82	Palbinone	17.78	$C_{22}H_{30}O_4$	357.2071 [M − H]$^-$	−1.7	357.2067,285.1906,241.1612	92.40%	PRA

Table 1. Cont.

No.	Compound	T_R (min)	Molecular Formula	Detected Mass (m/z) Ion Type	Mass Error (ppm)	MS/MS (m/z)	Purity Score	Source
83	SSn	17.83	$C_{48}H_{78}O_{18}$	987.5156 [M + HCOOH-H]$^-$	−0.3	941.5220, 779.4644	100.00%	BR
84	SSm/e	17.94	$C_{42}H_{68}O_{12}$	809.4682 [M + HCOOH-H]$^-$	−4.8	763.4729, 617.4095, 161.0454	86.50%	BR
85	SSa	18.11	$C_{42}H_{68}O_{13}$	825.4631 [M + HCOOH-H]$^-$	2.8	779.4587, 617.4059	100.00%	BR
86	SSb$_2$	18.25	$C_{42}H_{68}O_{13}$	825.4631 [M + HCOOH-H]$^-$	2.5	779.4587, 617.4059	100.00%	BR
87	Licoricesaponin K$_2$	18.35	$C_{42}H_{62}O_{16}$	821.3965 [M − H]$^-$	0.3	821.4064,351.0578,193.0350	72.00%	GRM
88	Licoricesaponin H$_2$	18.64	$C_{42}H_{62}O_{16}$	821.3965 [M − H]$^-$	−0.4	821.4067,351.0582	100.00%	GRM
89	Limonin	18.75	$C_{26}H_{30}O_8$	469.1368 [M − H]$^-$	−2.7	469.1872,229.1219,145.0650	90.20%	AFI
90	2''-O-Acetyl-SSa	18.82	$C_{44}H_{70}O_{14}$	867.4737 [M + HCOOH-H]$^-$	−0.3	821.4798,779.4684,617.4118	94.90%	BR
91	Nomilinic acid	18.85	$C_{28}H_{36}O_{10}$	531.2236 [M − H]$^-$	−1.2	489.2170,325.1799,59.0169	100.00%	AFI
92	Dipropyl phthalate	18.86	$C_{14}H_{18}O_4$	249.1132 [M − H]$^-$	3.0	149.0935,59.0177	85.70%	PRA
93	Licoricesaponin I$_2$	18.89	$C_{42}H_{64}O_{16}$	823.4122 [M − H]$^-$	0.1	823.4212,351.0575,193.0352	100.00%	GRM
94	SSg	18.98	$C_{42}H_{68}O_{13}$	825.4631 [M + HCOOH-H]$^-$	1.3	779.4665,617.4099	100.00%	BR
95	Nobiletin	19.04	$C_{21}H_{22}O_8$	403.1387 [M + H]$^+$	1.1	403.1383,373.0912,327.0860	77.80%	AFI
96	SSb$_1$	19.05	$C_{42}H_{68}O_{13}$	825.4631 [M + HCOOH-H]$^-$	1.1	779.4587,617.4059	100.00%	BR
97	3''-O-Acetyl-SSa	19.13	$C_{44}H_{70}O_{14}$	867.4737 [M + HCOOH-H]$^-$	0.2	821.4781,779.4662,617.4096	100.00%	BR
98	4''-O-Acetyl-SSa	19.28	$C_{44}H_{70}O_{14}$	867.4737 [M + HCOOH-H]$^-$	−0.7	821.4775,779.4658,617.4094	100.00%	BR
99	Licoricesaponin C$_2$	19.44	$C_{42}H_{62}O_{15}$	805.4016 [M − H]$^-$	0.1	805.4118,351.0568	100.00%	GRM
100	prosaikogenin f	19.49	$C_{36}H_{58}O_8$	663.4103 [M + HCOOH-H]$^-$	−0.6	617.4094,145.0499	77.80%	BR
101	SSe/m	19.59	$C_{42}H_{68}O_{12}$	809.4682 [M + HCOOH-H]$^-$	−1.3	763.4722,601.4170,161.0442	96.40%	BR
102	Licoricesaponin B$_2$	19.72	$C_{42}H_{64}O_{15}$	807.4·73 [M − H]$^-$	−0.6	807.4277,351.0574,193.0343	100.00%	GRM
103	6''-O-Acetyl-SSa	20.09	$C_{44}H_{70}O_{14}$	867.4737 [M + HCOOH-H]$^-$	−0.2	821.4780,779.4666,617.4095	100.00%	BR
104	Licoisoflavone a	20.27	$C_{20}H_{18}O_6$	353.1031 [M − H]$^-$	2.4	353.1056,285.1131,171.0446	74.90%	GRM
105	Glycycoumarin	20.40	$C_{21}H_{20}O_6$	367.1187 [M − H]$^-$	0.5	367.1188,309.0411,201.0187	89.90%	GRM
106	Prosaikogenin g	20.56	$C_{36}H_{58}O_8$	663.4103 [M + HCOOH-H]$^-$	−0.1	617.4060,145.0540	100.00%	BR
107	SSd	20.61	$C_{42}H_{68}O_{13}$	825.4631 [M + HCOOH-H]$^-$	2.5	779.4587,617.4059	100.00%	BR
108	Sinensitin	20.66	$C_{20}H_{20}O_7$	373.1282 [M + H]$^+$	1.1	373.1288,297.0766	79.80%	AFI
109	Diacetyl-SSd	21.03	$C_{46}H_{72}O_{15}$	909.4823 [M + HCOOH-H]$^-$	−0.7	863.4894,821.4782,761.4554	92.00%	BR
110	2''-O-Acetyl-SSd	21.04	$C_{44}H_{70}O_{14}$	867.4737 [M + HCOOH-H]$^-$	−0.4	821.4766,779.4660,617.4085	100.00%	BR
111	Liconeolignan	21.33	$C_{21}H_{22}O_5$	354.1467 [M − H]$^-$	−1.9	353.1020,297.0441,173.0224	80.30%	GRM
112	Diacetyl-SSd	21.61	$C_{46}H_{72}O_{15}$	909.4823 [M + HCOOH-H]$^-$	0.0	863.4896,821.4773,761.4552	100.00%	BR
113	3''-O-Acetyl-SSd	21.89	$C_{44}H_{70}O_{14}$	867.4737 [M + HCOOH-H]$^-$	0.3	821.4794,779.4683,617.4103	100.00%	BR
114	Acetyl-SSe	21.95	$C_{44}H_{70}O_{13}$	851.4788 [M + HCOOH-H]$^-$	−1.7	805.4838,763.4701,601.4155	91.00%	BR
115	Neoglycyrol	22.36	$C_{21}H_{18}O_6$	365.1031 [M − H]$^-$	0.3	365.1037,307.0250,207.0430	96.40%	GRM
116	Prosaikogenin d	22.42	$C_{36}H_{58}O_8$	663.4103 [M + HCOOH-H]$^-$	−1.9	617.408	72.80%	BR
117	6''-O-Acetyl-SSd	22.54	$C_{44}H_{70}O_{14}$	867.4737 [M + HCOOH-H]$^-$	−0.9	821.4770,779.4651,617.4087	100.00%	BR
118	Obacunon	22.74	$C_{26}H_{30}O_7$	453.1919 [M − H]$^-$	−4.2	453.2044,339.1957,149.0963	90.20%	AFI
119	Saikogenin e	22.78	$C_{30}H_{48}O_3$	455.3519 [M − H]$^-$	−2.5	455.3529, 325.1855, 152.9936	93.20%	BR
120	Diacetyl-SSd	23.06	$C_{46}H_{72}O_{15}$	909.4823 [M + HCOOH-H]$^-$	−3.0	863.4894,821.4774,617.4091	100.00%	BR
121	Diacetyl-SSd	23.24	$C_{46}H_{72}O_{15}$	909.4823 [M + HCOOH-H]$^-$	−2.7	863.4859,821.4747,761.4478	94.40%	BR
122	Saikogenin f	23.38	$C_{30}H_{48}O_4$	533.3473 [M + HCOOH-H]$^-$	−6.3	471.3452,453.1727,388.9749	90.10%	BR

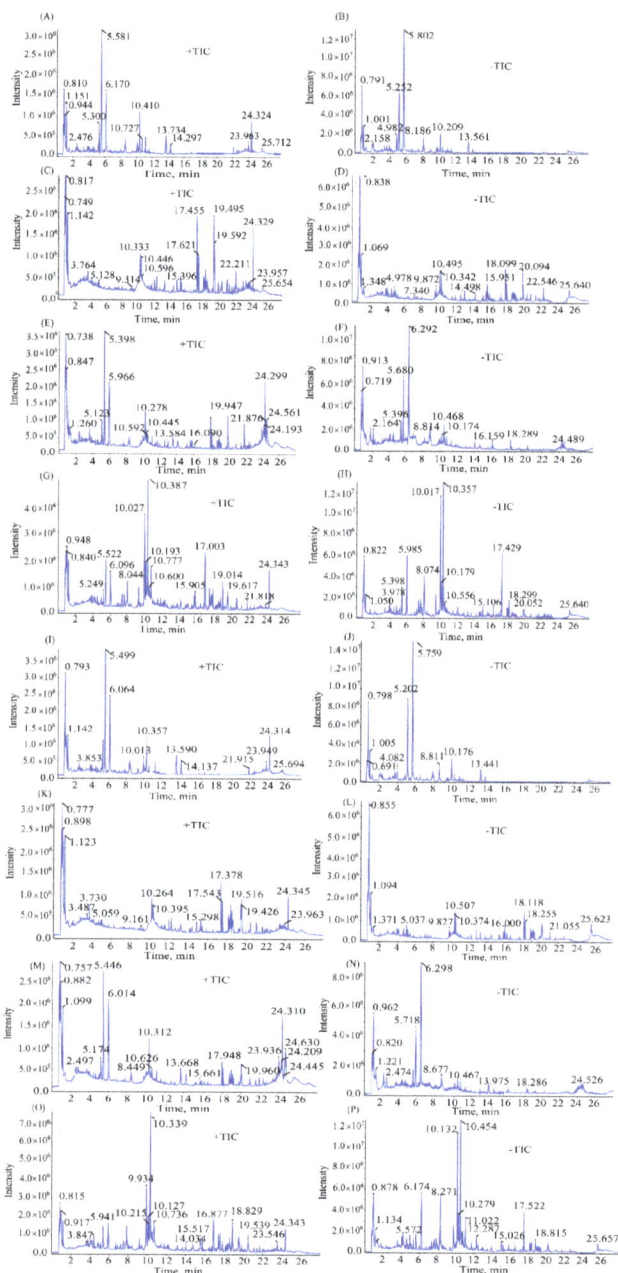

Figure 1. Typical total ion chromatograms (TICs) in positive ion mode of PRA (**A**), VPPRA (**I**), BR (**C**), VPBR (**K**), BR-PRA herb-pair (**E**), VPBR-VPPRA herb-pair (**M**), SNS (**G**), and SNS-containing VPBR and VPPRA (**O**). Typical total ion chromatograms (TICs) in negative ion mode of PRA (**B**), VPPRA (**J**), BR (**D**), VPBR (**L**), BR-PRA herb-pair (**F**), VPBR-VPPRA herb-pair (**N**), SNS (**H**), and SNS-containing VPBR and VPPRA (**P**).

2.2. Multivariate Data Analysis

Using MarkerView™ 1.2.1 data handling software, multivariate data analysis were completed. The principal component analysis (PCA) score plot in negative and positive ion modes were shown in Figure 2. The results showed that all crude and processed samples including individual herb, herb-pair, and complicated Chinese medicinal formula were successfully classified into two categories in both positive and negative ion modes.

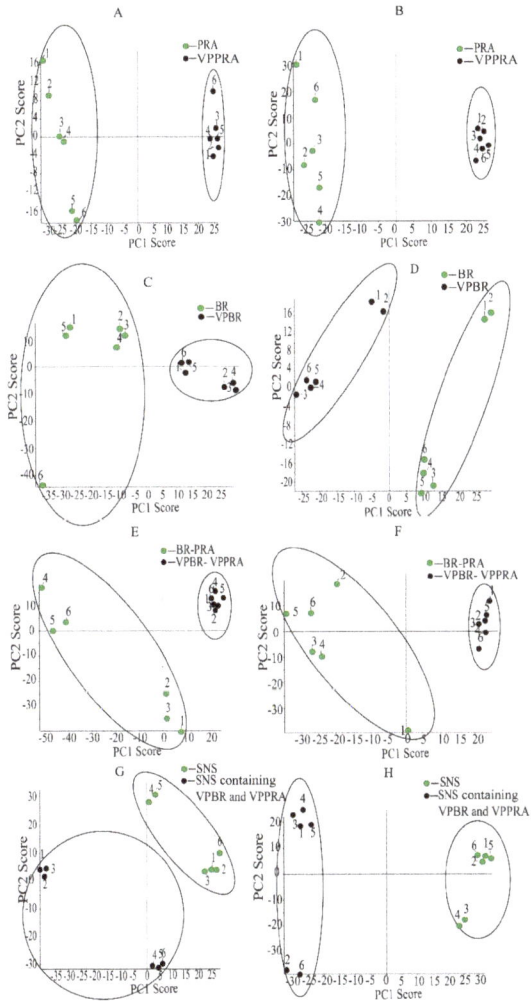

Figure 2. Principal component analysis (PCA) score plots in positive ion mode of PRA and VPPRA (**A**), BR and VPBR (**C**), BR-PRA herb-pair and VPBR-VPPRA herb-pair (**E**), SNS and SNS containing VPBR and VPPRA (**G**). PCA score plots in negative ion mode of PRA and VPPRA (**B**), BR and VPBR (**D**), BR-PRA herb-pair and VPBR-VPPRA herb-pair (**F**), and SNS and SNS-containing VPBR and VPPRA (**H**).

2.3. Compounds Changed after Processing and Formula Compatibility

The variations of components ($p < 0.05$) in the individual herb, herb-pair, and complicated Chinese herbal formula before and after processing were shown in Tables 2 and 3. For BR, 22 peaks were shown significant differences after processing. Comparing with BR, the intensity of seven peaks increased in VPBR; the other 15 peaks declined in VPBR. Taking compatibility into consideration, it was interesting to find that 14 peaks contributing to differentiate crude and processed individual herbs disappeared in herb-pair, while three new peaks (isorhamnetin-3-rutinoside, HOSSd, 2″-O-AcetylSSd) appeared. Additionally, prosaikogenin f decreased in individual herb but increased in herb-pair. Compatibility may be responsible for these changes. On the contrary, adonltol, SSh, SSi, SSg, SSb$_1$, 3″-O-AcetylSSa, and SSd all showed the same trend after processing of BR in the individual herb and herb-pair. Thus, it was hard to distinguish that the seven components were affected by processing, compatibility, or even their combination. Taking into further account the formula compatibility effect of AFI and GRM, eight peaks showing significant differences in herb-pair vanished in the formula, however seven new peaks (isorhamnetin, buddlejasaponin IV, acetylSSc, 4″-O-AcetylSSa, SSe, 6″-O-AcetylSSc, and 6″-O-AcetylSSd) appeared. Meanwhile SSg, 3″-O-AcetylSSa, and SSd showed the same tendency and this would result in the unidentifiable problem.

Table 2. Results of the *t*-test of 26 peaks from BR showing significant difference in individual herb, herb-pair, and complicated Chinese herbal formula before and after processing ($n = 6$).

	BR		Individual Herb	Herb-Pair	Herbal Formula
No.	T$_R$ (min)	Identified Compound	*p*-Value	*p*-Value	*p*-Value
1	0.82	Adonitol	0.00394 ↓ **	0.00011 ↓ **	____
11	4.18	Chlorogenic acid	0.00137 ↓ **	____	____
27	7.57	Rutin	0.00946 ↓ **	____	____
35	9.56	Isorhamnetin	0.04005 ↑ *	____	0.01029 ↑ *
36	9.65	Isorhamnetin-3-rutinoside	____	0.00055 ↓ **	____
59	12.79	HOSSd	____	0.00077 ↓ **	____
60	13.24	Buddlejasaponin IV	1.72×10^{-5} ↓ **	____	3.90×10^{-6} ↓ **
67	15.79	SSc	0.01180 ↓ *	____	____
68	15.9	SSi/h	0.00130 ↑ **	3.34×10^{-8} ↑ **	____
74	16.62	SSh/i	0.00017 ↑ **	0.00027 ↑ **	____
80	17.32	AcetylSSc	0.00089 ↓ **	____	0.01867 ↓ *
85	18.11	SSa	0.00475 ↓ **	____	____
86	18.25	SSb$_2$	0.03997 ↑ *	____	____
94	18.98	SSg	0.00577 ↑ **	1.90×10^{-6} ↑ **	0.04480 ↑ *
96	19.05	SSb$_1$	0.00656 ↑ **	4.85×10^{-5} ↑ **	____
97	19.13	3″-O-AcetylSSa	0.00016 ↑ **	4.18×10^{-6} ↑ **	0.002821 ↑ **
98	19.28	4″-O-AcetylSSa	____	____	0.001645 ↑ **
100	19.49	prosaikogenin f	0.00031 ↓ **	0.00281 ↑ **	____
101	19.59	SSe/m	0.00014 ↓ **	____	0.00626 ↓ **
103	20.09	6″-O-AcetylSSa	4.43×10^5 ↓ **	____	0.024542 ↓ *
107	20.61	SSd	0.00299 ↓ **	0.00078 ↓ **	0.04567 ↓ *
110	21.04	2″-O-AcetylSSd	____	0.00116 ↓ **	____
112	21.61	Diacetyl-SSd	0.03744 ↓ *	____	____
113	21.89	3″-O-AcetylSSd	9.31×10^{-7} ↓ **	____	____
117	22.54	6″-O-AcetylSSd	0.00053 ↓ **	____	0.04310 ↓ *
121	23.24	Diacetyl-SSd	1.06×10^{-8} ↓ **	____	____

Compared with BR, "↓" represents decrease in contents, "↑" represents increase in contents, * $p < 0.05$, ** $p < 0.01$.

Table 3. Results of *t*-test of 22 peaks from PRA showing significant difference in individual herb, herb-pair, and complicated Chinese herbal formula before and after processing ($n = 6$).

	PRA		Individual Herb	Herb-Pair	Herbal Formula
No.	T_R (min)	Identified Compounds	*p*-Value	*p*-Value	*p*-Value
2	0.83	Sucrose	0.00678 ↓ **	0.00852 ↓ **	——
4	1.97	Gallic acid	0.00250 ↓ **	——	——
5	2.39	1-O-β-D-glucopyranosyl-paeonisuffrone	0.02508 ↑ *	0.04461 ↑ *	——
6	3.16	6-O-β-D-glucopyranosyl lactinolide	——	0.03649 ↑ *	4.15×10^{-5} ↑ **
7	3.31	Mudanpioside f	0.00056 ↑ **	0.04576 ↑ *	0.00043 ↑ **
9	3.83	Oxypaeoniflora	2.79×10^{-6} ↑ **	——	0.00021 ↑ **
10	4.16	4''-Hydroxy-3''-methoxyalbiflorin	0.04610 ↑ *	——	——
13	4.40	Cianidanol	0.01515 ↑ *	0.00631 ↓ **	——
15	4.76	6'-O-β-D-glucopyranosylalbiflorin	0.02004 ↓ *	——	0.04757 ↓ *
18	5.13	Isomaltopaeoniflorin	1.28×10^{-9} ↓ **	2.58×10^{-6} ↓ **	——
19	5.49	Albiflorin	7.64×10^{-8} ↑ **	0.00303 ↑ **	0.01407 ↑ *
20	5.58	Paeoniflorigenone	8.60×10^{-10} ↑ **	0.02864 ↑ *	0.0168 ↑ *
21	5.61	Isomaltoalbiflorin	0.00062 ↑ **	0.00952 ↑ **	0.040769 ↑ *
23	5.98	Paeoniflorin	0.04235 ↓ *	——	——
24	6.70	Paeonol	2.80×10^{-7} ↑ **	0.00106 ↑ **	0.00418 ↑ **
39	10.08	Benzoic acid	5.34×10^{-5} ↓ **	0.00558 ↓ **	0.04072 ↓ *
41	10.18	Mudanpioside i	0.00050 ↑ **	——	——
42	10.19	Galloylpaeoniflorin	0.00260 ↓ **	——	0.00856 ↑ **
48	10.68	Lactiflorin	0.03681 ↑ *	——	0.00508 ↓ **
62	13.96	Benzoylpaeoniflorin	——	0.00078 ↑ **	——
63	14.09	Benzoylalbiflorin	2.40×10^{-5} ↑ **	——	0.02116 ↑ *
82	17.78	Palbinone	1.72×10^{-6} ↑ **	——	——

Compared with PRA, "↓" represents decrease in contents, "↑" represents increase in contents, * $p < 0.05$, ** $p < 0.01$.

For PRA, 20 peaks showed significant differences after processing. Comparing with PRA, the intensity of 13 peaks enhanced in VPPRA, the other seven peaks decreased in VPPRA. Considering compatibility, 10 of these 20 peaks disappeared in the herb-pair, at the same time, 6-O-β-D-glucopyranosyl lactinolide and benzoylpaeoniflorin appeared. Also, cianidanol enhanced in individual herb but decreased in herb-pair. These changes perhaps resulted from compatibility. Moreover, nine peaks had the same trend after processing of PRA in individual herb and herb-pair, and it was also hard to distinguish as BR. Under further influence of formula compatibility with AFI and GRM, five peaks showing significant differences in herb-pair vanished in formula; oppositely, five new peaks (oxypaeoniflora, 6'-O-β-D-glucopyranosylalbiflorin, galloylpaeoniflorin, lactiflorin, benzoylalbiflorin) appeared. Formula compatibility may be responsible for these changes. In addition, seven peaks (6-O-β-D-glucopyranosyl lactinolide, mudanpioside f, albiflorin, isomaltoalbiflorin, paeoniflorigenone, paeonol, and benzoic acid) displayed an identical trend; this still led to the unidentifiable problem. Figure 3 shows the comparison of the contents of the components identified with significant differences. Processing with vinegar and formula compatibility can both regulate the acidity and alkalinity of the solution and promote changes in chemical composition, such as hydrolysis reaction, isomerization reaction, etc., resulting in increased or decreased dissolution of some components. Finally, we found that processing of BR and PRA also had the impact on AFI and GRM, and the results were shown in Table 4.

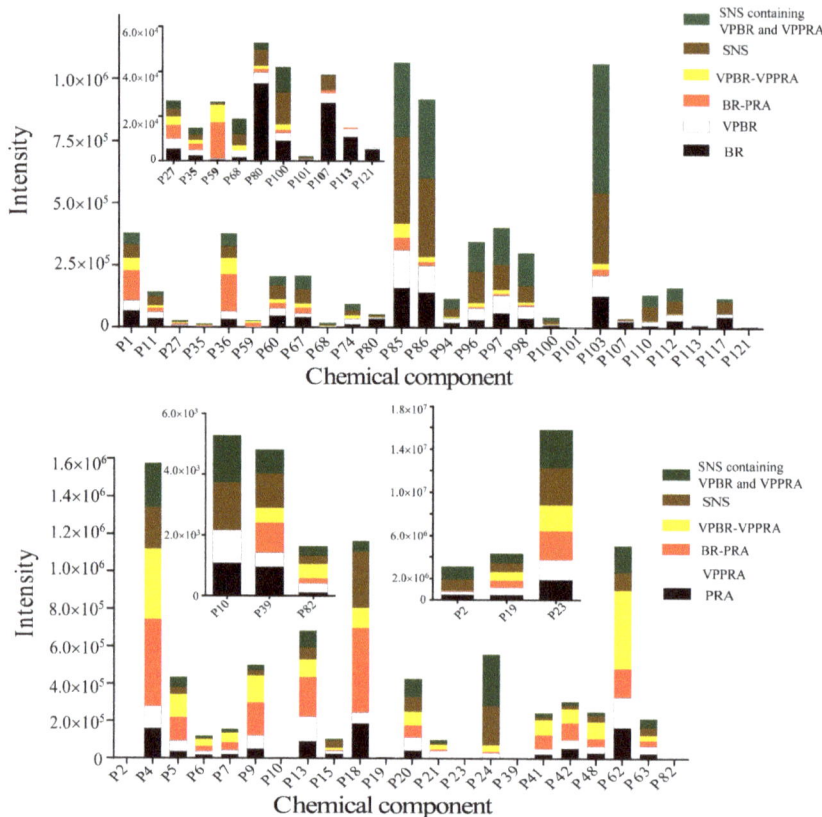

Figure 3. Contents of components identified with significant differences in individual herb, herb-pair, and complicated Chinese herbal formula of SNS.

Table 4. Results of t-test of 12 peaks from AFI and GRM showing significant difference ($n = 6$).

No.	T_R (min)	Identified Compound	t-Value	p-Value	Source
17	4.99	Lonicerin	2.44	0.03474 ↑ *	AFI
22	5.91	Schaftoside	−4.17	0.00193 ↓ **	AFI
29	7.93	Liquiritin	8.36	8.02×10^{-6} ↑ **	GRM
44	10.39	Hesperetin	−4.07	0.00361 ↓ **	AFI
49	10.83	Ononin	5.62	0.00050 ↑ **	GRM
58	12.65	5,4″-dihydroxy-3,7-dimethoxyflavone	−2.31	0.04979 ↓ *	GRM
64	14.83	Licoricesaponin A_3	−4.69	0.00085 ↓ **	GRM
70	16.42	Licoricesaponin G_2	−3.40	0.00677 ↓ **	GRM
72	16.55	Licoricesaponin E_2	3.53	0.00548 ↑ **	GRM
79	17.31	Formononetin	−3.28	0.01125 ↓ *	GRM
104	20.27	Licoisoflavone a	−4.16	0.00195 ↓ **	GRM
105	20.40	Glycycoumarin	5.93	0.00014 ↑ **	GRM

Compared with SNS, "↓" represents decrease in contents, "↑" represents increase in contents, * $p < 0.05$, ** $p < 0.01$.

As shown in Table 2, the intensity of paeonol significantly increased after stir-frying with vinegar. According to a previous report [16], adding acid could greatly improve the extraction efficiency of paeonol. Since the boiling point of paeonol is 154 °C, the use of slow fire (130 °C) controlled by infrared radiation thermometer during the processing minimized the loss of paeonol. In addition, acetic acid plays an important role to form intermolecular hydrogen bonds by Van der Waals' force with paeonol, resulting in the increase of dissolution rate. Modern researches indicate that paeonol has analgesic and antiphlogistic pharmacological activities [17,18] and is consistent with TCM theory that processing of medicinal herbs with vinegar can enhance the effects of promoting blood circulation and relieving pain. As an illustration, Figure 4 revealed the course of deducing fragmentation of paeonol.

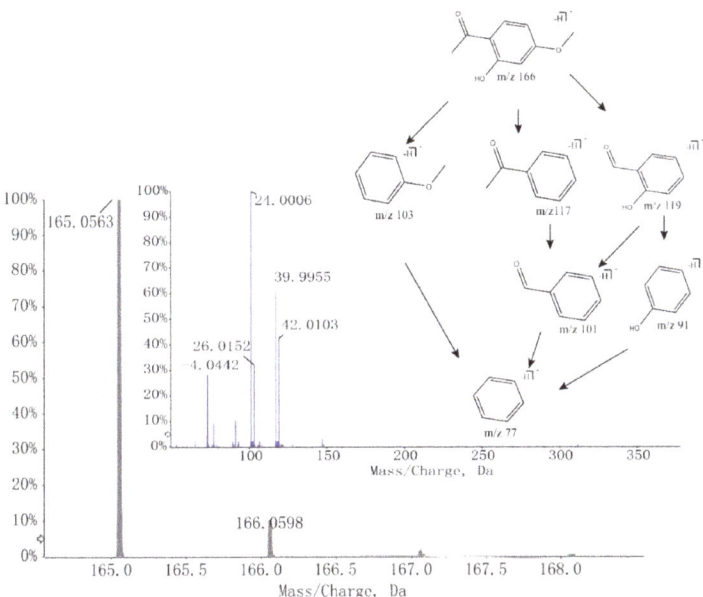

Figure 4. MS and tandem mass spectroscopy (MS/MS) spectra and fragmentation of Paeonol.

As shown in Table 3, we found that the intensity of SSa and SSd declined but the intensity of SSb_2 and SSb_1 increased in the BR. SSs, a kind of oleanane type triterpenoid saponin, could be divided into seven types according to their different aglycones. SSa, SSd, and SSc are epoxy-ether saikosaponins (type I), while SSb_2 and SSb_1 with a different aglycone, form a heterocyclic diene saikosaponin (type II) [19]. The glycosidic bond is very easily hydrolyzed in the acidic conditions or being heated [20,21]. Vinegar processing could promote the hydrolyzation from 13 to 28 allyl oxide linkage to its corresponding heteroannular diene structure, resulting in the aglycone accumulation. As shown in Figure 5, peak No. 94 was clearly observed in VPBR, VPBR-VPPRA herb-pair, SNS-containing VPBR and VPPRA, and SNS, and almost undetectable in BR and BR-PRA herb-pair. According to the fragmentations in both positive and negative ion modes and other reports [22–24], we suggested that peak No. 94 is SSg. SSg in SNS could be related to the acidic compounds of herbal formula, such as glycyrrhizic acid. Also, peak No. 68 (SSh/i), as the isomer of SSc, had the same change with SSg. Based on these, we hypothesized that SSa and SSd could be transformed to SSb_2, SSb_1, and SSg, while SSc could be converted to SSh and SSi after processing and formula compatibility.

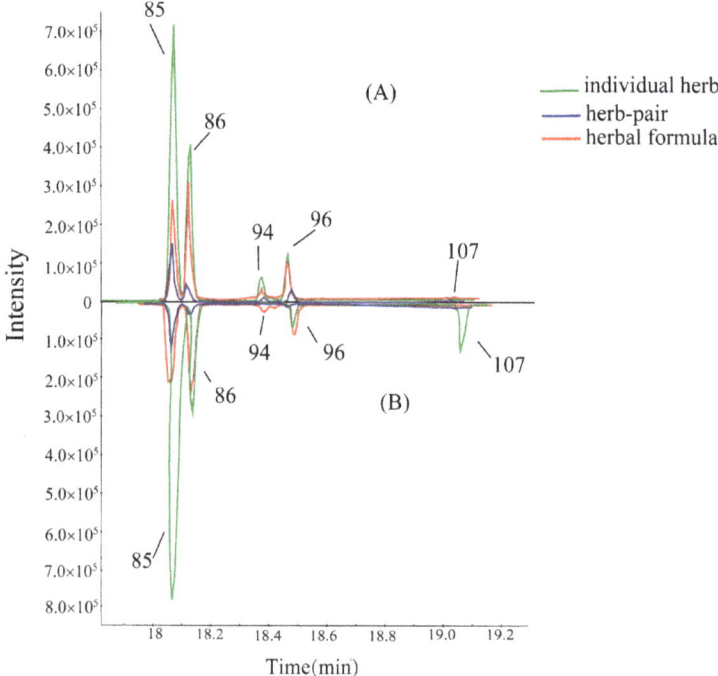

Figure 5. Comparison on intensity of five isomers of Saikosaponins in BR, BR-PRA herb-pair, and SNS (**B**). Comparison on intensity of five isomers of Saikosaponins in VPBR, VPBR-VPPRA herb-pair, and SNS-containing VPBR and VPPRA (**A**).

3. Materials and Methods

3.1. Materials and Reagents

Acetonitrile (Merck, Darmstadt, Germany) and formic acid from Anaqua Chemical Supply (ACS, Houston, TX, USA) of HPLC/MS-grade were purchased for UHPLC-Q-TOF/MS analysis. Deionized water was prepared using a Milli-Q system (Millipore, Molsheim, France). SPE columns (LC-C_{18}, 500 mg/mL) were purchased from ANPLE Scientific Instrument (Shanghai, China). Other reagents of analytical grade were purchased from Nanjing Chemical Reagent Co., Ltd. (Jiangsu, China).

BR, PRA, AFI, and GRM were obtained from different Chinese pharmacies and pharmaceutical factories, and authenticated by Professor Hao Cai. The quality of all collected samples was strictly evaluated and consistent with the regulations of Chinese Pharmacopoeia (Edition 2015, Part One). VPBR and VPPRA were prepared according to the processing standards described in Chinese Pharmacopoeia (Edition 2015, Part Four). The voucher specimens were deposited in School of Pharmacy, Nanjing University of Chinese Medicine (Nanjing, China).

3.2. Sample Preparation

The decoction of BR was prepared as follows. Eight grams of BR were extracted twice in a reflux water heating mantle in 48 mL and 32 mL of deionized water for 1.5 h and 1 h of reflux, respectively. The mixed solution was filtered through a four-layer mesh following the reflux. One milliliter of the solution was loaded onto a C_{18} RP SPE column and the gradient elution was performed as the following sequence. One milliliter of 20% acetonitrile in water (20:80, v/v), 1 mL of 40% acetonitrile in water (40:60, v/v), 1 mL of 60% acetonitrile in water (60:40, v/v), 1 mL of 80% acetonitrile in water

(80:20, v/v), and 1 mL of acetonitrile. After the sequent elution, the collected eluent was eddied for 2 min and centrifuged at 13,000 rpm for 5 min. Finally, the supernatant was collected as the injection solution. The decoctions of VPBR, PRA, and VPPRA were prepared according to the same procedures above.

The decoction of BR-PRA herb-pair consisted of 4 g of BR and 4 g of PRA, and prepared as the same procedures as individual herb described above. The decoction of VPBR-VPPRA herb-pair was prepared using the same procedures as the decoction of BR-PRA herb-pair. The decoction of SNS was consist of 2 g of BR, 2 g of PRA, 2 g of AFI, and 2 g of GRM, and prepared using the same procedures as individual herb. The decoction of SNS containing VPBR and VPPRA was prepared using the same procedures as the decoction of SNS.

3.3. Chromatographic Separation

Chromatographic analysis was performed using a UHPLC system (Shimadzu, Kyoto, Japan) consisting of an LC-30AD binary pump, an autosampler (Model SIL-30SD), an online degasser (DGU-20A5R), and a temperature controller for columns (CTO-30A). Separation was carried out on an extended C_{18} Column (2.1 mm × 100 mm, 1.8 µm; Agilent, Palo Alto, CA, USA) at 30 °C and the flow rate was 0.3 mL/min. The optimal mobile phase consisted of A (HCOOH/H_2O, 0.1:100, v/v) and B (C_2H_3N). The optimized UHPLC elution conditions were as follows 0–2 min, 3–15% B; 2–7 min, 15–20% B; 7–8 min, 20% B; 8–9 min, 20–30% B; 9–13 min, 30–32% B; 13–21 min; 32–54% B; 21–23 min, 54–100% B; 23–27 min, 100–3% B; and 27–28 min, 3% B. The injection volume was 2 µL.

3.4. MS and MS/MS Experiments

A triple TOF 5600$^+$ System (AB Sciex, Concord, CA, USA) equipped with an electrospray ionization (ESI) source was performed. The MS was operated in both positive and negative ion modes. Parameters were set as follows: ion spray voltage of +4500/−4500 V; turbo spray temperature of 550 °C; declustering potential (DP) of +60/−60 V; collision energy of +35/−45 V; nebulizer gas (gas 1) of 55 psi; heater gas (gas 2) of 55 psi and curtain gas of 35 psi. TOF MS and TOF MS/MS were scanned with the mass ranges of m/z 100–2000 and 50–1000, respectively. The experiments were run with 200 ms accumulation time for TOF MS and 80 ms accumulation time for TOF MS/MS. Continuous recalibration was performed at the intervals of 3 h. Dynamic background subtraction and information-dependent acquisition techniques were applied to reduce the impact of matrix interference and increase the efficiency of analysis.

3.5. MS and MS/MS Data Processing and Analysis

The raw data were obtained by the Analyst TF 1.6 software (AB Sciex, Concord, CA, USA). Before data processing, a database about chemical components of medicinal herbs in SNS, including names, molecular formulas, chemical structures, and accurate molecular weights, was established by searching relevant reported literature and database websites, including PubMed and SciFinder. The data were analyzed by using PeakView^{TM} 1.2 software (AB Sciex, Concord, CA, USA) for a perfect match with the information in the established database, according to fragmentations of the different peaks. The main parameters used were set as follows: retention time range of 0–28 min, mass range of 100 to 2000 Da, and mass tolerance of 10 ppm. By using the method of PCA with MarkerView^{TM} 1.2.1 software (AB Sciex, Concord, CA, USA) to check for outliers and variation trend, the gathered data were more intuitionistic. The Student's t-test was performed to find out a list of peaks that were finally defined as the main contributors to the significant difference between raw and processed medicinal herbs ($p < 0.05$).

4. Conclusions

A total of 122 constituents had been identified by creative global analysis in individual herb, herb-pair, and complicated Chinese herbal formula of SNS. Taking BR as an example, 29 kinds of

SSs had been identified, including some new discoveries in recent years, such as SSq, SSm, and so forth. Monoterpene glycosides (oxypaeoniflora, mudanpioside f, paeoniflorigenone, etc) showed a marked increase after processing of PRA. This is the first report of SSh/i and SSg being identified in SNS. Through three progressive levels of comparison, it suggests that processing herbal medicine and/or changing medicinal formula compatibility could alter herbal chemical constituents, resulting in different pharmaceutical effects. Herbal formula has always been the predicament of Chinese medicine research, and some scholars only employed SSd and paeoniflorin (the main components of BR and PRA) for research [25], whereas the effects between individual components and herbal formula containing individual components are quite different. We hope that the thoughts of this article would be some helpful for further research of herbal formula.

Author Contributions: J.Z., H.C., and Y.D. contributed to the design of the study. J.Z., S.T., Y.D., K.P., Y.X., J.L., and L.S. performed the laboratory experiments and data analysis. J.Z., H.C., Y.D., M.N., and Y.Z. wrote the manuscript. H.C., S.T., and Q.Z. revised the final manuscript. All authors reviewed the manuscript.

Funding: This research was financially supported by the National Natural Science Foundation of China (No. 81673600).

Conflicts of Interest: The authors declare no conflict of interest.

Abbreviations

AFI	Aurantii Fructus Immaturus
BR	Bupleuri Radix
GRM	Glycyrrhizae Radix et Rhizoma Praeparata Cum Melle
PRA	Paeoniae Radix Alba; SNS, Sinisan
SS	saikosaponin
TCM	traditional Chinese medicine
UHPLC-Q-TOF/MS	ultrahigh performance liquid chromatography coupled with electrospray ionization tandem quadrupole-time-of-flight mass spectrometry
VPBR	vinegar-processed Bupleuri Radix
VPPRA	vinegar-processed Paeoniae Radix Alba
PCA	principal component analysis

References

1. Shen, X.; Zhao, Z.Y.; Luo, X.; Wang, H.; Hu, B.X.; Guo, Z.H. Systems pharmacology based study of the molecular mechanism of SiNiSan formula for application in nervous and mental diseases. *Evid.-Based Complement. Altern. Med.* **2016**, *2016*, 9146378. [CrossRef] [PubMed]
2. Feng, D.D.; Tang, T.; Lin, X.P.; Yang, Z.Y.; Yang, S.; Xia, Z.A.; Wang, Y.; Zheng, P.; Wang, Y.; Zhang, C.H. Nine traditional Chinese herbal formulas for the treatment of depression: An ethnopharmacology, phytochemistry, and pharmacology review. *Neuropsych. Dis. Treat* **2016**, *12*, 2387–2402.
3. Li, Y.B.; Zhang, T.J.; Zhang, X.L.; Xu, H.Y.; Liu, C.X. Chemical figerprint analysis of Phellodendri Amurensis Cortex by ultra performance LC/Q-TOF-MS methods combined with chemometrics. *J. Sep. Sci.* **2015**, *33*, 3347–3353. [CrossRef] [PubMed]
4. Pei, K.; Duan, Y.; Cai, H.; Tu, S.C.; Qiao, F.X.; Song, X.Q.; Liu, X.; Cao, G.; Fan, K.L.; Cai, B.C. Ultra-high-performance liquid chromatography quadrupole/time of flight mass spectrometry combined with statistical analysis for rapidly revealing the influence of sulfur-fumigated Paeoniae Radix Alba on the chemical constituents of Si Wu Tang. *Anal. Methods* **2015**, *7*, 9442–9451. [CrossRef]
5. Guo, S.; Duan, J.A.; Qian, D.W.; Wang, H.Q.; Tang, Y.P.; Qian, Y.F.; Wu, D.W.; Su, S.L.; Shang, E.X. Hydrophilic interaction ultra-high performance liquid chromatography coupled with triple quadrupole mass spectrometry for determination of nucleotides, nucleosides and nucleobases in Ziziphus plants. *J. Chromatogr. A* **2013**, *1301*, 147–155. [CrossRef] [PubMed]
6. Li, C.Y.; Qi, L.W.; Li, P. Correlative analysis of metabolite profiling of Danggui Buxue Tang in rat biological fluids by rapid resolution LC-TOF/MS. *J. Pharm. Biomed.* **2011**, *55*, 146–160. [CrossRef] [PubMed]
7. Chen, J.M. *Materia Medica Companion*; People's Medical Publishing House: Beijing, China, 1988.

8. Chen, X.Z.; Yu, T.Y.; Chen, Z.X.; Zhao, R.Z.; Mao, S.R. Effect of saikosaponins and extracts of vinegar-baked Bupleuri Radix on the activity of β-glucuronidase. *Xenobiotica* **2014**, *44*, 785–791. [CrossRef] [PubMed]
9. Zhu, L.; Liang, Z.T.; Yi, T.; Ma, Y.; Zhao, Z.Z.; Guo, B.L.; Zhang, J.Y.; Chen, H.B. Comparison of chemical profiles between the root and aerial parts from three Bupleurum species based on a UHPLC-QTOF-MS metabolomics approach. *BMC Complement. Altern. Med.* **2017**, *17*, 305. [CrossRef] [PubMed]
10. Liu, J.; Chen, L.; Fan, C.R.; Li, H.; Huang, M.Q.; Xiang, Q.; Xu, W.; Xu, W.; Chu, K.D.; Lin, Y. Qualitative and quantitative analysis of major constituents of Paeoniae Radix Alba and Paeoniae Radix Rubra by HPLC-DAD-Q-TOF-MS/MS. *China J. Chin. Mater. Med.* **2015**, *40*, 1762–1770.
11. Li, P.; Zeng, S.L.; Duan, L.; Ma, X.D.; Dou, L.L.; Wang, L.J.; Li, P.; Bi, Z.M.; Liu, E.H. Comparison of Aurantii Fructus Immaturus and Aurantii Fructus based on multiple chromatographic analysis and chemometrics methods. *J. Chromatogr. A* **2016**, *1469*, 96–107. [CrossRef] [PubMed]
12. Ota, M.; Xu, F.; Li, Y.L.; Shang, M.Y.; Makino, T.; Cai, S.Q. Comparison of chemical constituents among licorice, roasted licorice, and roasted licorice with honey. *J. Nat. Med.* **2017**, *72*, 1–16. [CrossRef] [PubMed]
13. Yang, Y.Y.; Tang, Y.Z.; Fan, C.L.; Luo, H.T.; Guo, P.R.; Chen, J.X. Identification and determination of the saikosaponins in Radix bupleuri by accelerated solvent extraction combined with rapid-resolution LC-MS. *J. Sep. Sci.* **2010**, *33*, 1933–1945. [CrossRef] [PubMed]
14. Ni, F.Y.; Song, Y.L.; Liu, L.; Zhao, Y.W.; Huang, W.Z.; Wang, Z.Z.; Xiao, W. Preparation technology of isochlorogenic acids A, B, and C. *Chin. Tradit. Herb. Drugs* **2015**, *46*, 369–373.
15. Zhu, M.; Duan, J.A.; Tang, Y.P.; Guo, J.M.; Shang, E.X.; Zhu, Z.H. Identification of chemical constituents in SiWu decoction by UHPLC-DAD-TOF/MS. *Acta Chromatogr.* **2014**, *26*, 517–537. [CrossRef]
16. Gong, C.B.; Kang, H.X. Study on extraction of Paeonol from Cortex Moutan by steam distillation with the addition of acid and inorganic salt. *J. Shandong Univ. TCM* **2013**, *37*, 162–163.
17. Jin, X.; Wang, J.; Xia, Z.M.; Shang, C.H.; Chao, Q.L.; Liu, Y.R.; Fan, H.Y.; Chen, D.Q.; Qiu, F.; Zhao, F. Anti-inflammatory and anti-oxidative activities of Paeonol and its metabolites through blocking MAPK/ERK/p38 signaling pathway. *Inflammation* **2016**, *39*, 434–446. [CrossRef] [PubMed]
18. Meng, Y.J.; Wang, M.X.; Xie, X.J.; Di, T.T.; Zhao, J.X.; Lin, Y.; Xu, X.L.; Li, N.F.; Zhai, Y.T.; Wang, Y.; et al. Paeonol ameliorates imiquimod-induced psoriasis-like skin lesions in BALB/c mice by inhibiting the maturation and activation of dendritic cells. *Int. J. Mol. Med.* **2017**, *39*, 1101–1110. [CrossRef] [PubMed]
19. Lin, T.Y.; Chiou, C.Y.; Chiou, S.J. Putative genes involved in saikosaponin biosynthesis in Bupleurum species. *Int. J. Mol. Sci.* **2013**, *14*, 12806–12826. [CrossRef] [PubMed]
20. Li, J.; Jiang, H.; Zhang, Y.P.; Zhang, Q.; Xu, Y. Content change of saikosaponins during preparation of saiko decoction. *Chin. J. Exp. Tradit. Med. Formulae* **2012**, *18*, 155–158.
21. Li, J.; Shi, R.B.; Liu, B.; Jiang, H. Influence of different component combinations of Sini Powder on decocting quantity of saikosaponin-a and b_2. *J. Beijing Univ. Tradit. Chin. Med.* **2007**, *30*, 115–120.
22. Li, J.; Xu, Q.; Jiang, H. Identification and characterization of two new degradation products of saikosaponin A under acid hydrolytic conditions. *J. Lumin.* **2016**, *171*, 131–137. [CrossRef]
23. Yu, P.; Qiu, H.; Wang, M.; Tian, Y.; Zhang, Z.J.; Song, R. In vitro metabolism study of saikosaponin d and its derivatives in rat liver microsomes. *Xenobiotica* **2016**, *47*, 1–9. [CrossRef] [PubMed]
24. Yu, B.B.; Wang, L.; Yin, L.S.; Sun, R. Research on biotransformation of saikosaponin A in vitro based on HPLC-DAD-MS^n. *Chin. Tradit. Herb. Drugs* **2017**, *48*, 333–338.
25. Liang, G.W.; Chen, Y.C.; Wang, Y.; Wang, H.M.; Pan, X.Y.; Chen, P.H.; Niu, Q.X. Interaction between saikosaponin D, paeoniflorin, and human serum albumin. *Molecules* **2018**, *23*, 249. [CrossRef] [PubMed]

Sample Availability: Samples of Bupleuri Radix, Paeoniae Radix Alba, Aurantii Fructus Immaturus, and Glycyrrhizae Radix et Rhizoma Praeparata Cum Melle are available from the authors.

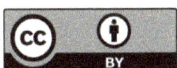

© 2018 by the authors. Licensee MDPI, Basel, Switzerland. This article is an open access article distributed under the terms and conditions of the Creative Commons Attribution (CC BY) license (http://creativecommons.org/licenses/by/4.0/).

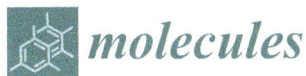

Communication

Optimization of the Extraction Conditions and Biological Evaluation of *Dendropanax morbifera* H. Lev as an Anti-Hyperuricemic Source

Seung-Sik Cho [1], Seung-Hui Song [1], Chul-Yung Choi [2], Kyung Mok Park [3], Jung-Hyun Shim [1,*] and Dae-Hun Park [4,*]

[1] Department of Pharmacy, College of Pharmacy, Mokpo National University, Muan, Jeonnam 58554, Korea; sscho@mokpo.ac.kr (S.-S.C.); tmdgml7898@naver.com (S.-H.S.)
[2] Jeonnam Institute of Natural Resources Research, Jangheung-gun, Jeonnam 57922, Korea; blockstar@hanmail.net
[3] Department of Parmaceutical Engineering, Dongshin University, Naju, Jeonnam 58245, Korea; parkkm@dsu.ac.kr
[4] Department of Nursing, Dongshin University, Naju, Jeonnam 58245, Korea
* Correspondence: s1004jh@gmail.com (J.-H.S.); dhj1221@hanmail.net (D.-H.P.); Tel.: +82-61-450-2684 (J.-H.S.); + 82-61-330-3587 (D.-H.P.)

Academic Editors: In-Soo Yoon and Hyun-Jong Cho
Received: 1 November 2018; Accepted: 13 December 2018; Published: 14 December 2018

Abstract: *Dendropanax morbifera* H. Lev is a medicinal plant native to South Korea, East Asia, and South America. Among some 75 species, one species grows in Korea. In previous studies, *D. morbifera* extracts with anti-oxidant, anti-inflammatory, anti-complementary and anti-cancer activities were reported. The present study aims to investigate optimization of extraction and evaluation of anti-hyperuricemic effects of *D. morbifera* leaf and the phytochemicals contained therein. Ethanol and hexane extract were found to display the best xanthine oxidase inhibition among six types of solvent and water extract. The antioxidant effect of the ethanol extract was superior to that of the hexane extract. The DPPH radical scavenging effect of the ethanol and hexane extracts were 81.52 ± 1.57% and 2.69 ± 0.16. The reducing power of the ethanol and hexane extracts were 9.71 ± 0.15 and 0.89 ± 0.01 mg/g equivalent of gallic acid. Total phenols of the ethanol and hexane extracts were 6.53 ± 0.16 and 0.63 ± 0.001 mg/g equivalent of gallic acid. In addition, we compared the two marker compounds from *D. morbifera*, chlorogenic acid and rutin, which were determined in the ethanol extract at 0.80 ± 0.03% and 0.52 ± 0.01%, respectively. We found that the ethanol extracts showed better xanthine oxidase inhibition than hexane extracts. Especially, ethanol extracts showed higher antioxidant activity than hexane extracts. Based on these results, we selected the ethanol extract as an effective xanthine oxidase inhibitor and confirmed whether ethanol extracts showed xanthine oxidase inhibition in animal experiments. The in vivo mouse study demonstrated that ethanol extract of *D. morbifera* leaf at the dose of 300 mg/kg could inhibit blood/hepatic xanthine oxidase activity and this result shows that the xanthine oxidase inhibitory activity in vitro is reproduced in vivo. The present study showed that ethanol extract was optimal xanthine oxidase inhibitor which can be applied to prevent diseases related to hyperuricemia.

Keywords: *Dendropanax morbifera* leaf; xanthine oxidase; hyperuricemia; HPLC

1. Introduction

Dendropanax morbifera (Aralicaceae), called ginseng tree, is a perennial tree that grows in forests in the southern regions in South Korea. The leaf, stem, and root of *D. morbifera* have been used in traditional medicine to treat infectious diseases, dermatopathy, dysmenorrhea and migraine [1,2]. To date, a few studies have been carried out investigating *D. morbifera* as a functional food and medicinal source [2]. This plant has been reported to exhibit various pharmacologic effects including antioxidant, anticancer, anti-inflammatory, anticomplementary, anti-amnesic, and antidiabetic activities [3–6]. However, systematic evaluation of pharmacological efficacy based on active constituents and the standardization of *D. morbifera* remains insufficient.

Recently, we found that the extract of *D. morbifera* leaf exhibited in vitro xanthine oxidase inhibitory activity, indicating that it could serve as a functional source for anti-hyperuricemia agents [2]. Hyperuricemia involves excessive uric acid levels in the blood, which are due to the abnormal intake of food with high purine content, and these excessive uric acid levels are consistently accompanied by gout and metabolic syndrome [7]. Uric acid is formed by the oxidation of hypoxanthine to xanthine and of xanthine to uric acid by xanthine oxidase (XO) [8]. High levels of uric acid by XO lead to hyperuricemia, which is a main cause of gout. Gout is a metabolic disorder that is strongly associated with high levels of uric acid in the body, and it can cause diabetic cardiomyopathy, arthritis, and nephrolithiasis [9].

In our recent study, the optimized extraction and analysis method of marker compounds in *D. morbifera* leaf was established [2]. Additionally, we identified the common components of *D. morbifera* leaf from four Korean production sites and compared the extraction yield and effective marker content by region [2]. In the present study, we investigated the optimum extraction of *D. morbifera* leaf as well as the biological activities of extracts from *D. morbifera* leaf to evaluate their feasibility as an anti-hyperuricemic source. The optimized extract from *D. morbifera* leaf was prepared and evaluated for its antioxidant and XO inhibitory activities of *D. morbifera* leaf extract in vivo.

2. Results and Discussion

2.1. In Vitro Xanthine Oxidase Inhibitory Activities of D. morbifera Extracts

The effects of the various solvent extracts on the XO inhibitory activity of *D. morbifera* are shown in Table 1. Allopurinol (ALP, positive control) at a concentration of 50 µg/mL significantly decreased the uric acid concentration (4.04 ± 1.49%). The XO inhibitory activities of the hexane and ethanol extracts were significantly higher than those of the other extracts at the concentration of 2 mg/mL (38.7 and 37.3% inhibition). According to previous reports, in the case of XO inhibition at 1 to 2 mg/mL, the plant extracts showed significant results in animal experiments [10]. We previously reported various plant sources as potential XO inhibitors [11]. Yoon et al. [10,12] reported that the extracts of *Corylopsis coreana* and *Camellia japonica* each inhibited XO activity by approximately 50% at a concentration of 2 mg/mL. Yoon et al. [11] also reported that *Quercus acuta* extract showed approximately 50% XO inhibitory activity at a concentration of 1 mg/mL, and that *Cudrania tricuspidata* extract inhibited XO by approximately 75% at a concentration of 2 mg/mL [13]. All of the above results showed in vitro and in vivo correlation of XO inhibition. However, further investigation on the clinical and biomedical relevance of our previous and present results is needed.

Table 1. In vitro xanthine oxidase inhibitory activity of various solvent extract.

Extract	Relative Activity (%)
Control	100 ± 10
ALP	4.04 ± 1.49
Ethyl acetate	67.2 ± 1.2
Hexane	61.3 ± 1.9
Acetone	66.8 ± 0.9
MeOH	77.6 ± 1.0
Water	96.2 ± 4.1
EtOH	62.7 ± 3.9

Therefore, we considered that the hexane and ethanol extracts would inhibit XO in animal models, and performed an antioxidant test to determine the optimal results in an animal model. The antioxidant activity of plant material is known to play important roles in hyperuricemia and gout. Thus, we compared the antioxidant capacities of the hexane and ethanol extracts and tested the best materials for an in vivo test.

2.2. Antioxidant Activity and Total Phenolic Contents of D. morbifera Extracts

According to previous reports, the antioxidant effects of plant extracts have curative benefits against conditions such as inflammation, oxidative stress, and other metabolic diseases such as hyperuricemia and gout arthritis [10,14,15]. Thus, we compared the antioxidant effects of the hexane and ethanol extracts. First, we compared the DPPH radical scavenging activities between the hexane and ethanol extracts. The ethanol extract showed an antioxidant activity 30 times higher than the hexane extract. Reducing power is one of the tools used to evaluate an antioxidant effect. The ethanol extract showed a reducing power 11 times higher than the hexane extract. Furthermore, phenolic-rich sources of phytochemicals with antioxidant activities have curative benefits against various metabolic diseases. In the present study, the ethanol extract showed total phenolic contents 10.3 times higher than the hexane extract (Table 2). Based on the antioxidant data, it was concluded that the ethanol extract had an antioxidant ability that was better by 10 times or more than the hexane extract. Considering that its xanthine oxidase inhibition activity is similar to that of the hexane extract, it is considered that the ethanol extract is excellent for the development of an anti-hyperuricemic material.

Table 2. Antioxidant activities of hexane and ethanol extract from D. morbifera leaf.

	DPPH Acavenging (%)	Reducing Power (mg/g eq GA)	Total Phenol (mg/g GA)	Total Flavonoid (mg/g QT)
Hexane ex	2.69 ± 0.16	0.89 ± 0.01	0.63 ± 0.00	ND *
Ethanol ex	81.5 ± 1.6	9.71 ± 0.15	6.53 ± 0.16	ND *

* ND (not detected).

2.3. Contents of Marker Compounds in D. morbifera Leaf Extracts

In a previous report, we identified chlorogenic acid and rutin as marker compounds of the extracts of D. morbifera leaves [2]. This finding could be important in industrial uses of this plant. Based on a chromatographic measurement, we found that the two indicator substances were not detected in the hexane extract, but rutin (0.52%) and chlorogenic acid (0.8%) were detected in the ethanol extract. Rutin and chlorogenic acid are known to have diverse pharmacological effects, such as antihyperuricemic and anti-inflammatory activities [16–19]. In the present study, we compared the rutin and chlorogenic acid contents between the ethanol and hexane extracts; rutin and chlorogenic acid were both found in the ethanol extract (Table 3). In our previous study, we set chlorogenic acid and rutin as indicators of D. morbifera. Two markers were set as markers for identification and quality control of D. morbifera extract [2]. In the present study, the presence of two substances in hexane extract could not be confirmed, however xanthine oxidase inhibition had activity similar to ethanol extract. This result implies that there is another xanthine oxidase inhibitor in the hexane extract. We will use a bioassay guided purification method in hexane extract as a further study to find another marker compound.

Table 3. Comparison of marker compounds of hexane and ethanol extract from D. morbifera leaf.

Extract	Chlorogenic Acid (%, v/v)	Rutin (%, v/v)
Hexane	ND *	ND *
Ethanol	0.80 ± 0.03	0.52 ± 0.01

* ND (not detected).

2.4. In Vivo XO Inhibitory and Antihyperuricemic Effects of Ethano Extract from D. morbifera Leaf

Figure 1 shows the effects of the ethanol extract on the hepatic and serum XO activities in potassium oxonate-induced hyperuricemic mice. The one-week oral administration of allopurinol (by 47%) and ethanol extract at a dose of 300 mg/kg (by 97%, respectively) significantly reduced hepatic XO activity in comparison to the hyperuricema group ($p < 0.05$). Similarly, the one-week oral administration of allopurinol (by 16%) and ethanol extract at a dose of 300 mg/kg (by 50%, respectively) significantly reduced plasma XO activity in comparison to the hyperuricemia group ($p < 0.05$). However, ethanol extract at a dose of 30 mg/kg did not show statistical significance as compared to the hyperuricemia group. Thus, the 300 mg/kg treatment of ethanol extract was considered to show XO inhibitory activity. In an in vitro test, the ethanol extract showed a significant XO inhibitory effect and a consistent XO inhibitory effect in an in vivo test.

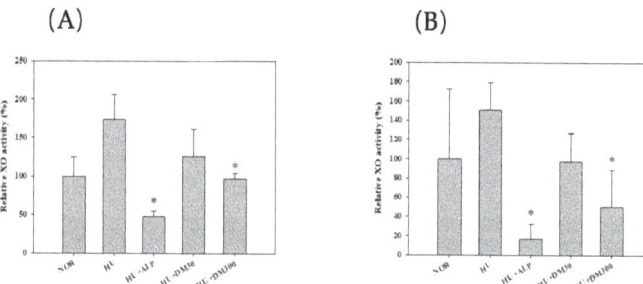

Figure 1. Relative activity of hepatic (**A**) and serum (**B**) xanthine oxidase (XO) after the oral administration of saline in normal mice (NOR) and after the oral administration of saline (HU), allopurinol at a dose of 10 mg/kg (HU + ALP), or DM at doses of 30 mg/kg (HU + DM30) and 300 mg/kg (HU + DM300) in hyperuricemic mice for 7 days. The rectangular bars and their error bars represent the means and standard deviations, respectively ($n = 5$). The asterisks indicate values that are significantly different from those of the HU group ($p < 0.05$).

Figure 2 shows the effects of the extract on the serum uric acid levels in the same animal model. Notable, the 300 mg/kg treatment of the extract exhibited a significant antihyperuricemic effect in an in vivo test.

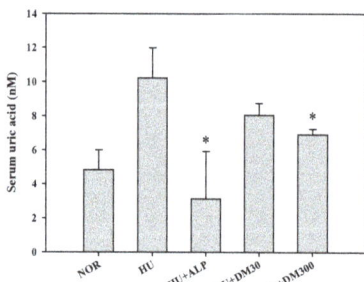

Figure 2. Serum uric acid levels after the oral administration of saline in normal mice (NOR) and after the oral administration of saline (HU), allopurinol at a dose of 10 mg/kg (HU + ALP), or DM at doses of 30 mg/kg (HU + DM30) and 300 mg/kg (HU + DM300) in hyperuricemic mice for 7 days. The rectangular bars and their error bars represent the means and standard deviations, respectively ($n = 5$). The asterisks indicate values that are significantly different from those of the HU group ($p < 0.05$).

We considered the oral intake of ethanol extract of 1.46 g daily to help in preventing hyperuricemia and gout. The oral dose for a human weighing 60 kg is 1460 mg/day (24.33 mg/kg/day). The conversion factor between humans and mice is known to be 12.33. Therefore, if the effective dose for mice is 300 mg/kg/day, the human equivalent dose is 1.46 g/60 kg/day of ethanol extract or 15.2 g/60 kg/day as dried leaf. Thus, we concluded that the oral intake of 1.46 g of the extract of *D. morbifera* leaves is beneficial for preventing and/or decreasing the possibility of the occurrence of hyperuricemia-related disease. Taken together, we found beneficial effects of the extract of *D. morbifera* leaves from the results of biological evaluation through the antioxidant assay and XO assay in vitro and in vivo. We optimized the basic extraction condition due to antioxidant and XO inhibitory activities and the contents of marker compounds as XO inhibitors (e.g., rutin and chlorogenic acid). In addition, we have applied optimized extracts to in vivo hyperuricemic mouse models and found that the XO in liver and plasma was inhibited. In previous reports, rutinwas shown to have the ability to draw out dose-dependent hypouricemic effects by exerting significant inhibitory effects on XO [20]. Meng et al. described that chlorogenic acid showed an anti-gout effect due to XO inhibition [18]. In addition, chlorogenic acid has shown an anti-inflammatory effect via the suppression of levels of proinflammatory cytokines such as interleukin (IL)-1β, IL-6, and tumor necrosis factor (TNF)-α induced by uric acid [18,19,21]. These results suggest that chlorogenic acid exerts dual effects in anti-gout and gout inflammatory diseases. Phenolic compounds are also known to be closely related to the prevention and treatment of diseases such as inflammation and gout. Phenolic contents are also associated with antioxidant and XO inhibition [10]. In the present study, we compared the antioxidant activity of hexane and ethanol extracts, and the ethanol extract showed higher phenolic content than the hexane extract. Therefore, it was thought that phenolic contents and antioxidant capacity were beneficial in XO inhibition, and our result was thought to confirm the results of animal experiments. Based on these results, it is necessary to study the function mechanism of XO and the single component from *D. morbifera* leaf that is inhibiting XO.

3. Experimental Section

3.1. Plant Materials

D. morbifera leaves were provided by the Jeollanamdo Wando provincial government in Jeonnam, Korea. A voucher specimen (MNUCSS-DM-02) was deposited in the Mokpo National University (Muan, Korea). The leaves were separated for the present study. The dried *D. morbifera* leaf (50 g) was extracted twice with each of hexane, ethyl acetate, acetone, methanol, ethanol, and hot water (250 mL, v/v) for 72 h. The yields of hexane, ethyl acetate, acetone, methanol, ethanol, and hot water extracts were 1.4, 1.8, 6, 9, 9.6 and 13% (w/w), respectively. Each resulting sample was filtered, the solvent was evaporated, and the water extract was freeze dried. For in vivo evaluation, *D. morbifera* leaf (200 g) was extracted twice with ethanol (2000 mL, v/v) at room temperature for 72 hours and evaporated in vacuo (50 °C). All samples were stored at 4 °C.

3.2. Animals

Male ICR mice (four-weeks old) were purchased from Samtaco Co. (Osan, Korea). The mice were kept in a clean room at a temperature of 20–23 °C with a relative humidity of 50 ± 5%. The mice were housed in ventilated mice cages (Tecniplast USA, Inc, West Chester, PA, USA) under filtered and pathogen-free air, with diet (Agribrands Purina Korea, Inc., Sungnam, Korea) and water available ad libitum. All animal experiments were carried out according to the Guidelines of the Animal Investigation Committee of Jeonnam Bioindustry Foundation (Naju, Korea) (approval number: JINR1503).

3.3. DPPH Free Radical Assay

The DPPH radical scavenging assay was evaluated to compare antioxidant activity of the extracts [10]. Briefly, sample solutions (0.5 mL) were mixed with 0.4 mM DPPH (0.5 mL) for 10 min. The absorbance at 517 nm was measured using a microplate reader (Perkin Elmer, Waltham, CT, USA). The radical scavenging activity was calculated in the form of a percentage using the following equation:

$$\text{DPPH radical scavenging activity (\%)} = [1 - (A_{sample}/A_{blank})] \times 100 \tag{1}$$

3.4. Reducing Power

The reducing power was used to evaluate the antioxidant activities of the extracts. Sample was mixed with 0.2 M sodium phosphate buffer and 1% potassium ferricyanide, followed by incubation at 50 °C for 20 min. Ten percent trichloroacetic acid solution was used and stop solution. Reaction mixture was centrifuged at 2000× g for 10 min, the supernatant was mixed with distilled water and 0.1% iron (III) chloride solution. Reaction mixture was measured at 700 nm. The reducing powers of the extracts were expressed as vitamin C equivalents [10].

3.5. Total Phenolic Content

The total phenolic content was determined using the Folin-Ciocalteu assay [10]. A sample and gallic acid (as standard) was mixed with 2% sodium carbonate and 10% Folin-Ciocalteu phenol reagent for 10 min. The absorbance of the mixture was then measured at 750 nm. The results were expressed as milligrams of gallic acid equivalents per gram of the sample

3.6. Chromatographic Conditions

Analysis of samples were performed using high performance liquid chromatography (Alliance 2695 HPLC system, Waters, Milford, CT, USA). A Zorbax RP C18 analytical column (5 µm, 150 mm × 5 mm) was used with a mobile phase consisting of a mixture of acetonitrile and 0.2% phosphoric acid. A gradient elution (from 10/90 to 80/20, v/v) at a flow rate of 0.8 mL/min was used under the same analytical conditions previously described [2].

3.7. Determination of In Vitro Xanthine Oxidase (XO) Inhibitory Activity

The XO inhibitory assay was performed as follows: the assay system consisted of phosphate buffer (0.6 mL, 100 mM; pH 7.4), various concentrations of extract (0.1 mL), XO (0.1 mL, 0.2 U/mL), and xanthine (0.2 mL, 1 mM; dissolved in 0.1 N NaOH). Each mixture was shaken for 15min and a stop buffer (0.2 mL, 1 M HCl) was added at 290 nm. Allopurinol was used as a positive control [22].

3.8. Preparation of Hyperuricemia Model and Drug Administration

The mice were divided into five groups; NOR: normal, HU: hyperuricemic mouse, ALP: allopurinol (10 mg/kg) treatment group, DM30: DM (ethanol extract of *D. morbifera* leaf) 30 mg/kg treatment group, DM300: DM 300 mg/kg treatment group (n = 5 for each group). Hyperuricemia was induced via an intraperitoneal injection of potassium oxonate [23]. Briefly, the DM (30, 300 mg/kg) or allopurinol (10 mg/kg) were dissolved in 0.3% carboxymethylcellulose sodium solution. The allopurinol and DMs were orally administered once per day for seven days. Food (but not water) was withdrawn from the mice at 1.5 h prior to the drug administration, and mice were intraperitoneally injected with potassium oxonate (300 mg/kg) at 1 h before the last drug treatment on the seventh day in order to make hyperuricemic mice. Blood samples were collected at 1 h after the last drug treatment on the seventh day. The blood samples were allowed to clot for approximately 1 h at room temperature, then centrifuged at 10,000× g for 15 min in order to obtain serum. The serum samples were stored at −80 °C until use. Serum uric acid concentration was measured using standard diagnostic kits (Abcam, Cambridge, UK). Each assay was performed in triplicate.

3.9. Determination of In Vivo Xanthine Oxidase (XO) Inhibitory Activity

The residual activity of XO in the mouse liver and plasma were determined as reported previously [8]. Mice livers (0.5 g) were homogenized in a 1 mL aliquot of 50 mM sodium phosphate buffer (pH 7.4). The homogenates were centrifuged at 3000× g for 10 min at 4 °C. The supernatant was centrifuged at 10,000× g for 60 min at 4 °C, and was used for determining XO residual activity and total protein. An aliquot of xanthine solution (0.12 mL, 250 mM) was added to a test tube containing liver homogenate (10 µL) and potassium oxonate solution (0.54 mL, 1 mM) in sodium phosphate buffer (50 mM, pH 7.4) that had been previously incubated at 35 °C for 15 min. The reaction was stopped by adding a 0.1 mL of 0.6 M HCl. Thereafter, the mixture was centrifuged at $3000\times g$ for 5 min and finally measured at 295 nm. The total protein concentration was determined through the Bradford method [24]. XO activity was expressed as micromoles of uric acid formed per minute (U) per milligram protein.

3.10. Statistical Analysis

A *p*-value less than 0.05 was considered to be statistically significant using a *t*-test between the two means for the unpaired data or an ANOVA (post hoc test: Tukey's multiple range test) among the three or more means for the unpaired data. All data were expressed as mean ± standard deviation and rounded to two decimal places.

4. Conclusions

In the present study, various solvent extracts of *D. morbifera* leaf were prepared. We selected hexane and ethanol extracts as XO inhibiting candidates, and their biological activities, such as antioxidant effects, XO inhibition, and contents of maker compounds were evaluated. The ethanol extract exhibited the most potent DPPH radical scavenging activity, reducing power, phenolic content, and XO inhibitory activity. Marker compounds such as chlorogenic acid and rutin were found in the ethanol extract as well. We confirmed the inhibition of XO in animal models, and found significant results on liver and plasma. Further investigation is warranted to confirm the in vivo mechanism study of *D. morbifera* extract, identify another XO, and assess the safe use of this plant.

Author Contributions: J.-H.S. and D.-H.P. conceived and designed the experiments. S.-S.C., S.-H.S., C.-Y.C. and K.M.P. performed the experiments and analyzed the data. J.-H.S. and D.-H.P. statistically analyzed the data.

Funding: This research was funded by National Research Foundation of Korea (NRF-2017R1C1B5015187) and Korea Forest Service (Project No. 2016014A00-1619-AB02) and Food and Rural Affairs (No. 116032-3).

Conflicts of Interest: The authors declare no conflict of interest.

References

1. Kim, M.; Park, Y.J.; Lim, H.S.; Lee, H.H.; Kim, T.H.; Lee, B. The clinical effects of *Dendropanax morbifera* on postmenopausal symptoms: Review article. *J. Menopausal. Med.* **2017**, *23*, 146–155. [CrossRef] [PubMed]
2. Choi, H.J.; Park, D.H.; Song, S.H.; Yoon, I.S.; Cho, S.S. Development and validation of a HPLC-UV method for extraction optimization and biological evaluation of hot-water and ethanolic extracts of *Dendropanax morbifera* leaves. *Molecules* **2018**, *23*, 650. [CrossRef] [PubMed]
3. Chung, I.M.; Song, H.K.; Kim, S.J.; Moon, H.I. Anticomplement activity of polyacetylenes from leaves of *Dendropanax morbifera* Leveille. *Phytother. Res.* **2011**, *25*, 784–786. [CrossRef] [PubMed]
4. Hyun, T.K.; Kim, M.O.; Lee, H.; Kim, Y.; Kim, E.; Kim, J.S. Evaluation of anti-oxidant and anti-cancer properties of *Dendropanax morbifera* Leveille. *Food Chem.* **2013**, *141*, 1947–1955. [CrossRef] [PubMed]
5. Hyun, T.K.; Ko, Y.-J.; Kim, E.-H.; Chung, I.-M.; Kim, J.-S. Anti-inflammatory activity and phenolic composition of *Dendropanax morbifera* leaf extracts. *Ind. Crop. Prod.* **2015**, *74*, 263–270. [CrossRef]
6. Hossen, M.J.; Kim, M.Y.; Kim, J.H.; Cho, J.Y. *Codonopsis lanceolata*: A review of its therapeutic potentials. *Phytother. Res.* **2016**, *30*, 347–356. [CrossRef] [PubMed]
7. Zhao, M.; Zhu, D.; Sun-Waterhouse, D.; Su, G.; Lin, L.; Wang, X.; Dong, Y. In vitro and in vivo studies on adlay-derived seed extracts: Phenolic profiles, antioxidant activities, serum uric acid suppression, and xanthine oxidase inhibitory effects. *J. Agric. Food Chem.* **2014**, *62*, 7771–7778. [CrossRef]
8. Lemos Lima Rde, C.; Ferrari, F.C.; de Souza, M.R.; de Sa Pereira, B.M.; de Paula, C.A.; Saude-Guimaraes, D.A. Effects of extracts of leaves from *Sparattosperma leucanthum* on hyperuricemia and gouty arthritis. *J. Ethnopharmacol.* **2015**, *161*, 194–199. [CrossRef]

9. Sharaf El Din, U.A.A.; Salem, M.M.; Abdulazim, D.O. Uric acid in the pathogenesis of metabolic, renal, and cardiovascular diseases: A review. *J. Adv. Res.* **2017**, *8*, 537–548. [CrossRef]
10. Seo, J.H.; Kim, J.E.; Shim, J.H.; Yoon, G.; Bang, M.A.; Bae, C.S.; Lee, K.J.; Park, D.H.; Cho, S.S. HPLC analysis, optimization of extraction conditions and biological evaluation of *Corylopsis coreana* Uyeki Flos. *Molecules* **2016**, *21*, 94. [CrossRef]
11. Yoon, I.S.; Park, D.H.; Bae, M.S.; Oh, D.S.; Kwon, N.H.; Kim, J.E.; Choi, C.Y.; Cho, S.S. In vitro and in vivo studies on *Quercus acuta* Thunb. (Fagaceae) extract: Active constituents, serum uric acid suppression, and xanthine oxidase inhibitory activity. *Evid. Based Complement. Alternat. Med.* **2017**, *2017*. [CrossRef] [PubMed]
12. Yoon, I.S.; Park, D.H.; Kim, J.E.; Yoo, J.C.; Bae, M.S.; Oh, D.S.; Shim, J.H.; Choi, C.Y.; An, K.W.; Kim, E.I.; et al. Identification of the biologically active constituents of *Camellia japonica* leaf and anti-hyperuricemic effect in vitro and in vivo. *Int. J. Mol. Med.* **2017**, *39*, 1613–1620. [CrossRef] [PubMed]
13. Song, S.H.; Ki, S.H.; Park, D.H.; Moon, H.S.; Lee, C.D.; Yoon, I.S.; Cho, S.S. Quantitative analysis, extraction optimization, and biological evaluation of *Cudrania tricuspidata* leaf and fruit extracts. *Molecules* **2017**, *22*, 1489. [CrossRef] [PubMed]
14. Chansiw, N.; Chotinuntakool, K.; Srichairatanakool, S. Anti-inflammatory and antioxidant activities of the extracts from leaves and stems of *Polygonum odoratum* Lour. *Anti-Inflamm. Anti-Allergy Agents Med. Chem.* **2018**. [CrossRef] [PubMed]
15. Mohammad, M.K.; Almasri, I.M.; Tawaha, K.; Issa, A.; Al-Nadaf, A.; Hudaib, M.; Alkhatib, H.S.; Abu-Gharbieh, E.; Bustanji, Y. Antioxidant, antihyperuricemic and xanthine oxidase inhibitory activities of *Hyoscyamus reticulatus*. *Pharm. Biol.* **2010**, *48*, 1376–1383. [CrossRef] [PubMed]
16. Shi, H.; Shi, A.; Dong, L.; Lu, X.; Wang, Y.; Zhao, J.; Dai, F.; Guo, X. Chlorogenic acid protects against liver fibrosis in vivo and in vitro through inhibition of oxidative stress. *Clin. Nutr.* **2016**, *35*, 1366–1373. [CrossRef] [PubMed]
17. Zatorski, H.; Salaga, M.; Zielinska, M.; Piechota-Polanczyk, A.; Owczarek, K.; Kordek, R.; Lewandowska, U.; Chen, C.; Fichna, J. Experimental colitis in mice is attenuated by topical administration of chlorogenic acid. *Naunyn-Schmiedebergs Arch. Pharmacol.* **2015**, *388*, 643–651. [CrossRef]
18. Meng, Z.-Q.; Tang, Z.-H.; Yan, Y.-X.; Guo, C.-R.; Cao, L.; Ding, G.; Huang, W.-Z.; Wang, Z.-Z.; Wang, K.D.G.; Xiao, W.; et al. Study on the anti-gout activity of chlorogenic acid: Improvement on hyperuricemia and gouty inflammation. *Am. J. Chin. Med.* **2014**, *42*, 1471–1483. [CrossRef]
19. Hwang, S.J.; Kim, Y.W.; Park, Y.; Lee, H.J.; Kim, K.W. Anti-inflammatory effects of chlorogenic acid in lipopolysaccharide-stimulated RAW 264.7 cells. *Inflamm. Res.* **2014**, *63*, 81–90. [CrossRef]
20. Zhu, J.X.; Wang, Y.; Kong, L.D.; Yang, C.; Zhang, X. Effects of *Biota orientalis* extract and its flavonoid constituents, quercetin and rutin on serum uric acid levels in oxonate-induced mice and xanthine dehydrogenase and xanthine oxidase activities in mouse liver. *J. Ethnopharmacol.* **2004**, *93*, 133–140. [CrossRef]
21. Kim, H.R.; Lee, D.M.; Lee, S.H.; Seong, A.R.; Gin, D.W.; Hwang, J.A.; Park, J.H. Chlorogenic acid suppresses pulmonary eosinophilia, IgE production, and Th2-type cytokine production in an ovalbumin-induced allergic asthma: Activation of STAT-6 and JNK is inhibited by chlorogenic acid. *Int. Immunopharmacol.* **2010**, *10*, 1242–1248. [CrossRef]
22. Arimboor, R.; Rangan, M.; Aravind, S.G.; Arumughan, C. Tetrahydroamentoflavone (THA) from *Semecarpus anacardium* as a potent inhibitor of xanthine oxidase. *J. Ethnopharmacol.* **2011**, *133*, 1117–1120. [CrossRef] [PubMed]
23. Huo, L.N.; Wang, W.; Zhang, C.Y.; Shi, H.B.; Liu, Y.; Liu, X.H.; Guo, B.H.; Zhao, D.M.; Gao, H. Bioassay-guided isolation and identification of xanthine oxidase inhibitory constituents from the leaves of *Perilla frutescens*. *Molecules* **2015**, *20*, 17848–17859. [CrossRef] [PubMed]
24. Bradford, M.M. A rapid and sensitive method for the quantitation of microgram quantities of protein utilizing the principle of protein-dye binding. *Anal. Biochem.* **1976**, *72*, 248–254. [CrossRef]

Sample Availability: Not available.

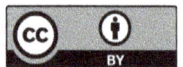

© 2018 by the authors. Licensee MDPI, Basel, Switzerland. This article is an open access article distributed under the terms and conditions of the Creative Commons Attribution (CC BY) license (http://creativecommons.org/licenses/by/4.0/).

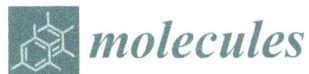

Article

Simultaneous Determination of N^ε-(carboxymethyl) Lysine and N^ε-(carboxyethyl) Lysine in Different Sections of Antler Velvet after Various Processing Methods by UPLC-MS/MS

Rui-ze Gong [1], Yan-hua Wang [1,2], Yu-fang Wang [1], Bao Chen [1,2], Kun Gao [1,2] and Yin-shi Sun [1,*]

[1] Institute of Special Animal and Plant Sciences, Chinese Academy of Agricultural Sciences, Changchun 130112, China; 82101172456@caas.cn (R.-z.G.); yhwangsdlc@126.com (Y.-h.W.); wangyufang_jl@163.com (Y.-f.W.); 15543598331@163.com (B.C.); 13356954028@163.com (K.G.)

[2] College of Chinese Material Medicine, Jilin Agricultural University, Changchun 130112, China

* Correspondence: sunyinshi2015@163.com; Tel.: +86-431-81919580; Fax: +86-431-81919580

Academic Editors: In-Soo Yoon and Hyun-Jong Cho
Received: 13 November 2018; Accepted: 12 December 2018; Published: 14 December 2018

Abstract: N^ε-(Carboxymethyl) lysine (CML) and N^ε-(carboxyethyl) lysine (CEL) are two typical advanced glycation end-products (AGEs) and are frequently used as markers of AGE formation. AGEs, such as CML and CEL, have harmful effects in the human body and have been closely linked to many diseases such as diabetes and uremia. However, details on the contents of CML and CEL after applying different antler velvet processing methods are lacking. In this research, a robust UPLC-MS/MS method has been developed for the simultaneous determination of CML and CEL in various sections of antler velvet processed with different methods. In addition, factors affecting the CML and CEL contents are discussed. The CML contents of antler velvet after freeze-drying, boiling, processing without blood, and processing with blood were 74.55–458.59, 119.44–570.69, 75.36–234.92, and 117.11–456.01 µg/g protein, respectively; the CEL contents were 0.74–12.66, 11.33–35.93, 0.00–6.75, and 0.00–23.41 µg/g protein, respectively. The different contents of CML and CEL in the different samples of antler velvet result from the different interactions of the protein and lysine at different temperatures. These data can be used to estimate the potential consumer intake of CML and CEL from antler velvet and for guiding producers on how to reduce the production of CML and CEL.

Keywords: advanced glycation end-products (AGEs); N^ε-(carboxymethyl) lysine (CML); N^ε-(carboxyethyl) lysine (CEL); antler velvet processing; UPLC-MS/MS

---

1. Introduction

Antler velvet is a representative animal medicinal material and dietary supplement that has been an important part of traditional Chinese medicine for thousands of years in China, Korea, and Southeast Asian countries [1–3]. It has various pharmacological effects, such as anti-oxidation and anti-osteoporosis properties [4–6]. Fresh antler velvet is rich in nutrients, such as proteins and amino acids; these are highly susceptible to spoilage if the antler velvet is not processed promptly. Based on the methods of processing and consumption, antler velvet can be classified as processed with blood or without blood, as boiled or freeze-dried, and as wax slices, powder slices, gauze slices, or bone slices. Different processing methods and sections of the antler velvet have different influences on the bioactive components and pharmacological activities [4–6]; therefore, the processing conditions are crucial for antler velvet's dietary and medical functions.

During the processing and storage of antler velvet, amino compounds (e.g., proteins, amino acids) react with carbonyl compounds (e.g., reducing sugars, lipid oxidation products) to randomly form advanced glycation end-products (AGEs) by the Maillard reaction [7]. AGEs have been shown to be detrimental to human health, being closely linked to many conditions such as diabetes, Alzheimer's disease, atherosclerosis, renal diseases, and aging [8–12]; with the accumulation of AGEs in the human body, the probability of people suffering the above-mentioned chronic degenerative diseases will increase greatly. Food is the main source of AGEs, especially high-fat and high-sugar foods [8,11,13], although human bodies can also produce some AGEs by themselves.

N^ε-(Carboxymethyl) lysine (CML) and N^ε-(carboxyethyl) lysine (CEL) are two typical AGEs and are frequently used as markers of AGE formation in foods [14–16]. However, the determination of CML and CEL in antler velvet has not been reported. The contents of CML and CEL in antler velvets are affected by the matrix and processing conditions [17,18]. Antler velvet rich in amino compounds and carbonyl compounds may contribute more CML and CEL than other foods [19,20]. Therefore, information on the CML and CEL contents in processed antler velvets is essential to estimate the potential consumer intake of AGEs from antler velvet.

Since CML and CEL have no UV absorption and fluorescence properties, enzyme-linked immunosorbent assay (ELISA), high-performance liquid chromatography (HPLC), gas chromatography–mass spectrometry (GC-MS), and high-performance liquid chromatography-mass spectrometry (HPLC-MS) techniques have previously been used to determine their contents [21–28]. The ELISA method requires specific antibodies, and the sensitivity is greatly affected by the matrix effect of the sample, which can cause large errors [21–23]. HPLC and GC-MS typically require pre-column derivatization, which is cumbersome and reduces sensitivity [24–26]. HPLC-MS has the advantages of simple operation, repeatability, and stability; therefore, HPLC-MS has usually been used to determine CML and CEL contents [14,16,27].

In this research, we have developed a robust UPLC-MS/MS method to simultaneously determine CML and CEL contents in various sections of antler velvet processed with different methods. The CML and CEL contents in the various samples were determined by a validated method, which may contribute to the assessment of AGEs in antler velvets. This study provides a foundation and valuable reference for safe antler velvet processing and provides a basis for the development of recommended antler velvet dosages.

2. Results and Discussion

2.1. Sample Pretreatment

Preparation of the antler velvet samples consisted of processing, segmenting, grinding, defatting, reduction, hydrolysis, and SPE. According to the processing method and consumption, antler velvet samples were classified as boiled or freeze-dried and processed with or without blood; samples were then divided into wax, powder, gauze, and bone slices. Because CML and CEL can be generated via peroxidation of the antler velvet lipid content, it was important to remove lipids from the antler velvet samples to prevent overestimation in the results. Before hydrolysis, 0.1 N sodium borohydride was applied for 12 h to reduce the amadori (e.g., fructose–lysine) and lipid oxidation products, thus preventing the formation of CML and CEL during acid hydrolysis [28]. The samples were subjected to SPE by using a C_{18} Sep-Pak cartridge (Sepax technology, Cork, Ireland; 500 mg, 6 mL), to remove impurities from the sample.

2.2. Optimization of Chromatography Conditions

CML and CEL are highly polar compounds and are difficult to retain in most reversed-phase columns. Researchers have usually analyzed these substances with a C18 column by using nonafluoropentanoic acid (NFPA) as the eluent. However, NFPA can lead to a low-pH (~2) mobile phase, which may result in deterioration of the reversed-phase column [29]. To avoid the use of NFPA, we developed a UPLC-MS/MS method to separate CML and CEL with a WATERS CORTECS HILIC UPLC column. HILIC uses the separation principle of affinity chromatography to maximize the retention and separation of highly polar compounds, relative to other columns. The elution effects of methanol and acetonitrile were assessed: acetonitrile/water (30:70 *v/v*) and methanol/water (30:70 *v/v*) mixtures were used as mobile phases, and the flow rate was 0.3 mL/min. In comparison to chromatograms with the methanol mobile phase, UPLC-MS chromatograms using water and acetonitrile as the eluent have better spectrum peak symmetries and fewer miscellaneous peaks.

The UPLC-MS chromatograms of standard solutions (a) and antler velvet samples (b) are shown in Figure 1. The retention times of CML and CEL in the antler velvet samples were consistent with those of the standard solutions, and no peak interference was observed. The column was very stable and robust without obvious shifts in the retention times throughout the experimental procedure.

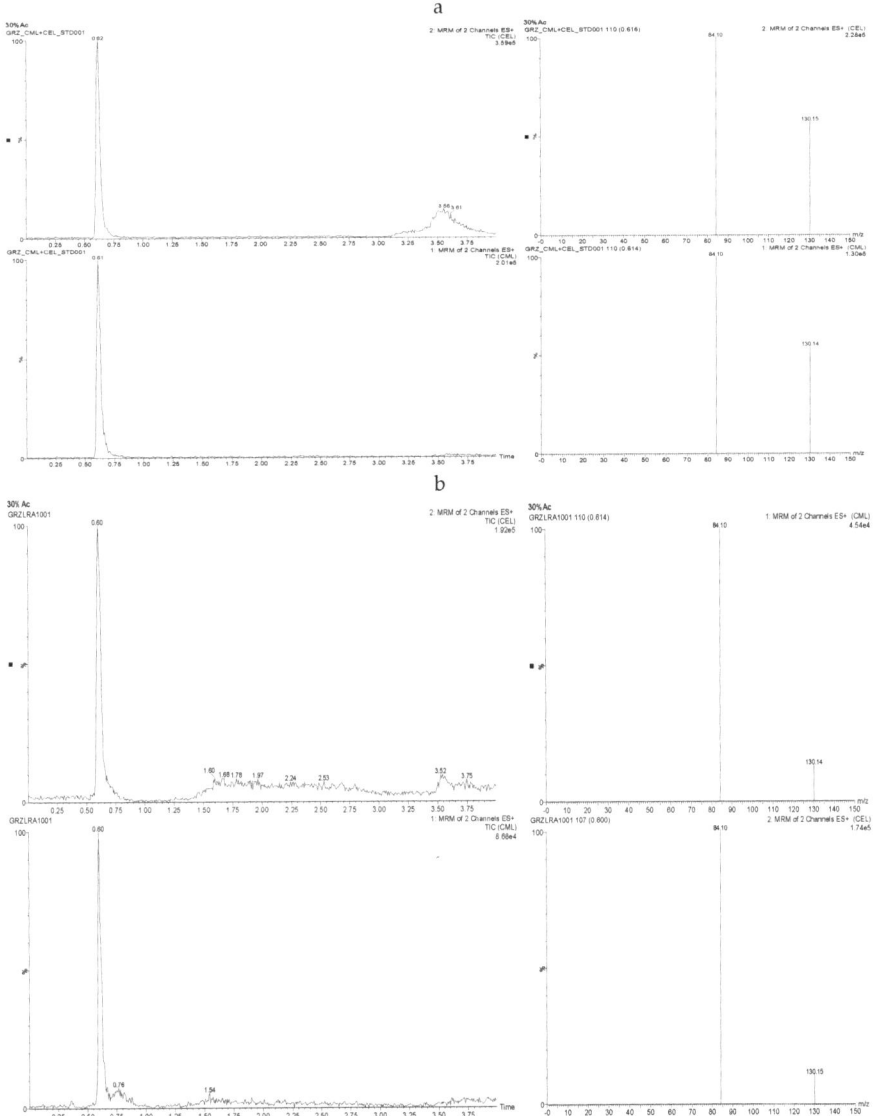

Figure 1. Total ion chromatogram and selected ion of N^ε-(Carboxymethyl) lysine (CML) and N^ε-(carboxyethyl) lysine (CEL) standard solutions (**a**) and antler velvet samples (**b**).

2.3. Method Validation

The developed method was validated by assessing the CML and CEL contents in antler velvet samples and considering the selectivity, linearity, precision, and accuracy. The fragmentation pattern of CML and CEL indicated two major product ions at m/z 84 and 130, with the most intense peak at m/z 130. The two sample ions were used for quantitation in MRM mode.

As shown in Table 1, the correlation coefficients (R^2) were both greater than 0.99. The linear range (20–3500 ng/mL) was sufficiently wide to assess the CML and CEL contents in the present antler velvet samples. The limit of detection (LOD) and limit of quantitation (LOQ) were defined as the concentrations (ng/g) at which the signal-to-noise ratios of the peaks of interest were 3 and 10, respectively (Table 1).

Table 1. Calibration, sensitivity and recovery in UPLC-MS/MS.

Compound	Calibration		Sensitivity		Recovery		
	Range (ng/mL)	R^2	LOD (ng/g)	LOQ (ng/g)	30 (ng/mL)	300 (ng/mL)	3000 (ng/mL)
CML	20–3500	0.9997	1.3	4.1	95.21 ± 1.22	93.22 ± 1.13	97.42 ± 1.21
CEL	20–3500	0.9987	1.4	4.3	95.43 ± 1.09	93.22 ± 1.24	91.84 ± 1.18

The antler velvet samples were extracted in triplicate and analyzed by using the developed UPLC-MS/MS method. The relative standard deviations of intra-day precision for CML and CEL were 3.32% and 3.08%, respectively, and those of inter-day precision were 3.14% and 3.53%, respectively. The coefficients of variation obtained for the reproducibility tests described above were less than 5%. The recoveries of exogenous CML and CEL added to antler velvet samples were determined at three concentrations (low, intermediate, and high): 30, 300, and 3000 ng/mL, respectively. Recovery experiments were conducted five times for each concentration, affording values for CML and CEL of 93.22–97.42% and 91.84–95.43%, respectively.

2.4. CML and CEL Contents in Processed Antler Velvet

2.4.1. CML Contents in Different Sections of Antler Velvet with Different Processing Methods

The CML contents in different sections of antler velvet processed with different methods are shown in Table 2. The CML contents in freeze-dried and boiled antler velvet were 74.55–458.59 and 119.44–570.69 µg/g protein, respectively. The CML contents in antler velvet processed without blood and with blood were 75.36–234.92 and 117.11–456.01 µg/g protein, respectively. These results indicate that antler velvet protein is glycosylated, to a considerable extent, relative to other processed foods such as fried chicken breast (12.34–90.52 µg/g protein) and processed meat and fish (44.53–167.60 µg/g protein) [15,16,30].

The CML contents of freeze-dried antler velvet were significantly lower than those of the corresponding sections of boiled antler velvet ($P < 0.01$). This suggests that temperature can affect the formation of CML; specifically, high-temperature processing can produce more CML. The high content of CML in freeze-dried antler velvet is endogenous. The CML contents of antler velvet processed without blood were significantly lower than those of the corresponding sections of antler velvet processed with blood ($P < 0.01$). The reason may be that the antler velvet processed without blood was subjected to physical centrifugal discharge of the blood. Blood contains many reducing sugars, amino acids, and proteins that can react to generate CML during processing.

Table 2. CML contents in different sections of antler velvet with different processing methods expressed per μg/g protein, μg/g, and μmol/mmol lysine.

Processing Methods	Sections	μg CML/g Protein [a]	μmol CML/mmol Lysine [b]	μg CML/g
freeze-dried	wax slices	458.59 ± 22.04	4.00 ± 1.23	328.15 ± 20.13
	powder slices	159.70 ± 11.67	1.71 ± 0.92	94.70 ± 8.72
	gauze slices	97.59 ± 9.22	0.98 ± 0.45	51.47 ± 5.33
	bone slices	74.55 ± 8.94	0.79 ± 0.33	37.51 ± 4.25
	entire	120.93 ± 10.28	1.14 ± 0.72	64.21 ± 6.56
boiled	wax slices	570.69 ± 34.74	6.07 ± 2.82	480.87 ± 31.22
	powder slices	198.64 ± 13.56	2.23 ± 1.42	122.21 ± 9.96
	gauze slices	130.24 ± 10.25	1.38 ± 0.72	71.01 ± 8.23
	bone slices	119.44 ± 10.12	1.18 ± 0.69	51.87 ± 6.09
	entire	141.41 ± 15.23	1.40 ± 0.71	80.09 ± 7.89
processed without blood	wax slices	234.92 ± 23.03	2.58 ± 1.44	200.25 ± 18.27
	powder slices	101.14 ± 12.31	1.59 ± 0.89	89.07 ± 8.93
	gauze slices	99.26 ± 9.18	1.11 ± 0.74	58.46 ± 6.04
	bone slices	75.36 ± 8.56	0.78 ± 0.41	39.13 ± 4.02
	entire	103.14 ± 9.88	1.29 ± 0.82	54.26 ± 5.78
processed with blood	wax slices	456.01 ± 24.32	5.16 ± 2.56	407.88 ± 30.42
	powder slices	167.70 ± 11.82	1.96 ± 0.98	86.79 ± 9.51
	gauze slices	129.02 ± 9.23	1.44 ± 0.74	62.94 ± 7.89
	bone slices	117.11 ± 11.23	1.19 ± 0.70	57.64 ± 6.33
	entire	124.73 ± 12.51	1.30 ± 0.83	73.30 ± 7.88

[a] Data were calculated using the protein contents quantified by combustion method. [b] Data were calculated using the amino acid concentration in the acid hydrolysates, quantified by amino acid analyze.

Wax pieces had the highest CML content, and bone pieces had the lowest. The differentiation capacity was faster closer to the top of the antler velvet; therefore, higher contents of reducing sugars, proteins, and amino acids may exist in the antler velvet to produce CML. Closer to the bottom of the antler velvet, the degree of ossification is higher; therefore, the reducing sugar, protein, and amino acid contents are lower and produce less CML.

In summary, by comparing the CML contents from different sections of antler velvet after different processing methods, the CML contents of freeze-dried antler velvet and antler velvet processed without blood were found to be lower than those of the corresponding areas of boiled antler velvet and antler velvet processed with blood; wax pieces were more likely to produce CML than other sections.

2.4.2. CEL Contents in Different Sections of Antler Velvet with Different Processing Methods

The CEL contents in different sections of antler velvet processed with different methods are shown in Table 3. The CEL contents in freeze-dried and boiled antler velvet were 0.74–12.66 and 11.33–35.93 μg/g protein, respectively. The CEL contents in antler velvet processed without blood and with blood were 0–6.75 and 0–23.41 μg/g protein, respectively. The results indicate that the CEL contents in antler velvet are similar to those in other processed foods such as bread [27].

Table 3. CEL contents in different sections of antler velvet with different processing methods, expressed per μg/g protein, μg/g, and μmol/mmol lysine.

Processing Methods	Sections	μg CEL/g Protein [a]	μmol CEL/mmol Lysine [b]	μg CEL/g
freeze-dried	wax slices	12.66 ± 1.33	0.11 ± 0.21	9.06 ± 1.12
	powder slices	10.99 ± 0.98	0.10 ± 0.14	6.28 ± 0.74
	gauze slices	1.83 ± 0.32	0.02 ± 0.07	0.96 ± 0.23
	bone slices	0.74 ± 0.12	0.01 ± 0.09	0.36 ± 0.11
	entire	10.84 ± 0.99	0.10 ± 0.11	6.17 ± 0.72
boiled	wax slices	35.93 ± 4.22	0.34 ± 0.23	29.19 ± 4.21
	powder slices	15.43 ± 2.01	0.15 ± 0.11	8.97 ± 1.05
	gauze slices	11.33 ± 1.23	0.13 ± 0.12	6.12 ± 0.72
	bone slices	12.70 ± 1.41	0.11 ± 0.09	6.49 ± 0.78
	entire	14.54 ± 1.47	0.14 ± 0.14	8.87 ± 1.22
processed without blood	wax slices	6.57 ± 0.74	0.06 ± 0.10	5.24 ± 0.56
	powder slices	—	—	—
	gauze slices	—	—	—
	bone slices	—	—	—
	entire	2.57 ± 0.33	0.03 ± 0.06	1.45 ± 0.21
processed with blood	wax slices	23.41 ± 3.01	0.23 ± 0.18	19.22 ± 2.53
	powder slices	2.24 ± 0.22	0.02 ± 0.06	1.37 ± 0.16
	gauze slices	0.03 ± 0.11	0.01 ± 0.04	0.02 ± 0.09
	bone slices	—	—	—
	entire	7.97 ± 0.92	0.08 ± 0.15	4.72 ± 0.52

[a] Data were calculated using the protein contents quantified by combustion method. [b] Data were calculated using the amino acid concentration in the acid hydrolysates, quantified by amino acid analyzer. — Indicates not detected.

In general, the variation tendency for CEL in different sections of antler velvet after different processing methods was similar to that for CML, despite the CEL contents of antler velvet being lower than the CML contents or undetected. The CEL contents in freeze-dried antler velvet were significantly lower than those in the corresponding sections of boiled antler velvet ($P < 0.01$); the CEL contents of antler velvet processed without blood were significantly lower than those of the corresponding sections of antler velvet processed with blood ($P < 0.01$). Wax pieces had the highest content of CEL, and bone pieces had the lowest. As described above for CML, the differences in temperature and contents of proteins, amino acids, and reducing sugars are the main reasons for the different CEL contents after different processing methods.

2.5. Protein and Lysine Contents in Processed Antler Velvet

The CML and CEL in antler velvet exist in the combined state and the free form, among which the combined state is the most common. The CML and CEL contents and protein contents of samples are closely related in the combined state [23]. Therefore, the CML and CEL contents can be expressed in units of protein. The Dumas combustion method was used to determine the protein contents in different sections of antler velvet after different types of processing; the results are shown in Table 4.

Table 4. Protein contents in different sections of antler velvet with different processing methods which were determined by combustion method.

Processing Methods	Sections	Protein Contents		Processing Methods	Sections	Protein Contents	
		Content (%)	Coefficient of Variation (%)			Content (%)	Coefficient of Variation (%)
freeze-dried	wax slices	81.56 ± 0.04	0.27	processed without blood	wax slices	79.81 ± 0.09	0.32
	powder slices	57.12 ± 0.03	0.25		powder slices	56.69 ± 0.11	0.28
	gauze slices	52.74 ± 0.10	0.78		gauze slices	58.88 ± 0.31	0.41
	bone slices	49.03 ± 0.25	0.22		bone slices	54.11 ± 0.24	0.33
	entire	56.93 ± 0.34	0.41		entire	56.43 ± 0.28	0.21
boiled	wax slices	81.25 ± 0.12	0.17	processed with blood	wax slices	82.09 ± 0.74	0.56
	powder slices	58.11 ± 0.18	0.14		powder slices	61.49 ± 0.33	0.42
	gauze slices	53.99 ± 0.33	0.21		gauze slices	61.45 ± 0.41	0.38
	bone slices	51.13 ± 0.25	0.25		bone slices	49.65 ± 0.56	0.52
	entire	60.99 ± 0.44	0.33		entire	59.25 ± 0.35	0.41

It was found that there was no significant difference ($P > 0.05$) in protein content between the same sections of freeze-dried and boiled antler velvet. Additionally, sections of antler velvet processed with blood had significantly higher protein contents than those processed without blood ($P < 0.05$), because the blood, which contains protein, had been retained during the processing.

The protein contents were different among the different sections. Wax pieces had significantly higher contents of protein than the other sections ($P < 0.01$). The reason may be that wax pieces from the antler tip had more meristem tissue, which promotes the expression of protein [20]. Protein is the Maillard reaction substrate, and its distribution in different sections of antler velvet subjected to different processing methods is a leading factor for the differences in the CML and CEL contents, consistent with the results in Section 2.4.

An automatic amino acid analyzer was used to determine the lysine contents in different sections of antler velvet processed differently; the results are shown in Table 5.

Table 5. Lysine contents in different sections of antler velvet with different processing methods which were determined by amino acid automatic analyzer.

Sample		Lysine Contents g/100 g	Sample		Lysine Contents g/100 g
Processing Methods	Sections		Processing Methods	Sections	
freeze-dried	wax slices	5.87 ± 0.20	processed without blood	wax slices	5.56 ± 0.11
	powder slices	3.96 ± 0.11		powder slices	4.01 ± 0.09
	gauze slices	3.76 ± 0.03		gauze slices	3.76 ± 0.11
	bone slices	3.41 ± 0.09		bone slices	3.58 ± 0.08
	entire	4.02 ± 0.12		entire	3.01 ± 0.15
boiled	wax slices	5.67 ± 0.22	processed with blood	wax slices	5.66 ± 0.12
	powder slices	3.92 ± 0.14		powder slices	4.86 ± 0.07
	gauze slices	3.69 ± 0.10		gauze slices	4.21 ± 0.02
	bone slices	3.15 ± 0.13		bone slices	3.48 ± 0.11
	entire	4.09 ± 0.17		entire	4.03 ± 0.14

No significant differences were observed in the lysine contents between the same sections of antler velvet processed with different methods ($P > 0.05$). The lysine contents in different sections of antler velvet were different. Wax slices had significantly higher lysine contents than the other sections ($P < 0.01$), and there was no significant difference among powder, gauze, and bone slices ($P > 0.05$). CML and CEL are two lysine derivatives; the contents of lysine can reflect the degree of reaction of different samples. The results are roughly consistent with the results for CML and CEL contents discussed in Section 2.4.

2.6. Factors Influencing CML and CEL Contents in Differently Processed Antler Velvets

The differences in CML and CEL contents in different sections of antler velvet with different processing methods are caused by different degrees of the Maillard reaction. Factors that affect the Maillard reaction include the processing temperature and the contents of reducing sugars, unsaturated fatty acids, amino acids, and protein [17,18,31]. In addition, vitamins and inorganic ions in food can inhibit or promote the Maillard reaction [32].

The study determined the contents of CML and CEL in different sections of antler velvet with different processing methods and found that antler velvet boiled at high temperature produced more CML and CEL than that freeze-dried at low temperature: high temperatures exacerbate the Maillard reaction and cause boiled antler velvet to produce more CML and CEL. The lysine and protein contents were different in different sections of antler velvet after different processing methods. Lysine and proteins are substrates for the Maillard reaction; therefore, their concentration determines the extent of the Maillard reaction. Relative to antler velvet processed without blood, antler velvet processed with blood, which is rich in lysine and protein, may produce more CML and CEL. Similarly, wax pieces rich in lysine and protein are more likely to produce CML and CEL than other sections.

According to the literature [32], the contents of vitamins and inorganic ions in food, such as vitamin B, vitamin C, and calcium, magnesium, and ferric ions, can affect the Maillard reaction and inhibit or promote the production of AGEs. Among these factors, vitamin B, vitamin C, calcium ions, and magnesium ions can inhibit the Maillard reaction, especially magnesium ions; ferric ions can promote the occurrence of this reaction. Therefore, the contents of vitamins and inorganic ions in different sections of antler velvet after different processing methods can also affect the CML and CEL contents.

To summarize, the differences in CML and CEL contents in different sections of antler velvet after different processing methods are the result of the combined action of lysine, proteins, vitamins, and inorganic ions at different temperatures.

3. Materials and Methods

3.1. Materials

CML, CEL, and trifluoroacetic acid (TFA) were purchased from Sigma-Aldrich (San Francisco, CA, USA). The purities of these standards were above 99%. Lysine, ninhydrin (NIN), and a citric acid buffer solution were purchased from Hitachi Inc. (Hitachi Co., Osaka, Japan). Acetonitrile, HPLC-grade, was purchased from Fisher-Scientific (Waltham, MA, USA). C_{18} Sep-Pak® SPE tubes were purchased from Sepax (Sepax technology, Cork, Ireland). Ultrapure water was obtained by using a super-pure water system (Water Purifier Co. Ltd., Chengdu, China). All other reagents were of analytical grade and were purchased from Sinopharm Chemical Reagent Co. Ltd (Beijing, China).

3.2. Sources and Preparation of Antler Velvet

Antler velvet (*Cervi Cornu Pantotrichum*) was collected in Shuangyang, Jilin Province, China, and identified by Dr. C.Y. Li from the Chinese Academy of Agricultural Sciences Institute of Special Animal and Plant Sciences.

3.3. Preparation of Processed Antler Velvet

In accord with the classification of commercially available antler velvet, boiling, freeze-drying, processing with blood, and processing without blood were chosen for this study. Six pairs of antler velvet samples were randomly selected and processed with blood or without blood for comparison, and another six pairs were randomly selected and processed by boiling or freeze-drying for comparison. Antler velvet was boiled for 1 min in boiled water, followed by high-temperature (75 °C) baking for multiple 2 h cycles until dry. During the freeze-drying process, the antler velvet was directly frozen to dryness. For the boiling process without blood, the antler velvet was prepared by removing the blood by centrifugation, whereas no blood removal was performed for the samples processed with blood.

3.4. Preparation of Antler Velvet Slices

Three pairs of antler velvet samples with blood and without blood were randomly selected for analysis, and three pairs of boiled and freeze-dried antler velvet were crushed whole. The remaining six pairs of antler velvet were divided into wax slices, powder slices, gauze slices, and bone slices based on morphological and microscopic characteristics (Figure 2) [20]; these samples were segmented, sliced, crushed, sieved, bagged, and labeled.

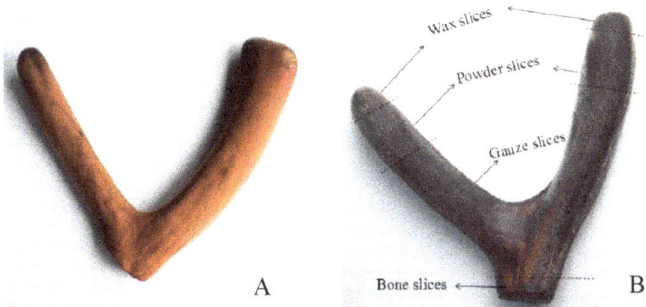

Figure 2. Schematic diagram of fresh antler velvet (**A**) and different sections of processed antler velvet (**B**). The processed antler velvet has a significant Maillard reaction browning compared to the fresh antler velvet. The processed antler velvet was divided into wax slices, powder slices, gauze slices, and bone slices based on morphological and microscopic characteristics.

3.5. Protein Content Analysis

The protein contents in antler velvet samples prepared by different processing methods and from different sections were determined on a Dumas nitrogen analyzer (Velp NDA 701-Monza, Brianza, Italy), according to a previous method with minor modifications [33]. The total nitrogen content was converted into the protein content by using a conversion factor of 6.25. The operating conditions of the NDA instrument were: O_2 gas at 400 mL/min, He gas at 195 mL/min, combustion reactor at 1030 °C, reduction reactor at 650 °C, and pressure at 88.1 kPa.

3.6. Lysine Content Analysis

An amino acid analyzer (L-8900 System; Hitachi Co., Osaka, Japan) equipped with a visible detector was used for amino acid analysis. Analytical 2622# (4.6 mm × 60 mm) and guard 2650# (4.6 mm × 40 mm) columns were used for amino acid determination. Immediately after sample injection into the columns, an auto-sampler was used for inline derivatization by NIN post-column derivatization. The NIN-derivatized lysine were detected at 570 nm. Lysine standards (Hitachi Co., Osaka, Japan) were used for identification and quantification (external standard method). Lysine content was expressed as g/100 g of antler velvet for the different processing methods and different sections of the antler velvet.

3.7. Preparation of Samples

The method of reference was slightly modified in this work [16,27]. Samples of 30 mg of antler velvet (equivalent to 20 mg of protein) were defatted twice by using n-hexane (5 mL) before being reduced for 12 h at 4 °C in 0.5 M sodium borate buffer (pH 9.2, 1 mL) and 2 M sodium borohydride (0.1 M sodium hydroxide, 0.5 mL). The proteins were isolated by using a chloroform:methanol mixture

(2:1 *v/v*, 1 mL), and the precipitates were mixed with 15 mL of 6 M hydrochloric acid and incubated at 110 °C for 24 h. The diluted acid hydrolysate (equivalent to approximately 600 µg of protein) was dried with a gas-blowing concentrator (Hengao, Tianjin, China) at 70 °C. The dried hydrolysate was dissolved in 1 mL ultra-pure water and then solid-phase extracted by using a C_{18} Sep-Pak® (Sepax Technology, Cork, Ireland) cartridge (500 mg, 6 mL). The solid-phase extraction (SPE) column was pretreated with 3 mL of methanol and 3 mL of 0.1 M TFA at a flow rate of 1 mL/min. The sample was loaded into the pretreated SPE column at a flow rate of 0.5 mL/min and washed with 6 mL of 0.1 M TFA. Finally, the sample was eluted with 3 mL of methanol at a flow rate of 0.5 mL/min. The eluate was dried by freezing, re-dissolved in 1 mL of ultra-pure water, filtered through a 0.22-µm membrane, and stored at −20 °C prior to UPLC-MS/MS analysis.

3.8. UPLC-MS/MS Analysis

CML and CEL concentrations in the hydrolysates were determined by UPLC-MS/MS. Protein hydrolysates (2 µg protein, 3 µL) were injected into a WATERS CORTECS HILIC UPLC column (2.1 mm × 50 mm, 1.6 µm; Waters, Cork, Ireland) housed in a column oven at 40 °C and operated in gradient-elution mode. Solvent A was water and solvent B was acetonitrile. Gradient elution was started at 100% solvent B for 1 min; this was followed by a linear gradient from 100% to 60% solvent B in 1.5 min, holding at 60% solvent B for 1.5 min, and then returning to 100% solvent B in 2 min. The analysis was performed by using a Waters Acquity UPLC instrument (Waters, Manchester, UK) coupled to a triple quadrupole MS operating in multiple reaction monitoring (MRM) mode. The flow rate was 0.3 mL/min. The MS instrument was operated in electrospray ionization positive mode. The optimized MRM conditions are shown in Table 6. CML and CEL were quantified by using standards and by reference to an external standard calibration curve. Data are reported as means ± standard deviation of triplicate experiments. CML and CEL contents in the samples are expressed as µmol/mmol lysine, µg/g protein, and µg/g sample.

Table 6. UPLC-MS settings for multiple reaction monitoring (MRM).

Compound	Precursor Ion (*m/z*)	Product Ion (*m/z*)	Cone Voltage (V)	Collision Energy (*ev*)	Dwell Time (*ms*)
CML	205	130	25	15	36
	205	84	25	25	36
CEL	219	130	25	15	36
	219	84	25	25	36

4. Conclusions

The CML and CEL contents in different sections of antler velvet subjected to different processing methods have been simultaneously determined for the first time. The CML contents of antler velvet after freeze-drying, boiling, processing without blood, and processing with blood were 74.55–458.59, 119.44–570.69, 75.36–234.92, and 117.11–456.01 µg/g protein, respectively; the corresponding CEL contents were 0.74–12.66, 11.33–35.93, 0.00–6.75, and 0.00–23.41 µg/g protein. The CML and CEL contents in the same sections of boiled antler velvet were significantly higher than those in freeze-dried antler velvet; high temperatures exacerbate the Maillard reaction, leading to boiled antler velvet producing more CML and CEL. Antler velvet processed with blood had obviously higher CML and CEL contents than antler velvet processed without blood; the antler velvet processed without blood was subjected to physical centrifugal discharge of the blood and therefore contains fewer substrates that can react to generate CML and CEL.

With the same processing methods, the CML and CEL contents were different in different sections of the antler velvet. Wax pieces had significantly higher CML and CEL contents than the types of antler velvet. Closer to the top of the antler velvet, there is a more rapid differentiation capacity and more substrates exist in the antler velvet to produce CML and CEL. Closer to the bottom of the antler velvet, there is a higher degree of ossification and fewer substrates so less CML and CEL is produced.

Through the detection and comparison of CML, CEL, lysine, and protein contents in antler velvet after different processing methods and from various sections, it was found that the different contents of CML and CEL in antler velvet samples are the result of the interaction of protein and lysine at different temperatures.

Author Contributions: Data curation, R.-z.G. and B.C.; Funding acquisition, Y.-s.S.; Methodology, Y.-f.W. (Yu-fang Wang); Resources, Y.-s.S.; Software, Y.-f.W (Yu-fang Wang). and B.C.; Validation, Y.-h.W. (Yan-hua Wang); Writing—original draft, R.-z.G. and K.G.; Writing—review and editing, R.-z.G., K.G. and Y.-s.S.

Funding: This work was financially supported by the Jilin Province Science and Technology Development Project (20170309002YY, 20170311027YY, and 20180201076YY), the Science and Technology Innovation Project of Chinese Academy of Agricultural Sciences (CAAS-ASTIP-2016-ISAPS) and the National Key Research and Development Program of China (2018YFC1706604 and 2018YFC1706605).

Conflicts of Interest: The authors declare no conflict of interest.

References

1. Jeon, B.; Kim, S.; Lee, S.; Park, P.; Sung, S.; Kim, J.; Moon, S. Effect of antler growth period on the chemical composition of velvet antler in sika deer (*Cervus nippon*). *Z. Saugetierkd.* **2009**, *74*, 374–380. [CrossRef]
2. Wu, F.; Li, H.; Jin, L.; Li, X.; Ma, Y.; You, J.; Li, S.; Xu, Y. Deer antler base as a traditional Chinese medicine: A review of its traditional uses, chemistry and pharmacology. *J. Ethnopharmacol.* **2013**, *145*, 403–415. [CrossRef] [PubMed]
3. Zhou, R.; Li, S. In vitro antioxidant analysis and characterisation of antler velvet extract. *Food Chem.* **2009**, *114*, 1321–1327. [CrossRef]
4. Sui, Z.; Yuan, H.; Liang, Z.; Zhao, Q.; Wu, Q.; Xia, S.; Zhang, L.; Huo, Y.; Zhang, Y. An activity-maintaining sequential protein extraction method for bioactive assay and proteome analysis of velvet antlers. *Talanta* **2013**, *107*, 189–994. [CrossRef] [PubMed]
5. Sui, Z.; Zhang, L.; Huo, Y.; Zhang, Y. Bioactive components of velvet antlers and their pharmacological properties. *J. Pharm. Biomed.* **2014**, *87*, 229–240. [CrossRef] [PubMed]
6. Tseng, S.H.; Sung, C.H.; Chen, L.G.; Lai, Y.J.; Chang, W.S.; Sung, H.C.; Wang, C.C. Comparison of chemical compositions and osteoprotective effects of different sections of velvet antler. *J. Ethnopharmacol.* **2014**, *151*, 352–360. [CrossRef] [PubMed]
7. Singh, R.; Barden, A.; Mori, T.; Beilin, L. Advanced glycation end-products: A review. *Diabetologia* **2001**, *2001*, 129–146. [CrossRef] [PubMed]
8. Vlassara, H.; Palace, M.R. Glycoxidation: The menace of diabetes and aging. *Mt Sinai J. Med.* **2003**, *70*, 232–241. [PubMed]
9. Drenth, H.; Zuidema, S.U.; Krijnen, W.P.; Bautmans, I.; van der Schans, C.; Hobbelen, H. Advanced glycation end-products are associated with the presence and severity of paratonia in early stage alzheimer disease. *J. Am. Med. Dir. Assoc.* **2017**, *18*, 636.e7–636.e12. [CrossRef] [PubMed]
10. de Vos, L.C.; Lefrandt, J.D.; Dullaart, R.P.; Zeebregts, C.J.; Smit, A.J. Advanced glycation end products: An emerging biomarker for adverse outcome in patients with peripheral artery disease. *Atherosclerosis* **2016**, *254*, 291–299. [CrossRef]
11. Henle, T. AGEs in foods: Do they play a role in uremia? *Kidney Int.* **2003**, *63*, S145–S147. [CrossRef] [PubMed]
12. Reynaert, N.L.; Gopal, P.; Rutten, E.P.; Wouters, E.F.; Schalkwijk, C.G. Advanced glycation end products and their receptor in age-related, non-communicable chronic inflammatory diseases; Overview of clinical evidence and potential contributions to disease. *Int. J. Biochem. Cell B.* **2016**, *81*, 403–418. [CrossRef] [PubMed]
13. Uribarri, J.; Woodruff, S.; Goodman, S.; Cai, W.; Chen, X.; Pyzik, R.; Yong, A.; Striker, G.E.; Vlassara, H. Advanced glycation end products in foods and a practical guide to their reduction in the diet. *J. Am. Diet. Assoc.* **2010**, *110*, 911–916. [CrossRef]
14. Troise, A.D.; Fiore, A.; Wiltafsky, M.; Fogliano, V. Quantification of N^{ε}-(2-Furoylmethyl)-L-lysine (furosine), N^{ε}-(Carboxymethyl)-L-lysine(CML), N^{ε}-(Carboxyethyl)-L-lysine(CEL) and total lysine through stable isotope dilution assay and tandem mass spectrometry. *Food Chem.* **2015**, *188*, 357–364. [CrossRef]

15. Goldberg, T.; Cai, W.; Peppa, M.; Dardaine, V.; Baliga, B.S.; Uribarri, J.; Vlassara, H. Advanced glycoxidation end products in commonly consumed foods. *J. Am. Diet. Assoc.* **2004**, *104*, 1287–1291. [CrossRef]
16. Hull, G.L.J.; Woodside, J.V.; Ames, J.M.; Cuskelly, G.J. N^ε-(carboxymethyl)lysine content of foods commonly consumed in a Western style diet. *Food Chem.* **2012**, *131*, 170–174. [CrossRef]
17. Trevisan, A.J.; de Almeida Lima, D.; Sampaio, G.R.; Soares, R.A.; Markowicz Bastos, D.H. Influence of home cooking conditions on Maillard reaction products in beef. *Food Chem.* **2016**, *196*, 161–169. [CrossRef] [PubMed]
18. Jiao, Y.; He, J.; Li, F.; Tao, G.; Zhang, S.; Zhang, S.; Qin, F.; Zeng, M.; Chen, J. N^ε-(carboxymethyl)lysine and N^ε-(carboxyethyl)lysine in tea and the factors affecting their formation. *Food Chem.* **2017**, *232*, 683–688. [CrossRef] [PubMed]
19. Lu, C.; Wang, M.; Mu, J.; Han, D.; Bai, Y.; Zhang, H. Simultaneous determination of eighteen steroid hormones in antler velvet by gas chromatography-tandem mass spectrometry. *Food Chem.* **2013**, *141*, 1796–1806. [CrossRef] [PubMed]
20. Li, C.; Zhao, H.; Liu, Z.; McMahon, C. Deer antler—A novel model for studying organ regeneration in mammals. *Int. J. Biochem. Cell B.* **2014**, *56*, 111–122. [CrossRef]
21. Vay, D.; Vidali, M.; Allochis, G.; Cusaro, C.; Rolla, R.; Mottaran, E.; Bellomo, G.; Albano, E. Antibodies against advanced glycation end product N^ε-(carboxymethyl)lysine in healthy controls and diabetic patients. *Diabetologia* **2000**, *43*, 1385–1388. [CrossRef] [PubMed]
22. Dittrich, R.; Hoffmann, I.; Stahl, P.; Müller, A.; Beckmann, M.W.; Pischetsrieder, M. Concentrations of N^ε-Carboxymethyllysine in human breast milk, infant formulas, and urine of infants. *J. Agr. Food Chem.* **2006**, *54*, 6924–6928. [CrossRef] [PubMed]
23. Tareke, E.; Forslund, A.; Lindh, C.H.; Fahlgren, C.; Östman, E. Isotope dilution ESI-LC-MS/MS for quantification of free and total N^ε-(1-Carboxymethyl)-L-Lysine and free N^ε-(1-Carboxyethyl)-L-Lysine: Comparison of total N^ε-(1-Carboxymethyl)-L-Lysine levels measured with new method to ELISA assay in gruel samples. *Food Chem.* **2013**, *141*, 4253–4259.
24. Naila, A.; Argirov, O.K.; Minhas, H.S.; Cordeiro, C.A.A.; Thornalley, P.J. 5. Assay of advanced glycation endproducts (AGEs): Surveying AGEs by chromatographic assay with derivatization by 6-aminoquinolyl-N-hydroxysuccinimidyl-carbamate and application to N^ε-carboxymethyl-lysine and N^ε-(1-carboxyethyl)lysine-modified al. *Biochem. J.* **2002**, *364*, 1–14.
25. Charissou, A.; Ait-Ameur, L.; Birlouez-Aragon, I. Evaluation of a gas chromatography-mass spectrometry method for the quantification of carboxymethyllysine in food samples. *J. Chromatogr. A* **2007**, *1140*, 189–194. [CrossRef] [PubMed]
26. Petrovic, R.; Futas, J.; Chandoga, J.; Jakus, V. Rapid and simple method for determination of N^ε-(carboxymethyl)lysine and N^ε-(carboxyethyl)lysine in urine using gas chromatography/mass spectrometry. *Biomed. Chromatogr.* **2010**, *19*, 649–654. [CrossRef]
27. He, J.; Zeng, M.; Zheng, Z.; He, Z.; Chen, J. Simultaneous determination of N^ε-(carboxymethyl) lysine and N^ε-(carboxyethyl) lysine in cereal foods by LC–MS/MS. *Eur. Food Res. Technol.* **2014**, *238*, 367–374. [CrossRef]
28. Assar, S.H.; Moloney, C.; Lima, M.; Magee, R.; Ames, J.M. Determination of N^ε-(carboxymethyl)lysine in food systems by ultra performance liquid chromatography-mass spectrometry. *Amino Acids.* **2009**, *2009*, 317–326. [CrossRef]
29. Schettgen, T.; Tings, A.; Brodowsky, C.; Müller-Lux, A.; Musiol, A.; Kraus, T. Simultaneous determination of the advanced glycation end product N^ε-carboxymethyllysine and its precursor, lysine, in exhaled breath condensate using isotope-dilution– hydrophilic-interaction liquid chromatography coupled to tandem mass spectrometry. *Anal. Bioanal. Chem.* **2007**, *387*, 2783–2791. [CrossRef]
30. Niquet-Léridon, C.; Tessier, F.J. Quantification of N^ε-carboxymethyl-lysine in selected chocolate-flavoured drink mixes using high-performance liquid chromatography–linear ion trap tandem mass spectrometry. *Food Chem.* **2011**, *126*, 655–663. [CrossRef]
31. Xu, X.B.; Ma, F.; Yu, S.J.; Guan, Y.G. Simultaneous analysis of N^ε-(carboxymethyl)lysine, reducing sugars, and lysine during the dairy thermal process. *J. Dairy Sci.* **2013**, *96*, 5487–5493. [CrossRef] [PubMed]

32. Voziyan, P.A.; Metz, T.O.; Baynes, J.W.; Hudson, B.G. A Post-Amadori Inhibitor Pyridoxamine Also Inhibits Chemical Modification of Proteins by Scavenging Carbonyl Intermediates of Carbohydrate and Lipid Degradation. *J. Biol. Chem.* **2002**, *277*, 3397–3403. [CrossRef] [PubMed]
33. Juhaimi, F.A.L.; Ghafoor, K.; Ozcan, M.M. Physical and chemical properties, antioxidant activity, total phenol and mineral profile of seeds of seven different date fruit (*Phoenix dactylifera* L.) varieties. *Int. J. Food Sci. Nutr.* **2012**, *63*, 84–89. [CrossRef] [PubMed]

Sample Availability: Samples of the compounds N^ε-(carboxymethyl) lysine, N^ε-(carboxyethyl) lysine and lysine are available from the authors.

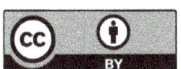

© 2018 by the authors. Licensee MDPI, Basel, Switzerland. This article is an open access article distributed under the terms and conditions of the Creative Commons Attribution (CC BY) license (http://creativecommons.org/licenses/by/4.0/).

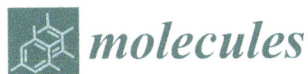

Communication

Phytochemical Constituents and the Evaluation Biological Effect of *Cinnamomum yabunikkei* H.Ohba Leaf

Seung-Yub Song [1], Seung-Hui Song [1], Min-Suk Bae [2] and Seung-Sik Cho [1,*]

1. Department of Pharmacy, College of Pharmacy, Mokpo National University, Muan, Jeonnam 58554, Korea; tgb1007@naver.com (S.-Y.S.); tmdgml7898@naver.com (S.-H.S.)
2. Department of Environmental Engineering, Mokpo National University, Muan, Jeonnam 58554, Korea; minsbae@hotmail.com
* Correspondence: sscho@mokpo.ac.kr; Tel.: +82-61-450-2687

Academic Editors: In-Soo Yoon and Hyun-Jong Cho
Received: 13 December 2018; Accepted: 24 December 2018; Published: 27 December 2018

Abstract: *Cinnamomum yabunikkei* H.Ohba leaf is known as a traditional medicinal material in Korea. However, no scientific identification of the components or efficacy of *C.yabunikkei* H.Ohba leaf has been reported. In the present study, we prepared various solvent extracts of *C.yabunikkei* H.Ohba leaf to understand its basic properties and evaluated the antioxidant, xanthine oxidase inhibitory, and elastase inhibitory activities of hexane, ethyl acetate, acetone, methanol, ethanol, and water extracts for the first time. The antioxidant properties were evaluated based on 1,1-diphenyl-2-picrylhydrazyl (DPPH) free radical scavenging activity, reducing power, and total phenolic contents. The hot water extract showed the highest DPPH radical scavenging activity and total phenolic contents, and the reducing power was the highest in the water extract. The hexane extract showed an excellent elastase inhibitory effect compared to control (phosphoramidone) and the highest xanthine oxidase inhibitory activity. These results present basic information for the possible uses of the hot water and hexane extracts from *C. yabunikkei* leaf for the treatment of diseases caused by oxidative imbalance. In the present study, individual extracts exhibited different effects. Therefore, it is hypothesized that the applicability of *C. yabunikkei* will depend on the extraction method and nature of the extract. The hot water and hexane extracts could be used as antioxidants, and as anti-gout and anti-wrinkle materials respectively. Several biologically active substances present in hexane extract of *C. yabunikkei* have been analyzed by GCMS and demonstrated to possess antioxidant and xanthine oxidase inhibitory activity. To the best of our knowledge, this is the first study that reports the chemical profiling and biological effects of various *C. yabunikkei* leaf extracts, suggesting their potential use in food therapy, cosmetics or alternative medicine.

Keywords: *Cinnamomum yabunikkei* leaf; antioxidant; xanthine oxidase; elastase

1. Introduction

Cinnamomum yabunikkei H.Ohba is a species of camphor tree native to the southern coast and Jeju Island in South Korea and can be seen in southern China and Taiwan. Leaves have been used as a bath material or tea and berries as a source of oil. In addition, the bark has traditionally been used for the treatment of various diseases related to pain and blood circulation.

Due to the acceleration in global warming, the southern part of South Korea has experienced the cultivation of *C.yabunikkei* H.Ohba, hence studies dealing with the possibilities of using *C.yabunikkei* H.Ohba for various purposes are necessitated.

Until now, the components of the leaves of *C.yabunikkei* have not been identified and biological activity studies have not been conducted. To the best of our knowledge, this is the first report to understand the composition and biological activity of the *C.yabunikkei* leaf.

In the present study, various extracts of the *C.yabunikkei* leaf using hexane, ethyl acetate, acetone, ethanol, methanol, and hot water were prepared to determine the optimal extraction solvent with respect to biological activity and phytochemical profiles. Gas chromatography-mass spectrometry (GC-MS) was used for the chemical profiling of hexane extracts. Subsequently, antioxidant, xanthine oxidase inhibitory, and elastase inhibitory activity of the leaf extracts were examined. The antioxidant activity was confirmed by measuring 1,1-diphenyl-2-picrylhydrazyl (DPPH) radical scavenging activity, reducing power, and reducing total phenolic contents.

2. Results and Discussion

2.1. Antioxidant Activity and Total Phenolic Contents of C.yabunikkei Extracts

The antioxidant potential of various extracts of the *C.yabunikkei* leaf was determined by measuring 2,2-diphenyl-1-picrylhydrazyl (DPPH) scavenging activity, reducing power assay and reducing total phenolics. The DPPH scavenging assay is a fast and easy method for evaluating the free radical scavenging capacity of given samples. The antioxidant effects of extracts are generally related to the phenolic contents, and phenolic-rich sources of phytochemicals with antioxidant activity have curative benefits against conditions such as inflammation, oxidative stress, and other metabolic diseases [1]. The antioxidative properties of the test plant extracts were closely correlated with the composition of active compounds such as phenolics.

Therefore, we compared the phenolic contents (mg/g as gallic acid) of various *C.yabunikkei* leaf extracts. The DPPH radicalscavenging activity is shown in Figure 1. The hot water, methanol, and ethanol extracts showed the highest DPPH radical scavenging activity (81.4 ± 0.8%, 80.6 ± 2.1%, 82.89 ± 3.1%) at the concentration of 0.5 mg/mL. Ascorbic acid (Vit C, 20 µg/mL) was used as positive control.

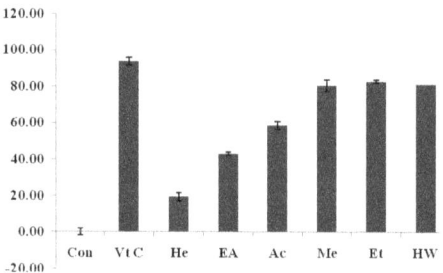

Figure 1. DPPH scavenging activity of solvent extracts of *C.yabunikkei* leaf (extract cont: 0.5 mg/mL, Ascorbic acid: 20 µg/mL). The asterisk represents a value significantly different from the other groups ($p < 0.05$). Values were the mean ± standard deviation (n = 3) Vt C; ascorbic acid, He; hexane ex, EA; ethylacetate ez, Ac; acetone ex, Me; methanol ex, Et; ethanol ex, HW; hot water ex.

The reducing power assay is useful for evaluating the antioxidant activity. In the present study, the reductive capability of extract samples was tested by measuring the reduction of Fe^{3+}. The hot water extract exhibited the highest activity compared to the other extracts (Table 1). The reductive activity expressed as vitamin C equivalents was 3.27 ± 0.052 µg/100 µg as the extract.

The total phenolic content was determined by Folin–Ciocalteu method [1], and the data was reported as gallic acid equivalents by referencing the standard curve ($r^2 > 0.999$), as shown in Table 1. The phenolic content of the hot water extract was higher than that of the other extracts (16.39 ± 0.28 mg/g as gallic acid equivalents). Taken together, the results indicate that the DPPH radical scavenging activity, power reduction, and phenolic contents reduction were significantly higher in the hot water extract as compared to other extracts.

Table 1. Reducing power and total phenolic contents of *C.yabunikkei* leaf extracts.

Extract	Reducing Power (Ascorbic Acid eq. µg/100 µg Extract)	Total Phenolic Content (Gallic Acid eq. mg/g)
He	0.25 ± 0.002	0.06 ± 0.00
EA	0.55 ± 0.003	0.98 ± 0.00
Ace	1.28 ± 0.018	6.18 ± 0.19
Me	2.73 ± 0.068	9.24 ± 0.17
Et	2.05 ± 0.034	13.89 ± 0.45
HW	3.27 ± 0.052	16.39 ± 0.28

2.2. Xanthine Oxidase Inhibitory Activity of C.yabunikkei Leaf Extracts

The effect of various solvent extracts on the xanthine oxidase inhibitory activity of the *C.yabunikkei* leaf is shown in Figure 2. Allopurinol (ALP, positive control) at a concentration of 50 µg/mL significantly inhibited xanthine oxidase activity (94.54%). The xanthine oxidase inhibitory activity of the hexane extract was significantly higher than other extracts at the concentration of 1 mg/mL (19.93%). Previously, we reported four different botanical extracts as potential xanthine oxidase inhibitors [2]. Yoon et al. [3,4] reported that the optimized extracts of *Corylopsis coreana* and *Camellia japonica* inhibited xanthine oxidase activity by approximately 50% at a concentration of 2 mg/mL. Additionally, Yoon et al. [2] demonstrated that Quercus acuta extract showed approximately 50% xanthine oxidase inhibitory activity at a concentration of 1 mg/mL. *Cudrania tricuspidata* extract inhibited xanthine oxidase by approximately 75% at a concentration of 2 mg/mL [5]. Previously, we have screened four kinds of xanthine oxidase inhibiting sources in five hundred Korean plant extracts (data not shown). The activities of hexane extract were similar to the extracts of *Corylopsis coreana* and *Camellia japonica*, but about 2.5 times lower than Quercus acuta extract and about 1.8 times lower than *Cudrania tricuspidata* extract. The plant extracts with XO inhibitory activity at 1 and 2 mg/mL demonstrated consistent effects in the in vivo animal disease model. Thus, it is plausible that the hexane extract of *C.yabunikkei* leaves could be developed as a candidate anti-hyperuricemic agent.

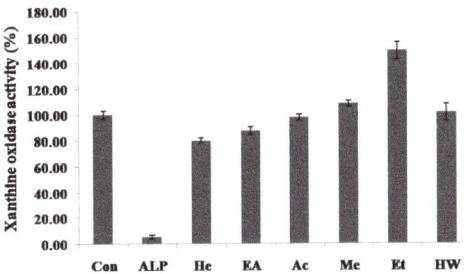

Figure 2. Xanthine oxidase inhibitory activities in various solvent extracts of *C.yabunikkei* leaves (1 mg/mL) and allopurinol (ALP, 50 µg/mL). ALP; allopurinol, He; hexane, EA; ethylacetate, Ac; acetone, Me; methanol, Et; ethanol, HW; hot water extract. Values were the mean ± standard deviation ($n = 3$).

2.3. Elastase Inhibitory Activity of C.yabunikkei Leaf Extracts

The effect of various solvent extracts on the elastase inhibitory activity of *C.yabunikkei* leaf is shown in Figure 3. Phosphoramidon (PPRM, positive control) at a concentration of 0.5 mg/mL significantly inhibited elastase activity (56.12 ± 1.53%). The elastase inhibitory activity of the hexane extract was significantly higher than other extracts and positive control at the concentration of 0.5 mg/mL (75.65 ± 3.5%).

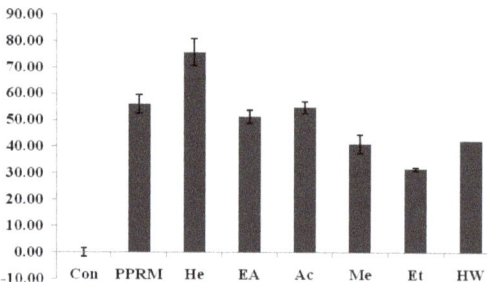

Figure 3. Elastase inhibitory activities in various solvent extracts of *C.yabunikkei* leaves (0.5 mg/mL) and Phospharamidon (PPRM, 0.5 mg/mL), He; hexane, EA; ethylacetate, Ac; acetone, Me; methanol, Et; ethanol, HW; hot water extract. Values were the mean ± standard deviation (n = 3).

2.4. Identification of Some Active Constituents

In the present study, several candidates of extracts of *C.yabunikkei* were analyzed and it was confirmed that several compounds' were present as common constituents inthe *C.yabunikkei* leaves. This finding is of significance in the use of the plant for industrial purposes.

None of the studies reported so far state the diverse activities and constituents of extracts of *C.yabunikkei* leaves. Thus, to the best of our knowledge, our present study is the first to report the optimization of the extraction process of pharmaceutically active indicators from *C.yabunikkei* leaves and the comparison of the antioxidant, xanthine oxidase inhibitory and elastase activities of various extracts.

GC-MS analyses were performed to identify the active constituents from *C.yabunikkei* leaf with antioxidant, xanthine oxidase inhibitory and elastase inhibitory activities. Typical GC-MS chromatograms of phytochemical contents and their retention times are shown in Table 2. Eight compounds [i.e., α-Linolenic acid (16.1%), Hexadecanoic acid (11.48%), Neophytadiene (2.05%), D-(−)-Fructofuranose (2.03%), α-Tocopherol (1.65%), Phytol (1.36%), β-Eudesmol (0.94%), Guaiol (0.86%), and D-(−)-Fructofuranose (0.68%)] were mainly identified by GC-MS analysis (Figure 4). As shown in Table 2, several components associated with antioxidant efficacy and xanthine oxidase inhibition were referenced. α-Linolenic acid and α-Tocopherol were typical substances with both antioxidant effect and xanthine oxidase inhibition. In Table 2, it is considered that the activity of hexane extract is due to the synergistic effect of various substances since a number of active substances are involved in the process of antioxidant and xanthine oxidase inhibition.

Table 2. Identified substances from the hexane extracts of *C.yabunikkei*.

RT (min)	Hit Name	Quality	M.W.	Composition (%)	Antioxidant Activity [reference]	Xanthine Oxidase Inhibition [reference]
19.681	Methyleugenol	95	178	0.34%		
22.885	Dodecanoic acid	99	272	0.27%		
23.251	Guaiol	91	294	0.86%	[6]	
24.001	β-Eudesmol	91	294	0.94%	[7]	
24.51	D-(−)-Fructofuranose (isomer 2)	91	540	2.03%	[8]	
24.59	D-(−)-Fructofuranose (isomer 1)	93	540	0.68%	[8]	
24.653	D-(−)-Fructopyranose (isomer 1)	93	540	0.65%		
24.956	Neophytadiene	97	278	2.05%	[9]	
25.048	Myristic acid	97	300	0.48%		
25.443	α-D-Mannopyranose	94	540	1.21%		
26.272	β-D-Glucopyranose	95	540	2.59%		
27.039	Hexadecanoic acid	99	328	11.48%	[10]	
27.811	Oleyl alcohol	99	340	0.22%		
27.937	Heptadecanoic acid	96	342	0.49%		
28.109	9(E),11(E)-Conjugated linoleic acid	99	308	0.59%		
28.189	Phytol	96	368	1.36%	[11]	
28.63	α-Linolenic acid	99	350	16.10%	[12]	[13]
28.819	Octadecanoic acid	99	356	1.07%	[14]	
31.605	1-Monopalmitin	93	474	0.26%		
33.03	Glycerol monostearate	95	502	0.70%		
35.982	α-Tocopherol	99	502	1.65%	[15]	[15]
37.298	Campesterol	99	472	0.67%		
38.449	β-Sitosterol	99	486	6.78%		

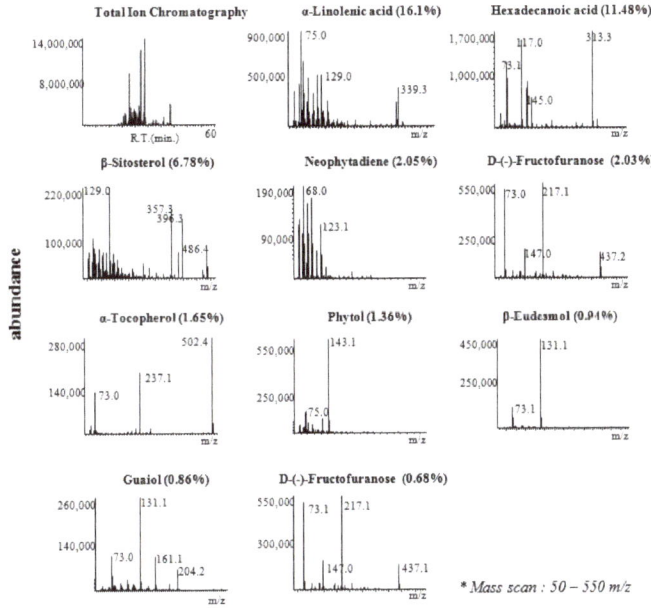

Figure 4. Representative GC-MS chromatogram of extracts of *C.yabunikkei* leaf.

3. Experimental Section

3.1. Plant Material and Extract Preparation

C.yabunikkei leaves were supplied by Wando Arboretum (Wando, Korea). A voucher specimen (MNUCSS-CY-01) was deposited at the Mokpo National University (Muan, Korea). Air-dried and powdered *C.yabunikkei* leaves (20 g) were subjected to extraction twice with hexane, ethyl acetate, acetone, ethanol, and methanol (100 mL) at room temperature for 48 h or subjected to extraction with hot water (100 °C) for 4 h. The resultant solution was evaporated, dried, and stored at −20 °C for further experiments.

3.2. DPPH Free Radical Assay

Antioxidant activity of the sample was determined following a 2,2-diphenyl-1-picrylhydrazyl (DPPH) radical scavenging assay. Briefly, sample solution (1 mL) containing 1 to 20 mg of sample was added to 0.4 mM DPPH sample solution (1 mL) and mixed. The mixture was allowed to react at room temperature in the dark for 10 min. Absorbance value at 517 nm was measured using a microplate reader (Perkin Elmer, Waltham, MA, USA). The DPPH free radical scavenging activities of samples were compared in terms of their IC_{50} (µg/mL) values [5].

3.3. Reducing Power

The reducing power of the sample was determined following a modified reducing power assay method. The sample (0.1 mL) was added to 0.2 M sodium phosphate buffer (0.5 mL) and 1% potassium ferricyanide (0.5 mL) followed by incubation at 50 °C for 20 min. Subsequently, 10% trichloroacetic acid solution (0.5 mL) was added to the reaction mixture followed by centrifugation at 12,000 rpm for 10 min. The supernatant was mixed with distilled water (0.5 mL) and 0.1% iron (III) chloride solution (0.1 mL). The absorbance value of the resulting solution was measured at 700 nm. Reducing powers of samples were expressed as vitamin C equivalents [5].

3.4. Determination of Total Phenolic Content

The total phenolic content was determined using Folin-Ciocalteu assay [5]. Sample (1 mL) containing 5 mg of sample or standard was mixed with 1 mL of 2% sodium carbonate solution and 1 mL of 10% Folin-Ciocalteu's phenol reagent. After incubating the mixture at room temperature for 10 min, the absorbance was measured at 750 nm using a microplate reader (Perkin Elmer, Waltham, MA, USA) and compared with the calibration curve of gallic acid. Results were expressed as milligrams of gallic acid equivalents per gram of sample [5].

3.5. Determination of Xanthine Oxidase Inhibitory Activity

Xanthine oxidase inhibitory activity was measured by monitoring uric acid formation in the xanthine oxidase system as described previously [5]. The assay system consisted of 0.6 mL phosphate buffer (100 mM; pH 7.4), 0.1 mL sample, 0.1 mL xanthine oxidase (0.2 U/mL), and 0.2 mL xanthine (1 mM; dissolved in 0.1 N NaOH). The reaction was initiated by adding the enzyme with or without inhibitors. A 0.2 mL aliquot of 1 N HCl was used to stop the enzymatic reaction. Allopurinol was used as a positive control. The absorbance of the reaction mixture was measured at 290 nm using a microplate reader (Perkin Elmer, Waltham, MA, USA).

3.6. Determination of Elastase Inhibitory Activity

The assay was modified and performed according to the method of Chiocchio et al. [16]. Briefly, 10 µL elastase from porcine pancreas (10 µg/mL) was mixed with 90 of 0.2M Tris-HCl, 100 uL of STANA (2.5 mM, N-Succinyl-Ala-Ala-Ala-p-nitroanilide), and 50 µL of sample at 37 °C for 30 min. After completion of the reaction, the supernatant was centrifuged at 15,000 rpm for 10 min. The absorbance of the reaction mixture was measured at 405 nm using a microplate reader (Perkin Elmer, Waltham, MA, USA). Phosphoramidon was used as a positive control.

3.7. Chemical Profiling by GC-MS Analysis

The molecular mass fragmental scanning of active constituents from *C.yabunikkei* leaf using GC-MS was performed based on a previously reported method with moderate modifications [14]. Briefly, Agilent 7890 gas chromatography (GC) and Agilent 5975 quadrupole mass spectrometry (MS) system (Agilent Technologies, Palo Alto, CA, USA) was utilized to analyze molecular mass fragments (50–550 amu) of *C.yabunikkei* leaf. The mass fragments were ionized under electron ionization (EI) conditions after an Agilent HP-5MS fused silica capillary column (30 mm *l.* × 0.25 mm *i.d.*, 0.25-µm film thickness). GC oven was thermally programmed as isothermal at 65 °C for 10 min and 10 min^{-1} to 300 with helium (He) as a carrier gas. All the scanned mass spectra were compared with the data system library (NIST 2017).

4. Conclusions

The present study reveals that hot water extract of *C.yabunikkei* leaf possesses antioxidant activity and hexane extract possesses xanthine oxidase and elastase inhibitory activities. In addition, it is hypothesized that the photochemicals present in the *C.yabunikkei* leaf might be responsible for the biological activities. The results of this study provide an excellent foundation for the future development of *C.yabunikkei* leaf-based dietary or medicinal preparations.

Author Contributions: S.Y.-S., M.-S.B. and S.-H.S. performed the experiments and S.-S.C. statistically analyzed the data.

Funding: This research was funded the National Research Foundation of Korea (NRF) grant funded by the Korea government (MSIP; Ministry of Science, ICT & Future Planning) (No. NRF-2017R1C1B5015187) and Wando county (2017120B312–00).

Conflicts of Interest: The authors declare no conflict of interest.

References

1. Seo, J.H.; Kim, J.E.; Shim, J.H.; Yoon, G.; Bang, M.A.; Bae, C.S.; Lee, K.J.; Park, D.H.; Cho, S.S. HPLC Analysis, Optimization of Extraction Conditions and Biological Evaluation of *Corylopsis coreana* Uyeki Flos. *Molecules* **2016**, *21*, 94. [CrossRef] [PubMed]
2. Yoon, I.S.; Park, D.H.; Bae, M.S.; Oh, D.S.; Kwon, N.H.; Kim, J.E.; Choi, C.Y.; Cho, S.S. In vitro and in vivo studies on *Quercus acuta* Thunb. (Fagaceae) extract: Active constituents, serum uric acid suppression, and xanthine oxidase inhibitory activity. *Evid.-Based Complement. Altern. Med.* **2017**, *2017*, 4097195. [CrossRef] [PubMed]
3. Yoon, I.S.; Park, D.H.; Kim, J.E.; Yoo, J.C.; Bae, M.S.; Oh, D.S.; Shim, J.H.; Choi, C.Y.; An, K.W.; Kim, E.I.; et al. Identification of the biologically active constituents of *Camellia japonica* leaf and anti-hyperuricemic effect in vitro and in vivo. *Int. J. Mol. Med.* **2017**, *39*, 1613–1620. [CrossRef] [PubMed]
4. Yoon, I.S.; Park, D.H.; Ki, S.H.; Cho, S.S. Effects of extracts from *Corylopsis coreana* Uyeki (Hamamelidaceae) flos on xanthine oxidase activity and hyperuricemia. *J. Pharm. Pharmacol.* **2016**, *68*, 1597–1603. [CrossRef] [PubMed]
5. Song, S.H.; Ki, S.H.; Park, D.H.; Moon, H.S.; Lee, C.D.; Yoon, I.S.; Cho, S.S. Quantitative analysis, extraction optimization, and biological evaluation of *Cudrania tricuspidata* leaf and fruit extracts. *Molecules* **2017**, *22*, 1489. [CrossRef] [PubMed]
6. Pino, J.A.; Regalado, E.L.; Rodriguez, J.L.; Fernandez, M.D. Phytochemical analysis and in vitro free-radical-scavenging activities of the essential oils from leaf and fruit of *Melaleuca leucadendra* L. *Chem. Biodivers.* **2010**, *7*, 2281–2288. [CrossRef] [PubMed]
7. Larayetan, R.A.; Okoh, O.O.; Sadimenko, A.; Okoh, A.I. Terpene constituents of the aerial parts, phenolic content, antibacterial potential, free radical scavenging and antioxidant activity of *Callistemon citrinus* (Curtis) Skeels (Myrtaceae) from Eastern Cape Province of South Africa. *BMC Complement. Altern. Med.* **2017**, *17*, 292. [CrossRef] [PubMed]
8. Zhang, C.R.; Aldosari, S.A.; Vidyasagar, P.S.; Nair, K.M.; Nair, M.G. Antioxidant and anti-inflammatory assays confirm bioactive compounds in Ajwa date fruit. *J. Agric. Food Chem.* **2013**, *61*, 5834–5840. [CrossRef] [PubMed]
9. Cheng, M.C.; Chang, W.H.; Chen, C.W.; Li, W.W.; Tseng, C.Y.; Song, T.Y. Antioxidant Properties of Essential Oil Extracted from *Pinus morrisonicola* Hay Needles by Supercritical Fluid and Identification of Possible Active Compounds by GC/MS. *Molecules* **2015**, *20*, 19051–19065. [CrossRef] [PubMed]

10. Henry, G.E.; Momin, R.A.; Nair, M.G.; Dewitt, D.L. Antioxidant and cyclooxygenase activities of fatty acids found in food. *J. Agric. Food Chem.* **2002**, *50*, 2231–2234. [CrossRef] [PubMed]
11. Santos, C.C.; Salvadori, M.S.; Mota, V.G.; Costa, L.M.; de Almeida, A.A.; de Oliveira, G.A.; Costa, J.P.; de Sousa, D.P.; de Freitas, R.M.; de Almeida, R.N. Antinociceptive and Antioxidant Activities of Phytol In Vivo and In Vitro Models. *Neurosci. J.* **2013**, *2013*, 949452. [CrossRef] [PubMed]
12. Fagali, N.; Catala, A. Antioxidant activity of conjugated linoleic acid isomers, linoleic acid and its methyl ester determined by photoemission and DPPH techniques. *Biophys. Chem.* **2008**, *137*, 56–62. [CrossRef] [PubMed]
13. Songur, A.; Sarsilmaz, M.; Sogut, S.; Ozyurt, B.; Ozyurt, H.; Zararsiz, I.; Turkoglu, A.O. Hypothalamic superoxide dismutase, xanthine oxidase, nitric oxide, and malondialdehyde in rats fed with fish omega-3 fatty acids. *Prog. Neuropsychopharmacol. Biol. Psychiatry* **2004**, *28*, 693–698. [CrossRef] [PubMed]
14. Zheng, X.; Wang, H.; Zhang, P.; Gao, L.; Yan, N.; Li, P.; Liu, X.; Du, Y.; Shen, G. Chemical Composition, Antioxidant Activity and alpha-Glucosidase Inhibitory Activity of *Chaenomeles Speciosa* from Four Production Areas in China. *Molecules* **2018**, *23*, 2518. [CrossRef] [PubMed]
15. Mohd Fahami, N.A.; Ibrahim, I.A.; Kamisah, Y.; Ismail, N.M. Palm vitamin E reduces catecholamines, xanthine oxidase activity and gastric lesions in rats exposed to water-immersion restraint stress. *BMC Gastroenterol.* **2012**, *12*, 54. [CrossRef] [PubMed]
16. Chiocchio, I.; Mandrone, M.; Sanna, C.; Maxia, A.; Tacchini, M.; Poli, F. Screening of a hundred plant extracts as tyrosinase and elastase inhibitors, two enzymatic targets of cosmetic interest. *Ind. Crop. Prod.* **2018**, *122*, 498–505. [CrossRef]

Sample Availability: Samples of the compounds are not available from the authors.

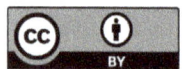

© 2018 by the authors. Licensee MDPI, Basel, Switzerland. This article is an open access article distributed under the terms and conditions of the Creative Commons Attribution (CC BY) license (http://creativecommons.org/licenses/by/4.0/).

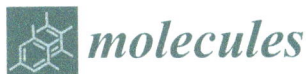

Article

Identification and Extraction Optimization of Active Constituents in *Citrus junos* Seib ex TANAKA Peel and Its Biological Evaluation

Jung-hyun Shim [1], Jung-il Chae [2],* and Seung-sik Cho [1],*

[1] Department of Pharmacy, College of Pharmacy, Mokpo National University, Muan, Jeonnam 58554, Korea; s1004jh@gmail.com
[2] Department of Dental Pharmacology, School of Dentistry and Institute of Oral Bioscience, BK21 Plus, Chonbuk National University, Jeonju 56443, Korea
* Correspondence: jichae@jbnu.ac.kr (J.-i.C.); sscho@mokpo.ac.kr (S.-s.C.); Tel.: +82-61-450-2687 (S.-s.C.)

Academic Editors: In-Soo Yoon, Hyun-Jong Cho and Derek J. McPhee
Received: 27 January 2019; Accepted: 13 February 2019; Published: 14 February 2019

Abstract: *Citrus junos* Seib ex TANAKA possesses various biological effects. It has been used in oriental remedies for blood circulation and the common cold. Recently, biological effects of *C. junos* peel have been reported. However, optimization of the biological properties of *C. junos* peel preparations has yet to be reported on. We developed a high-performance liquid chromatography (HPLC) method for quantification of the active constituents in *C. junos* peel. Hot water and ethanolic extracts of *C. junos* peel were prepared and their chemical profiles and biological activities were evaluated. The 80% ethanolic extract demonstrated the greatest antioxidant activity and phenolic content, while the 100% ethanolic extract had the greatest xanthine oxidase inhibitory activity. Elastase inhibition activity was superior in aqueous and 20% ethanolic extracts. The contents of two flavonoids were highest in the 100% ethanolic extract. We postulated that the antioxidant and anti-aging effects of *C. junos* peel extract could be attributed to phenolics such as flavonoids. Our results suggest that the flavonoid-rich extract of *C. junos* may be utilized for the treatment and prevention of metabolic disease and hyperuricemia while the water-soluble extract of *C. junos* could be used as a source for its anti-aging properties.

Keywords: *Citrus junos* Seib ex TANAKA; antioxidant; xanthine oxidase; elastase

1. Introduction

Citrus junos Seib ex TANAKA, a species of the family Rutaceae, is native to the southern coast and Jeju Island in Korea and China [1]. *C. junos* has been used in traditional medicine, cosmetics, and edible foods [2–4]. *C. junos* fruit has been traditionally used to improve blood circulation and treat the common cold [5]. It has been reported that *C. junos* contains many bioactive compounds such as vitamins, flavonoids, and limonoids that show anti-inflammatory and/or antioxidant activities [6]. The extract of *C. junos* can inhibit platelet aggregation, prevent ventricular dysfunction, and exert an antidiabetic effect [1,5,6]. Its fruits have been used as tea and its peels have been used as a source of essential oil. The *C. junos* peel has been dried and used as a raw material for tea. Recently, the biological effects of *C. junos* peel have been reported. Nakajima et al. have reported that *Citrus junos* peel can attenuate dextran sulfate sodium-induced murine experimental colitis and that its anti-inflammatory effect is related to its bioactive components such as hesperidin and naringin [7]. Shin et al. have found that 70% ethanolic extract of *C. junos* peel can reduce oleic acid-induced hepatic lipid accumulation in HepG2 cells with hypocholesterolemic effect in high-cholesterol diet mice models [8]. However, Shin et al. did not give reasons for or show active markers about why 70% ethanol extract was used in their experiment. Kim et al. have also reported the anti-diabetic effect of *C. junos* extract and its biomarkers such as rutin, hesperidin, quercetin [5].

On the other hand, there are no reports about optimization or the biological properties of *C. junos* peel extracts. Thus, the objective of this study was to investigate the active compounds and the biological activities of *C. junos* peel extracts for the development of natural medicine and as a source for cosmetics. Extraction optimization and standard analytical methods for quality control in plant sources utilization were important steps. Isolation and separation techniques were used to aid the identification of plant sources [9].

However, there is no standard profile for *C. junos* peel. Thus, in the present study, we established the quality control method using HPLC to separate and quantify hesperidin and naringin. We also investigated the optimum extraction of *C. junos* peel and the biological activities of these extracts. The optimized extract from *C. junos* peel was prepared and evaluated for its antioxidant, xanthine inhibitory, and elastase inhibitory activities in vitro.

2. Results and Discussion

2.1. Antioxidant Activity of C. junos Peel Extracts

Antioxidant potentials of hot water and ethanolic extracts of *C. junos* peels were determined by measuring 2,2-diphenyl-1-picrylhydrazyl (DPPH) scavenging activity, reducing power, and total phenolics. DPPH scavenging assay is a simple method for evaluating the free radical scavenging capacity of *C. junos* peel extracts. The antioxidant activities of natural sources are closely related to their phenolic components. Phenolic-rich sources from plant materials with antioxidant activity have diverse benefits against conditions such as oxidative imbalance and other metabolic diseases [9]. Thus, the antioxidant capacity of *C. junos* peel will provide important basic data for the development of medicinal and cosmetic materials.

Measured DPPH radical scavenging activity is shown in Table 1. The 80% ethanol extract showed the highest DPPH radical scavenging activity (IC_{50}: 1042.37 µg/mL). A low IC_{50} value indicates strong antioxidant activity of a sample. The scavenging effects based on IC_{50} data of DPPH radicals were in the following order: 80% EtOH extract (1042.37 µg/mL) > 60% ethanol extract (1226.76 µg/mL) > 40% ethanol extract (1329.41 µg/mL) > 100% ethanol extract (1754.14 µg/mL) > hot water extract (2160.89 µg/mL) > 20% ethanol extract (2560.64 µg/mL).

Table 1. DPPH radical scavenging effect of extracts from *C. junos* peel (IC_{50} value).

	DPPH Scavenging Activity IC_{50} (µg/mL)
Vitamin C	8.09
Hot water	2160.89
20% EtOH ex	2560.64
40% EtOH ex	1329.41
60% EtOH ex	1226.76
80% EtOH ex	1042.37
100% EtOH ex	1754.14

We tested the reducing power of various extracts. The reducing power assay is a method of measuring the reducing power of an extract using ferrous ions. The 80% ethanolic extract exhibited the highest activity among all extracts (Table 2). The reductive activity expressed as vitamin C equivalents was 24.99 ± 0.35 µg/100 µg ex as extract. Reducing ability expressed as vitamin C equivalents was in the order: 80% ethanol extract (24.99 ± 0.35 µg/100 µg ex) > 60% ethanol extract (23.32 ± 0.27 µg/100 µg ex) > 40% ethanol extract (22.90 ± 0.28 µg/100 µg ex) > 20% ethanol extract (22.21 ± 0.46 µg/100 µg ex) > 100% ethanol extract (21.75 ± 0.38 µg/100 µg ex) > hot water extract (18.22 ± 0.20 µg/100 µg ex).

Total phenol content is tested using the reaction of Folin–Ciocalteu solution and phenolic compound [10]. Results are reported as gallic acid equivalents by referencing to a standard curve

($r^2 > 0.999$) as shown in Table 2. Phenolic content in 80% ethanolic extract was higher than that in other extracts (25.44 ± 0.46 mg/g as gallic acid equivalents). Taken together, these results indicate that DPPH radical scavenging activity, reducing power, and phenolic contents were significantly higher in the 80% ethanolic extract than in other extracts.

Table 2. Reducing power and total phenolic contents of *C. junos* peel extracts.

Extract	Reducing Power (Ascorbic Acid eq. µg/100 µg Extract)	Total Phenolic Content (Gallic Acid eq. mg/g)
Hot water	18.22 ± 0.20	17.22 ± 0.27
20% EtOH ex	22.21 ± 0.46	20.43 ± 0.23
40% EtOH ex	22.90 ± 0.28	21.67 ± 0.4
60% EtOH ex	23.32 ± 0.27	22.81 ± 0.58
80% EtOH ex	24.99 ± 0.35	25.44 ± 0.46
100% EtOH ex	21.75 ± 0.38	24.77 ± 0.21

In our previous report, we found that 80% ethanol was a more efficient solvent in the extraction of phenolic compounds from *C. coreana*. However, the contents of four main markers such as bergenin, quercetin, quercitrin, and isosalipurposide were increased when they were extracted with ethanol [9]. Thus, we concluded that phenolic extraction might be affected by solvent combinations. In the present study, 80% ethanolic extract showed the most excellent antioxidant activities.

2.2. Xanthine Oxidase Inhibitory Activity of C. junos Peel Extracts

Xanthine oxidase inhibitory activities of various solvent extracts of *C. junos* peel are shown in Figure 1. Allopurinol (Allo) at a concentration of 50 µg/mL significantly inhibited xanthine oxidase activity (99.75%). The xanthine oxidase inhibitory activity of the 100% ethanolic extract was significantly higher than that of other extracts at a concentration of 1 mg/mL (55.74%). Previously, we have reported that various botanical extracts are potential xanthine oxidase inhibitors [11]. Yoon et al. [12,13] have found that extracts of *Corylopsis coreana* and *Camellia japonica* inhibit xanthine oxidase activity (by 50%) at a concentration of 2 mg/mL. Yoon et al. [11] have reported that *Quercus acuta* extract shows approximately 50% xanthine oxidase inhibition at a concentration of 1 mg/mL. Optimized extract *Cudrania tricuspidata* showed xanthine oxidase inhibition by approximately 75% at a concentration of 2 mg/mL [9]. Activities of 100% ethanolic extract were two times stronger than extracts of *Corylopsis coreana* and *Camellia japonica*, but similar to *Quercus acuta* extract. Plant extracts with xanthine oxidase inhibitory activity at 1 and 2 mg/mL demonstrated consistent effects in a hyperuricemic mouse model. Thus, it is plausible that the 100% ethanolic extract of *C. junos* peel could be developed as a candidate anti-gout (anti-hyperuricemic) agent.

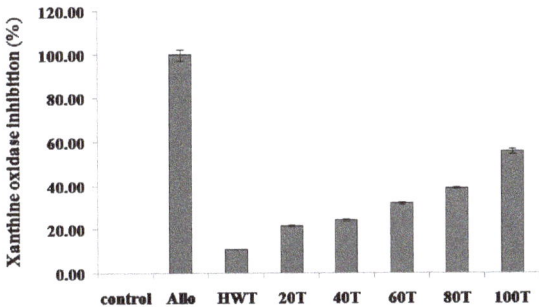

Figure 1. Xanthine oxidase inhibitory activities in extracts of *C. junos* peel (1 mg/mL) and allopurinol (Allo, 50 µg/mL). Allo; allopurinol, HWT; hot water, 20T; 20% EtOH ex, 40T; 40% EtOH ex, 60T; 60% EtOH ex, 80T; 80% EtOH ex, 100T; 100% EtOH ex, Values were the mean ± standard deviation (n = 3).

2.3. Elastase Inhibitory Activity of C. junos Peel Extracts

Elastase is a protease enzyme that degrades elastin. Inhibition of elastase can prevent skin aging [14]. An anti-elastase assay was performed to determine the ability of phytochemicals to inhibit elastase activity. Elastase inhibitory activities of various solvent extracts of *C. junos* peels are shown in Figure 2. Phosphoramidon (PPRM, positive control) at a concentration of 0.5 mg/mL significantly inhibited elastase activity (57.6 ± 8.33%). Elastase inhibitory activities of 20% ethanolic extract and hot water extract were significantly higher than those of other extracts at concentration of 1.0 mg/mL (61.4 ± 0.26% and 56.3 ± 0.6%, respectively).

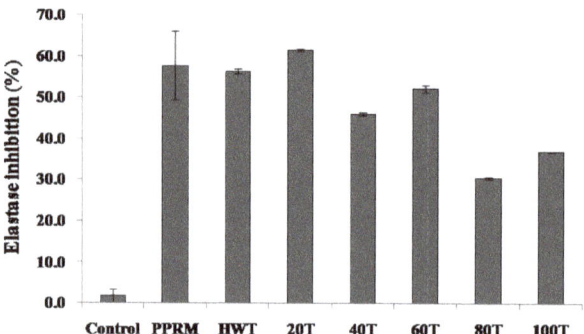

Figure 2. Elastase inhibitory activities in various solvent extracts of *C. junos* peel (1.0 mg/mL) and Phosphoramidon (PPRM, 0.5 mg/mL), HWT; hot water, 20T; 20% EtOH ex, 40T; 40% EtOH ex, 60T; 60% EtOH ex, 80T; 80% EtOH ex, 100T; 100% EtOH ex, Values were the mean ± standard deviation (n = 3).

Elastase inhibition of *C. junos* peel extract showed an opposite trend of antioxidant ability. Antioxidant activity was higher for ethanol extracts whereas elastase inhibition activity was higher for aqueous extracts. Elastase inhibitors are associated with anti-wrinkle and anti-aging properties. They can be developed into cosmetic materials [14]. An assessment of the anti-elastase activity of a plant extract can be a useful indicator of its potential application in cosmetic agents. Hot water and 20% ethanolic extract of *C. junos* peel exhibited more anti-elastase activity compared to other extracts (56.3 and 61%). However, this anti-elastase activity of the hot water extract could not be attributed to the presence of phenolics as reported in previous studies showing that phenolics such as flavonoids and tannins exhibited significant elastase inhibitory properties [15,16]. Therefore, studies on elastase inhibitory compounds of *C. junos* peel need to be conducted in the future.

2.4. Optimization of the Chromatographic Conditions and Contents of Marker Compounds from C. junos Extracts

In the present study, we investigated the analysis condition to separate two flavonoids such as naringin and hesperidin. A gradient program was used to separate the naringin and hesperidin in a single run within a practical period of time (Table 3). Chromatograms of standards and sample solutions are shown in Figure 3.

Information on retention time (RT) and quantification range, limit of detection (LOD) and limitation of quantification (LOQ) are summarized in Table 4. Limitation of detection of an individual analytical procedure is the lowest amount of an analyte in a sample that can be detected but not necessarily quantified. The limitation of quantification of an individual analytical procedure is the lowest amount of analyte in a sample that can be determined with suitable precision and accuracy. LODs for naringin and hesperidin were found to be 0.78 and 6.09 µg/mL, respectively. LOQ values for naringin and hesperidin were found to be 2.57 and 20.11 µg/mL, respectively (Table 4).

Table 3. Analytical conditions of HPLC system for analyzing markers.

Parameters	Conditions		
Column	Zorbax extended-C18 (C18, 4.6 mm × 150 mm, 5 μm)		
Flow rate	0.8 mL/min		
Injection volume	10 μL		
UV detection	280 nm		
Run time	55 min		
	Time (min)	A (%)	B (%)
Gradient	0	15	85
	45	15	85
	50	100	0
	51	15	85
	55	15	85

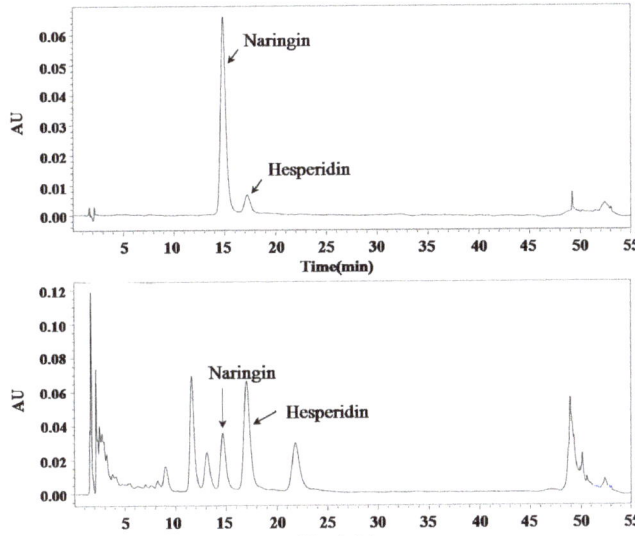

Figure 3. Bioactive constituent profiles of *C. junos* peel using HPLC.

Table 4. HPLC data for the calibration graphs and limit of quantification of naringin and hesperidin.

Analyte	Retention Time (min)	r^2	Linear Range (μg/mL)	LOQ (μg/mL)	LOD (μg/mL)
Naringin	15.3	0.9999	6.25–100	2.57	0.78
Hesperidin	17.7	0.9999	6.25–100	20.11	6.09

In previous reports, several extracts of *C. junos* peel were analyzed and several compounds were confirmed to be present in *C. junos* peel as marker compounds [4]. This finding is of significance in the use of this plant for industrial purposes. Two main peaks were identified as hesperidin and naringin in chromatographic profiles of extracts of *C. junos* peel. Kim et al. have previously reported that *C. junos* peel contains hesperidin and naringin, in agreement with our results [5]. We compared contents of these two active compounds in extracts of *C. junos* peel. Contents of these two compounds were found to be the highest in the 100% ethanolic extract (Table 5). The contents of hesperidin and naringin in the 100% ethanolic extract were 7.48 ± 0.04% and 0.63 ± 0.002%, respectively.

Table 5. Contents of naringin and hesperidin from *C. junos* peel extracts.

	Naringin (%)	Hesperidin (%)
Water	0.35 ± 0.006	4.67 ± 0.01
20% EtOH	0.44 ± 0.02	5.15 ± 0.09
40% EtOG	0.47 ± 0.003	5.92 ± 0.01
60% EtOH	0.44 ± 0.01	5.64 ± 0.01
80% EtOH	0.55 ± 0.01	7.07 ± 0.04
100% EtOH	0.63 ± 0.002	7.48 ± 0.04

Hesperidin is a well-known flavonoid with anti-oxidant [17], anti-inflammatory [18], and immune modulatory activities [19]. Recently, Lee et al. have reported that hesperidin can inhibit UVB-induced increase of skin thickness, wrinkle formation, and collagen fiber loss in male hairless mice. Hesperidin significantly inhibited the increase of epidermal thickness and epidermal hypertrophy and suppressed expression levels of MMP-9 and pro-inflammatory cytokines. These results indicate that hesperidin has anti-photoaging activity in UVB-irradiated hairless mice [20]. Contents of hesperidin in *C. junos* peel extract was 4.67 to 7.48%. Kim et al. have reported that hesperidin and naringin concentrations in 70% extract of *C. junos* peel are 0.03% and 0.01% (w/w), respectively [5]. In the present study, flavonoid-rich extracts containing hesperidin and naringin (7.48 and 0.63%, w/w respectively) were obtained.

Naringin (flavanone-7-O-glycoside) is known to have antioxidative, neuroprotective, and anti-inflammatory activities [21–23]. Naringin is also thought to contribute to anti-aging effects of the skin. Ren et al. have found that naringin can effectively protect skin against UVB-induced keratinocyte apoptosis and damage via inhibition of ROS (reactive oxygen species) production and COX-2 overexpression [24]. Additionally, Candhare et al. have reported that naringin ointment exerts wound healing potential via down-regulating expression levels of inflammatory factors, factors, and up-regulating expression of growth factors [25].

In previous reports on naringin and hesperidin, the DPPH radical scavenging activity of naringin was reported to be over 100 µg/mL [26]. Monica et al. described that naringin reduced Fe in a concentration dependent manner from 5 mM to 0.5 mM/mL to 15 mM at 0.1 mg/mL [27].

Srimathi et al. reported the antioxidant effects of hesperidin. IC_{50} of DPPH radical scavenging activity of hesperidin was 41.55 µg/mL. The reducing power of hesperidin was found to be 47.46 µg/mL while the standard antioxidant ascorbic acid was of 35.35 µg/mL [28]. The amount of hesperidin in the 80% extract was calculated to be 33.54 µg/100 µg extract eq based on the reducing power prescribed by Srimathi et al. However, the hesperidin content of the 80% extract was calculated to be 7.48% (7.48 µg/100 µg extract w/w), and actually, hesperidin contributes to the reducing power of the 20% portion. Therefore, naringin and hesperidin were not considered to be the major influencing factors for the antioxidant ability of *C. junos* peel extract. Thus, naringin and hesperidin are markers of *C. junos* peel, but various other antioxidants should be identified as marker/active compounds.

Both hesperidin and naringin are thought to be suitable as anti-oxidant and anti-inflammatory markers, as well as anti-aging markers of *C. junos* peel extract. *C. junos* peel is considered suitable as anti-aging material because all extract samples show elastase inhibitory activity. As shown in Figure 2, the elastase inhibitory activity was the highest in the hot water extract and 20% ethanolic extract. Besides, hesperidin and naringin as good antioxidant and anti-inflammatory agents showed the highest contents in 100% ethanol extract. Therefore, hesperidin and naringin are anti-aging markers in *C. junos* peel extract. Other water-soluble elastase inhibitors might be present in the hot water extract and 20% ethanolic extract. Thus, studies on elastase inhibitory compounds of water-soluble fraction from *C. junos* peel need to be conducted in the future.

Taken together, these results suggest that 80% ethanolic extract is suitable as an antioxidant while 100% ethanolic extract is suitable as an xanthine oxidase inhibitor. Meanwhile, hot water extract and 20% ethanolic extract are suitable as cosmetic materials showing an anti-aging effect.

None of previous studies reported so far have stated diverse activities and constituents of extracts of *C. junos* peel. To the best of our knowledge, our present study is the first to report the optimization of the extraction process of pharmaceutically and/or cosmetically active indicators from *C. junos* peel and to compare the antioxidant, xanthine oxidase inhibitory, and elastase activities of various extracts of *C. junos* peel.

3. Materials and Methods

3.1. Plant Material and Extract Preparation

C. junos peel was supplied from Korea Yuju Inc. (Gwangju, Korea). A voucher specimen (MNUCSS-CJ-01) was deposited at the Mokpo National University (Muan, Korea). Peels were dried and extracted for the present study. These air-dried and powdered *C. junos* peels (10 g) were extracted with 20%, 40%, 60%, 80%, and 100% ethanol (100 mL) at room temperature for 3 days. The 0% extract was prepared using hot water extraction (100 °C, 4 h). After filtration, the residual part was evaporated, freeze-dried and then stored at -70 °C before analysis.

3.2. DPPH Free Radical Assay

Antioxidant activity of the sample was determined using 2,2-diphenyl-1-picrylhydrazyl (DPPH) radical scavenging assay. Briefly, sample solution (1 mL) containing extract was added to DPPH sample solution (0.4 mM, 1 mL) and mixed at room temperature for 10 min. Absorbance was recorded at 517 nm using a microplate reader (Perkin Elmer, Waltham, MA, USA). DPPH free radical scavenging activities of samples were compared based on their IC_{50} (μg/mL) values [10].

3.3. Reducing Power

The reducing power of extracts was determined following a modified reducing power assay method. The sample (0.1 mL) was mixed with sodium phosphate buffer (0.2 M, 0.5 mL) and potassium ferricyanide (1%, 0.5 mL) followed by incubation at 50 °C for 20 min. Subsequently, trichloroacetic acid solution (10%, 0.5 mL) was added to the reaction mixture. Reaction mixture was centrifuged at 12,000 rpm for 10 min. The supernatant was mixed with distilled water (0.5 mL) and iron (III) chloride solution (0.1%, 0.1 mL) The absorbance was recorded at 700 nm. Reducing powers of extracts were expressed as vitamin C equivalents [10].

3.4. Determination of Total Phenolic Content

Folin–Ciocalteu assay was used for the quantifcation of the total phenolic content [10]. Sample or standard (1 mL) was mixed with sodium carbonate solution (2%, 1 mL) and Folin–Ciocalteu's phenol reagent (10%, 1 mL) followed by incubation at room temperature for 10 min. Absorbance was measured at 750 nm using a microplate reader (Perkin Elmer, Waltham, MA, USA) and compared with a calibration curve of gallic acid. Results were expressed as milligrams of gallic acid equivalents per gram of sample [10].

3.5. Determination of Xanthine Oxidase Inhibitory Activity

Xanthine oxidase assay is a method to measure the amount of uric acid produced by xanthine oxidase as described previously [10]. Phosphate buffer (100 mM; pH 7.4, 0.6 mL), sample (0.1 mL), xanthine oxidase (0.2 U/mL, 0.1 mL), and xanthine (1 mM; dissolved in 0.1 N NaOH, 0.2 mL) was mixed at 37 °C for 30 min and HCl (1 N, 0.2 mL) was added to finish the reaction. Allopurinol was used as a positive control. The absorbance was measured at 290 nm using a microplate reader (Perkin Elmer, Waltham, MA, USA).

3.6. Determination of Elastase Inhibitory Activity

The elastase inhibitory assay was used with a slight modification of the method described by Chiocchio et al. [29]. Briefly, elastase from porcine pancreas (10 µg/mL, 10 µL) was mixed with Tris-HCl (0.2 M, 90 µL), STANA (2.5 mM, *N*-Succinyl-Ala-Ala-Ala-*p*-nitroanilide, 100 µL), and sample (50 µL) at 37 °C for 30 min. After completion of the reaction, the supernatant was centrifuged at 15,000 rpm for 10 min. The absorbance was measured at 405 nm using a microplate reader (Perkin Elmer, Waltham, MA, USA). Phosphoramidon was used as a positive control.

3.7. Chemical Profiling by HPLC Analysis

All analyses were performed using an Alliance 2695 HPLC system (Waters, Milford, MA, USA). A reverse phase C18 column (5-µm, 150 mm × 5 mm) was used with a mobile phase consisting of a mixture of solvent A (acetonitrile) and B (0.2% phosphoric acid). The gradient was programmed as follows: 0–45 min: 15% A; 45–50 min: a linear gradient from 15 to 100% A; 50–51 min: a linear gradient from 100 to 15%; 51–55 min: 15% A. The flow rate was 0.8 mL/min. The UV detector was set at 280 nm.

4. Conclusions

The present study reveals both that the 80% ethanolic extract of *C. junos* peel possesses antioxidant activity and that the 100% ethanolic extract possesses a xanthine oxidase inhibitory effect. Hot water extract and 20% ethanolic extract possess elastase inhibitory activities. In addition, it is hypothesized that the photochemicals present in the *C. junos* peel might be responsible for biological activities of its extracts. Results of this study provide an excellent foundation for future development of *C. junos* peel-based medicinal and/or cosmetic preparations.

Author Contributions: J.-h.S. performed the experiments and J.-i.C., S.-s.C. statistically analyzed the data and design manuscript.

Funding: This Research was supported by the Research Funds of Mokpo National University in 2018.

Conflicts of Interest: The authors declare no conflicts of interest.

References

1. Yu, H.Y.; Park, S.W.; Chung, I.M.; Jung, Y.S. Anti-platelet effects of yuzu extract and its component. *Food Chem. Toxicol.* **2011**, *49*, 3018–3024. [CrossRef] [PubMed]
2. Hirota, R.; Roger, N.N.; Nakamura, H.; Song, H.S.; Sawamura, M.; Suganuma, N. Anti-inflammatory effects of limonene from yuzu (*Citrus junos* Tanaka) essential oil on eosinophils. *J. Food Sci.* **2010**, *75*, H87–H92. [CrossRef] [PubMed]
3. Sawamura, M.; Wu, Y.; Fujiwara, C.; Urushibata, M. Inhibitory effect of yuzu essential oil on the formation of N-nitrosodimethylamine in vegetables. *J. Agric. Food Chem.* **2005**, *53*, 4281–4287. [CrossRef] [PubMed]
4. Yoo, K.M.; Lee, K.W.; Park, J.B.; Lee, H.J.; Hwang, I.K. Variation in major antioxidants and total antioxidant activity of Yuzu (*Citrus junos* Sieb ex Tanaka) during maturation and between cultivars. *J. Agric. Food Chem.* **2004**, *52*, 5907–5913. [CrossRef] [PubMed]
5. Kim, S.H.; Hur, H.J.; Yang, H.J.; Kim, H.J.; Kim, M.J.; Park, J.H.; Sung, M.J.; Kim, M.S.; Kwon, D.Y.; Hwang, J.T. *Citrus junos* Tanaka Peel Extract Exerts Antidiabetic Effects via AMPK and PPAR-gamma both In Vitro and In Vivo in Mice Fed a High-Fat Diet. *Evid. Based Complement. Alternat. Med.* **2013**, *2013*, 921012. [PubMed]
6. Yu, H.Y.; Ahn, J.H.; Park, S.W.; Jung, Y.S. Preventive effect of yuzu and hesperidin on left ventricular remodeling and dysfunction in rat permanent left anterior descending coronary artery occlusion model. *PLoS ONE* **2015**, *10*, e110596. [CrossRef] [PubMed]
7. Abe, H.; Ishioka, M.; Fujita, Y.; Umeno, A.; Yasunaga, M.; Sato, A.; Ohnishi, S.; Suzuki, S.; Ishida, N.; Shichiri, M.; et al. Yuzu (*Citrus junos* Tanaka) Peel Attenuates Dextran Sulfate Sodium-induced Murine Experimental Colitis. *J. Oleo. Sci.* **2018**, *67*, 335–344. [CrossRef]

8. Shin, E.J.; Park, J.H.; Sung, M.J.; Chung, M.Y.; Hwang, J.T. *Citrus junos* Tanaka peel ameliorates hepatic lipid accumulation in HepG2 cells and in mice fed a high-cholesterol diet. *BMC Complement. Altern. Med.* **2016**, *16*, 499. [CrossRef]
9. Seo, J.H.; Kim, J.E.; Shim, J.H.; Yoon, G.; Bang, M.A.; Bae, C.S.; Lee, K.J.; Park, D.H.; Cho, S.S. HPLC Analysis, Optimization of Extraction Conditions and Biological Evaluation of *Corylopsis coreana* Uyeki Flos. *Molecules* **2016**, *21*, 94. [CrossRef]
10. Song, S.H.; Ki, S.H.; Park, D.H.; Moon, H.S.; Lee, C.D.; Yoon, I.S.; Cho, S.S. Quantitative Analysis, Extraction Optimization, and Biological Evaluation of *Cudrania tricuspidata* Leaf and Fruit Extracts. *Molecules* **2017**, *22*, 1489. [CrossRef]
11. Yoon, I.S.; Park, D.H.; Bae, M.S.; Oh, D.S.; Kwon, N.H.; Kim, J.E.; Choi, C.Y.; Cho, S.S. In vitro and in vivo studies on *Quercus acuta* Thunb. (Fagaceae) extract: Active constituents, serum uric acid suppression, and xanthine oxidase inhibitory activity. *Evid. Based Complement. Alternat. Med.* **2017**, *2017*, 4097195. [CrossRef]
12. Yoon, I.S.; Park, D.H.; Kim, J.E.; Yoo, J.C.; Bae, M.S.; Oh, D.S.; Shim, J.H.; Choi, C.Y.; An, K.W.; Kim, E.I.; et al. Identification of the biologically active constituents of *Camellia japonica* leaf and anti-hyperuricemic effect in vitro and in vivo. *Int. J. Mol. Med.* **2017**, *39*, 1613–1620. [CrossRef] [PubMed]
13. Yoon, I.S.; Park, D.H.; Ki, S.H.; Cho, S.S. Effects of extracts from *Corylopsis coreana* Uyeki (Hamamelidaceae) flos on xanthine oxidase activity and hyperuricemia. *J. Pharm. Pharmacol.* **2016**, *68*, 1597–1603. [CrossRef] [PubMed]
14. Kalyana Sundaram, I.; Sarangi, D.D.; Sundararajan, V.; George, S.; Sheik Mohideen, S. Poly herbal formulation with anti-elastase and anti-oxidant properties for skin anti-aging. *BMC Complement. Altern. Med.* **2018**, *18*. [CrossRef] [PubMed]
15. Kanashiro, A.; Souza, J.G.; Kabeya, L.M.; Azzolini, A.E.; Lucisano-Valim, Y.M. Elastase release by stimulated neutrophils inhibited by flavonoids: Importance of the catechol group. *Z. Naturforsch. C* **2007**, *62*, 357–361. [CrossRef] [PubMed]
16. Hrenn, A.; Steinbrecher, T.; Labahn, A.; Schwager, J.; Schempp, C.M.; Merfort, I. Plant phenolics inhibit neutrophil elastase. *Planta. Med.* **2006**, *72*, 1127–1131. [CrossRef] [PubMed]
17. Bhargava, P.; Verma, V.K.; Malik, S.; Khan, S.I.; Bhatia, J.; Arya, D.S. Hesperidin regresses cardiac hypertrophy by virtue of PPAR-gamma agonistic, anti-inflammatory, antiapoptotic, and antioxidant properties. *J. Biochem. Mol. Toxicol.* **2019**, e22283. [CrossRef] [PubMed]
18. Moon, P.D.; Kim, H.M. Antiinflammatory effects of traditional Korean medicine, JinPi-tang and its active ingredient, hesperidin in HaCaT cells. *Phytother. Res.* **2012**, *26*, 657–662. [CrossRef]
19. Camps-Bossacoma, M.; Franch, A.; Perez-Cano, F.J.; Castell, M. Influence of Hesperidin on the Systemic and Intestinal Rat Immune Response. *Nutrients* **2017**, *9*, 580. [CrossRef]
20. Lee, H.J.; Im, A.R.; Kim, S.M.; Kang, H.S.; Lee, J.D.; Chae, S. The flavonoid hesperidin exerts anti-photoaging effect by downregulating matrix metalloproteinase (MMP)-9 expression via mitogen activated protein kinase (MAPK)-dependent signaling pathways. *BMC Complement. Altern. Med.* **2018**, *18*, 39. [CrossRef]
21. Cui, J.; Wang, G.; Kandhare, A.D.; Mukherjee-Kandhare, A.A.; Bodhankar, S.L. Neuroprotective effect of naringin, a flavone glycoside in quinolinic acid-induced neurotoxicity: Possible role of PPAR-gamma, Bax/Bcl-2, and caspase-3. *Food Chem. Toxicol.* **2018**, *121*, 95–108. [CrossRef] [PubMed]
22. El-Desoky, A.H.; Abdel-Rahman, R.F.; Ahmed, O.K.; El-Beltagi, H.S.; Hattori, M. Anti-inflammatory and antioxidant activities of naringin isolated from *Carissa carandas* L.: In vitro and in vivo evidence. *Phytomedicine* **2018**, *42*, 126–134. [CrossRef]
23. Li, C.; Zhang, J.; Lv, F.; Ge, X.; Li, G. Naringin protects against bone loss in steroid-treated inflammatory bowel disease in a rat model. *Arch. Biochem. Biophys.* **2018**, *650*, 22–29. [CrossRef] [PubMed]
24. Ren, X.; Shi, Y.; Zhao, D.; Xu, M.; Li, X.; Dang, Y.; Ye, X. Naringin protects ultraviolet B-induced skin damage by regulating p38 MAPK signal pathway. *J. Dermatol. Sci.* **2016**, *82*, 106–114. [CrossRef] [PubMed]
25. Kandhare, A.D.; Alam, J.; Patil, M.V.; Sinha, A.; Bodhankar, S.L. Wound healing potential of naringin ointment formulation via regulating the expression of inflammatory, apoptotic and growth mediators in experimental rats. *Pharm. Biol.* **2016**, *54*, 419–432. [CrossRef] [PubMed]
26. De Martino, L.; Mencherini, T.; Mancini, E.; Aquino, R.P.; De Almeida, L.F.; De Feo, V. In vitro phytotoxicity and antioxidant activity of selected flavonoids. *Int. J. Mol. Sci.* **2012**, *13*, 5406–5419. [CrossRef] [PubMed]

27. Cavia-Saiz, M.; Busto, M.D.; Pilar-Izquierdo, M.C.; Ortega, N.; Perez-Mateos, M.; Muniz, P. Antioxidant properties, radical scavenging activity and biomolecule protection capacity of flavonoid naringenin and its glycoside naringin: A comparative study. *J. Sci. Food Agric.* **2010**, *90*, 1238–1244. [CrossRef]
28. Srimathi Priyanga, K.; Vijayalakshmi, K. Investigation of antioxidant potential of quercetin and hesperidin: An in vitro approach. *Asian J. Pharm. Clin. Res.* **2017**, *10*, 83–86. [CrossRef]
29. Chiocchio, I.; Mandrone, M.; Sanna, C.; Maxia, A.; Tacchini, M.; Poli, F. Screening of a hundred plant extracts as tyrosinase and elastase inhibitors, two enzymatic targets of cosmetic interest. *Ind. Crop. Prod.* **2018**, *122*, 498–505. [CrossRef]

Sample Availability: Samples of the compounds are not available from the authors.

© 2019 by the authors. Licensee MDPI, Basel, Switzerland. This article is an open access article distributed under the terms and conditions of the Creative Commons Attribution (CC BY) license (http://creativecommons.org/licenses/by/4.0/).

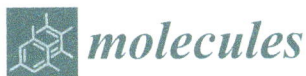

Article

Bioactivity Determination of a Therapeutic Recombinant Human Keratinocyte Growth Factor by a Validated Cell-based Bioassay

Wenrong Yao [1,2,†], Ying Guo [1,†], Xi Qin [1,†], Lei Yu [1], Xinchang Shi [1], Lan Liu [1], Yong Zhou [1], Jinpan Hu [1], Chunming Rao [1,*] and Junzhi Wang [1,*]

1. National Institutes for Food and Drug Control, No. 2, Tiantan Xili, Dongcheng District, Beijing 100050, China; yz1322@126.com (W.Y.); guoying@nifdc.org.cn (Y.G.); qinxi@nifdc.org.cn (X.Q.); yulei@nifdc.org.cn (L.Y.); shixc@nifdc.org.cn (X.S.); liulan@nifdc.org.cn (L.L.); zhouyong@nifdc.org.cn (Y.Z.); 13716691086@163.com (J.H.)
2. Institutes of Process Engineering, Chinese Academy of Sciences, 1 North 2nd Street, Zhongguancun, Haidian District, Beijing 100190, China
* Correspondence: raocm@nifdc.org.cn (C.R.); wangjz_nifdc2014@163.com (J.W.); Tel.: +8610-67095380 (C.R.); +8610-67095782 (J.W.)
† They contributed equally to this work.

Academic Editors: In-Soo Yoon and Hyun-Jong Cho
Received: 19 January 2019; Accepted: 13 February 2019; Published: 15 February 2019

Abstract: The therapeutic recombinant human keratinocyte growth factor 1 (rhKGF-1) was approved by the FDA for oral mucositis resulting from hematopoietic stem cell transplantation for hematological malignancies in 2004. However, no recommended bioassay for rhKGF-1 bioactivity has been recorded in the U.S. Pharmacopoeia. In this study, we developed an rhKGF-1-dependent bioassay for determining rhKGF-1 bioactivity based on HEK293 and HaCat cell lines that stably expressed the luciferase reporter driven by the serum response element (SRE) and human fibroblast growth factor receptor (FGFR2) IIIb. A good responsiveness to rhKGF-1 and rhKGF-2 shared by target HEK293/HaCat cell lines was demonstrated. Our stringent validation was completely focused on specificity, linearity, accuracy, precision, and robustness according to the International Council for Harmonization (ICH) Q2 (R1) guidelines, AAPS/FDA Bioanalytical Workshop and the Chinese Pharmacopoeia. We confirmed the reliability of the method in determining rhKGF bioactivity. The validated method is highly timesaving, sensitive, and simple, and is especially valuable for providing information for quality control during the manufacture, research, and development of therapeutic rhKGF.

Keywords: rhKGF-1; rhKGF-2; bioactivity; cell-based bioassay; method validation

1. Introduction

Keratinocyte growth factor (KGF) was originally isolated from human embryonic lung fibroblast-conditioned medium, and it is a member of the fibroblast growth factor (FGF) family [1,2]. The FGF family is composed of 23 members and classified into six subfamilies in mammals [3]. Among these, FGF7 (also called KGF-1) [1] and FGF10 (also called KGF-2) [4] belong to the FGF7 subfamily. The human *Fgf7* gene was mapped to chromosome 15q21.2, and its 582 bp open reading frame (ORF), which consisted of four exons, could encode a native 194 amino acid monomeric polypeptide with approximately 25–30 kDa [1,5,6]. The chromosomal localization of human *Fgf10* gene was in p12-p13 region of chromosome 5. The complete ORF sequence with three exons encoded a protein of 208 amino acids. The observed molecular mass of the recombinant human FGF10 expressed in *E.coli* was approximately 19 kDa [7,8]. The conserved region of human KGF-2, i.e., amino acid 60–205, had the highest homology with that of KGF-1, sharing 54% amino acid identity. Based on the evolutionary relationship, KGF-2 is closest to KGF-1. Additionally, the specificity of mitogenic activity of KGF-2 is similar to that of KGF-1 [2,7,8].

Given the biological functions, KGF-1 and KGF-2 are considered paracrine factors, and regulate embryonic development by binding to their specific FGF receptor 1 (FGFR1) and FGFR2. FGFR2, which is expressed exclusively on epithelial cells, is a high affinity receptor for KGF-1 and KGF-2 [9–13]. It must be emphasized that KGF-1 and KGF-2 preferentially activate the IIIb splice variant of FGFR2 (FGFR2 IIIb), and KGF-2 also activates the IIIb splice variant of FGFR1 (FGFR1 IIIb) [14,15]. Upon binding to their receptors, the activated FGFR1 and FGFR2 (especially FGFR2 IIIb), autophosphorylate tyrosine residues, phosphorylate the intracellular domains of other kinases, and subsequently induce mitogen-activated protein kinases (MAPKs), the phosphoinositide 3-kinase (PI3K)/AKT/mammalian target of rapamycin (mTOR) pathway, and the phospholipase Cγ (PLCγ) intracellular signaling pathway [3,16–18].

Through its intracellular signal transduction, KGF induces its biological activity in keratinocytes and in the development and morphogenesis of multiple epithelial cell lineages within the skin, lung, and reproductive tract [19,20]. Therefore, KGF may have potential therapeutic benefits in the growth and development of related tissues and in wound healing [21]. In 2004, palifermin, a recombinant human KGF-1 (rhKGF-1, developed by Amgen, Thousand Oaks, CA, USA), was approved by the FDA for the treatment of severe oral mucositis in adult patients receiving myeloablative radiochemotherapy for hematological malignancies and requiring autologous hematopoietic stem cell transplants [22,23]. Palifermin has further been investigated as concomitant chemotherapy for the treatment of colorectal cancers and head/neck cancers in recent years [24]. In comparison to endogenous KGF-1, palifermin is more stable due to its removal of 23 amino acids from the N-terminal end [2,25,26]. Palifermin binds to FGFR2 IIIb, thereby inducing the proliferation, differentiation, and migration of epithelial cells. It also inhibits apoptosis of epithelial cells and repairs damaged epithelium [23,27]. Nowadays, repifermin (recombinant human KGF-2) demonstrated mixed results in a clinical trial of topical treatment for healing of chronic venous leg ulcers [9].

Understanding the biological activity of therapeutic rhKGF-1 is critical for clinical safety and efficacy, especially prior to its use in humans. However, bioassays of rhKGF-1 have not been recorded in the U.S. Pharmacopoeia, although palifermin was approved for the therapeutical use. Previous studies had shown that KGF-1 promoted mitogenic activity by a [^{3}H] thymidine incorporation assay in human FGFR2b-expressing BaF3 cells and type II alveolar cells [15,18,28]. Recently, the MTT assay showed that rhKGF-1 had a significant proliferative effect on the NIH3T3, A549b, and MCF7 cell lines [26]. However, the aforementioned bioassay is time-consuming and tedious (88 h–160 h per experimental procedure) and high variability with low signal-noise-ratio (SNR). Reporter gene assays (RGAs) are Mechanism of Action (MOA)-related, less variable, higher sensitive and labor-saving. They have been increasingly adopted as quality control of biopharmaceuticals [29,30].

Herein, an RGA for determining the bioactivity of therapeutic rhKGF was developed based on HEK293 and HaCat cell lines stably transfected with luciferase reporter gene controlled by the serum response element (SRE) promoter and human FGFR2 IIIb. Upon rhKGF binding to FGFR2 IIIb and subsequent intracellular signaling cascades, the interaction between the transcription factor and SRE drives downstream luciferase gene expression. The bioactivity of rhKGF was determined by measuring relative luciferase units (RLU) driven by SRE. The new method was then optimized and fully validated with respect to specificity, linearity, accuracy, and precision based on the regular requirements as stated in the (ICH) Q2 (R1) guidelines, AAPS/FDA Bioanalytical Workshop and the Chinese Pharmacopoeia. The desired results of this validation were obtained and provide invaluable information for quality control during the manufacture, research, and development of therapeutic rhKGF-1 and rhKGF-2.

2. Results

2.1. Identification of Cells Responsive to rhKGF-1

To develop responsive cell lines for rhKGF-1bioactivity, transformed HEK293 and HaCat cells bearing an SRE-luciferase reporter and human FGFR2 IIIb were constructed. By limiting dilutions, we produced nine HEK293 clonal cell lines and six HaCat clonal cell lines from single cells. All of these clones were responsive to rhKGF-1 stimulation and were hygromycin B/puromycin resistant. Of the nine HEK293-Luc clonal cell lines, a representative cell line, 1C1, was chosen and characterized in terms of its rhKGF-1-dependence. This cell line had the highest SNR, and it was more sensitive to rhKGF-1 stimulation than the other cell lines; that is, it had a lower EC_{50} value (Figure 1). Clonal cell line 1A6 from the HaCat-Luc cells was demonstrated to produce a typical sigmoidal curve much like the HEK293-Luc cell line did (Figure S1). Clones 1C1 and 1A6 were selected for further method validation.

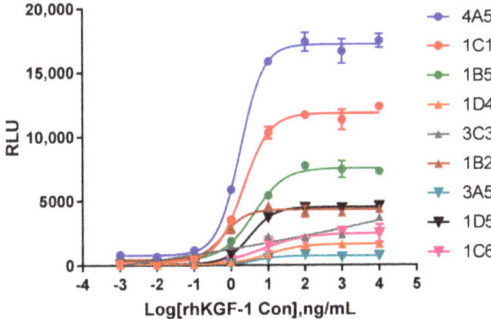

Figure 1. The establishment of HEK293-Luc cell lines responsive to rhKGF-1. The nine clones of single-cell dilutions of HEK293-Luc cells bearing luciferase and human KGFR2 IIIb were evaluated by their luciferase activity with rhKGF-1 stimulation (initial concentration of 10,000 ng/mL, dilution ratio of 1:10). The curves were calculated in a four-parameter model. RLU = Relative Luciferase Units. The mean ± SD is shown on each curve.

2.2. Optimization Procedure

To obtain optimal sensitivity and stable results with HEK293-Luc cells, the optimal initial concentration of rhKGF-1, heparin concentration in the assay media, number of cells per well, and incubation time were investigated. Additionally, the cells were routinely cultured in DMEM-10% FBS media, which caused increased background luciferase values (Figure S2A). The SNR of 9.30 seen in this media was significantly lower than that seen in DMEM-0.5% FBS, which had an SNR of 38.07. In the experiment we designed, we optimized one parameter by changing it while keeping the others constant.

2.2.1. Optimal initial rhKGF-1 concentration

As shown in Figure S3, luciferase activity dose-dependently increased with increasing rhKGF-1, and the sigmoidal curve drew close to its bottom asymptote and top asymptote between 0.02 ng/mL and 137 ng/mL of rhKGF-1. Thus, an optimized assay was subsequently designed, with different initial concentrations with three dilution factors. Figure 2A illustrated dose-dependent curves of luciferase activity at all of the initial concentrations. The points of the top and bottom asymptotes of 100 ng/mL and 120 ng/mL as initial concentrations met the experimental demand, although all of the curves were similar. Here, the recommended concentration in the bioassay was 120 ng/mL.

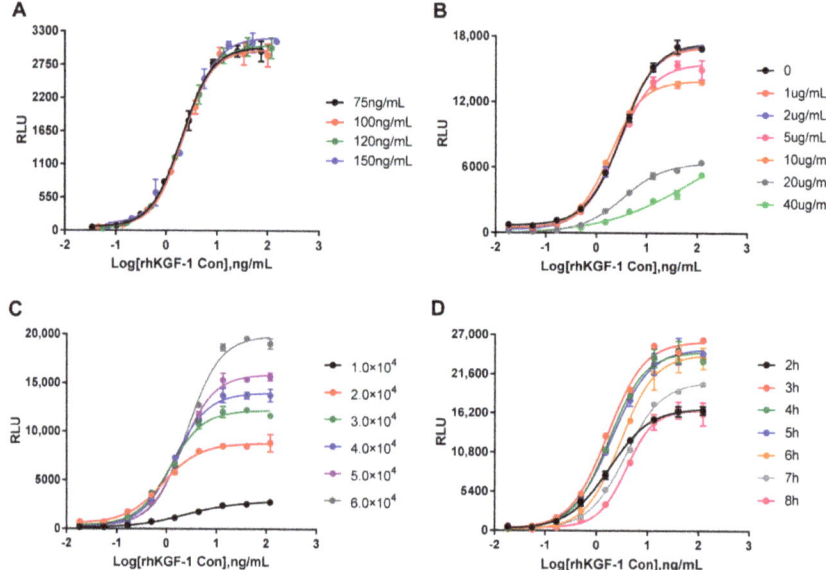

Figure 2. Optimization of parameters using responsive HEK293-Luc cells for determination of rhKGF-1 bioactivity. (**A**) The initial concentration of rhKGF-1. HEK293-Luc cells were stimulated at initial concentrations of 75, 100, 120 and 150 ng/mL with three dilution factors. (**B**) Heparin concentration in the assay medium. (**C**) Different numbers of HEK293-Luc cells per well added to a 96-well plate. (**D**) Incubation time after the rhKGF-1 was added to the HEK293-Luc cells. The curves were calculated in a four-parameter model. In each experiment, every dilution point was tested in three wells of cells. RLU = Relative Luciferase Units. The mean ± SD is shown on each curve.

2.2.2. Optimization of Heparin Concentration in Assay Media

To achieve a possibly higher sensitivity, we thought it might be necessary to supplement the assay media with heparin. We determined the suitable concentration of heparin by investigating the EC_{50} value and the SNR. As shown in Figure 2B, we found that the three curves overlapped and probably were equivalent at 0, 1 and 2 μg/mL of heparin in assay media. The RLUs at the top asymptote resulting from all but the above three concentrations were decreased gradually with increasing heparin concentrations, and the sigmoidal curves were not significant at 20 and 40 μg/mL of heparin. Based on the EC_{50} values (3.96, 3.57 and 3.58 ng/mL at 0, 1 and 2 μg/mL of heparin, respectively) and SNR's (25.2, 35.1, and 52.7, respectively), we concluded that 2 μg/mL of heparin was superior to other heparin concentrations.

2.2.3. Optimization of Cell Numbers and Incubation Time

For optimizing the number of cells per well, freshly trypsinized HEK293-Luc cells were added in various numbers to a 96-well plate. Although the RLU of the top asymptote was increased with increasing cell numbers, no significant differences in the SNR were observed. Due to the lower EC_{50} value, 4×10^4 cells per well were used in the subsequent assay (Figure 2C). Finally, the highest magnitude of RLU was found between 3 h and 5 h. The curves and EC_{50} values were nearly identical for 3 h to 5 h, indicating that 3 h to 5 h was a good incubation period under the given conditions (Figure 2D). The decline in RLU between 6 h and 8 h was probably associated with a lack of rhKGF-1. Considering the ease of operation and sensitivity of the bioassay, we therefore chose a 4 h incubation as the optimal time.

2.3. Validation of Bioactivity Procedures

In this study, the HEK293-Luc cells responsive to rhKGF-1 were further validated according to the ICH Q2 (R1) guidelines, AAPS/FDA Bioanalytical Workshop and the Chinese Pharmacopoeia. In particular, the following typical validation parameters were considered.

2.3.1. Specificity

As mentioned in the ICH Q2 (R1), degradants are one of the typically investigation of specificity. Here, forced degradation of rhKGF-1 was induced through thermal stress. An rhKGF-1 sample was subjected to 37 °C for different days to induce specific forced degradation. Figure 3A,B summarized the results of specificity with the forced degradation study. Compared to an in-house rhKGF-1 reference and the untreated sample (0 day), the RLU of degraded rhKGF-1 (37 °C for 1 d, 3 d and 5 d) did not reach the top asymptote (Figure 3A). A gradual decrease in relative bioactivity was observed, from 0.98 of the untreated sample to 0.03 of the degraded rhKGF-1 for 5 days (Figure 3B).

Furthermore, the specificity of the new bioassay was elaborated in another assay. Four other therapeutic cytokines, i.e., rhEGF, rhEPO, rhbFGF, and NGF were treated with the rhKGF-1 bioactivity procedure, and we then determined the luciferase activity by adding to HEK293-Luc cells. The results demonstrated that HEK293-Luc cells responded to rhKGF-1 in a dose-dependent activity, but did not respond to rhEPO, rhbFGF, and NGF. For rhEGF, a slight curve appeared, but the RLU of the top asymptote was significantly lower than that for rhKGF-1 (Figure 3C). It is also worth highlighting that the HEK293-Luc cells responded to rhKGF-2 in a dose-dependent manner. This response to rhKGF-2 occurred at a higher initial concentration (300 ng/mL) and lower sensitivity (with an EC_{50} value of 6.28 ng/mL) than the response to rhKGF-1 (Figure 3D).

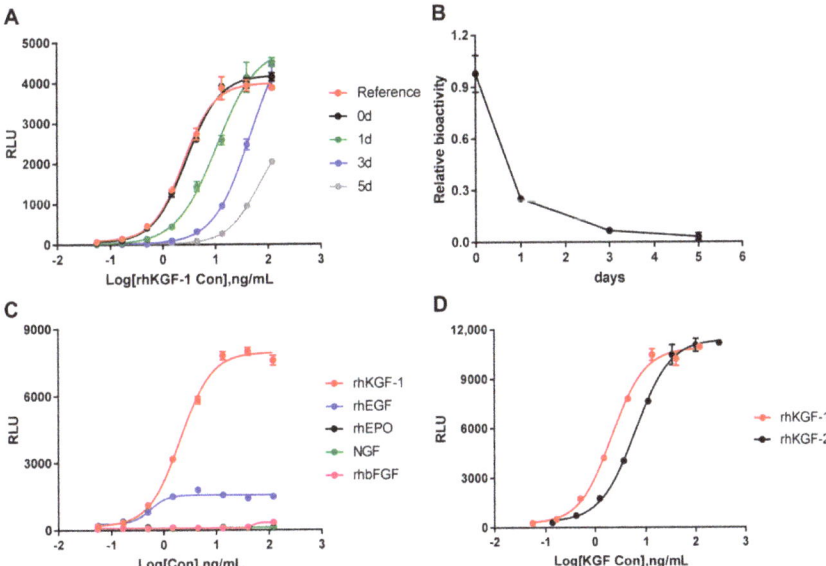

Figure 3. The specificity of rhKGF-1 bioassay. (**A**) The sigmoidal curves of untreated and forced degradation of rhKGF-1. The forced degradation was induced by 37 °C incubation for 1 d, 3 d and 5 d. (**B**) The relative bioactivity of forcibly degraded rhKGF-1. The relative bioactivities were decreased gradually with time of degradation. (**C**) The responsiveness of cells to rhKGF-1 and to the therapeutic cytokines rhEGF, rhEPO, NGF, and rhbFGF. (**D**). The responsiveness of cells to rhKGF-1 and rhKGF-2. RLU = Relative Luciferase Units. The mean ± SD is shown in each curve.

2.3.2. Linearity

The linearity of an analytical method is its ability to give test results which are directly proportional to the concentration of analyte in the sample. For linearity validation, the percentage of relative bioactivity from five concentrations in the range of 50% to 150% of optimized initial concentration, i.e., 120 ng/mL, were determined by the EC_{50} value of an in-house reference at five different concentrations. The data were obtained three times per experiment in four independent experiments executed on four different days and were analyzed using a linear regression model. The CV of measured bioactivity for five different concentrations was calculated to be 0.44% to 4.96%, which was < 5% (Table S1). The measured bioactivity versus expected bioactivity indicated a good linearity ($R^2 > 0.9954$ in each experiment), suggesting excellent linearity of the established method (Figure 4A).

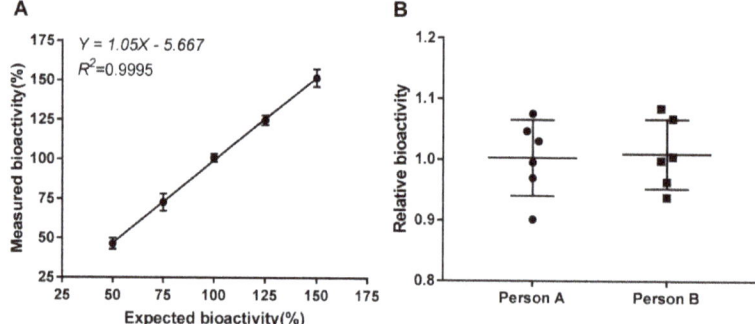

Figure 4. The results of the linearity and intermediate precision tests. (**A**) Linearity plot for the expected bioactivity against the measured bioactivity. Each point indicates the mean of three replicates. (**B**) Intermediate precision. Tests of six batches of rhKGF-1 were performed by two persons on different days. The mean ± SD and representative linear regression of four independent experiments is shown.

2.3.3. Accuracy

According to the ICH Q2 (R1) PART II, the accuracy of a method should be reported as the rate of recovery of a known added amount of analyte in a sample. So, we verified the percentage of an rhKGF-1 in-house reference recovered from our rhKGF-1 samples by analysis of three repeated assays each day on four different days. As shown in Table 1, satisfactory results for intra-day CV values for the final rhKGF-1 were obtained. These values ranged from 3.92% to 7.51%, and the inter-day CV was 6.91%. The average recovery rate was 92.75%, and the 95% confidence intervals (CI) of reference recovery were 88.68% to 96.82%. Thus, the acceptance recovery rate was satisfactory, and the method demonstrated sufficient accuracy.

Table 1. The recovery rate in the final rhKGF-1 sample.

	Recovery Rate (%)			Intra-day CV (%)	Mean	SD
	1	2	3			
1	97.13	91.17	100.70	5.00	96.33	4.82
2	94.80	95.90	101.90	3.92	97.53	3.82
3	82.40	88.27	95.70	7.51	88.79	6.67
4	92.82	90.86	81.35	6.94	88.34	6.13
Inter-day CV (%)		6.91				
Mean		92.75				
SD		6.41				

2.3.4. Precision

The precision of an analytical method may be investigated by the method's repeatability (also termed intra-day precision) and intermediate precision, given as the CV. The repeatability was estimated from the results of relative bioactivity on four different days and in triplicate on each day for each sample. A batch of the final product and a bulk batch of rhKGF-1 were used for this purpose. As shown in Table 2, the maximum intra-day and inter-day CV values were lower than 5.00%. To assess the intra-plate precision, five repeated final product tests were performed in the same plate, and the resulting CV was 4.85% (data not shown).

Table 2. The repeatability of final and bulk rhKGF-1 samples.

Sample	Intra-day CV (%)				Inter-day CV (%)	95% CI of Relative Bioactivity
	1	2	3	4		
rhKGF-1	1.49	3.09	1.73	3.75	2.82	1.05–1.10
rhKGF-1 bulk	4.62	0.90	3.62	0.52	4.75	1.01–1.08

To validate the variations within laboratories, intermediate precision was determined on different days by two operators [31]. Six different batches of rhKGF-1 (final products and bulk batches) were involved in this test. The mean relative bioactivities were 1.003 for person A and 1.009 for person B. Overall, the statistical indifference of the results suggested that the new bioassay was characterized by consistent performance and a good intermediate precision (Figure 4B).

2.3.5. Stability of the HEK293-Luc Cell Line

The stability of the HEK293-Luc cell line and the response to rhKGF-1 are crucial for the cells to be used in the bioassay. Stability was evaluated by comparing EC_{50} value and SNR in response to rhKGF-1 at three different passages. We obtained parallel dose-response curves, indicating the consistency of the cell line between passage 5 and passage 42 (Figure 5A). The SNR showed a moderate tendency to increase with increasing cell passage number, from 39.35 at passage 5 to 45.39 at passage 42, but no significant difference was observed between three different passages (Figure 5B). However, the EC_{50} values associated with the sensitivities of passage 16 and passage 42 were significantly higher than that of passage 5, having changed from 1.24 to 1.61. Even so, the EC_{50} of passage 16 and passage 42 were the same as each other, 1.61 (Figure 5C). Therefore, the responsiveness of the HEK293-Luc cell line to rhKGF-1 was proven to be highly stable, especially between passage 16 and passage 42.

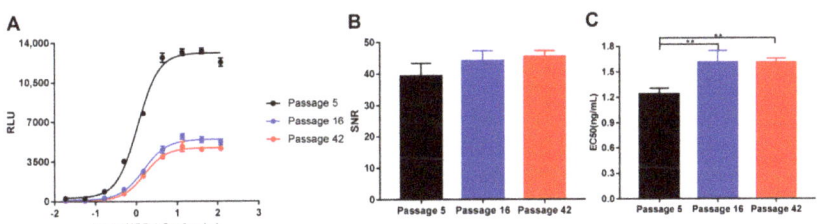

Figure 5. Stability of HEK293-Luc cell lines. (**A**) The responsiveness of HEK293-Luc cells to rhKGF-1 at different passages. (**B**) SNR of HEK293-Luc cells at three passages. (**C**) EC_{50} of HEK293-Luc cells at three passages. RLU = Relative Luciferase Units. SNR = Signal-Noise-Ratio. The mean ± SD is shown on each curve. ** $p < 0.001$.

2.3.6. Comparison of Responsiveness to rhKGF-1 between HEK293-Luc and HaCat-Luc Cell Lines

As shown in Figure 6 and Table S2, the CV values of method validation, recovery rates, and relative bioactivity were compared between HEK293-Luc and HaCat-Luc cell lines responding to rhKGF-1. Concordance between HEK293-Luc and HaCat-Luc cell lines was demonstrated with the CV values of the linearity (Figure 6A), accuracy (Figure 6C), and precision (Figure 6D). In comparing the recovery rates, the HaCat-Luc cell line showed a significantly higher rate (107.70%) than did the HEK293-Luc cell line (92.75%) (Figure 6B). Additionally, equivalent relative bioactivity with final rhKGF-1 and bulk rhKGF-1 was observed between the two cell lines (Figure 6E,F). In summary, when considering the concordance levels, only the recovery rate had a difference, whereas the CV and relative bioactivity supported a conclusion of greater agreement between the HEK293-Luc and HaCat-Luc cell lines.

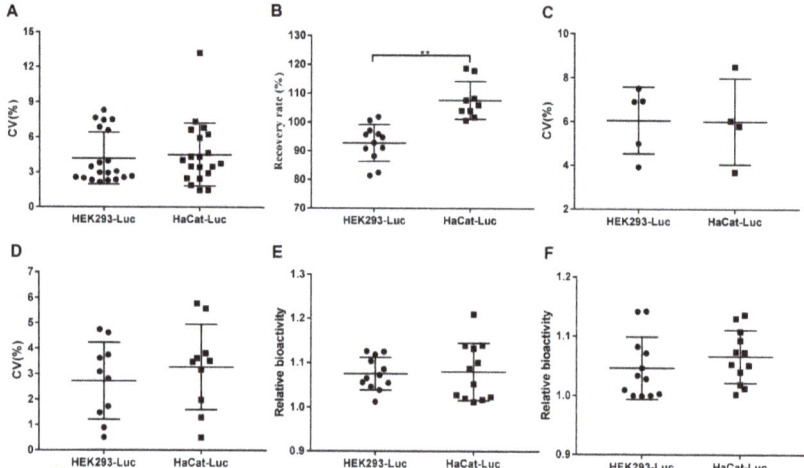

Figure 6. Comparison of validation between the HEK293-Luc and HaCat-Luc cell lines responding to rhKGF-1. Validation of bioactivity procedures is depicted in detail in the Results section. (**A**) CV of linearity validation (n = 20). (**B**) Recovery rate (n = 12 for the HEK293-Luc cell line and n = 9 for the HaCat-Luc cell line), $p = 0.0057$. (**C**) CV of accuracy validation (n = 5 for the HEK293-Luc cell line and n = 4 for the HaCat-Luc cell line). (**D**) CV of precision validation (n = 10). (**E**) Relative bioactivity of the final rhKGF-1 product (n = 12). (**F**) Relative bioactivity of bulk rhKGF-1 (n = 12). The mean ± SD is shown. ** $p < 0.01$.

3. Discussion

KGF is a member of the FGF family and is an epithelial-specific growth factor. Studies have indicated that KGF can induce cell proliferation and mitogenic responses in various cell types by binding to the KGF receptor (KGFR) [3]. The KGFR is cell surface FGFR2 IIIb, a splice variant of the FGFR2 gene that belongs to the receptor tyrosine kinase (RTK) family [11]. *KGFR* mRNA has been detected in almost all of the examined tissues, yet KGFR is expressed exclusively in epithelial cells. It confers the characteristics of proliferation and differentiation with KGF stimulation [2,13]. A previous study indicated that *Fgfr2* gene expression in embryonic kidney tissue was one of the most relevant aspects of renal development [32]. Therefore, we proposed HEK293 and HaCat cell lines as candidates in the subsequent study, as the former was derived from human embryonic kidney, and the HaCat cell line was derived from a human keratinocyte cell line spontaneously immortalized from a primary culture of keratinocytes, and widely used as a model to study keratinocyte differentiation [33,34]. Furthermore, the HEK293 and HaCat cell lines are robust enough to be handled and cultured.

FGFR2 IIIb plays a critical role in the MAPK, PI3K/AKT/mTOR, and PLCγ intracellular signaling pathways, and it contributes to the biological activity of KGF involved in proliferation, differentiation, and migration [3,35]. In the MAPK pathway, the KGF-KGFR complex induces autophosphorylation of KGFR's tyrosine kinase domains and phosphorylation of its intracellular domain. These changes assemblages opportunities for FGFR substrate 2α (frs2α) docking protein, which then sequentially activates Raf, MEK, and ERK. Finally, the activated ERK translocates to the nucleus, where it activates transcription factors and induces cell proliferation [14,36]. In this study, we suggest that SRE response element can drive expression of the luciferase reporter gene in response to activation of the MAPK/ERK signaling pathway. Furthermore, we describe a new bioassay to determine the bioactivity of rhKGF-1 based on the luciferase reporter gene driven by SRE in HEK293 and HaCat cells bearing FGFR2 IIIb. The two target cell lines were labeled with HEK293-Luc and HaCat-Luc.

It is well known that heparan sulfate (HS) in the extracellular matrix and proteoglycans on the surfaces of cells act as obligatory co-receptors, facilitating the binding of FGF to FGFR. This confers FGF dimerization, increases receptor binding affinity, and stabilizes the FGF-FGFR complex [21,25,36,37]. Moreover, KGF-1 and KGF-2 have been shown to bind to HS. In the optimized procedure, heparin, a proxy HS, was investigated in assay media. We found that the RLU value of top asymptote of 0–2 μg/mL of heparin was higher than that of 5–40 μg/mL of heparin, and a better SNR was appeared in 2 μg/mL of heparin in assay media.

The method validation was in line accordance with the regular requirements as stated in the ICH Q2 (R1) guidelines, AAPS/FDA Bioanalytical Workshop and the Chinese Pharmacopoeia. Typical validation which should be considered are specificity, linearity, accuracy, precision, and robustness [38,39]. The new bioassay described was based on double-transfected cells harboring the full-length FGFR2 IIIb and luciferase-SRE, which were obtained from Promega with an improved synthetically derived luciferase reporter gene (luc2P). First we found that the validated method produced a better SNR and sensitivity than cells without the FGFR2 IIIb but having the luciferase-SRE vector (data not shown). Second, the specificity was assessed using other therapeutic cytokines (Figure 3C). We found that rhKGF-1 appeared to exhibit absolute specificity for FGFR2 IIIb, whereas rhKGF-2 exhibits similar ability to bind to FGFR2 IIIb but also binds FGFR1 IIIb [2]. We think that a slight responsiveness to rhEGF is probably due to the same signaling pathway as seen in KGF, and HEK293 cells expressing EGF receptor. Therefore, to improve responsiveness to KGF, specific FGFR2 IIIb was stably transfected into cells. Non-responsiveness to rhbFGF (rhFGF2) was seen, which was the expected result, because its specific receptors, i.e., FGFR1c, FGFR3c, FGFR2c, FGFR1b, and FGFR4, are different from FGFR2 IIIb [9]. This also showed that there is high sensitivity in detecting the bioactivity of degraded rhKGF-1.

As for the acceptance criteria of CV values in analytical method validation, we followed the AAPS/FDA Bioanalytical Workshop acceptance criteria for precision and accuracy, i.e., the acknowledged CV values of 15% to 20% [40]. Actually, in our study, all of the CV values had an advantage over the acceptance criteria. Thereinto, the CV values of repeatability and linearity were less than 5%; the CV values of accuracy were lower than 8.00%. Additionally, a clear recovery rates and stability for desired HEK293-Luc cells were demonstrated, as the recovery rates ranged from 81.35% to 101.90%, and there was stability of the sensitivity and SNR between passage 16 and passage 42.

We have optimized and characterized two cell lines to measure the bioactivity of rhKGF-1. Although concordance between HEK293-Luc and HaCat-Luc cells (except in the recovery rate) was shown, the HEK293-Luc cell line was preferentially chosen compared to HaCat-Luc cell line because of its increased sensitivity and a higher SNR to rhKGF-1 treatment. Regarding the recovery rate, it is not essential to have 100% recovery, but it is important that the recovery be reproducible [41]. Moreover, the parallelism of the dose-response curves and the similarity of SNR and EC_{50} between RPMI 1640 media and cell culture plate obtained from Thermo Fisher indicated the consistency and robustness of the HEK293-Luc cell line in determining the bioactivity of rhKGF-1 (Figure S2B).

4. Materials and Methods

4.1. Cells and Materials

The HEK293 cell line (CRL-1573™) was obtained from the American Type Culture Collection (Manassas, VA, USA). The HaCat cell line (3111C0001CCC00037) was purchased from National Infrastructure of Cell Line Resource (Beijing, China). All of the cells were maintained in DMEM containing 10% fetal bovine serum (FBS) at 37 °C in a humidified 5% CO_2 incubator. DMEM, RPMI1640, FBS, puromycin, and hygromycin B were purchased from Gibco (Grand Island, NY, USA). pGL4.33[luc2p/SRE/Hygro] firefly luciferase reporter plasmid and ViaFect™ transfection reagent were obtained from Promega (Madison, WI, USA). Lentivirus production for the human FGFR2 IIIb gene (GenBank No: NM_022970) was completed by the Genechem Company (Shanghai, China). The Britelite Plus Reporter Gene Assay System was obtained from PerkinElmer (Waltham, MA, USA). An in-house rhKGF reference, rhKGF1, rhKGF2, recombinant human epidermal growth factor (rhEGF), recombinant human basic fibroblast growth factor (rhbFGF), recombinant human erythropoietin (rhEPO), and nerve growth factor (NGF) were archived therapeutic drugs that had been preserved at 4 °C or −80 °C in our laboratory.

4.2. Preparation of Desired Responsive Cells to rhKGF-1

The serum response element (SRE)-luciferase reporter plasmid was transfected into exponentially dividing HEK293 and HaCat cells using ViaFect™ transfection reagent according to the manufacturer's instructions. The transfected cells received regular changes of DMEM-10% FBS with hygromycin B (300 μg/mL), and were continuously cultured for 3–4 weeks. For FGFR2 IIIb, hygromycin B-resistant HEK293 and HaCat cells were then infected with lentivirus containing the human FGFR2 IIIb gene as per the manufacturer's recommendations. Following a change of media with hygromycin B and puromycin (3 μg/mL), the two cell lines were incubated for an additional 72–120 h. Then, a clonal cell line derived from a single cell was produced by limiting dilution in a 96-well plate, using 0.8 cells per well from the stably transfected cells. After isolating the clones, clone scale-up and screening assessments (responsive to rhKGF-1 stimulation) were performed. We desired cells that would be highly responsive to rhKGF-1, and obtained such cells and named them HEK293-Luc and HaCat-Luc. The target cell lines were maintained in DMEM-10% FBS with 200 μg/mL of hygromycin B and 1.5 μg/mL puromycin. Hereafter this media is referred to as growth media.

4.3. Bioactivity Assay

A cell-based bioassay was performed as described previously with moderate modifications [29,30]. In brief, 4×10^4 cells in 60 μL assay media (DMEM with 0.5% FBS and 2 μg/mL heparin) were added to each well of a 96-well cell plate (3903, Costar, New York, NY, USA) and were incubated for 16–18 h in a humidified 5% CO_2 incubator at 37 °C.

An in-house rhKGF-1 reference and rhKGF-1 were diluted by serial 3-fold dilutions with assay media, starting from initial concentrations of 240 ng/mL on the HEK293-Luc cells and 600 ng/mL on the HaCat-Luc cells. Then, 60 μL of serially diluted rhKGF-1 was added to each well. It should be noted that the final concentrations of rhKGF-1 were 120 ng/mL for HEK293-Luc and 300 ng/mL for HaCat-Luc. After incubation for 4–5 h at 37 °C, with 5% CO_2, the supernatant was removed from each well, followed by addition of 60 μL Britelite Plus Reporter Gene Assay reagent. After 5 min of incubation at room temperature in the dark, the luciferase activity was determined by a Luminoscan Ascent plate reader (SpectraMax M5, Molecular Devices, San Jose, CA, USA).

4.4. Preparation of Forced Degradation from rhKGF-1

The specificity of the bioassay was assessed by the presence of degraded components of rhKGF-1. It is known that with increasing temperature, proteins may undergo conformational changes, subsequently leading to other degradation reactions [42]. Therefore, forced degradation of rhKGF-1 was induced through thermal stress. That is, the reconstitution of freeze-dried rhKGF-1 was incubated at 37 °C for 1 d, 3 d, and 5 d. The relative bioactivity for the stressed samples was compared with the bioactivity of samples that had not undergone degradation treatment. We performed this bioactivity assay using HEK293-Luc cells under the same conditions as described above.

4.5. Data Analysis and Statistics

All of the statistical analyses were performed using SoftMaxPro (Molecular Devices) and GraphPad Prism 7.0 (GraphPad Software Inc., San Diego, CA, USA). The sigmoidal curve and the concentration for 50% maximal effect (EC_{50}) were calculated through a four-parameter model (dose-response-stimulation). The relative bioactivity of rhKGF-1 is shown as the ratio of the EC_{50} values of an in-house reference to the EC_{50} values of the samples. The SNR is indicated by the ratio of the top asymptote to the bottom asymptote. Comparisons between two groups were performed using a two-tailed Mann-Whitney test, and multiple comparisons were performed using a Kruskal-Wallis test with Dunn's multiple comparisons. p-values < 0.05 were deemed to be statistically significant.

5. Conclusions

In summary, we describe a highly timesaving, sensitive, and simple bioassay. This is the first use of an SRE-dependent reporter gene assay to determine rhKGF bioactivity. This bioassay has a superior specificity, linearity, accuracy, precision, and robustness, and could provide invaluable information for quality control during the manufacture, research, and development of therapeutic rhKGF.

Supplementary Materials: The following are available online, Figure S1: The establishment of responsive HaCat-Luc cells for rhKGF-1 bioactivity, Figure S2: The robustness of assays on rhKGF-1 bioactivity, Figure S3: Determination of the quantitation range of rhKGF-1, Table S1: Statistical evaluation of linearity studies, Table S2: Statistical data of linearity, recovery and precision studies between HEK293-Luc and HaCat-Luc cell lines.

Author Contributions: Conceptualization, W.Y., C.R. and J.W.; Data Curation, X.S., Formal Analysis, X.S., Funding Acquisition, Y.Z., Investigation, X.Q. and L.Y., Methodology, W.Y., Resources, Y.G. and L.L., Validation, J.H., Writing-Original Draft Preparation, W.Y., Writing-Review & Editing, C.R. and J.W., Supervision, C.R. and J.W.

Funding: This work was supported by MOST of China (Grant number 2018ZX09101001); and Improvement of drug quality standards of Chinese Pharmacopoeia (Grant number 2018S001).

Conflicts of Interest: The authors declare that they have no conflict of interest

References

1. Rubin, J.S.; Osada, H.; Finch, P.W.; Taylor, W.G.; Rudikoff, S.; Aaronson, S.A. Purification and characterization of a newly identified growth factor specific for epithelial cells. *Proc. Natl. Acad. Sci. USA* **1989**, *86*, 802–806. [CrossRef] [PubMed]
2. Farrell, C.L.; Scully, S.; Danilenko, D.M. *Keratinocyte Growth Factor*; Elservier Science Ltd.: Amsterdam, The Netherlands, 2002; pp. 1–16. [CrossRef]
3. Nakao, Y.; Mitsuyasu, T.; Kawano, S.; Nakamura, N.; Kanda, S.; Nakamura, S. Fibroblast growth factors 7 and 10 are involved in ameloblastoma proliferation via the mitogen-activated protein kinase pathway. *Int. J. Oncol.* **2013**, *43*, 1377–1384. [CrossRef] [PubMed]
4. Yamasaki, M.; Miyake, A.; Tagashira, S.; Itoh, N. Structure and expression of the rat mRNA encoding a novel member of the fibroblast growth factor family. *J. Biol. Chem.* **1996**, *271*, 15918–15921. [CrossRef] [PubMed]
5. Aaronson, S.A.; Bottaro, D.P.; Miki, T.; Ron, D.; Finch, P.W.; Fleming, T.P.; Ahn, J.; Taylor, W.G.; Rubin, J.S. Keratinocyte growth factor. A fibroblast growth factor family member with unusual target cell specificity. *Ann. N. Y. Acad. Sci.* **1991**, *638*, 62–77. [CrossRef] [PubMed]
6. Finch, P.W.; Rubin, J.S.; Miki, T.; Ron, D.; Aaronson, S.A. Human KGF is FGF-related with properties of a paracrine effector of epithelial cell growth. *Science* **1989**, *245*, 752–755. [CrossRef] [PubMed]
7. Emoto, H.; Tagashira, S.; Mattei, M.G.; Yamasaki, M.; Hashimoto, G.; Katsumata, T.; Negoro, T.; Nakatsuka, M.; Birnbaum, D.; Coulier, F.; et al. Structure and expression of human fibroblast growth factor-10. *J. Biol. Chem.* **1997**, *272*, 23191–23194. [CrossRef] [PubMed]

8. Igarashi, M.; Finch, P.W.; Aaronson, S.A. Characterization of recombinant human fibroblast growth factor (FGF)-10 reveals functional similarities with keratinocyte growth factor (FGF-7). *J. Biol. Chem.* **1998**, *273*, 13230–13235. [CrossRef]
9. Hui, Q.; Jin, Z.; Li, X.; Liu, C.; Wang, X. FGF Family: From Drug Development to Clinical Application. *Int. J. Mol. Sci.* **2018**, *19*, 1875. [CrossRef]
10. Radtke, M.L.; Kolesar, J.M. Palifermin (Kepivance) for the treatment of oral mucositis in patients with hematologic malignancies requiring hematopoietic stem cell support. *J. Oncol. Pharm. Pract.* **2005**, *11*, 121–125. [CrossRef]
11. Moghadasi, M.; Ilghari, D.; Sirati-Sabet, M.; Amini, A.; Asghari, H.; Gheibi, N. Structural characterization of recombinant human fibroblast growth factor receptor 2b kinase domain upon interaction with omega fatty acids. *Chem. Phys. Lipids* **2017**, *202*, 21–27. [CrossRef]
12. Dell, K.R.; Williams, L.T. A novel form of fibroblast growth factor receptor 2. Alternative splicing of the third immunoglobulin-like domain confers ligand binding specificity. *J. Biol. Chem.* **1992**, *267*, 21225–21229. [PubMed]
13. Belleudi, F.; Purpura, V.; Torrisi, M.R. The receptor tyrosine kinase FGFR2b/KGFR controls early differentiation of human keratinocytes. *PLoS ONE* **2011**, *6*, e24194. [CrossRef] [PubMed]
14. Ornitz, D.M.; Itoh, N. The Fibroblast Growth Factor signaling pathway. *Wiley Interdiscip. Rev. Dev. Biol.* **2015**, *4*, 215–266. [CrossRef] [PubMed]
15. Zhang, X.; Ibrahimi, O.A.; Olsen, S.K.; Umemori, H.; Mohammadi, M.; Ornitz, D.M. Receptor specificity of the fibroblast growth factor family. The complete mammalian FGF family. *J. Biol. Chem.* **2006**, *281*, 15694–15700. [CrossRef] [PubMed]
16. Turner, N.; Grose, R. Fibroblast growth factor signalling: from development to cancer. *Nat. Rev. Cancer* **2010**, *10*, 116–129. [CrossRef] [PubMed]
17. Desai, A.; Adjei, A.A. FGFR Signaling as a Target for Lung Cancer Therapy. *J. Thorac. Oncol.* **2016**, *11*, 9–20. [CrossRef] [PubMed]
18. Portnoy, J.; Curran-Everett, D.; Mason, R.J. Keratinocyte growth factor stimulates alveolar type II cell proliferation through the extracellular signal-regulated kinase and phosphatidylinositol 3-OH kinase pathways. *Am. J. Respir. Cell Mol. Biol.* **2004**, *30*, 901–907. [CrossRef] [PubMed]
19. Geer, D.J.; Swartz, D.D.; Andreadis, S.T. Biomimetic Delivery of Keratinocyte Growth Factor upon Cellular Demand for Accelerated Wound Healing in Vitro and in Vivo. *Am. J. Pathol.* **2005**, *167*, 1575–1586. [CrossRef]
20. Terakawa, J.; Rocchi, A.; Serna, V.A.; Bottinger, E.P.; Graff, J.M.; Kurita, T. FGFR2IIIb-MAPK Activity Is Required for Epithelial Cell Fate Decision in the Lower Mullerian Duct. *Mol. Endocrinol.* **2016**, *30*, 783–795. [CrossRef] [PubMed]
21. Osslund, T.D.; Syed, R.; Singer, E.; Hsu, E.W.; Nybo, R.; Chen, B.L.; Harvey, T.; Arakawa, T.; Narhi, L.O.; Chirino, A.; et al. Correlation between the 1.6 A crystal structure and mutational analysis of keratinocyte growth factor. *Protein Sci.* **1998**, *7*, 1681–1690. [CrossRef] [PubMed]
22. Yuan, A.; Sonis, S. Emerging therapies for the prevention and treatment of oral mucositis. *Expert Opin. Emerg. Drugs* **2014**, *19*, 343–351. [CrossRef] [PubMed]
23. Oronsky, B.; Goyal, S.; Kim, M.M.; Cabrales, P.; Lybeck, M.; Caroen, S.; Oronsky, N.; Burbano, E.; Carter, C.; Oronsky, A. A Review of Clinical Radioprotection and Chemoprotection for Oral Mucositis. *Transl. Oncol.* **2018**, *11*, 771–778. [CrossRef] [PubMed]
24. Sonis, S.T. Efficacy of palifermin (keratinocyte growth factor-1) in the amelioration of oral mucositis. *Core Evid.* **2010**, *4*, 199–205. [CrossRef] [PubMed]
25. Athar, U.; Gentile, T.C. Keratinocyte growth factor. *Expert Opin. Biol. Ther.* **2009**, *9*, 779–787. [CrossRef]
26. Bahadori, Z.; Kalhor, H.R.; Mowla, S.J. Producing functional recombinant human keratinocyte growth factor in Pichia pastoris and investigating its protective role against irradiation. *Enzyme Microb. Technol.* **2018**, *111*, 12–20. [CrossRef] [PubMed]
27. Wu, J.C.; Beale, K.K.; Ma, J.D. Evaluation of current and upcoming therapies in oral mucositis prevention. *Future Oncol.* **2010**, *6*, 1751–1770. [CrossRef] [PubMed]
28. Ornitz, D.M.; Xu, J.; Colvin, J.S.; McEwen, D.G.; MacArthur, C.A.; Coulier, F.; Gao, G.; Goldfarb, M. Receptor specificity of the fibroblast growth factor family. *J. Biol. Chem.* **1996**, *271*, 15292–15297. [CrossRef]

29. Yang, Y.; Zhou, Y.; Yu, L.; Li, X.; Shi, X.; Qin, X.; Rao, C.; Wang, J. A novel reporter gene assay for Recombinant Human Erythropoietin (rHuEPO) pharmaceutical products. *J. Pharm. Biomed. Anal.* **2014**, *100*, 316–321. [CrossRef]
30. Larocque, L.; Bliu, A.; Xu, R.; Diress, A.; Wang, J.; Lin, R.; He, R.; Girard, M.; Li, X. Bioactivity Determination of Native and Variant Forms of Therapeutic Interferons. *J. Biomed. Biotechnol.* **2011**, *2011*, 1–11. [CrossRef]
31. Li, Y.; Igne, B.; Drennen, J.K., 3rd; Anderson, C.A. Method development and validation for pharmaceutical tablets analysis using transmission Raman spectroscopy. *Int. J. Pharm.* **2016**, *498*, 318–325. [CrossRef]
32. Bates, C.M. Role of fibroblast growth factor receptor signaling in kidney development. *Am. J. Physiol. Renal Physiol.* **2011**, *301*, F245–F251. [CrossRef]
33. Capone, A.; Visco, V.; Belleudi, F.; Marchese, C.; Cardinali, G.; Bellocci, M.; Picardo, M.; Frati, L.; Torrisi, M.R. Up-modulation of the expression of functional keratinocyte growth factor receptors induced by high cell density in the human keratinocyte HaCaT cell line. *Cell Growth Differ.* **2000**, *11*, 607–614.
34. Boukamp, P.; Petrussevska, R.T.; Breitkreutz, D.; Hornung, J.; Markham, A.; Fusenig, N.E. Normal keratinization in a spontaneously immortalized aneuploid human keratinocyte cell line. *J. Cell Biol.* **1988**, *106*, 761–771. [CrossRef] [PubMed]
35. Zhang, Y.M.; Zhang, Z.Q.; Liu, Y.Y.; Zhou, X.; Shi, X.H.; Jiang, Q.; Fan, D.L.; Cao, C. Requirement of Galphai1/3-Gab1 signaling complex for keratinocyte growth factor-induced PI3K-AKT-mTORC1 activation. *J. Invest. Dermatol.* **2015**, *135*, 181–191. [CrossRef] [PubMed]
36. Price, C.A. Mechanisms of fibroblast growth factor signaling in the ovarian follicle. *J. Endocrinol.* **2016**, *228*, R31–R43. [CrossRef]
37. Xu, R.; Rudd, T.R.; Hughes, A.J.; Siligardi, G.; Fernig, D.G.; Yates, E.A. Analysis of the fibroblast growth factor receptor (FGFR) signalling network with heparin as coreceptor: Evidence for the expansion of the core FGFR signalling network. *FEBS J.* **2013**, *280*, 2260–2270. [CrossRef] [PubMed]
38. ICH. *International Conference on Harmonization (ICH) Guidelines ICH Q2(R1), Validation of Analytical Procedures: Text and Methodology*; ICH: Geneva, Switzerland, 2005.
39. Chinese Pharmacopoeia Commission. *Chinese Pharmacopoeia*, 4th ed.; People's Medical Publishing House: Beijing, China, 2015.
40. Viswanathan, C.T.; Bansal, S.; Booth, B.; DeStefano, A.J.; Rose, M.J.; Sailstad, J.; Shah, V.P.; Skelly, J.P.; Swann, P.G.; Weiner, R. Quantitative bioanalytical methods validation and implementation: best practices for chromatographic and ligand binding assays. *Pharm. Res.* **2007**, *24*, 1962–1973. [CrossRef]
41. Booth, B.; Arnold, M.E.; DeSilva, B.; Amaravadi, L.; Dudal, S.; Fluhler, E.; Gorovits, B.; Haidar, S.H.; Kadavil, J.; Lowes, S.; et al. Workshop report: Crystal City V–quantitative bioanalytical method validation and implementation: the 2013 revised FDA guidance. *AAPS J.* **2015**, *17*, 277–288. [CrossRef] [PubMed]
42. Hawe, A.; Wiggenhorn, M.; van de Weert, M.; Garbe, J.H.O.; Mahler, H.-C.; Jiskoot, W. Forced Degradation of Therapeutic Proteins. *J. Pharm. Sci.* **2012**, *101*, 895–913. [CrossRef] [PubMed]

Sample Availability: Samples of the compounds rhKGF1 and rhKGF2 are available from the authors.

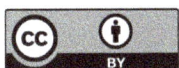

© 2019 by the authors. Licensee MDPI, Basel, Switzerland. This article is an open access article distributed under the terms and conditions of the Creative Commons Attribution (CC BY) license (http://creativecommons.org/licenses/by/4.0/).

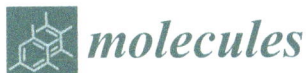

Article

Two Approaches for Evaluating the Effects of Galangin on the Activities and mRNA Expression of Seven CYP450

Yin-Ling Ma [1,2], Feng Zhao [1], Jin-Tuo Yin [1], Cai-Juan Liang [1], Xiao-Li Niu [2], Zhi-Hong Qiu [2] and Lan-Tong Zhang [1,*]

1. Department of Pharmaceutical Analysis, School of Pharmacy, Hebei Medical University, Shijiazhuang 050017, China; maling-shz@163.com (Y.-L.M.); zhaofeng-37@163.com (F.Z.); yinjintuo@163.com (J.-T.Y.); caijuanliang@126.com (C.-J.L.)
2. National Clinical Drug Monitoring Center, Department of Pharmacy, Hebei Province General Center, Shijiazhuang 050051, China; niuxl0327@163.com (X.-L.N.); 15930818866@126.com (Z.-H.Q.)
* Correspondence: zhanglantong@263.net; Tel.: +86-0311-86266419

Academic Editors: In-Soo Yoon and Hyun-Jong Cho
Received: 1 March 2019; Accepted: 22 March 2019; Published: 25 March 2019

Abstract: Galangin is a marker compound of honey and *Alpinia officinarum* Hance that exhibits great potential for anti-microbial, anti-diabetic, anti-obesity, anti-tumour and anti-inflammatory applications. Galangin is frequently consumed in combination with common clinical drugs. Here, we evaluated the effects of galangin on cytochrome P450 (CYP)-mediated metabolism, using two different approaches, to predict drug–drug interactions. Male Sprague Dawley rats were administered galangin daily for 8 weeks. A "cocktail-probes" approach was employed to evaluate the activities of different CYP450 enzymes. Blood samples of seven probe drugs were analysed using liquid chromatography-tandem mass spectrometry in positive and negative electrospray-ionisation modes. Pharmacokinetic parameters were calculated to identify statistical differences. CYP mRNA-expression levels were investigated in real-time quantitative polymerase chain reaction experiments. The galangin-treated group showed significantly decreased $AUC_{0-\infty}$ and C_{max} values for CYP1A2, and CYP2B3. The galangin-treated group showed significantly increased $AUC_{0-\infty}$ and C_{max} values for CYP2C13 and CYP3A1. No significant influences were observed in the pharmacokinetic profiles of CYP2C11, CYP2D4 and CYP2E1. The mRNA-expression results were consistent with the pharmacokinetic results. Thus, CYP450 enzyme activities may be altered by long-term galangin administration, suggesting galangin to be a promising candidate molecule for enhancing oral drug bioavailability and chemoprevention and reversing multidrug resistance.

Keywords: CYP450 enzyme; cocktail probe drug; RT-PCR; LC-MS/MS; galangin

1. Introduction

Cytochrome P450 (CYP450) is a phase I metabolic enzyme that is expressed in multiple biological organs. It is mainly responsible for transforming endogenous and exogenous substances, including drugs, in vivo. When the activity of cytochrome P450 is disturbed, it can affect the metabolic links of corresponding substrates and cause various biological effects [1]. By evaluating the activity of CYP450, we can predict possible drug–drug interactions, drug–food interactions and the compatibility mechanisms of Chinese herbs in vivo, and provide valuable clinical information for drug combinations and compatibility with the daily diet.

Galangin, a natural flavonoid, is a marker compound of honey and *Alpinia officina rum* Hance (Zingiberaceae family) [2], which exhibits great potential in terms of its anti-microbial [3], anti-diabetic [4], anti-obesity [5], anti-tumour [6], anti-inflammatory properties [7], anti-oxidant [8], anti-osteoporosis [9] and lipid regulating effects [10]. Based on the wide application of galangin in food, medicine and health care products, and the lack of research on the biological interactions of galangin, this study was designed to investigate the effects of galangin on the CYP1A2, CYP2B3, CYP2C11, CYP2C13, CYP2D4, CYP2E1 and CYP3A1 enzymes in rats. First, liquid chromatography/tandem mass spectrometry (LC-MS/MS) was used to establish a method for simultaneously probing the levels of seven drugs in rat plasma samples: phenacetin, bupropion, diclofenac acid, omeprazole, dextromethorphan, chlorzoxazone and midazolam. Then, probes were used to study the effects of galangin on the activities of seven metabolic enzymes. Finally, real-time fluorescence quantitative polymerase chain reaction (PCR)was used to evaluate galangin mRNA expression. The effects of galangin on the expression of seven metabolic enzymes in rats were comprehensively analysed, and potential interactions between galangin and drug combinations were predicted.

2. Results and Discussion

2.1. High-Performance Liquid Chromatography–Tandem Mass Spectrometry (HPLC-MS/MS) Method Development

Different HPLC-MS/MS methods for simultaneous quantitative determination of probe drugs have been published [11,12]. However, only four methods employed simultaneous quantitative assays with multiple probes [11–14]. Lu et al. [11] established an HPLC-MS/MS method for evaluating the activity of seven CYP isoenzymes (CYP1A2, 2B6, 2C9, 2C19, 2D6, 2E1 and 3A4) in rats, but negative-ionization mode is not sensitive enough for probing drugs such as phenacetin, bupropion and omeprazole. Kim et al. [12] used a gradient elution method to detect most metabolites in positive electrospray ionisation (ESI) mode. Li et al. [13] adopted two methods combining different HPLC systems, namely, one method that coupled a high-pressure chemical-ionization interface with MS, with the other method being negative ESI mode. Nevertheless, previous investigators [12,13] concluded that matrix effects were absent. The matrix effect is an important issue in LC-MS method development. The method by De Bock et al. [14] adopted the approach of monitoring and detecting CYP activity in either positive or negative ESI mode, which has a certain practical value. Nevertheless, two runs, one in positive-ionisation mode and one in negative-ionisation mode, were necessary in order to detect all metabolites.

Recently, we used an LC-MS method to quantify seven probe drugs. A more intense and stable signal for the seven probe drugs and the internal standard (IS) was observed by ESI, in positive and negative ion-switching mode. The precursor and daughter ions were selected and the MS/MS parameters were optimized to give the highest response in multiple-reaction monitoring (MRM) mode (Figure 1 and Table 1). A Wonda Cract ODS-2 C18 Column was employed to provide better performance for the peaks of the seven analytes in this study. A mobile phase consisting of water fortified with 0.1% formic acid enhanced the response and improved the peak shape. Considering the chemical diversity in the structures of the metabolites, a mobile phase with a gradient elution was employed to obtain better peak shapes and a shorter run time for the seven analytes and the IS, using water containing 0.1% formic acid as eluent B. Eluent A (methanol + 0.1% formic acid) was increased gradually from 45% to 90% during the course of 17.5 min, using a flow rate of 1.0 mL/min. A column temperature of 25 °C was selected to obtain a symmetric peak shape. A chromatogram in both ionization modes is shown in Figure 2. All peaks were baseline-separated.

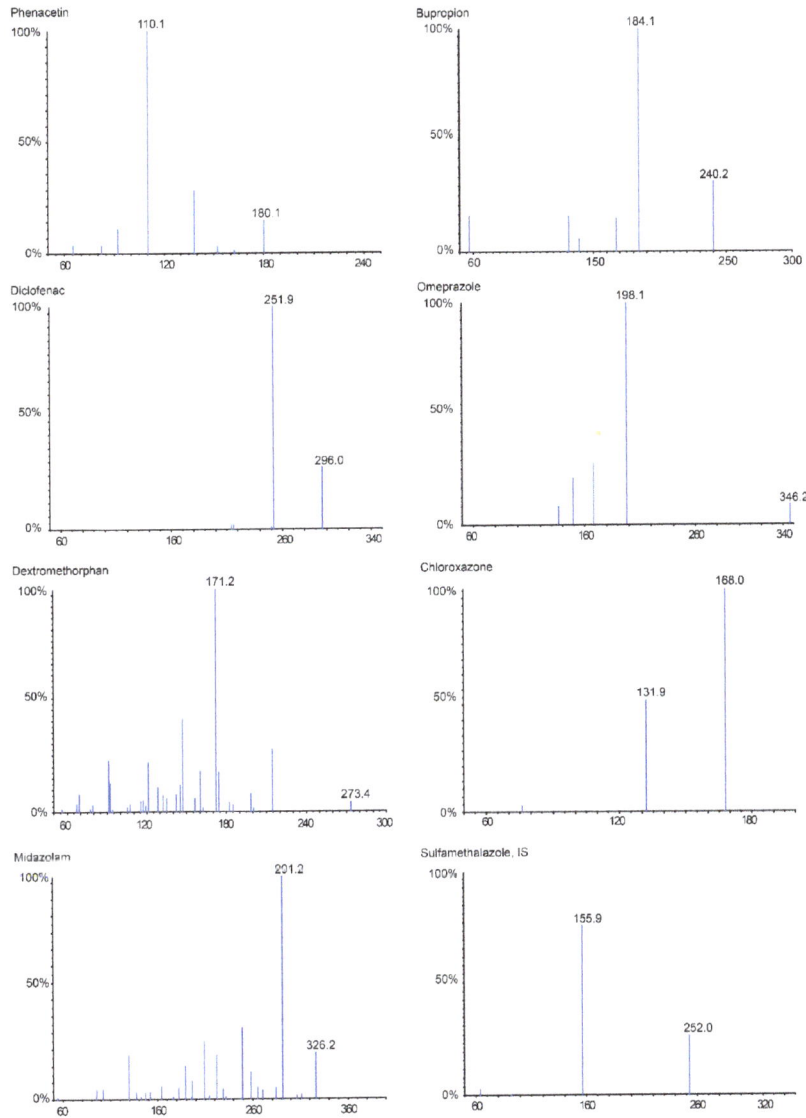

Figure 1. The MS/MS spectra of seven analytes and IS in positive and negative ion mode.

Table 1. MRM parameters for probe drugs and internal standards.

Enzyme Isoform	Probe Drug	Retention Time (min)	C (Probe Drug μmol/L)	MRM Condition			
				Precursor-Ion (m/z)	Daughter-Ion (m/z)	Fragment Energy (V)	Collision Energy (eV)
CYP1A2	Phenacetin	9.01	5	180.1	110.1	57.56	27.71
CYP2B3	Bupropion	6.29	10	240.2	184.1	64.64	17.15
CYP2C11	Diclofenac	16.68	5	296.0	251.9	−24.50	−16.50
CYP2C13	Omeprazole	11.31	10	346.2	198.1	31.38	15.29
CYP2D4	Dextromethor-phan	10.87	5	273.4	172.1	77.95	50.72
CYP2E1	Chloroxazone	14.79	10	168.0	131.9	−65.05	−27.00
CYP3A1	Midazolam	8.63	5	326.2	291.2	71.86	36.50
Internal standard	Sulfamethalaz-ole	3.99	-	252.0	155.9	−30.00	−20.00

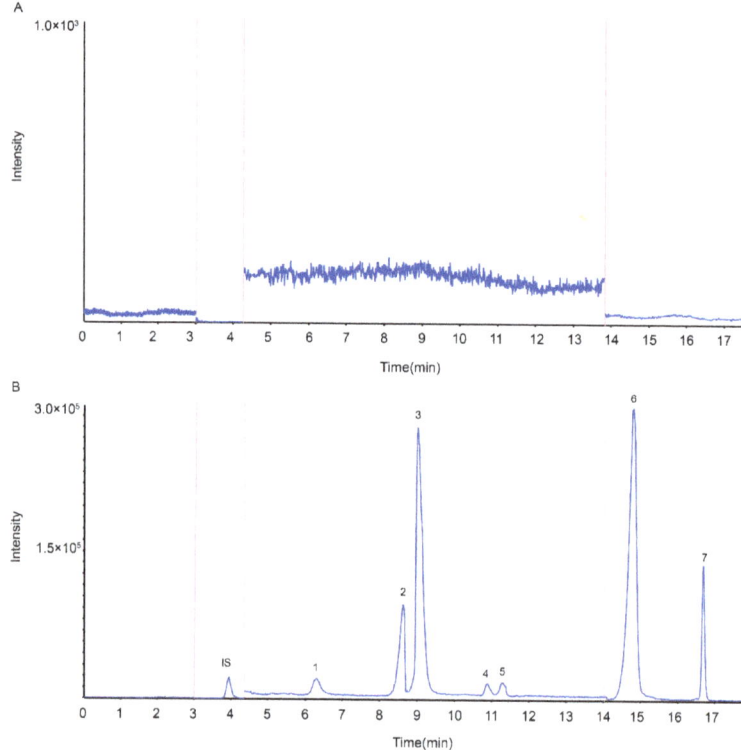

Figure 2. Chromatograms of the analytes and IS in positive ion mode. Note: (**A**) blank plasma; (**B**) sample plasma 1 h after administration of cocktail solution; (1) bupropion; (2) omeprazole; (3) phenacetin; (4) midazolam; (5) dextromethorphan; (6) chlorzoxazone; (7) diclofenac and IS.

2.2. Method Validation

A sensitive, rapid, simple and economical HPLC-MS/MS method was developed and validated for the simultaneous quantification of seven probe drugs. The method-validation procedure was based on the Guidance for Industry Bioanalytical Method Validation of the European Medicines Agency and the U.S. Food and Drug Administration (FDA) [15]. The probe drugs for phenacetin (CYP1A2), bupropion (CYP2B3), diclofenac (CYP2C11), omeprazole (CYP2C13), dextromethorphan (CYP2D4), chlorzoxazone (CYP2E1) and midazolam (CYP3A1) together with the IS sulfamethoxazole (STZ), were separated at 25 °C on a Wonda Cract ODS-2 C18 column (4.6 mm × 150 mm, inside diameter [i.d.], 5.0 μm). A gradient elution (total run time of 17.5 min) was performed, using methanol containing 0.1% (v/v) formic acid (A) and water containing 0.1% (v/v) formic acid (B) at a flow rate of 1.0 mL/min.

Calibration curves showed good linearity over the range of 1.006–2414.4 ng/mL for phenacetin ($r = 0.9933$), 0.801–403.2 ng/mL for bupropion ($r = 0.9902$), 1.01–808ng/mL for diclofenac ($r = 0.9892$), 1.1015–812 ng/mL for omeprazole ($r = 0.9918$), 0.99–247.5 ng/mL for dextromethorphan ($r = 0.9952$), 1.287–514.8 ng/mL for chlorzoxazone ($r = 0.9904$), and 2.005–6416 ng/mL for midazolam ($r = 0.9967$). The lower limits of detection of phenacetin, bupropion, diclofenac, omeprazole, dextromethorphan, chlorzoxazone, and midazolam were 1.006, 0.801, 1.01, 1.015, 0.99, 1.287 and 2.005 ng/mL, respectively. The concentrations of phenacetin, bupropion, diclofenac, omeprazole, dextromethorphan, chlorzoxazone, and midazolam in rat plasma were simultaneously determined using an HPLC-MS/MS method (Figure 2). As shown in Table 2, the intra-day and inter-day precision of the method were within 9.7%, and the accuracy ranged from 91.9% to 113.2%. The extraction recoveries for the analytes were greater than 81.4% (Table 3). All variations in the matrix effect were within the range of 84.3% to 111.1% (Table 3). The lower limit of quantification (LLOQ) was consistent with the intended application, and no relative matrix effects were observed. In addition, the sample extracts were stable under various storage conditions (Table 4). The feasibility of this method was demonstrated by calculating the pharmacokinetic parameters of the probe and CYP450 activities.

Table 2. Intra- and inter-day precision and accuracy values for probe drugs in rat plasma at LLOQ, low, medium and high concentrations ($n = 6$).

Compounds	Concentration (ng/mL)	Precision RSD (%)		Accuracy (%)	
		Intra-Day	Inter-Day	Intra-Day	Inter-Day
Phenacetin	1.006	8.21	7.06	4.12	6.23
	2.012	5.96	4.51	−2.34	−4.04
	201.20	7.35	6.30	8.41	11.79
	1609.6	4.79	4.66	3.23	5.34
Bupropion	0.801	2.91	6.43	3.52	9.23
	2.034	7.34	5.25	6.14	9.35
	20.34	6.16	2.71	5.65	7.11
	203.4	2.44	3.55	−2.47	−3.76
Diclofenac	1.01	2.80	8.34	4.98	5.92
	2.02	1.21	5.26	6.90	9.45
	20.20	4.37	4.91	7.04	8.61
	202.00	3.55	4.27	4.93	5.85
Omeprazole	1.015	2.89	3.55	11.71	12.13
	2.03	4.10	2.78	7.26	6.41
	20.30	3.62	4.40	5.85	8.28
	406	1.23	6.05	2.92	8.66
Dextromethorphan	0.99	6.41	7.03	−4.16	−6.84
	1.98	5.12	6.31	6.97	12.02
	9.9	4.75	2.26	8.77	9.52
	99	3.69	1.85	8.55	10.61
Chloroxazone	1.287	5.81	4.53	6.83	7.13
	2.574	2.33	3.75	6.32	9.06
	12.87	2.69	5.97	2.91	4.75
	257.4	5.13	4.32	5.45	8.27
Midazolam	2.005	2.01	7.08	5.86	7.85
	4.01	1.89	4.93	−3.7.83	−8.33
	401	1.13	6.12	3.39	4.27
	4010	0.71	0.63	4.11	8.31

Table 3. The mean extraction recoveries and matrix effect of the seven analytes and IS in rats plasma at low and high concentration ($n = 6$).

Compounds	Spiked Conc. (ng/mL)	Extraction Recovery (%)		Matrix Effect (%)	
		Mean ± SD	RSD (%)	Intra-Day	Inter-Day
Phenacetin	2.01	81.48 ± 5.97	7.33	102.33 ± 7.45	7.22
	1609.60	90.01 ± 3.26	3.62	92.25 ± 4.27	4.64
Bupropion	2.03	88.95 ± 6.84	7.61	93.51 ± 6.30	6.56
	203.40	94.92 ± 3.40	3.22	111.13 ± 4.16	3.77
Diclofenac	2.02	92.74 ± 4.25	3.67	85.63 ± 4.65	4.84
	404	90.20 ± 4.58	8.98	89.02 ± 8.03	3.99
Omeprazole	2.03	91.66 ± 5.25	4.51	85.64 ± 10.13	6.89
	406	93.49 ± 5.75	8.76	91.21 ± 4.63	4.56
Dextromethorphan	1.98	93.54 ± 3.68	12.58	95.23 ± 54.0	5.34
	99	94.61 ± 4.33	10.31	97.04 ± 6.21	6.30
Chloroxazone	2.574	93.52 ± 5.46	3.82	88.01 ± 7.82	5.46
	257.4	101.24 ± 5.17	9.82	86.84 ± 6.74	6.47
Midazolam	4.01	93.33 ± 5.06	4.63	84.34 ± 4.96	2.66
	4010.00	92.43 ± 2.36	6.36	89.16 ± 4.03	4.40

Table 4. Stability of seven probe drugs in rat plasma under various storage conditions ($n = 3$).

Compounds	Spiked conc. (ng/mL)	Blood Sample Stored at RT for 2 h		Blood Sample Stored at −80 °C for 15 Days		Blood Sample for Freeze-Thawing 3 Cycles		Post–Preparative Sample Stored at 4 °C for 24 h		Post–Preparative Sample Stored at RT for 4 h	
		Calc. conc (ng/mL)	Accuracy (%)	Calc. conc (ng/mL)	Accuracy (%)	Calc. conc (ng/mL)	Accuracy (%)	Calc. conc (ng/mL)	Accuracy (%)	Calc. conc (ng/mL)	Accuracy (%)
Phenacetin	10.08	9.79 ± 0.20	−2.9	9.85 ± 1.51	−2.25	9.73 ± 0.24	−3.5	9.97 ± 0.28	0.28	9.77 ± 0.50	−2.26
	201.2	203.6 ± 6.66	1.22	205.00 ± 12.53	1.89	192.30 ± 5.20	−4.42	196.96 ± 5.13	−2.12	195.72 ± 17.41	−2.73
	1609.6	1630.19 ± 61.37	1.28	1560.30 ± 12.44	−3.06	1564.93 ± 32.09	−2.78	1576.26 ± 38.13	−2.07	1561.74 ± 35.53	−2.97
Bupropion	2.3	2.42 ± 0.28	4.91	2.38 ± 0.23	3.33	2.22 ± 0.39	−3.33	2.35 ± 0.26	2.17	2.25 ± 0.35	−2.32
	20.34	20.47 ± 1.92	0.62	20.55 ± 1.92	1.02	20.98 ± 2.57	3.13	20.54 ± 0.18	0.97	19.93 ± 1.45	−2.02
	203.4	198.67 ± 12.84	−2.32	212.26 ± 22.29	4.36	196.30 ± 17.49	−3.49	206.79 ± 30.07	1.67	201.45 ± 29.70	−0.96
Diclofenac	2.02	1.95 ± 0.19	−3.63	1.99 ± 0.43	−1.65	2.05 ± 0.27	1.32	2.07 ± 0.12	2.64	2.06 ± 0.20	2.15
	20.2	19.75 ± 2.76	−2.22	20.52 ± 1.06	1.6	20.58 ± 1.42	1.88	20.45 ± 3.53	1.25	19.75 ± 2.76	−2.22
	404	401.17 ± 19.48	−0.7	404.99 ± 50.97	0.24	409.20 ± 29.18	1.29	406.63 ± 39.90	0.65	395.24 ± 14.96	−2.17
Omeprazole	2.03	2.09 ± 0.31	2.79	2.05 ± 0.34	0.99	2.00 ± 0.33	−1.48	2.07 ± 0.10	1.81	1.99 ± 0.24	−1.97
	203	205.96 ± 35.04	1.46	202.63 ± 30.88	−0.18	209.66 ± 29.66	3.1	202.63 ± 30.88	−0.18	200.91 ± 35.05	−1.02
	406	392.14 ± 32.82	−3.41	397.14 ± 35.26	−2.18	400.47 ± 38.99	−1.36	403.81 ± 23.84	−0.54	401.22 ± 31.33	−1.52
Dextromethorp–han	1.98	1.96 ± 0.16	−1.04	1.99 ± 0.12	0.67	1.93 ± 0.13	−2.53	2.01 ± 0.14	1.51	1.95 ± 0.33	−1.52
	9.9	9.88 ± 0.22	−0.24	10.03 ± 0.23	1.31	9.99 ± 2.02	0.88	9.76 ± 0.45	−1.45	9.65 ± 0.22	−2.49
	99	99.92 ± 2.14	0.93	97.2 ± 2.56	−1.82	97.87 ± 5.15	−1.14	97.55 ± 4.77	−1.99	100.38 ± 12.69	1.39
Chloroxazone	2.574	2.57 ± 0.37	−1.18	2.56 ± 0.13	0.43	2.53 ± 0.20	−0.54	2.59 ± 0.22	1.83	2.45 ± 0.31	−3.93
	12.87	12.99 ± 0.44	−1.63	13.12 ± 0.71	1.97	12.79 ± 0.44	−0.6	12.79 ± 1.24	−0.6	12.53 ± 1.43	−2.67
	257.4	250.20 ± 2.88	0.96	252.73 ± 17.27	−1.82	251.16 ± 10.37	−2.42	254.5 ± 16.71	−1.13	253.83 ± 17.43	−1.39
Midazolam	4.01	3.98 ± 0.29	−0.75	3.96 ± 0.27	−1.33	3.94 ± 0.35	−1.75	399.03 ± 11.57	2.16	4.08 ± 0.17	1.75
	401	395.70 ± 22.26	−1.32	405.7 ± 26.34	1.17	405.70 ± 25.59	1.17	399.03 ± 11.57	−0.49	406.67 ± 15.79	1.41
	4010	3969.06 ± 233.65	−1.02	4062.30 ± 108.90	1.3	4095.64 ± 87.80	2.14	3962.30 ± 66.21	−1.18	3995.64 ± 112.78	−0.36

2.3. Selection of CYP450 Isozymes

The liver is the most important scavenging organ for drugs and exogenous substances. Drugs are mainly metabolized by CYP enzymes in the liver. In the human body, the main CYP enzymes involved in drug metabolism include CYP1A2, CYP2B6, CYP2C9, CYP2C19, CYP2D6, CYP3A4 and CYP2E1, among which CYP2C9, CYP2D6 and CYP3A4 account for approximately 50% of the total liver CYP enzyme levels and can metabolize nearly 80% of all clinical drugs [16]. Human CYP1A2, CYP2B6, CYP2C9, CYP2C19, CYP2D6, CYP3A4 and CYP2E1 share high homology with rat CYP1A2, CYP2B3, CYP2C11, CYP2C13, CYP2D4, CYP3A1 and CYP2E1, respectively [17]. CYP1A2 is mainly distributed in the liver, accounting for 13% of the total CYP450. CYP1A2 is the main metabolic enzyme of warfarin, theophylline, clozapine, haloperidol and other drugs with a narrow therapeutic window [18]. The activity of CYP1A2 may change the exposure level of the above drugs in vivo and cause serious adverse drug reactions. CYP2B3 participates in the metabolism of approximately 7% of clinical drugs in vivo, including the anti-cancer drugs cyclophosphamide and tamoxifen, the anti-HIV drug Faviron, the anti-depressant imipramine, the intravenous anaesthetics propofol and ketamine, and the analgesic pethidine. CYP2B3 is also involved in the metabolism of carcinogens and environmental toxicants [19], making it an important exogenous metabolic enzyme. CYP3A4 is one of the most abundant CYP450 isoenzymes in the human body. Macrolactone antibiotics, antifungal agents, 3-hydroxy-3-methyl-glutaryl-coenzyme A (HMG-CoA) inhibitors, benzodiazepines, proton pump inhibitors, calcium channel blockers and other common clinical drugs are metabolized through CYP3A4 [20]. The CYP2E1 isoenzyme is a potent source for oxidative stress. Oxidative stress is critical for the pathogenesis of diseases and CYP2E1 is a major contributor to oxidative stress. When taking the above-mentioned medications, it is possible to take Chinese herbal medicine or dietary supplements containing galangin or related ingredients at the same time to induce or inhibit metabolic enzymes, which may lead to fluctuations of the therapeutic effect or an increase in metabolite concentrations and subsequent adverse reactions. In this study, seven rat-related isoenzymes were selected: CYP1A2, CYP2B3, CYP2C11, CYP2C13, CYP2D4, CYP3A1, and CYP2E1. The activities of the seven main CYP450 enzymes were determined using a sensitive, accurate, and reliable probe method.

2.4. Effect of Galangin on the Activities of Rat Liver CYPs

The plasma samples were collected and determined using the established method. The plasma concentration at each time point was calculated based on the standard curve. Average drug–time curves of the blank group and the drug-delivery group for the seven probe drugs were drawn using GraphPad prism 7.0.0 software (Figure 3). Pharmacokinetic parameters were calculated and analysed using DAS 3.2.4 and SPSS 21.0 software, respectively (Table 5). Compared with the control group, the CYP isoenzymes of the galangin group showed significant changes after 8 weeks of galangin administration.

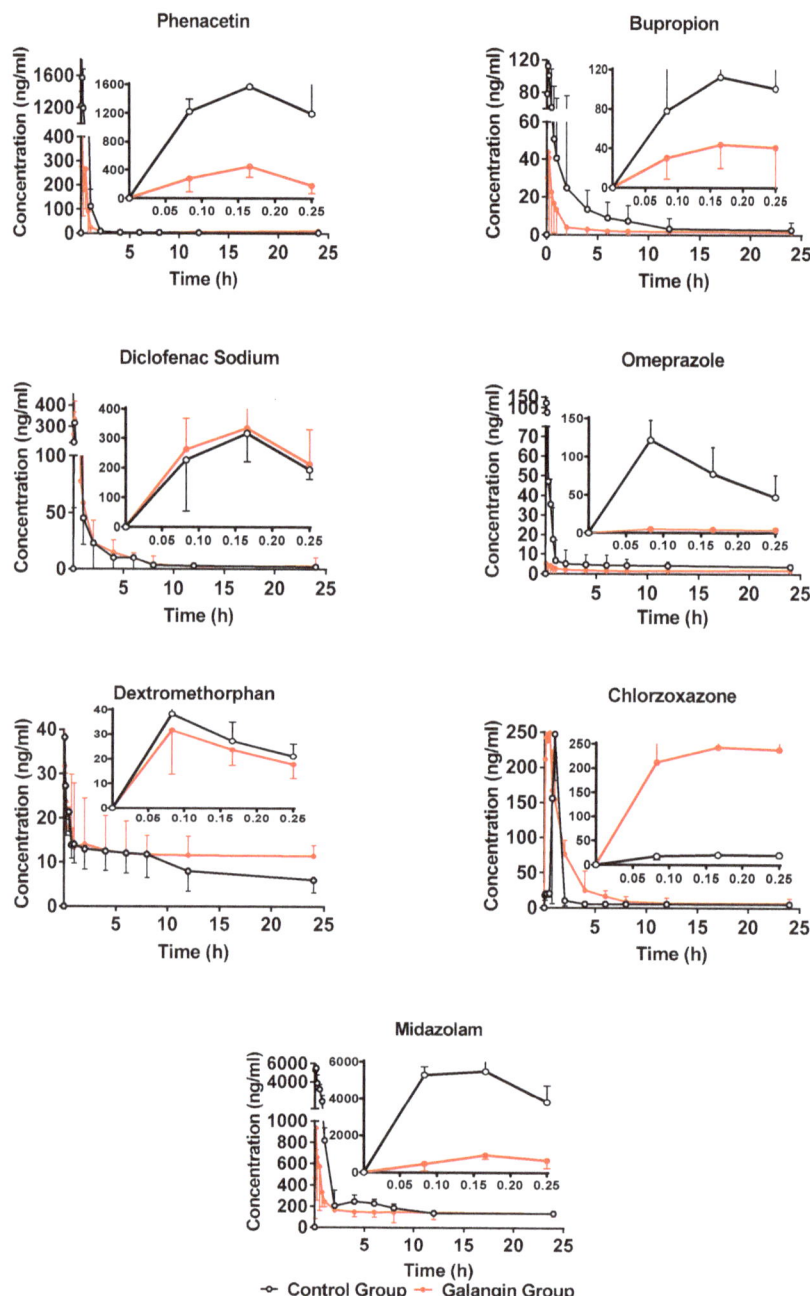

Figure 3. Mean plasma concentration–time curves of seven analytes in rats (mean ± SD, n = 6).

Table 5. Pharmacokinetic parameters of seven analytes in rat plasma after a single oral administration of a probe drugs solution in rats ($n = 6$).

Analytes	Group	$AUC_{(0-t)}$ (µg·h/L)	$AUC_{(0-\infty)}$ (µg·h/L)	C_{max} (ug/L)	T_{max} (h)	$T_{1/2}$ (h)
Phenacetin	Blank	1194.97 ±620.95	1276.56 ±617.86	1442.54 ±250.87	0.14 ±0.04	2.46 ±0.94
	Treat	327.63 ** ±228.18	353.22 ** ±224.12	433.42 ** ±147.95	0.16 ±0.06	1.38 * ±1.45
Bupropion	Blank	165.25 ±2.94	201.94 ±24.20	101.5 ±14.49	0.22 ±0.04	3.25 ±1.18
	Treat	51.13 ** ±14.68	64.91 ** ±17.01	57.97 ** ±18.09	0.19 ±0.05	4.05 ±1.42
Diclofenac	Blank	386.52 ±132.62	400.40 ±127.67	425.78 ±124.74	0.12 ±0.04	1.38 ±0.46
	Treat	397.96 ±18.43	430.27 ±238.07	354.53 ±84.72	0.15 ±0.03	2.01 ±0.630
Omeprazole	Blank	75.30 ±12.22	129.70 ±23.10	95.76 ±35.93	0.083 ±0.01	10.86 ±4.08
	Treat	126.86 * ±29.32	165.33 * ±29.54	159.49 * ±58.26	0.081 ±0.01	3.76 * ±1.72
Dextrometho-rphan	Blank	298.32 ±8.06	463.11 ±88.17	32.76 ±19.27	0.14 ±0.04	22.57 ±8.07
	Treat	399 ±46.39	758.12 ±599.98	61.47 ±62.32	0.32 ±0.38	23.39 ±7.91
Chloroxazone	Blank	218 ±274.51	306.99 ±399.66	380.06 ±499.13.	0.50 ±0.52	2.38 ±0.78
	Treat	302 ±124.51	496.20 ±192.58	232.33 ±100.08	0.23 ±0.21	2.84 ±3.19
Midazolam	Blank	6454.1 ±1345.7	11194.82 ±6581.06	5252.44 ±654.62	0.11 ±0.04	3.61 ±1.62
	Treat	1558.15 * ±732.44	4712.50 * ±1748.06	903.98 ** ±255.58	0.15 ±0.03	17.74 ** ±6.22

Values are expressed as mean ± SD, $n = 6$. $AUC_{(0-\infty)}$—area under concentration-time curve extrapolated to infinity, $T_{1/2}$—elimination half-time, T_{max}—time to maximum concentration, C_{max}—maximum concentration. * $p < 0.05$ vs. control. * $p < 0.05$ = significant difference in comparison to the control group (t-test). ** $p < 0.01$ = significant difference in comparison to the control group (t-test).

2.4.1. Effect of Galangin on Rat Hepatic CYP1A2

The pharmacokinetic profiles of phenacetin after long-term galangin treatments were used to describe the activity of CYP1A2. The pharmacokinetic parameters of phenacetin in the galangin-treatment groups in rats are shown in Table 5. The mean plasma concentration–time curves of phenacetin in two groups are presented in Figure 3. Compared with the control group, the AUC_{0-t} of phenacetin decreased significantly in the experimental group after 8 weeks of continuous gavage with galangin. Compared with the control group, the $AUC_{0-\infty}$, C_{max}, and $T_{1/2}$ values decreased by 72.33% ($p < 0.01$), 70% ($p < 0.01$) and 0.56-fold ($p < 0.05$), and CL_Z/F increased by 5.27-fold ($p < 0.01$). Thus, galangin significantly induced the activity of CYP1A2. Therefore, when taking warfarin, theophylline, clozapine or haloperidol, attention should be paid to the combination with galangal or its components.

2.4.2. Effect of Galangin on Rat Hepatic CYP2B3

Compared with the control group, the AUC_{0-t} of amphetazone decreased significantly in the experimental group after 8 weeks of continuous gavage of galangin. Compared with the control group, the $AUC_{0-\infty}$ and C_{max} values decreased by 67.86% ($p < 0.01$) and 42.89% ($p < 0.01$), respectively. The CL_Z/F increased by 3.2-fold ($p < 0.01$). These results suggest that continuous administration of galangin can induce the CYP2B3 enzyme in the rat liver and accelerate drug metabolism.

2.4.3. Effect of Galangin on Rat Hepatic CYP2C13

Compared with the control group, the $AUC_{0-\infty}$ value of omeprazole in the experimental group decreased significantly. Compared with the control group, the $AUC_{0-\infty}$ value increased 1.27-fold ($p < 0.05$), the C_{max} increased 1.66-fold ($p < 0.05$), and the $T_{1/2}$ value decreased to 34.6% of the control group ($p < 0.05$) (Table 5). These results suggest that continuous administration of galangin can inhibit CYP2C13 enzyme activity in the rat liver, thereby slowing down drug metabolism.

2.4.4. Effect of Galangin on Rat Hepatic CYP3A1

Compared with the control group, the AUC_{0-t} value of the drug–time curve of midazolam in the experimental group was significantly lower than that in the control group after 8 weeks of continuous gavage with galangin. Compared with the control group, the $AUC_{0-\infty}$ and C_{max} values decreased by 0.42-fold ($p < 0.05$) and 17.21% ($p < 0.01$), respectively, while the $T_{1/2}$ and CL_Z/F increased by 4.91-fold ($p < 0.05$) and 2-fold ($p < 0.05$), respectively. These results suggest that continuous administration of galangin can induce CYP3A1 enzyme activity in the rat liver and accelerate drug metabolism.

When taking drugs, such as macrolide antibiotics, antifungal agents, HMG-CoA reductase inhibitors, benzodiazepines, proton pump inhibitors or calcium channel blockers, it is possible to accelerate the metabolism of the corresponding medicines by consuming galangin or dietary supplements containing galangin or Chinese herbal medicines at the same time, which may lead to fluctuations in the therapeutic effect or increasing metabolite concentrations (causing adverse reactions), which should be paid close attention to.

2.4.5. Effect of Galangin on Rat Hepatic CYP2C11, CYP2D4, and CYP2E1

Compared with the control group, the drug–time curves of diclofenac, dextromethorphan and chlorzoxazone in the experimental group were similar to those in the control group after 8 weeks of continuous gavage with galangin. Compared with the control group, the $AUC_{0-\infty}$, C_{max}, T_{max}, CL_Z/F and $T_{1/2}$ values were not significantly different ($p > 0.05$), indicating that galangin had no significant effect on the activities of CYP2C11, CYP2D4 and CYP2E1.

2.5. Effects of Galangin on Rat Liver CYP mRNA-Expression Levels

Flavonoids can activate the aromatic hydrocarbon receptor (AhR) [21], pregnane X receptor (PXR) [22] and constitutive androstane receptor (CAR) [23], thereby inducing CYP1A, CYP2B and CYP3A, and the corresponding CYP450 gene-expression level and protein-synthesis level are up-regulated accordingly, thus showing an inductive effect. Some flavonoids [24] showed strong cytotoxicity and inhibition, while some [24] had almost no effect on CYP gene-expression levels and enzyme activities. Therefore, it is speculated that galangin also induces expression of the CYP1A2, CYP2B1 and CYP3A1 genes by activating nuclear receptors. There are two main induction mechanisms of metabolic enzymes: the first is related to nuclear receptor-mediated transcription, and the second is related to mRNA or enzyme stability of mRNA after gene transcription. The mRNA expression of tumor necrosis factor-α (TNF-α)and transforming growth factor-β1(TGF-β1)were significantly increased in the fructose diet-fed rats, and galangin supplementation to fructose diet-fed rats downregulated the expression of these genes [8]. Apart from its antioxidant action, galangin has anti-inflammatory effects by affecting gene expression. This could be attributed to the fact that flavones and hydroxyflavones can inhibit the phosphorylation of proteins involved in the signal transduction [25].

Quantitative PCR was used to detect the effects of galangin on expression of the rat liver genes CYP1A2, CYP2B3, CYP2C11, CYP2C13, CYP2D4, CYP2E1 and CYP3A1 (Figure 4). Compared with the control group, the experimental group showed significantly increased expression of CYP1A2 and CYP2B3 gene ($p < 0.01$), which were up-regulated 2.54-fold and 1.68-fold in the experimental group, respectively. However, continuous administration of galangin did not significantly affect the expression of CYP2D4, CYP2C11 or CYP2E1 in rat livers ($p > 0.05$). Compared with the control group, the expression levels of CYP2C13 and CYP3A1 in the experimental group were down-regulated by 0.59-fold ($p < 0.05$) and 0.46-fold ($p < 0.05$), respectively.

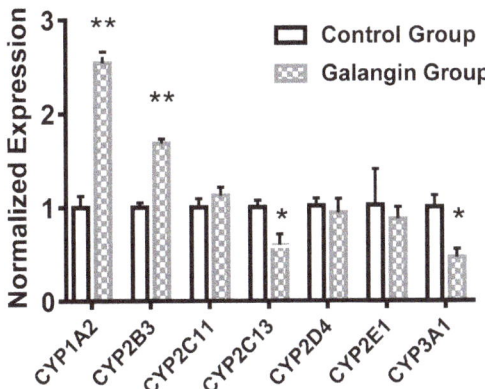

Figure 4. Effect of galangin on mRNA expression of CYP450 in rats ($n = 4$). * $p < 0.05$ versus control, ** $p < 0.01$ versus control.

These quantitative PCR results were consistent with those of the cocktail method.

3. Materials and Methods

3.1. Chemicals and Reagents

Galangin (98.3% purity) was obtained from Nanjing Plant Origin Biological Technology (Nanjing, China). Omeprazole (94.7% purity), chlorzoxazone (99.9% purity), and the IS sulfamethoxazole (99.6% purity) were purchased from National Institute for the Control of Pharmaceutical and Biological Products (Beijing, China). Dextromethorphan (98.4% purity) and bupropion (98.3% purity) were supplied by Dalian Meilun Biotechnology (Dalian, China). Phenacetin (98.5% purity) and diclofenac (98.5% purity) were purchased from Shanghai Macklin Biochemical Co., Ltd. (Shanghai, China). Midazolam (98.5% purity), and methanol and formic acid (LC-MS grade) were purchased from Sigma (St. Louis, MO, USA). Ultra-pure water was acquired from Wahaha Group Co., Ltd. (Hangzhou, China). Total RNA was extracted using the TRIzol reagent (Invitrogen, Carlsbad, CA, USA) and used for reverse transcription. Quantitative reverse transcription-polymerase chain reaction (PCR) analysis was performed with the ABI 7500 real-time PCR system (Applied Biosystems, Foster City, CA, USA). A Total RNA Kit was purchased from Tiangen Biotech Co., Ltd. (Beijing, China). PrimeScript™ RT Master Mix was obtained from Takara Bio, Inc. (Kusatsu, Japan).

3.2. Animals and Experimental Design

Male Sprague Dawley rats (220–230 g, 8 weeks of age) were acquired from the Experimental Animals Center of Hebei Medical University (Shijiazhuang, China, animal certificate number: SCXK (Ji) 2018-003). The animal study was conducted based on the Guide for Care and Use of Laboratory Animals published by the National Institutes of Health (NIH publication no. 85–23, revised in 1985). Animals were maintained with ad libitum access to standard laboratory food (Diet composition: corn starch 60.0 g/100 g, casein (fat free) 20.0 g/100 g, methionine 0.7 g/100 g, groundnut oil 5.0 g/100 g, wheat bran 10.6 g/100 g, salt mixture 3.5 g/100 g, vitamin mixture 0.2 g/100 g) [8] and water in a breeding room with an ambient temperature 24 °C, a relative humidity of 60% and 12-h dark/light cycle (lights on from 08:00 to 20:00).

An 8 mg·kg^{-1}·day^{-1} dose of galangin [26] was selected as an optimum dose to improve the antioxidant status and reduce hyperglycaemia in streptozotocin-induced diabetic rats. Twelve rats were assigned randomly to two groups of 6 animals each, namely the blank control group (CON) and the galangin-treated group (TRE). The CON group was treated with only 0.5% sodium carboxymethyl cellulose (CMC-Na) for 8 weeks. The TRE group was intragastrically treated 8 mg·kg^{-1}·day^{-1} of galangin by using a ball-tipped incubation steel needle placed on a graded disposable syringe for 8 weeks in succession.

3.3. Pharmacokinetic Study

Twenty-four hours after the last administration of galangin, a cocktail solution, which contained phenacetin, diclofenac, dextromethorphan, midazolam (5 mg/kg), bupropion, omeprazole, and chlorzoxazone (10 mg/kg) in 0.5% CMC-Na solution, were administered orally to all rats in each group. Blood samples of each rat were collected from the posterior orbital veins at pre-dose (0 h), 0.08, 0.17, 0.25, 0.5, 0.75, 1, 2, 4, 6, 8, 12 and 24 h after oral administration. The blood samples (0.3 mL) were immediately transferred to heparinized tubes. Then 100 μL plasma were prepared from blood samples by centrifuging (4200 rpm, 15 min) and stored at −80°C until LC-MS/MS analysis.

3.4. Sample Preparation

Each 100 μL plasma sample was mixed with 20 μL of the IS working solution via vortexing for 1 min in a 1.5-mL centrifuge tube, after which 300 μL of methanol was added. Then, the resulting solution was extracted via vortexing for 3 min.

After centrifuging at 15,000 rpm at 4 °C for 10 min, the organic phase was transferred to another tube and evaporated to dryness under a gentle stream of N$_2$ stream at 30 °C. The dried residue was reconstituted in 100 μL of methanol and vortexed for 1 min before being transferred to an autosampler vial for analysis. Drug and Statistics (DAS) software (version 3.2.4, Chinese Pharmacology Society, Shanghai, China) was employed to analyse the pharmacokinetics parameters.

3.5. Preparation of Calibration Curves and Quality Control (QC) Samples

Stock solutions of phenacetin, bupropion, diclofenac, omeprazole, dextromethorphan, chlorzoxazone, midazolam and the IS (each 100 μg/mL) were individually prepared in methanol.

The calibration standards solutions were serially diluted with methanol by blank plasma to concentrations of 1.006, 2.012, 10.06, 40.24, 402.4, 804.8, 1609.6 and 2414.4 ng/mL for phenacetin; 0.801, 2.034, 20.34, 101.7, 203.4 and 406.8 ng/mL for bupropion; 1.01, 2.02, 20.2, 202, 404 and 808 ng/mL for diclofenac; 1.015, 2.03, 10.15, 20.30, 203, 406 and 812 ng/mL for dextromethorphan; 1.287, 2.574, 12.87, 128.7, 257.4 and 514.8 ng/mL for chlorzoxazone; and 2.005, 4.01, 40.1, 401, 1604, 4010 and 6416 ng/mL for midazolam. The final concentration of the IS was 20 ng/mL.

QC samples were prepared by individually spiking blank rat plasma at three concentrations: low, medium or high (2.012, 201.2 or 1609.6 ng/mL for phenacetin; 2.304, 20.34 or 203.4 ng/mL for bupropion; 2.02, 20.2 or 202 ng/mL for diclofenac; 2.03, 20.3 or 406 ng/mL for omeprazole; 1.98, 9.9 or 99 ng/mL for dextromethorphan; 2.574, 12.87 or 257.4 ng/mL for chlorzoxazone; 4.01, 401 or 4010 ng/mL for midazolam). All solutions were prepared during the day prior to beginning the animal study and stored at 4 °C until analysis.

3.6. LC-MS Analytical Conditions

Samples were analysed on an Agilent 1200 series HPLC system (Agilent Technologies, Foster City, CA, USA), consisting of an autosampler, a degasser, a column compartment and a quaternary solvent delivery system. HPLC separations were carried out on a Wonda Cract ODS-2 C18 column (4.6 mm × 150 mm, i.d., 5.0 μm; SHIMADZU-GL, Kyoto City, Japan) at 25 °C. Linear gradient elution was performed using methanol containing 0.1% (v/v) (A) and water containing 0.1% (v/v) formic acid (B) as mobile phases, processed at a flow rate of 1.0 mL/min as follows: 0–11 min, 45% A;

11–12 min, 45%–90% A (linear); 12–17.5 min, 90% A; and then back to the initial A:B ratio of 45:55 (v/v). The injected volume for all samples was 10 µL.

For detection and quantification, MS detection was performed using an API 3200 Qtrap™ system (AB SCIEX, Foster City, CA, USA) equipped with Turbo V sources and a turbo ion spray interface. The ion spray voltages were set to 5500 V or −4500 V, the source temperature was maintained at 650 °C, the ion source gas (gas 1) pressure was 60 psi, the ion source gas (gas 2) pressure was 65 psi, the curtain gas (nitrogen) pressure was 30 psi, the collision cell-exit potentials were 5.0/−5.0 V, and the entrance potentials were 10.0/−10.0 V. The MS instrument was operated in MRM mode. Two ions were monitored for each molecule. The dwell time of each ion pair was held constant at 50 ms. The declustering potential and collision energy of the quantitative-optimization mode for the probe drugs and the IS sulfamethoxazole are described in Table 1. Analyst™ software (version 1.6.2 AB SCIEX, Foster City, CA, USA) was used for data acquisition and processing.

3.7. Method Validation

The method-validation procedure was based on the Guidance for Industry Bioanalytical Method Validation of the European Medicines Agency and the U.S. FDA [12]. Selectivity was determined by analysing twelve blank plasma samples in MRM to check for signals that might interfere with detection of the probe drug or the IS. In addition, two zero samples (blank samples including the IS) were analysed.

Twelve analyte-free plasma samples from different sources were analysed and checked for peaks interfering with the detection of the probe drug or the IS. The plasma samples did not contain any of the analytes.

Calibration curves were constructed at the different concentration ranges with a weighted ($1/x^2$) least-squares linear regression, using the peak-area ratio (y) of each probe drug to that of the IS versus the concentrations (x). The percent deviation of the relative error (RE) from the nominal concentration (a measure of accuracy) and the relative standard deviation (RSD, a measure of precision) of the concentration defined as the LLOQ (considered as the lowest calibration standard) had to be <20%.

The intra- and inter-day precision and accuracy of the method were evaluated with QC samples and LLOQ samples at three different concentrations (six replicates each) on three consecutive days. The criteria for acceptable data included an accuracy within ±15% RE from the nominal values and a precision of within ±15% of the RSD. The RSD was acceptable if it was less than 20% of the LLOQ concentration.

The extraction recovery was investigated by comparing the mean peak areas of six samples spiked with low- and high-concentration QC samples for each probe drug before the extraction process with those obtained from samples spiked after the extraction.

The matrix effect was calculated by comparing analytes spiked into blank plasma extracts with the peak areas of the analytes in the mobile phase at an equivalent concentration.

The stability in plasma was evaluated by processing QC samples at three different concentrations in different conditions; long-term stability was evaluated after storage at −80°C for 15 days; short-term stability was evaluated after storage at room temperature for 2 h; freeze-thaw stability was evaluated after three freeze-thaw cycles from −80 °C to room temperature; post-preparative stability was evaluated by comparing QC samples analysed immediately after preparation and after 24 h at 4 °C or at room temperature for 4 h.

3.8. Effects of Galangin on mRNA Expression of CYP Enzymes in Rats

Galangin-treated and control animals were euthanised via decapitation at 48 h after the last administration (without fasting), after which livers were excised quickly, perfused with ice-cold 0.9% (w/v) sodium chloride to remove blood residue, weighted and stored at −80°C. Total RNA was extracted from rat liver samples with the Trizol Reagent (Invitrogen) in accordance with the manufacturer's protocol. The RNA concentration was determined, and the quality of the isolated

RNA was assessed based on the 260/280 nm absorbance ratio (1.8–2.0 indicates a highly pure sample). Subsequently, 5 µg of RNA for each sample was reverse transcribed to cDNA using a PrimeScript™ RT Reagent Kit with gDNA Eraser (Kusatsu, Japan). The total RNA concentration of each reaction was 45 µg/mL. The reverse transcription conditions were as follows: gDNA was removed from the samples at 42 °C for 2 min, incubated at 4 °C for 10 min, reacted at 37 °C for 15 min, denatured at 85 °C for 5 s and held at 4 °C for 10 min. The obtained products were stored at −20°C. Reactions were performed in a final volume of 10 µL, according to the protocol recommended for the Power Up™ SYBR™ Green Master Mix Kit (Thermo Fisher Scientific, Vilnius, Lithuania). The amplification conditions were as follows: UDG enzyme activation at 50 °C for 2 min, and initial denaturation at 95 °C for 2 min followed by denaturation at 95 °C for 15 s, annealing at 60 °C for 15 s, extension at 72 °C for 1 min. Forty cycles were carried out. The relative mRNA-expression levels in the control and treated groups were calculated using the $2^{-\Delta\Delta CT}$ method. In this study, *GAPDH* was selected as the internal reference gene, and *CYP1A2, CYP2B3, CYP2C11, CYP2C13, CYP2D4, CYP2E1, CYP3A1* and *GAPDH* mRNA sequences were identified by searching National Center for Biotechnology Information (NCBI) NCBI's Nucleotide database and some references. The sequences of the forward and reverse primers are shown in Table 6.

Table 6. Sequences of primers for RT-PCR analyses.

CYPs	Forward Primer Sequence	Reverse Primer Sequence
1A2	GTCACCTCAGGGAATGCTGTG	GTTGACAATCTTCTCCTGAGG
2B3	AGGACCCCGTCCCTTACC	CCGGCCAGAGAAAGCCTC
2C11	CTGCTGCTGCTGAAACACG	TTTCATGCAGGGGCTCCG
2C13	TGGTCCACGAGGTTCAGAGATACA	GGTTGGGAAACTCCTTGCTGTCAT
2D4	TGCGAGAGGCACTGGTGA	CGTGGTCCAAAGCCCGAC
2E1	GACCTTTCCCTCTTCCCATCCTTG	GTAGCACCTCCTTGACAGCCTTG
3A1	GGCAAACCTGTCCCTGTGAAAGA	CTGGCGTGAGGAATGGAAAGAGT
GAPDH	TGCTGAGTATGTCGTGGAG	GTCTTCTGAGTGGCAGTGAT

3.9. Statistical Processing Method

The data were analysed using SPSS software, version 21.0 (SPSS InC., Chicago, IL, USA). The pharmacokinetic parameters were calculated using DAS software, version 3.2.4 (version 3.2.4, Chinese Pharmacology Society, Shanghai, China). The average drug–time curves were drawn using GraphPad prism 7.0.0 software for Windows (GraphPad Software Inc., La Jolla, CA, USA). The parameters of the drug-treated groups were compared with those of the blank-control group using a t test and the non-parametric rank–sum test. A p-value < 0.05 was considered to reflect a statistically significant difference.

4. Conclusions

Enzyme induction and inhibition have significant effects on the drug treatment of galangin, especially the combination of drugs. When galangin is combined with drugs mainly metabolised by the CYP1A2 and CYP2B3 enzymes, the blood concentrations of these drugs may be reduced. When galangin is combined with drugs mainly metabolised by the CYP2C13 and CYP3A1 enzymes, the metabolism of these drugs will be slowed down, the active time will be prolonged, and the pharmacological activity or toxic side effects will be enhanced. The results of this study may provide more reliable experimental data and scientific explanations for the rational clinical application of related herbal (dietary supplement)–drug interactions.

Author Contributions: Conceptualization: L.-T.Z. and Y.-L.M.; investigation: Y.-L.M., F.Z., J.-T.Y., C.-J.L., X.-L.N., Z.-H.Q. and L.-T.Z.; formal analysis: Y.-L.M. and F.Z.; writing—original draft preparation, review, and editing: Y.-L.M. and F.Z. All authors read and approved the final manuscript.

Funding: This work was funded by the National Natural Science Foundation of China, grant number 81473180; the Natural Science Foundation of Hebei Province, grant number H2017206158; and the Key Project of Hebei Medical Science, grant number 20170472.

Conflicts of Interest: The authors declare no conflict of interest.

References

1. Nebert, D.W.; Russell, D.W. Clinical importance of the cytochromes P450. *Lancet* **2002**, *360*, 1155–1162. [CrossRef]
2. Lee, J.J.; Lee, J.H.; Yim, N.H.; Han, J.H.; Ma, J.Y. Application of galangin, an active component of *Alpinia officinarum* Hance (Zingiberaceae), for use in drug-eluting stents. *Sci. Rep.* **2017**, *7*, 8207. [CrossRef]
3. Cushnie, T.P.; Hamilton, V.E.; Chapman, D.G.; Taylor, P.W.; Lamb, A.J. Aggregation of *Staphylococcus aureus* following treatment with the antibacterial flavonol galangin. *J. Appl. Microbiol.* **2007**, *103*, 1562–1567. [CrossRef] [PubMed]
4. Aloud, A.A.; Veeramani, C.; Govindasamy, C.; Alsaif, M.A.; El Newehy, A.S.; Al-Numair, K.S. Galangin, a dietary flavonoid, improves antioxidant status and reduces hyperglycemia-mediated oxidative stress in streptozotocin-induced diabetic rats. *Redox Rep.* **2017**, *22*, 290–300. [CrossRef] [PubMed]
5. Kumar, S.; Alagawadi, K.R. Anti-obesity effects of galangin, a pancreatic lipase inhibitor in cafeteria diet fed female rats. *Pharm. Biol.* **2013**, *51*, 607–613. [CrossRef] [PubMed]
6. Heo, M.Y.; Sohn, S.J.; Au, W.W. Anti-genotoxicity of galangin as a cancer chemopreventive agent candidate. *Mutat. Res.* **2001**, *488*, 135–150. [CrossRef]
7. Matsuda, H.; Ando, S.; Kato, T.; Morikawa, T.; Yoshikawa, M. Inhibitors from the rhizomes of Alpinia officinarum on production of nitric oxide in lipopolysaccharide-activated macrophages and the structural requirements of diarylheptanoids for the activity. *Bioorgan. Med. Chem.* **2006**, *14*, 138–142. [CrossRef]
8. Sivakumar, A.S.; Anuradha, C.V. Effect of galangin supplementation on oxidative damage and inflammatory changes in fructose-fed rat liver. *Chem. Biol. Interact.* **2011**, *193*, 141–148. [CrossRef]
9. Su, Y.; Chen, Y.; Liu, Y.; Yang, Y.; Deng, Y.; Gong, Z.; Chen, J.; Wu, T.; Lin, S.; Cui, L. Antiosteoporotic effects of Alpinia officinarum Hance through stimulation of osteoblasts associated with antioxidant effects. *J. Orthop. Transl.* **2016**, *4*, 75–91. [CrossRef]
10. Morello, S.; Vellecco, V.; Alfieri, A.; Mascolo, N.; Cicala, C. Vasorelaxant effect of the flavonoid galangin on isolated rat thoracic aorta. *Life. Sci.* **2006**, *78*, 825–830. [CrossRef]
11. Lu, Y.Y.; Du, Z.Y.; Li, Y.; Wang, J.L.; Zhao, M.B.; Jiang, Y.; Guo, X.Y.; Tu, P.F. Effects of Baoyuan decoction, a traditional Chinese medicine formula, on the activities and mRNA expression of seven CYP isozymes in rats. *J. Ethnopharmacol.* **2018**, *225*, 327–335. [CrossRef] [PubMed]
12. Kim, M.J.; Kim, H.; Cha, I.J.; Park, J.S.; Shon, J.H.; Liu, K.H.; Shin, J.G. High-throughput screening of inhibitory potential of nine cytochrome P450 enzymes in vitro using liquid chromatography/tandem mass spectrometry. *Rapid Commun. Mass Spectrom.* **2005**, *19*, 2651–2658. [CrossRef]
13. Li, X.; Chen, X.; Li, Q.; Wang, L.; Zhong, D. Validated method for rapid inhibition screening of six cytochrome P450 enzymes by liquid chromatography-tandem mass spectrometry. *J. Chromatogr. B Analyt. Technol. Biomed. Life Sci.* **2007**, *852*, 128–137. [CrossRef] [PubMed]
14. De Bock, L.; Boussery, K.; Colin, P.; De Smet, J.; T'Jollyn, H.; Van Bocxlaer, J. Development and validation of a fast and sensitive UPLC-MS/MS method for the quantification of six probe metabolites for the in vitro determination of cytochrome P450 activity. *Talanta* **2012**, *89*, 209–216. [CrossRef]
15. US Food and Drug Administration, Guidance for Industry: Bioanalytical Method Validation. 2001. Available online: http://www.fda.gov/downloads/Drugs/Guidance/ucm070107.pdf (accessed on 10 January 2017).
16. Zanger, U.M.; Schwab, M. Cytochrome P450 enzymes in drug metabolism: Regulation of gene expression, enzyme activities, and impact of genetic variation. *Pharmacol. Ther.* **2013**, *138*, 103–141. [CrossRef]
17. Wang, X.S.; Hu, X.C.; Chen, G.L.; Yuan, X.; Yang, R.N.; Liang, S.; Ren, J.; Sun, J.C.; Kong, G.Q.; Gao, S.G.; Feng, X.S. Effects of vitexin on the pharmacokinetics and mRNA expression of CYP isozymes in rats. *Phytother. Res.* **2015**, *29*, 366–372. [CrossRef]
18. Dorne, J.L.; Walton, K.; Renwick, A.G. Uncertainty factors for chemical risk assessment. human variability in the pharmacokinetics of CYP1A2 probe substrates. *Food Chem. Toxicol.* **2001**, *39*, 681–696. [CrossRef]

19. Mo, S.L.; Liu, Y.H.; Duan, W.; Wei, M.Q.; Kanwar, J.R.; Zhou, S.F. Substrate specificity, regulation, and polymorphism of human cytochrome P450 2B6. *Curr. Drug Metab.* **2009**, *10*, 730–753. [CrossRef] [PubMed]
20. Zhou, S.F.; Xue, C.C.; Yu, X.Q.; Li, C.; Wang, G. Clinically important drug interactions potentially involving mechanism-based inhibition of cytochrome p450 3A4 and the role of therapeutic drug monitoring. *Ther. Drug Monit.* **2007**, *29*, 687–710. [CrossRef]
21. Mohammadi-Bardbori, A.; Bengtsson, J.; Rannug, U.; Rannug, A.; Wincent, E. Quercetin, resveratrol, and curcumin are indirect activators of the aryl hydrocarbon receptor (AHR). *Chem. Res. Toxicol.* **2012**, *25*, 1878–1884. [CrossRef]
22. Okada, N.; Murakami, A.; Urushizaki, S.; Matsuda, M.; Kawazoe, K.; Ishizawa, K. Extracts of immature orange (*Aurantii fructus immaturus*) and citrus unshiu peel (*Citri unshiu pericarpium*) induce P-glycoprotein and cytochrome P450 3A4 expression via upregulation of pregnane X receptor. *Front. Pharmacol.* **2017**, *8*, 84. [CrossRef]
23. Carazo Fernandez, A.; Smutny, T.; Hyrsova, L.; Berka, K.; Pavek, P. Chrysin, baicalein and galangin are indirect activators of the human constitutive androstane receptor (CAR). *Toxicol. Lett.* **2015**, *233*, 68–77. [CrossRef] [PubMed]
24. Cheng, L.; Li, L.A. Flavonoids exhibit diverse effects on CYP11B1 expression and cortisol synthesis. *Toxicol. Appl. Pharmacol.* **2012**, *258*, 343–350. [CrossRef] [PubMed]
25. Baeuerle, P.A.; Henkel, T. Function and Activation of NF-κB in the Immune System. *Annu. Rev. Immunol.* **1994**, *12*, 141–179. [CrossRef] [PubMed]
26. Aloud, A.A.; Chinnadurai, V.; Chandramohan, G.; Alsaif, M.A.; Al-Numair, K.S. Galangin controls streptozotocin-caused glucose homeostasis and reverses glycolytic and gluconeogenic enzyme changes in rats. *Arch. Physiol. Biochem.* **2018**, 1–6. [CrossRef] [PubMed]

Sample Availability: Samples of compounds used in this study are available from the authors.

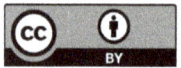

© 2019 by the authors. Licensee MDPI, Basel, Switzerland. This article is an open access article distributed under the terms and conditions of the Creative Commons Attribution (CC BY) license (http://creativecommons.org/licenses/by/4.0/).

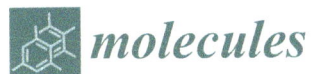

Article

Quantification of Furosine (N$^\varepsilon$-(2-Furoylmethyl)-L-lysine) in Different Parts of Velvet Antler with Various Processing Methods and Factors Affecting Its Formation

Rui-ze Gong [1], Yan-hua Wang [1,2], Kun Gao [1,2], Lei Zhang [1], Chang Liu [1], Ze-shuai Wang [1], Yu-fang Wang [1] and Yin-shi Sun [1,*]

[1] Institute of Special Animal and Plant Sciences, Chinese Academy of Agricultural Sciences, Changchun 130112, China; 82101172456@caas.cn (R.-z.G.); yhwangsdlc@126.com (Y.-h.W.); 13356954028@163.com (K.G.); leizhang0102@163.com (L.Z.); liuchang@caas.com (C.L.); 13091716585@163.com (Z.-s.W.); wangyufang_jl@163.com (Y.-f.W.)

[2] College of Chinese Material Medicine, Jilin Agricultural University, Changchun 130118, China

* Correspondence: sunyinshi2015@163.com; Tel.: +86-431-81919580; Fax: +86-431-81919876

Academic Editors: In-Soo Yoon and Hyun-Jong Cho
Received: 3 March 2019; Accepted: 28 March 2019; Published: 31 March 2019

Abstract: Furosine (N$^\varepsilon$-(2-furoylmethyl)-L-lysine) is formed during the early stages of the Maillard reaction from a lysine Amadori compound and is frequently used as a marker of reaction progress. Furosine is toxic, with significant effects on animal livers, kidneys, and other organs. However, reports on the formation of furosine in processed velvet antler are scarce. In this study, we have quantified the furosine content in processed velvet antler by using UPLC-MS/MS. The furosine contents of velvet antler after freeze-drying, boiling, and processing without and with blood were 148.51–193.93, 168.10–241.22, 60.29–80.33, and 115.18–138.99 mg/kg protein, respectively. The factors affecting furosine formation in processed velvet antler, including reducing sugars, proteins, amino acids, and process temperature, are discussed herein. Proteins, amino acids, and reducing sugars are substrates for the Maillard reaction and most significantly influence the furosine content in the processed velvet antler. High temperatures induce the production of furosine in boiled velvet antler but not in the freeze-dried samples, whereas more furosine is produced in velvet antler processed with blood, which is rich in proteins, amino acids, and reducing sugars, than in the samples processed without blood. Finally, wax slices rich in proteins, amino acids, and reducing sugars produced more furosine than the other parts of the velvet antler. These data provide a reference for guiding the production of low-furosine velvet antler and can be used to estimate the consumer intake of furosine from processed velvet antler.

Keywords: affecting factors; amadori compound; furosine; Maillard reaction; velvet antler processing

1. Introduction

Velvet antler is an important ingredient in traditional Chinese medicine that has been used for thousands of years in China, Korea, and Southeast Asian countries [1–3]. Velvet antler contains anti-oxidants and other compounds associated with immunity, anti-osteoporosis, and other pharmacological effects [4–6]. Fresh velvet antler is rich in blood, amino acids, and proteins, and is highly susceptible to spoilage if it is not processed promptly. Based on current processing methods and consumption patterns, velvet antler is mainly boiled or freeze-dried. It can be processed with or without blood and separated into wax, powder, gauze, and bone slices by segmentation. The various velvet antler processing techniques have different impacts on the bioactive components and pharmacological activities [4–6]. Therefore, the processing conditions are crucial for the resulting composition of the velvet antler.

Velvet antler is rich in amino- and carbonyl-containing compounds, which can produce advanced glycation end products (AGEs) via the Maillard reaction during processing [7]. Some AGEs have been associated with a variety of diseases, including diabetes, Alzheimer's disease, atherosclerosis, renal dysfunction, and aging [8–17]. Our group has reported the content of N^ε-(carboxymethyl) lysine (CML) and N^ε-(carboxyethyl) lysine (CEL) in different parts of velvet antler, processed by using different methods [18]. The contents of CML and CEL in boiled velvet antler and samples processed with blood were significantly higher than those in freeze-dried velvet antler and samples processed without blood, indicating that different processing methods can significantly affect the degree to which the Maillard reaction occurs. However, pre-treatment methods for CML and CEL in processed velvet antler are cumbersome and the compounds have no UV absorption or fluorescence characteristics, thereby necessitating LC-MS analysis [19–21].

Furosine (N^ε-(2-furoylmethyl)-L-lysine or N6-[2-(2-furanyl)-2-oxoethyl]-L-lysine, $C_{12}H_{18}N_2O_4$, Mw 254.12, FML) is a product of lysine Amadori compounds, its formation pathway, which is a part of the early stages of the Maillard reaction, as shown in Figure 1 [22]. Furosine can further react to form AGEs and can be used as a marker of Maillard reaction progress [23]. Li et al. [24] showed that furosine has strong toxic effects on animal livers, kidneys, and other organs. High doses of furosine cause adverse effects on health by inducing cell apoptosis and activation of inflammatory necrosis. Furosine has maximum UV absorption at 280 nm and is easily detected. However, furosine is a trace substance in foods and drugs. As LC-MS has better sensitivity and selectivity than UV measurements, LC-MS is now usually used to detect furosine in foods and drugs [19]. Furosine has been used to evaluate the shelf life and freshness of foods, including milk and honey [25,26]. However, data regarding furosine in processed velvet antler have not been reported to date. The furosine content in processed velvet antler is significantly influenced by the matrix and processing conditions [27,28]. Therefore, information regarding the furosine content in processed velvet antler is required to evaluate the quality of processed velvet antler.

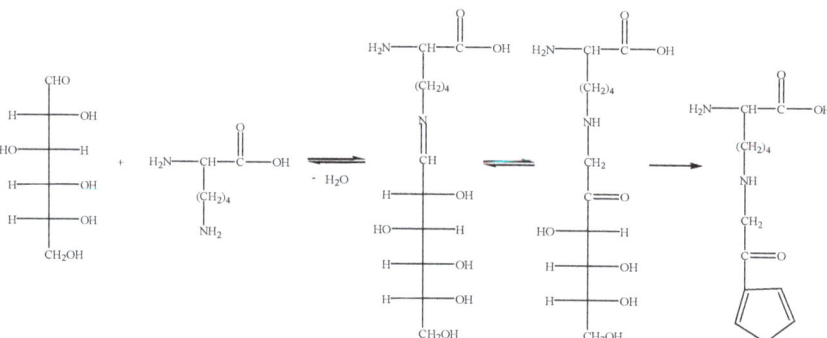

Figure 1. Reaction pathway for conversion of glucose and lysine into furosine via the Maillard reaction.

This study was performed to determine the furosine content in processed velvet antler by UPLC-MS/MS and to explore the factors affecting the content by measuring the contents of furosine, amino compounds (proteins and amino acids), and carbonyl compounds (reducing sugars) in different parts of the velvet antler, processed using various methods. In addition, the conditions affecting the production of furosine in the Maillard reaction during processing were analyzed. This study provides a solid theoretical basis for improving the processing technology of velvet antler and for controlling the degree of processing and production of furosine. This study also provides a reference for consumers to control their furosine intake from processed velvet antler.

2. Results and Discussion

2.1. Sample Pre-Treatment and Chromatography Conditions

Preparation of the velvet antler samples consisted of processing, segmenting, grinding, hydrolysis, and solid-phase extraction (SPE). Unlike the sample pre-treatment for CML and CEL, the pre-treatment method for detecting furosine does not involve defatting or reduction and is relatively simple. The samples were subjected to SPE by using a C18 Sep-Pak® cartridge (Sepax technology, Cork, Ireland; 500 mg, 6 mL) to remove impurities.

Furosine is a highly polar compound and is not well retained by most reversed-phase columns. Researchers have usually analyzed furosine by using a C18 column with nonafluoropentanoic acid (NFPA) and trifluoroacetic acid (TFA) as eluents to improve peak patterns and reduce tailing. However, NFPA and TFA can result in poor mass spectra and reduce the service life of the instrument [29]. To avoid using NFPA and TFA, we developed a UPLC-MS/MS method to separate furosine with an Acquity HSS T3 UPLC column. The HSS T3 column is a reverse-reverse column with excellent retention of highly polar compounds, relative to other commonly used columns. It relies on ion exchange and hydrophobic interactions between the stationary phase and furosine to achieve separation. In comparison with the HILIC column, the HSS T3 column stationary phase is compatible with 100% water and has a wider elution range. The elution effects of methanol and acetonitrile were assessed by using acetonitrile/water (80:20 v/v) and methanol/water (80:20 v/v) mixtures as mobile phases, with a flow rate of 0.3 mL/min. In comparison with the chromatograms obtained by using a methanol mobile phase, UPLC-MS chromatograms obtained by using water and acetonitrile as eluents yielded better spectrum peak symmetries and fewer miscellaneous peaks.

The UPLC-MS chromatograms of the furosine standard and a sample of powder slices of boiled velvet antler are shown in Figure 2a,b. In the Supplementary Materials, we provide a UV determination of furosine standards and powder slices of boiled velvet antler samples. The same retention time, UV measurement, and total ion chromatograms for furosine in the processed velvet antler samples were consistent with those of the furosine standard and no peak interference was observed.

2.2. Method Validation

The developed method was validated by assessing the furosine content in processed velvet antler samples and considering the resulting selectivity, linearity, precision, and accuracy. Figure 2c shows the fragmentation pattern of furosine, with three major product ions at m/z 84, 130, and 192, with the most intense peak at m/z 130. The three product ions were used for quantitation in multiple reaction monitoring (MRM) mode. Figure 2e shows the assignment of the furosine fragmentation pattern.

The correlation coefficient (R^2) of furosine was >0.9998 and the linear range (20–3500 ng/mL) was sufficiently wide to assess the furosine content in the processed velvet antler samples. The reference solution was diluted stepwise with ultrapure water. The limit of detection (LOD) and limit of quantitation (LOQ) were defined as the concentrations at which the signal-to-noise ratios of the furosine peak were 3 and 10, respectively. The LOD and LOQ values for furosine were 1.9 ng/g and 5.7 ng/g, respectively.

The processed velvet antler samples were extracted in triplicate and analyzed by using the developed UPLC-MS/MS method. The relative standard deviations of the intra-day and inter-day precision for furosine were 3.12 and 4.28%, respectively. The coefficients of variation obtained from the reproducibility tests were <5%. The recoveries of exogenous furosine added to the velvet antler samples were determined at three concentrations (low, intermediate, and high, corresponding to 30, 300, and 3000 ng/mL, respectively). Recovery experiments were performed five times for each concentration, affording values ranging from 93.22 to 95.43%.

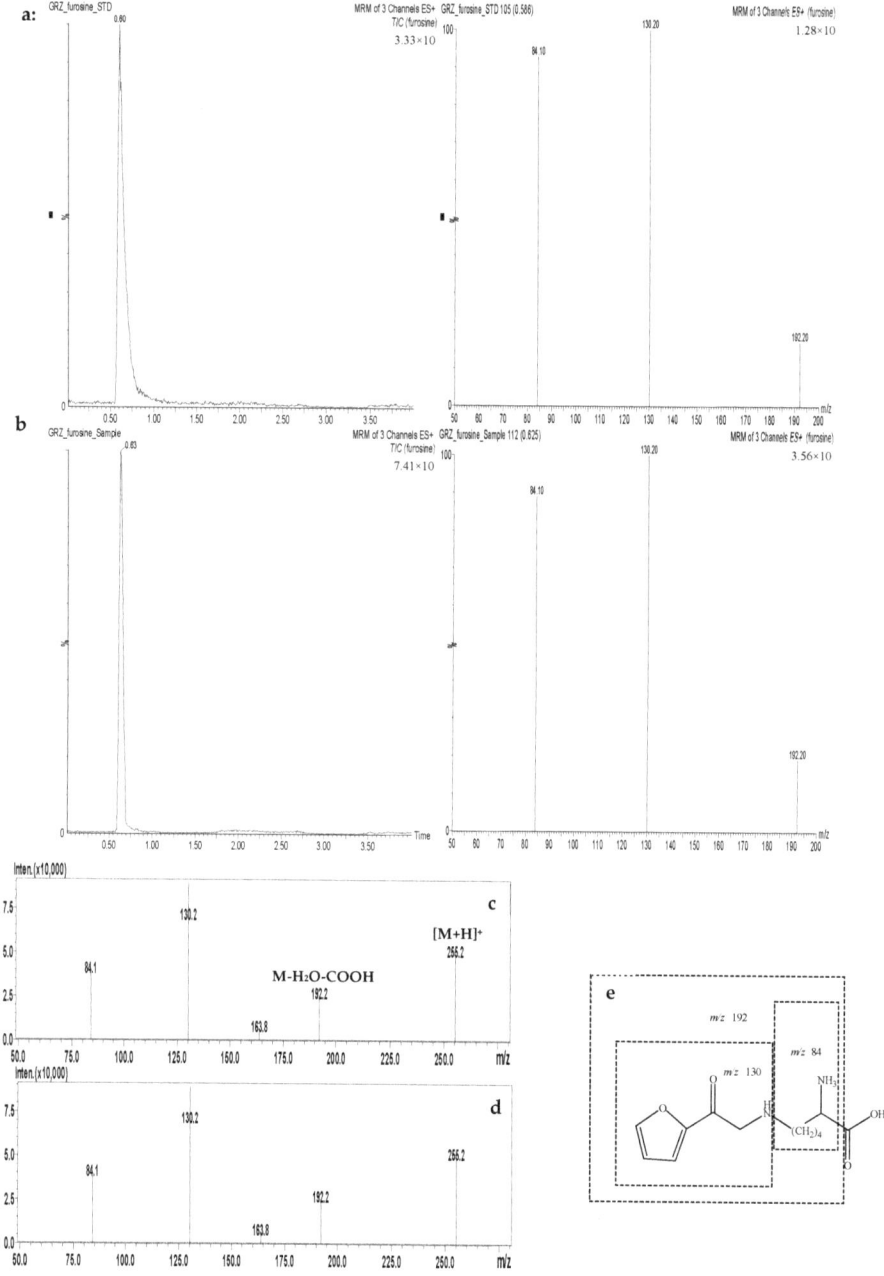

Figure 2. Total ion chromatograms and selected ion intensities for the furosine standard (**a**) and a sample of powder slices of boiled velvet antler (**b**). Mass spectrum fragmentation pattern of the furosine standard (**c**) and a sample of powder slices of boiled velvet antler (**d**). Assignment of the fragmentation pattern of the furosine standard (**e**).

2.3. Furosine Content in the Processed Velvet Antler

The furosine contents in the different parts of the velvet antler processed by using various methods are shown in Table 1. The furosine contents in the freeze-dried and boiled velvet antler samples were 148.51–193.94 and 168.10–241.22 mg/kg protein, respectively, whereas they were 60.29–80.33 and 115.18–139.88 mg/kg protein for the processed velvet antler without blood and with blood, respectively. These results suggest that the processed velvet antler protein is glycosylated to a considerable extent relative to that in processed foods, such as milk (150–300 mg/kg protein) [30] and processed meat (120 mg/kg protein) [31]. Comparing the contents of furosine, CML, and CEL in different parts of velvet antler processed by various methods [18], we found that the content of furosine in processed velvet antler is between that of CML and CEL. In other words, the CML content is the highest, the furosine content is second, and the CEL content is the lowest in the processed velvet antler.

Table 1. Furosine contents in the processed velvet antler, expressed per mg/kg protein, mg/kg, and mmol/mol lysine ($\bar{x} \pm SD$, $n = 3$).

Processing Methods	Parts	mg FML/kg Protein [a]	mmol FML/mol Lysine [b]	mg FML/kg
freeze-dried	wax slices	193.94 ± 1.21	0.53 ± 0.14	138.77 ± 1.78
	powder slices	155.05 ± 1.43	0.50 ± 0.09	88.56 ± 1.84
	gauze slices	154.69 ± 1.19	0.49 ± 0.21	81.58 ± 1.23
	bone slices	153.68 ± 1.98	0.50 ± 0.16	75.35 ± 1.42
	entire	148.51 ± 1.85	0.47 ± 0.20	84.54 ± 1.53
boiled	wax slices	241.22 ± 2.13	0.79 ± 0.23	155.35 ± 1.68
	powder slices	226.21 ± 1.98	0.67 ± 0.22	137.27 ± 1.72
	gauze slices	202.98 ± 1.84	0.62 ± 0.19	109.59 ± 1.66
	bone slices	155.02 ± 1.78	0.57 ± 0.24	79.26 ± 2.03
	entire	168.10 ± 1.22	0.56 ± 0.26	102.54 ± 1.22
processed without blood	wax slices	80.33 ± 1.25	0.26 ± 0.12	64.11 ± 2.04
	powder slices	61.65 ± 1.31	0.20 ± 0.14	34.96 ± 1.75
	gauze slices	49.26 ± 1.43	0.17 ± 0.21	29.01 ± 2.10
	bone slices	50.35 ± 1.13	0.17 ± 0.19	27.24 ± 1.45
	entire	60.29 ± 1.46	0.25 ± 0.17	34.02 ± 1.58
processed with blood	wax slices	139.88 ± 1.87	0.44 ± 0.22	106.62 ± 1.95
	powder slices	126.42 ± 1.54	0.42 ± 0.19	83.89 ± 1.63
	gauze slices	122.46 ± 1.44	0.41 ± 0.25	75.25 ± 1.39
	bone slices	129.15 ± 1.32	0.35 ± 0.17	64.13 ± 1.88
	entire	115.18 ± 2.13	0.38 ± 0.14	68.24 ± 1.21

[a] Data were calculated using the protein contents quantified by combustion method. [b] Data were calculated using the amino acid concentration in the acid hydrolysates, quantified by an amino acid analyzer.

The furosine contents of the freeze-dried velvet antler were significantly lower than those of the corresponding parts of the boiled samples ($p < 0.01$). This suggests that the processing temperature can significantly affect the formation of furosine. High-temperature processing increased furosine production, whereas the high content in the freeze-dried velvet antler was endogenous. The furosine contents of the velvet antler processed without blood were significantly lower than those of the corresponding parts processed with blood ($p < 0.01$). This may be because the velvet antler processed without blood underwent physical centrifugation to remove the blood. Blood contains many reducing sugars, amino acids, and proteins that can generate furosine during processing. The wax slices exhibited the highest furosine content, whereas the bone slices showed the lowest content. Closer to the top of the antler, more protein, lysine, and reducing sugars were present; these are the precursors of furosine [32,33].

In summary, by comparing the furosine contents in the various parts of velvet antler processed with different methods, we discovered that the furosine contents of freeze-dried velvet antler processed without blood were lower than those of the corresponding parts of boiled velvet antler processed with blood. Wax pieces were more likely to contain furosine than other parts of the velvet antler. Comparing the furosine, CML, and CEL contents in processed velvet antler, we found that the effects of the different processing methods and different parts on the furosine contents in processed velvet antler are similar to those for the CML and CEL contents [18]. Therefore, furosine can be considered as a marker for evaluating the degree of the Maillard reaction and AGE content in processed velvet antler.

2.4. Factors Influencing the Furosine Content in the Processed Velvet Antler

The differences in furosine contents between various parts of the velvet antler processed with different methods arise from the occurrence of different degrees of the Maillard reaction. Factors influencing the Maillard reaction include the carbonyl (reducing sugars) and amino (amino acids, proteins) contents, as well as the processing temperature [27,28,34]. Therefore, further investigation of the above-mentioned molecules was performed for different parts of the velvet antler samples processed with the various methods.

2.4.1. Protein and Amino Acid Contents in the Processed Velvet Antler

The protein content of the processed velvet antler samples was determined by using the Dumas combustion method and the related results are shown in Table 2. The protein contents of wax, powder, gauze, and bone slices of the freeze-dried velvet antler were 49.03–81.56%. The protein contents of the boiled velvet antler ranged from 51.13 to 81.25%. For the samples processed without and with blood, the protein contents were 54.11–79.81% and 49.65–82.09%, respectively.

Table 2. Protein, total amino acids, and lysine contents in the processed velvet antler ($\bar{x} \pm SD$, $n = 3$).

Processing Methods	Parts	Protein/%	Total Amino Acids/g/100 g	Lysine/g/100 g
freeze-dried	wax slices	81.56 ± 0.04	88.64 ± 3.30	5.87 ± 0.20
	powder slices	57.12 ± 0.03	62.51 ± 1.84	3.96 ± 0.11
	gauze slices	52.74 ± 0.10	61.75 ± 0.90	3.76 ± 0.03
	bone slices	49.03 ± 0.25	58.20 ± 1.17	3.41 ± 0.21
	entire	56.93 ± 0.34	68.00 ± 1.23	4.02 ± 0.13
boiled	wax slices	81.25 ± 0.12	87.48 ± 1.78	5.67 ± 0.22
	powder slices	58.11 ± 0.18	62.29 ± 0.82	3.92 ± 0.14
	gauze slices	53.99 ± 0.33	60.97 ± 0.28	3.69 ± 0.10
	bone slices	51.13 ± 0.25	55.62 ± 1.74	3.15 ± 0.12
	entire	60.99 ± 0.44	67.59 ± 1.82	4.09 ± 0.29
processed without blood	wax slices	79.81 ± 0.09	86.74 ± 0.18	5.56 ± 0.11
	powder slices	56.69 ± 0.11	66.65 ± 0.74	4.01 ± 0.09
	gauze slices	58.88 ± 0.31	62.35 ± 0.48	3.76 ± 0.11
	bone slices	54.11 ± 0.24	52.34 ± 0.72	3.01 ± 0.12
	entire	56.43 ± 0.28	63.55 ± 0.82	3.58 ± 0.15
processed with blood	wax slices	82.09 ± 0.74	91.02 ± 0.46	5.66 ± 0.12
	powder slices	61.49 ± 0.33	74.06 ± 0.34	4.81 ± 0.02
	gauze slices	61.45 ± 0.41	66.94 ± 0.49	4.26 ± 0.07
	bone slices	49.65 ± 0.56	61.06 ± 0.46	3.48 ± 0.15
	entire	59.25 ± 0.35	64.31 ± 0.56	4.03 ± 0.17

No significant differences ($p > 0.05$) in protein contents were observed between the same parts of the freeze-dried and boiled velvet antler samples. In addition, the parts of the processed velvet antler with blood showed a significantly higher protein content than those processed without blood ($p < 0.05$). This is because the blood (which contains protein) was removed from those samples processed without blood. Significant differences in protein contents between the different parts of the processed velvet antler were observed. The wax slices exhibited significantly higher protein contents than the other parts ($p < 0.01$). This is probably because the wax slices from the antler tip contain an increased amount of meristem tissue, which promotes protein expression [33].

The protein contents of the samples processed with blood are higher than those processed without blood and the protein contents of the wax slices are higher than those of the other parts. Since protein is a substrate for the Maillard reaction, the furosine contents in the samples processed with blood are significantly higher than those in the same parts processed without blood and the furosine contents in the wax slices were significantly higher than those of the other parts.

An automatic amino acid analyzer was used to determine the contents of seventeen amino acids in the various parts of velvet antler processed using different methods. The results of the total amino acid and lysine analyses are summarized in Table 2 and the specific content of all seventeen amino acids is provided in the supplementary material.

The total amino acid and lysine contents in boiled velvet antler were slightly lower than those observed in the same parts of the freeze-dried velvet antler. Heat treatment exacerbates the consumption of amino acids by the Maillard reaction, resulting in significantly higher furosine contents in the boiled velvet antler than those in the corresponding parts of freeze-dried velvet antler. The total amino acid and lysine contents in the samples processed with blood are slightly higher than those processed without blood. The blood in the samples is preserved during the processing and contains a large amount of amino acids, providing a sufficient amount of substrate for the Maillard reaction. Therefore, the furosine contents in the samples processed with blood are significantly higher than those of the corresponding parts processed without blood.

The total amino acid and lysine contents in the various parts of the velvet antler differed significantly. The total amino acid and lysine contents of the wax slices were significantly higher those of the other parts ($p < 0.01$). No significant differences were observed between the powder, gauze, and bone slices ($p > 0.05$). This is probably the result of the wax slices from the antler tip containing more meristem tissue, which increases amino acid demand. Wax slices contain more Maillard reaction substrate amino acids and, therefore, produce more furosine than the other parts.

2.4.2. Reducing Sugar Content in the Processed Velvet Antler

The reducing sugar content of the processed velvet antler was determined by using pre-column derivatization UPLC. The related chromatogram is shown in Figure 3 and the values are listed in Table 3. Eight monosaccharides were detected in the various parts of velvet antler processed with different methods, namely mannose, glucosamine, ribose, glucuronic acid, galacturonic acid, aminogalactose, glucose, and galactose.

The reducing sugar contents of the freeze-dried velvet antler were significantly higher than those of the corresponding parts of the boiled velvet antler ($p < 0.05$). High temperatures promote the Maillard reaction, so the sugars were consumed to produce furosine. The reducing sugar contents of the samples processed without blood were significantly lower than those of the corresponding parts processed with blood, except for the glucosamine and amino galactose contents ($p < 0.05$). Blood contains large amounts of carbohydrates and its removal by centrifugation decreases the reducing sugar content. Therefore, the samples processed without blood contain less reducing sugar and produce less furosine than the corresponding samples processed with blood.

The wax slices contained significantly higher amounts of reducing sugar than the other parts ($p < 0.01$). The reducing sugar contents in the powder, gauze, and bone slices were gradually reduced ($p < 0.05$). The reason for this is the different amounts of cartilage tissue in the various parts of the velvet antler and the different requirements for sugars [33]. As a consequence of the differential distribution of the Maillard reaction substrates, the furosine content varied in the different parts of the processed velvet antler.

In summary, differences in the furosine content of various parts of velvet antler processed using different methods are caused by the combined effects of reducing sugars, amino acids, proteins, and processing temperature.

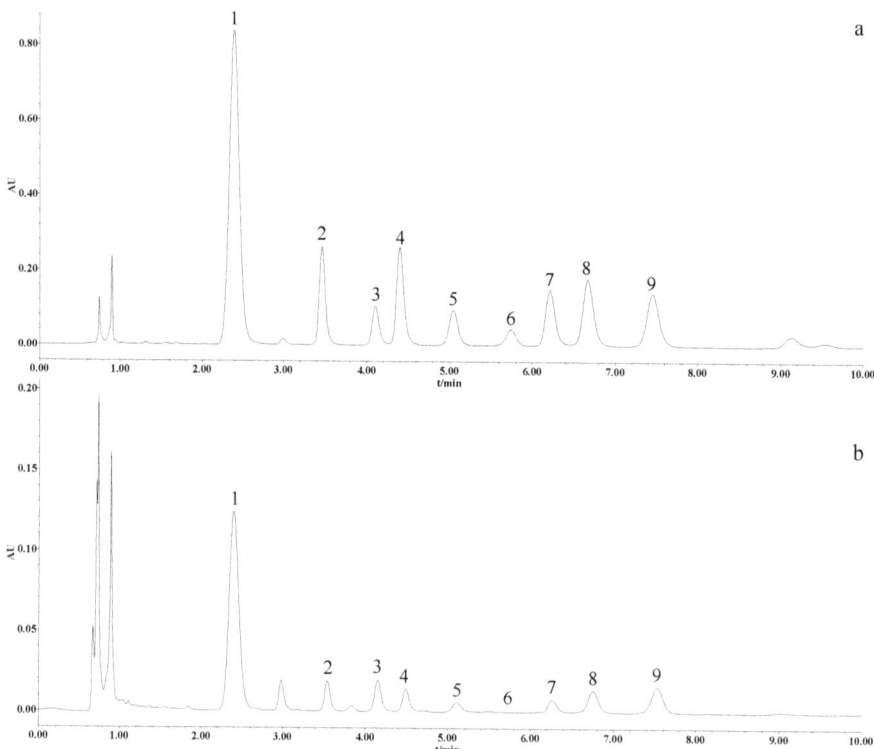

Figure 3. Chromatograms of the eight monosaccharides in (**a**) the mixed standard and (**b**) gauze slices of freeze-dried velvet antler. Peak numbers 1–9 represent 1-phenyl-3-methyl-5-pyrazolone, mannose, glucosamine, ribose, glucuronic acid, galacturonic acid, aminogalactose, glucose, and galactose, respectively.

Table 3. Eight monosaccharides contents in processed velvet antler, expressed per mg/kg ($\bar{x} \pm$ SD, $n = 3$).

Compound	Freeze-Dried				Boiled			
	Wax Slices	Powder Slices	Gauze Slices	Bone Slices	Wax Slices	Powder Slices	Gauze Slices	Bone Slices
mannose	13.31 ± 1.01	9.49 ± 0.78	9.75 ± 0.65	7.66 ± 0.55	10.10 ± 0.98	6.32 ± 0.42	5.86 ± 0.45	4.31 ± 0.33
glucosamine	70.21 ± 2.03	60.32 ± 1.84	58.45 ± 1.21	48.04 ± 1.97	66.34 ± 2.33	56.30 ± 1.04	51.75 ± 1.32	44.04 ± 1.74
ribose	14.16 ± 1.21	9.37 ± 0.96	7.94 ± 1.01	6.60 ± 0.95	7.63 ± 1.04	5.52 ± 0.97	4.07 ± 0.87	3.58 ± 0.74
glucuronic acid	20.02 ± 1.19	16.51 ± 1.20	12.09 ± 0.98	7.46 ± 0.77	15.34 ± 1.04	13.74 ± 0.96	8.05 ± 0.81	6.18 ± 0.77
galacturonic acid	3.55 ± 0.94	2.64 ± 0.81	1.26 ± 0.72	0.27 ± 0.18	2.75 ± 0.55	1.52 ± 0.53	1.29 ± 0.19	0.20 ± 0.12
aminogalactose	18.36 ± 1.32	15.77 ± 1.09	11.39 ± 0.75	3.96 ± 0.63	16.98 ± 0.94	11.32 ± 1.02	9.88 ± 0.91	2.39 ± 0.74
glucose	18.10 ± 1.52	13.46 ± 1.04	11.95 ± 1.22	10.13 ± 1.09	16.25 ± 1.43	10.86 ± 1.51	9.24 ± 1.06	7.13 ± 1.33
galactose	28.89 ± 1.82	26.54 ± 2.07	26.58 ± 1.67	22.33 ± 1.33	22.93 ± 1.47	16.62 ± 1.83	16.75 ± 1.42	19.43 ± 1.17

Compound	Processed with Blood				Processed without Blood			
	Wax Slices	Powder Slices	Gauze Slices	Bone Slices	Wax Slices	Powder Slices	Gauze Slices	Bone Slices
mannose	11.20 ± 1.07	9.60 ± 1.21	6.30 ± 0.97	5.83 ± 0.84	9.22 ± 1.07	7.15 ± 0.92	4.77 ± 0.67	3.22 ± 0.54
glucosamine	52.34 ± 2.07	35.47 ± 2.22	31.34 ± 1.98	28.11 ± 2.13	57.36 ± 2.45	38.11 ± 1.56	33.71 ± 1.42	30.13 ± 1.08
ribose	5.63 ± 0.71	4.78 ± 0.63	3.22 ± 0.58	2.10 ± 0.41	4.17 ± 0.51	3.90 ± 0.35	2.48 ± 0.24	1.16 ± 0.16
glucuronic acid	15.14 ± 0.74	13.83 ± 0.81	11.62 ± 0.53	5.01 ± 0.37	13.55 ± 1.02	8.76 ± 0.91	7.01 ± 0.87	3.65 ± 0.54
galacturonic acid	2.55 ± 0.32	1.90 ± 0.28	1.62 ± 0.17	0.82 ± 0.19	2.19 ± 0.23	1.72 ± 0.31	1.60 ± 0.22	0.20 ± 0.12
aminogalactose	16.78 ± 0.79	12.92 ± 0.82	9.46 ± 0.77	7.06 ± 0.54	20.24 ± 0.86	16.77 ± 0.72	12.34 ± 0.83	0.57 ± 0.14
glucose	16.25 ± 0.44	12.68 ± 0.58	9.21 ± 0.79	7.38 ± 0.88	13.65 ± 0.92	9.50 ± 0.77	7.62 ± 0.81	5.91 ± 0.69
galactose	22.73 ± 1.07	18.23 ± 0.98	16.44 ± 1.21	13.07 ± 0.78	18.08 ± 1.23	17.59 ± 1.42	15.22 ± 1.33	12.04 ± 0.79

3. Materials and Methods

3.1. Materials

Furosine and TFA were purchased from Sigma–Aldrich (San Francisco, CA, USA). Mannose, glucosamine, ribose, glucuronic acid, galacturonic acid, aminogalactose, glucose, and galactose were purchased from Yuan-ye Biotechnology Co., Ltd. (Shanghai, China). The purity of these reagents was >99%. A total of 17 amino acid standards, ninhydrin (NIN), and a citric acid buffer solution were purchased from Hitachi Inc. (Hitachi Co., Osaka, Japan). HPLC-grade acetonitrile was purchased from Fisher Scientific (Waltham, MA, USA), and C18 Sep-Pak® SPE tubes were purchased from Sepax (Sepax technology, Cork, Ireland). Ultrapure water was obtained by using a super-pure water system (Sichuan, China). All other reagents used in this study were of analytical grade and were purchased from Sinopharm Chemical Reagent Co. Ltd. (Beijing, China).

3.2. Sources and Preparation of the Velvet Antler

Velvet antler (*Cervi cornu pantotrichum*) was collected in Shuangyang, Jilin Province (China) and was identified by Dr. C.Y. Li from the Chinese Academy of Agricultural Sciences Institute of Special Animal and Plant Sciences.

3.3. Preparation of the Different Processed Velvet Antler Slices

According to the classification of commercially available velvet antler, samples that were boiled, freeze-dried, processed with blood, and processed without blood were chosen for this study. A total of six pairs of velvet antler samples were randomly selected to be processed with blood and without blood, for comparison, and another six pairs were randomly selected and processed by boiling and freeze-drying. The boiled velvet antler was boiled for 1 min in boiling water and then baked at a high temperature (75 °C) for 2 h. This operation was repeated several times until dryness was achieved. The freeze-dried velvet antler was directly frozen to dryness. The velvet antler processed without blood was prepared by removing the blood by physical centrifugation, whereas no blood removal was performed for the samples processed with blood. The blood content in velvet antler processed with blood is about 8% by measurement.

Three pairs of boiled and freeze-dried velvet antler samples and three pairs of velvet antler processed with and without blood were randomly selected and crushed whole for subsequent analysis. The remaining six pairs of velvet antler were divided into wax, powder, gauze, and bone slices, on the basis of their morphological and microscopic characteristics (Figure 4) [34]. These parts were segmented, sliced, crushed, sieved, bagged, and labelled for analysis.

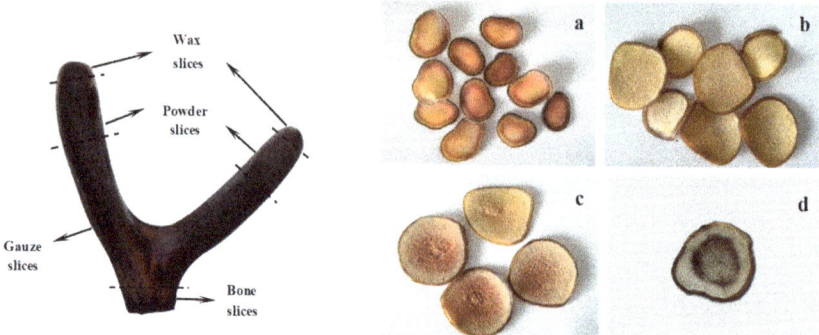

Figure 4. Schematic diagram of different parts of processed velvet antler. The processed velvet antler was divided into wax slices (**a**), powder slices (**b**), gauze slices (**c**), and bone slices (**d**) on the basis of morphological and microscopic characteristics.

3.4. Sample Preparation

Pieces of processed velvet antler samples equivalent to 30 mg were mixed with 8 M hydrochloric acid (HCl) and incubated at 110 °C for 24 h. The diluted acid hydrolysate (equivalent to approximately 600 μg of protein) was dried under a nitrogen stream at 70 °C by using a pressured gas-blowing concentrator. The dried hydrolysate was then dissolved in 1 mL of ultra-pure water and solid-phase extracted by using a C18 Sep-Pak® (Sepax Technology, Cork, Ireland) cartridge (500 mg, 6 mL). The SPE column was pre-treated with 3 mL of methanol and 0.1 M TFA at a flow rate of 1 mL/min. The sample was loaded onto the pre-treated SPE column washed with 6 mL of 0.1 M TFA. Finally, the sample was eluted with 3 mL of methanol at a flow rate of 0.5 mL/min. The eluate was dried by freezing, re-dissolved in 1 mL of ultra-pure water, and filtered through a 0.22-μm membrane prior to UPLC-MS/MS analysis.

3.5. Quantification of Furosine

The furosine concentration in the hydrolysates was determined by UPLC-MS/MS [35]. Briefly, the protein hydrolysates (2 μg protein, 3 μL) were injected into an Acquity HSS T3 UPLC column (2.1 × 100 mm, 1.8 μm) housed in a column oven at 40 °C and operated in gradient-elution mode. Solvent A was water and solvent B was acetonitrile. Gradient elution began at 80% solvent B for 1 min, followed by a linear gradient from 80% to 30% solvent B over 1.5 min, holding at 30% solvent B for 0.5 min, and then returning to 80% solvent B for 1 min. Analysis was performed by using a Waters Acquity UPLC instrument (Waters, Manchester, UK) coupled to a triple-quadrupole MS operating in MRM mode at a flow rate of 0.3 mL/min. The MS instrument was operated in electrospray-ionization positive mode. The optimized MRM conditions are listed in Table 4. The furosine was quantified by using a pure standard and by reference to an external standard calibration curve. The data are reported as the mean ± standard deviation of triplicate experiments. The furosine content in the samples was expressed as μmol/mmol lysine, μg/g protein, and μg/g sample.

Table 4. UPLC-MS settings for multiple reaction monitoring (MRM).

Compound	Precursor Ion (m/z)	Product Ion (m/z)	Cone Voltage (V)	Collision Energy (ev)	Dwell Time (ms)
furosine	255	192	25	15	36
	255	130	25	15	36
	255	84	25	25	36

3.6. Protein Content Analysis

The protein content of the processed velvet antler was determined by using a Dumas nitrogen analyzer (Velp NDA 701-Monza, Brianza, Italy) according to a previously described method, with minor modifications [29]. The total nitrogen content was converted into the protein content by using a conversion factor of 6.25. The operating conditions of the NDA instrument were as follows: O_2 gas at 400 mL/min, He gas at 195 mL/min, combustion reactor at 1030 °C, reduction reactor at 650 °C, and pressure of 88.1 kPa.

3.7. Amino Acid Content Analysis

An amino acid analyzer (L-8900 System; Hitachi Co., Osaka, Japan) equipped with a visible light detector was used for amino acid analysis. Analytical 2622# (4.6 × 60 mm) and guard 2650# (4.6 × 40 mm) columns were used for the determination of 17 amino acids. Immediately after injection of the sample into the columns, an auto-sampler was used for in-line derivatization by NIN post-column derivatization. NIN-derivatized proline was detected at 440 nm and the other amino acids were detected at 570 nm. Standards of the 17 amino acids were used for identification and quantification (external standard method) and their contents were expressed as g/100 g of processed velvet antler.

3.8. Reducing Sugar Content Analysis

The reducing sugars in the processed velvet antler samples were measured with UPLC by using the method reported by Teixeria et al. [36], with minor modifications. The velvet antler samples were boiled with ultra-pure water for 2 h and the reaction was performed with 1 mL of the extract, 0.5 mL of 0.3 M NaOH, and 0.5 mL of 0.3 M 1-phenyl-3-methyl-5-pyrazolone derivatization solution. The reaction mixture was heated in a water bath at 70 °C for 30 min, 0.5 mL of 0.3 M HCl was added to terminate the reaction, and the resultant solution was filtered through a 0.22 μm membrane prior to UPLC analysis. A UPLC instrument equipped with an Acquity UPLC BEH C18 column (100 × 2.1 mm, 1.7 μm) was used. Solvent A was 0.1 M phosphate buffer (pH 7.0) and solvent B was acetonitrile, with a gradient elution of 18% solvent B for 10 min, and a flow rate of 0.3 mL/min. The injection volume was 2 μL and the detection wavelength was 254 nm.

4. Conclusions

In the future, analysis of velvet antler and other biological samples from horny drugs, such as nails [37,38], will be a widespread concern. In this study, we established a method for the detection of furosine content in processed velvet antler, which was used for actual sample detection and evaluation of the degree of the Maillard reaction in processed velvet antler. The furosine contents in boiled velvet antler were significantly higher than those in freeze-dried samples. Velvet antler processed with blood exhibited significantly higher levels of furosine than the corresponding parts processed without blood.

Velvet antler boiled at high temperatures produced more furosine than the samples freeze-dried at low temperatures. The contents of Maillard reaction substrates, that is, carbonyl (reducing sugars) and amino (amino acids, proteins) compounds, were determined. The differing contents of these key molecules are the main reason behind the observed differences in furosine contents. For the same parts of processed velvet antler, boiling led to a certain amount of lysine and reducing sugars being consumed to produce more furosine than that in the freeze-dried samples. The samples processed with blood contained more proteins, amino acids, and reducing sugars than those processed without blood, which promoted furosine formation. Similarly, the wax slices contained more proteins, lysine, and reducing sugars and, thus, produced more furosine than the other parts of the velvet antler. The differences in furosine content between the various velvet antler parts, processed by using different methods, were a result of the combined action of the reducing sugars, amino acids, and proteins, as well as the processing temperature.

These data can be used to evaluate the degree of Maillard reaction that has occurred in processed velvet antler samples and can guide the production of low-furosine velvet antler for consumers through optimized processing. In addition, these data can also be used to estimate the furosine intake from velvet antler and educate consumers about how to reduce their furosine intake.

Supplementary Materials: The supplementary materials are available online.

Author Contributions: Data curation, R.-z.G. and Y.-h.W.; Funding acquisition, Y.-s.S., L.Z., and C.L.; Methodology, Y.-h.W.; Resources, Y.-s.S.; Software, Y.-f.W.; Validation, Y.-h.W.; Writing—original draft, R.-z.G., Z-s.W. and K.G.; Writing—review and editing, R.-z.G., K.G. and Y.-s.S.

Funding: This work was financially supported by the National Key Research and Development Program of China (2018YFC1706604 and 2018YFC1706605), the Jilin Province Science and Technology Development Project (20180201076YY), and the Science and Technology Innovation Project of the Chinese Academy of Agricultural Sciences (CAAS-ASTIP-2016-ISAPS).

Conflicts of Interest: The authors declare no conflict of interest.

References

1. Jeon, B.; Kim, S.; Lee, S.; Park, P.; Sung, S.; Kim, J.; Moon, S. Effect of antler growth period on the chemical composition of velvet antler in sika deer (*Cervus nippon*). *Z. Saugetierkd.* **2009**, *74*, 374–380. [CrossRef]

2. Wu, F.; Li, H.; Jin, L.; Li, X.; Ma, Y.; You, J.; Li, S.; Xu, Y. Deer antler base as a traditional Chinese medicine: A review of its traditional uses, chemistry and pharmacology. *J. Ethnopharmacol.* **2013**, *145*, 403–415. [CrossRef]
3. Zhou, R.; Li, S. In vitro antioxidant analysis and characterisation of antler velvet extract. *Food Chem.* **2009**, *114*, 1321–1327. [CrossRef]
4. Sui, Z.; Yuan, H.; Liang, Z.; Zhao, Q.; Wu, Q.; Xia, S.; Zhang, L.; Huo, Y.; Zhang, Y. An activity-maintaining sequential protein extraction method for bioactive assay and proteome analysis of velvet antlers. *Talanta* **2013**, *107*, 189–194. [CrossRef] [PubMed]
5. Sui, Z.; Zhang, L.; Huo, Y.; Zhang, Y. Bioactive components of velvet antlers and their pharmacological properties. *J. Pharm. Biomed.* **2014**, *87*, 229–240. [CrossRef]
6. Tseng, S.H.; Sung, C.H.; Chen, L.G.; Lai, Y.J.; Chang, W.S.; Sung, H.C.; Wang, C.C. Comparison of chemical compositions and osteoprotective effects of different sections of velvet antler. *J. Ethnopharmacol.* **2014**, *151*, 352–360. [CrossRef]
7. Singh, R.; Barden, A.; Mori, T.; Beilin, L. Advanced glycation end-products: A review. *Diabetologia* **2001**, *2001*, 129–146. [CrossRef]
8. Reynaert, N.L.; Gopal, P.; Rutten, E.P.A.; Wouters, E.F.M.; Schalkwijk, C.G. Advanced glycation end products and their receptor in age-related, non-communicable chronic inflammatory diseases; Overview of clinical evidence and potential contributions to disease. *Int. J. Biochem. Cell Biol.* **2016**, *81*, 403–418. [CrossRef]
9. Kuhla, A.; Ludwig, S.C.; Kuhla, B.; Münch, G.; Vollmar, B. Advanced glycation end products are mitogenic signals and trigger cell cycle reentry of neurons in Alzheimer's disease brain. *Neurobiol. Aging* **2015**, *36*, 753–761. [CrossRef] [PubMed]
10. de Vos, L.C.; Lefrandt, J.D.; Dullaart, R.P.; Zeebregts, C.J.; Smit, A.J. Advanced glycation end products: An emerging biomarker for adverse outcome in patients with peripheral artery disease. *Atherosclerosis* **2016**, *254*, 291–299. [CrossRef] [PubMed]
11. Drenth, H.; Zuidema, S.U.; Krijnen, W.P.; Bautmans, I.; Schans, C.V.D.; Hobbelen, H. Advanced glycation end-products are associated with the presence and severity of paratonia in early stage Alzheimer disease. *J. Am. Med. Dir. Assoc.* **2017**, *18*, 636.e7–636.e12. [CrossRef] [PubMed]
12. Gautieri, A.; Passini, F.S.; Silván, U.; Guizar-Sicairos, M.; Carimati, G.; Volpi, P.; Moretti, M.; Redaelli, A.; Berli, M.; Snedeker, J.G. Advanced glycation end-products: Mechanics of aged collagen from molecule to tissue. *Matrix Biol.* **2016**, *59*, 95–108. [CrossRef]
13. Vlassara, H.; Palace, M.R. Glycoxidation: The menace of diabetes and aging. *Mt. Sinai J. Med.* **2003**, *70*, 232–241.
14. Chuang, Y.C.; Wu, M.S.; Wu, T.H.; Su, Y.K.; Lee, Y.M. Pyridoxamine ameliorates the effects of advanced glycation end products on subtotal nephrectomy induced chronic renal failure rats. *J. Funct. Foods* **2012**, *4*, 679–686. [CrossRef]
15. Buraczynska, M.; Zaluska, W.; Buraczynska, K.; Markowska-Gosik, D.; Ksiazek, A. Receptor for advanced glycation end products (RAGE) gene polymorphism and cardiovascular disease in end-stage renal disease patients. *Hum. Immunol.* **2015**, *76*, 843–848. [CrossRef]
16. Hashimoto, K.; Kunikata, H.; Yasuda, M.; Ito, A.; Aizawa, N.; Sawada, S.; Kondo, K.; Satake, C.; Takano, Y.; Nishiguchi, K.M. The relationship between advanced glycation end products and ocular circulation in type 2 diabetes. *J. Diabetes Complicat.* **2016**, *30*, 1371–1377. [CrossRef] [PubMed]
17. Moriya, S.; Yamazaki, M.; Murakami, H.; Maruyama, K.; Uchiyama, S. Two soluble isoforms of receptors for advanced glycation end products (RAGE) in carotid Atherosclerosis: The difference of soluble and endogenous secretory RAGE. *J. Stroke Cerebrovasc.* **2014**, *23*, 2540–2546. [CrossRef] [PubMed]
18. Gong, R.Z.; Wang, Y.; Wang, Y.F.; Chen, B.; Gao, K.; Sun, Y.S. Simultaneous Determination of N^ε-(carboxymethyl) lysine and N^ε-(carboxyethyl) lysine in different sections of antler velvet after various processing methods by UPLC-MS/MS. *Molecules* **2018**, *23*, 3316. [CrossRef]
19. Troise, A.D.; Fiore, A.; Wiltafsky, M.; Fogliano, V. Quantification of N^ε-(2-Furoylmethyl)-L-lysine (furosine), N^ε-(Carboxymethyl)-L-lysine (CML), N^ε-(Carboxyethyl)-L-lysine (CEL) and total lysine through stable isotope dilution assay and tandem mass spectrometry. *Food Chem.* **2015**, *188*, 357–364. [CrossRef]
20. He, J.; Zeng, M.; Zheng, Z.; He, Z.; Chen, J. Simultaneous determination of N^ε-(carboxymethyl) lysine and N^ε-(carboxyethyl) lysine in cereal foods by LC–MS/MS. *Eur. Food Res. Technol.* **2014**, *238*, 367–374. [CrossRef]
21. Hull, G.L.J.; Woodside, J.V.; Ames, J.M.; Cuskelly, G.J. N^ε-(carboxymethyl)lysine content of foods commonly consumed in a Western style diet. *Food Chem.* **2012**, *131*, 170–174. [CrossRef]

22. Erbersdobler, H.F.; Somoza, V. Forty years of furosine—Forty years of using Maillard reaction products as indicators of the nutritional quality of foods. *Mol. Nutr. Food Res.* **2010**, *51*, 423–430. [CrossRef] [PubMed]
23. Harris, C.; Beaulieu, L.P.; Fraser, M.H.; Mcintyre, K.; Owen, P.; Martineau, L.; Cuerrier, A.; Johns, T.; Haddad, P.S.; Bennett, S.A.L.; et al. Inhibition of advanced glycation end product formation by medicinal plant extracts correlates with phenolic metabolites and antioxidant activity. *Planta Med.* **2010**, *77*, 196–204. [CrossRef] [PubMed]
24. Li, H.Y.; Xing, L.; Wang, J.Q.; Zheng, N. Toxicology studies of furosine in vitro/in vivo and exploration of the related mechanism. *Toxicol. Lett.* **2018**, *291*, 101–111. [CrossRef] [PubMed]
25. Bosch, L.; Alegrı, A.A.; Farré, R.; Clemente, G. Effect of storage conditions on furosine formation in milk–cereal based baby foods. *Food Chem.* **2008**, *107*, 1681–1686. [CrossRef]
26. Villamiel, M.; Castillo, M.D.D.; Corzo, N.; Olano, A. Presence of furosine in honeys. *J. Sci. Food Agric.* **2001**, *81*, 790–793. [CrossRef]
27. Trevisan, A.J.; de Almeida Lima, D.; Sampaio, G.R.; Soares, R.A.; Markowicz Bastos, D.H. Influence of home cooking conditions on Maillard reaction products in beef. *Food Chem.* **2016**, *196*, 161–169. [CrossRef] [PubMed]
28. Jiao, Y.; He, J.; Li, F.; Tao, G.; Zhang, S.; Zhang, S.; Qin, F.; Zeng, M.; Chen, J. N^ε-(carboxymethyl)lysine and N^ε-(carboxyethyl)lysine in tea and the factors affecting their formation. *Food Chem.* **2017**, *232*, 683–688. [CrossRef]
29. Schettgen, T.; Tings, A.; Brodowsky, C.; Müller-Lux, A.; Musiol, A.; Kraus, T. Simultaneous determination of the advanced glycation end product N^ε-carboxymethyllysine and its precursor, lysine, in exhaled breath condensate using isotope-dilution-hydrophilic-interaction liquid chromatography coupled to tandem mass spectrometry. *Anal. Bioanal. Chem.* **2007**, *387*, 2783–2791. [CrossRef]
30. Renterghem, R.V.; Block, J.D. Furosine in consumption milk and milk powders. *Int. Dairy J.* **1996**, *6*, 371–382. [CrossRef]
31. Yamaguchi, K.; Nomi, Y.; Homma, T.; Kasai, M.; Otsuka, Y. Determination of furosine and fluorescence as markers of the Maillard reaction for the evaluation of meat products during actual cooking conditions. *Food Sci. Technol. Res.* **2012**, *18*, 67–76. [CrossRef]
32. Dittrich, R.; Hoffmann, I.; Stahl, P.; Müller, A.; Beckmann, M.W.; Pischetsrieder, M. Concentrations of N^ε-carboxymethyllysine in human breast milk, infant formulas, and urine of infants. *J. Agric. Food Chem.* **2006**, *54*, 6924–6928. [CrossRef]
33. Li, C.; Zhao, H.; Liu, Z.; Mcmahon, C. Deer antler—A novel model for studying organ regeneration in mammals. *Int. J. Biochem. Cell Biol.* **2014**, *56*, 111–122. [CrossRef]
34. Xu, X.B.; Ma, F.; Yu, S.J.; Guan, Y.G. Simultaneous analysis of N^ε-(carboxymethyl)lysine, reducing sugars, and lysine during the dairy thermal process. *J. Dairy Sci.* **2013**, *96*, 5487–5493. [CrossRef] [PubMed]
35. Li, Y.; Liu, X.; Meng, L.; Wang, Y. Qualitative and quantitative analysis of furosine in fresh and processed ginsengs. *J. Ginseng Res.* **2018**, *42*, 21–26. [CrossRef] [PubMed]
36. Teixeira, R.S.S.; Silva, A.S.A.D.; Bon, E.P.D.S. Amino acids interference on the quantification of reducing sugars by the 3,5-dinitrosalicylic acid assay mislead carbohydrase activity measurements. *Carbohydr. Res.* **2012**, *363*, 33–37. [CrossRef] [PubMed]
37. Busardò, F.P.; Gottardi, M.; Tini, A.; Mortali, C.; Giorgetti, R.; Pichini, S. Ultra-high-performance liquid chromatography tandem mass spectrometry assay for determination of endogenous GHB and GHB-glucuronide in nails. *Molecules* **2018**, *10*, 2686. [CrossRef] [PubMed]
38. Takahashi, F.; Kobayashi, M.; Kobayashi, A.; Kobayashi, K.; Asamura, H. High-frequency heating extraction method for sensitive drug analysis in human nails. *Molecules* **2018**, *12*, 3231. [CrossRef]

Sample Availability: Samples of the compounds furosine, mannose, glucosamine, ribose, glucuronic acid, galacturonic acid, aminogalactose, glucose, galactose and 17 amino acid standards are available from the authors.

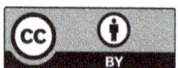

© 2019 by the authors. Licensee MDPI, Basel, Switzerland. This article is an open access article distributed under the terms and conditions of the Creative Commons Attribution (CC BY) license (http://creativecommons.org/licenses/by/4.0/).

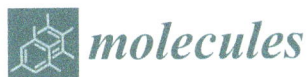

Article

Identification and Determination of Seven Phenolic Acids in Brazilian Green Propolis by UPLC-ESI-QTOF-MS and HPLC

Shengwei Sun [1], Meijuan Liu [1], Jian He [1], Kunping Li [2], Xuguang Zhang [1] and Guangling Yin [1,*]

1. Science and Technology Centre, By-Health Co. Ltd., No. 3 Kehui 3rd Street, No. 99 Kexue Avenue Central, Science City, Luogang District, Guangzhou 510000, China; ssw0929@163.com (S.S.); liumeijuan@by-health.com (M.L.); 13662340638@139.com (J.H.); zhangxg2@by-health.com (X.Z.)
2. School of Pharmacy, Guangdong Pharmaceutical University, Guangzhou 510006, China; kunping_china@gdpu.edu.cn
* Correspondence: yingl@by-health.com; Tel./Fax: +86-020-2895-6788

Academic Editors: In-Soo Yoon and Hyun-Jong Cho
Received: 2 April 2019; Accepted: 9 May 2019; Published: 9 May 2019

Abstract: Brazilian green propolis is a complex mixture of natural compounds that is difficult to analyze and standardize; as a result, controlling its quality is challenging. In this study, we used the positive and negative modes of ultra-performance liquid chromatography coupled with electrospray ionization quadrupole time of flight mass spectrometry in conjunction with high-performance liquid chromatography for the identification and characterization of seven phenolic acid compounds in Brazilian green propolis. The optimal operating conditions for the electrospray ionization source were capillary voltage of 3500 V and drying and sheath gas temperatures of 320 °C and 350 °C, respectively. Drying and sheath gas flows were set to 8 L/min and 11 L/min, respectively. Brazilian green propolis was separated using the HPLC method, with chromatograms for samples and standards measured at 310 nm. UPLC-ESI-QTOF-MS was used to identify the following phenolic compounds: Chlorogenic acid, caffeic acid, isochlorogenic acid A, isochlorogenic acid B, isochlorogenic acid C, caffeic acid phenethyl ester (CAPE), and artepillin C. Using a methodologically validated HPLC method, the seven identified phenolic acids were then quantified among different Brazilian green propolis. Results indicated that there were no significant differences in the content of a given phenolic acid across different Brazilian green propolis samples, owing to the same plant resin sources for each sample. Isochlorogenic acid B had the lowest content (0.08 ± 0.04) across all tested Brazilian green propolis samples, while the artepillin C levels were the highest (2.48 ± 0.94). The total phenolic acid content across Brazilian green propolis samples ranged from 2.14–9.32%. Notably, artepillin C quantification is an important factor in determining the quality index of Brazilian green propolis; importantly, it has potential as a chemical marker for the development of better quality control methods for Brazilian green propolis.

Keywords: Brazilian green propolis; phenolic acids; UPLC-ESI-QTOF-MS; HPLC; quantitation; methodological verification

1. Introduction

Propolis is a type of fragrant, gelatinous substance obtained by bees collecting the bud secretions and resins of pine trees, poplars, and other plants. After collection, propolis forms from the mixing of these secretions and resins with beeswax and its parotid secretions [1]. Studies have shown that propolis has a wide range of beneficial biological effects, including antibacterial, anti-inflammatory, anti-viral, anti-tumor, and anti-oxidative properties, as well as the ability to regulate blood lipids and blood sugar. As a result, it has gradually become a hot spot in nutrition research [2].

The propolis deriving from Southeastern Brazil is known as green propolis, owing to both its color and the most important botanical source of propolis: *Baccharis dracunculifolia* (Asteraceae) [3,4]. The composition of propolis is complex and may be affected by plant strain and the geographical environment of the collection; in turn, this complexity is closely related to ultimate biological properties. According to the current literature, there are at least 300 compounds of Brazilian green propolis [5]. Within these, phenolic acids (e.g., caffeic, ferulic, p-coumaric, and cinnamic acids) are its main compounds [6–9]. Recent years have seen increasing research on the pharmacological activity of propolis, which as driven expansion in its market scale. Advances in the identification and characterization of phenolic compounds are expected to provide reliable quality control metrics for Brazilian green propolis. More specifically, characterization of a single phenolic acid obtained from Brazilian green propolis is important for the selection and production of a bee product that has the highest possible levels of health-promoting compounds.

In recent years, global efforts have been made using different analytical methods to characterize phenols in propolis. Among these, high-performance liquid chromatography (HPLC) combined with mass spectrometry (MS), ultraviolet spectroscopy (UV), or photodiode array detection remain the most important analytical methods [10–13]. liquid chromatography- mass spectrometry (LC-MS) is a powerful method for the analysis of natural compounds. Given their high sensitivity and accuracy, MS analytical methods offer the potential to discover new secondary components that are difficult to obtain using conventional approaches. More detailed structural information can also be obtained by facilitating the use of tandem mass spectrometry (MS/MS), which allows for the identification of unknown compounds; critically, this identification can occur even without reference to standards [14]. For example, 40 kinds of Portuguese propolis ethanol extracts were extensively analyzed using liquid chromatography (LC), in which diode array detection was combined with electrospray ionization tandem mass spectrometry (LC-DAD-ESI-MS) [15]. The polyphenol fraction of propolis was characterized rapidly and qualitatively by chromatographic electrospray ionization tandem mass spectrometry (HPLC-ESI-MS/MS). The most recent method of HPLC-MS technology is that twelve compounds with antioxidant activities were identified in fermented A. dahurica (FAD) by an high-performance liquid chromatography method coupled with photodiode array detection and electro spray ionization ion trap-time of flight mass spectrometry and 2,2-azino-bis-(3-ethylbenzothiazoline-6-sulfonic acid) diammonium salt (HPLC-PDA-Triple-TOF-MS/MS-ABTS) method [16]. In the present study, high-efficiency, ultra-performance liquid chromatography (UPLC) was combined with HPLC. This combined approach was easy for methodological development in the context of research on phenolic acids in propolis. Importantly, there have been few reports thus far regarding either the use of UPLC-ESI-QTOF-MS to identify phenolic compounds in Brazilian green propolis or the use of HPLC to determine the exact content of identified phenolic acid compounds.

Over the past decade, the increased use and demand for propolis in a variety of products has made its effective quality control a pressing issue. In this study, we present the results of extensive research on phenolic compounds obtained from different Brazilian green propolis samples obtained from different manufacturers. These compounds were identified using accurate-mass, UPLC coupled with UPLC-ESI-QTOF-MS in both the positive and negative modes; these compounds were then characterized using HPLC. This two-fold approach was taken in an attempt to establish the Brazilian green propolis phenolic profile and lay the groundwork for its future use as a quality control strategy. Methodological analysis of HPLC was also conducted, with the aim of performing a scientific assessment of the established analytical method.

2. Results and Discussion

2.1. Identification of Phenolic Acids Compounds in Brazilian Green Propolis

Brazilian green propolis is collected by bees from bean sprouts, tree exudates, and other plant parts and further modified in beehives. This results in an incredibly complex chemical composition of the resulting propolis. After optimization, our UPLC-ESI-QTOF-MS method was successfully used to identify phenolic acids in Brazilian green propolis. The biggest advantage of UPLC was the quick separation of Brazilian green propolis alcohol extracts, which greatly improved the efficiency of the test. The combination of positive and negative ESI modes was chosen as the ionization method. The QTOF-MS detector allowed for more accurate measurements and higher resolution. Characteristic, common peaks were identified by comparing their chromatographic behavior, UV spectra, and MS information either to those of reference compounds or to reference-related studies [17,18]. Thirty-one compounds were isolated from Brazilian green propolis; of these, 10 phenolic compounds were obtained for later LC-MS analysis [19,20]. Total phenol content was quantified spectrophotometrically and 30 phenolic compounds were identified by HPLC-ESI-MS/MS analysis [21]. The pseudo-molecular ions $(M + Na)^+$ and $(M - H)^-$ of green propolis were detected in both positive and negative ESI mode. These phenolic acid compounds were then separated using the chromatographic conditions indicated in the experimental section.

Chlorogenic acid (1) with $(M + Na)^+$ at *m/z* 377 and $(M - H)^-$ at *m/z* 353 was eluted after 2.39 min, whereas caffeic acid (2) with $(M + Na)^+$ at *m/z* 203 and $(M - H)^-$ at *m/z* 179, isochlorogenic acid B (3) with $(M + Na)^+$ at *m/z* 539 and $(M - H)^-$ at *m/z* 515, isochlorogenic acid A (4) with $(M + Na)^+$ at *m/z* 539 and $(M - H)^-$ at *m/z* 515, isochlorogenic acid C (5) with $(M + Na)^+$ at *m/z* 539 and $(M - H)^-$ at *m/z* 549, caffeic acid phenethyl ester (6) with $(M + Na)^+$ at *m/z* 307 and $(M - H)^-$ at *m/z* 283, artepillin C (7) with $(M + Na)^+$ at *m/z* 323 and $(M - H)^-$ at *m/z* 299 appeared at 5.16, 7.53, 7.81, 9.82, 25.95 and 33.08 min, respectively. These compounds were identified by their total ion chromatogram (TIC) (as shown in Figure 1) and primary mass spectrum (Figure 2). The data were consistent with previous research [22] and are reported in Table 1.

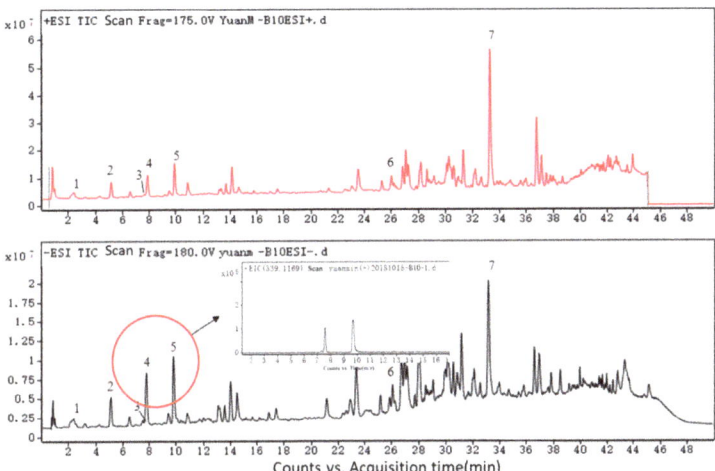

Figure 1. Chlorogenic acid (1), caffeic acid (2), isochlorogenic acid B (3), isochlorogenic acid A (4), isochlorogenic acid C (5), caffeic acid phenethyl ester (6) and artepillin C (7) were identified by ultra-high performance liquid chromatography(UHPLC)-electrospray ionization quadrupole time of flight mass spectrometry (ESI-QTOF-MS), appeared at 2.39, 5.16, 7.53, 7.81, 9.82, 25.95 and 33.08 min, respectively. The absorption of the seven peaks in TIC was similar in both positive and negative ESI modes. However, compound diversity in positive mode was greater than that in negative mode from 24 to 40 min.

Chlorogenic acid

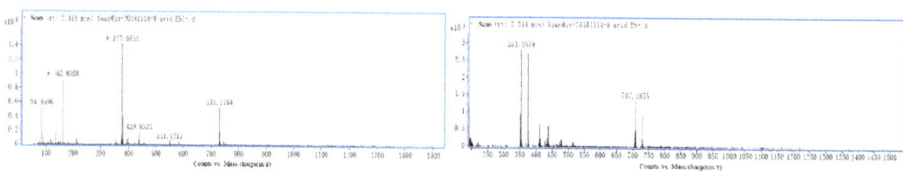

Caffeic acid

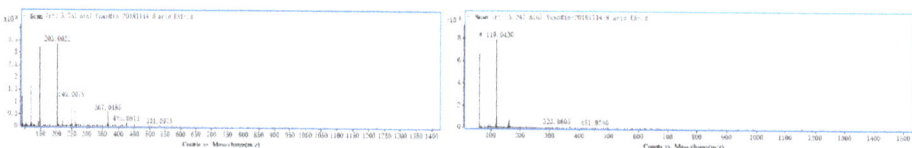

Isochlorogenic acid B

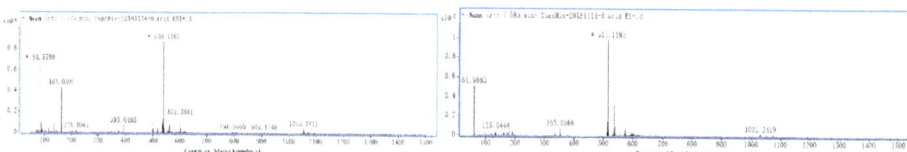

Isochlorogenic acid A

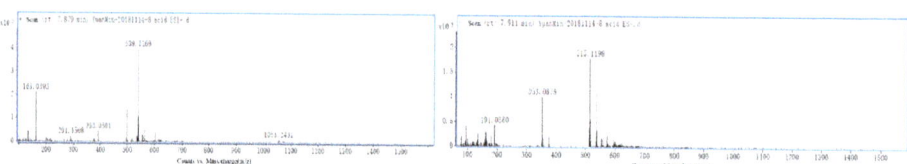

Isochlorogenic acid C

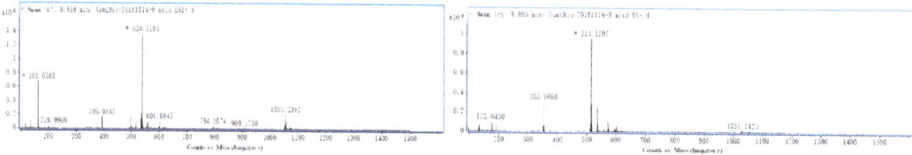

Caffeic acid phenethylester

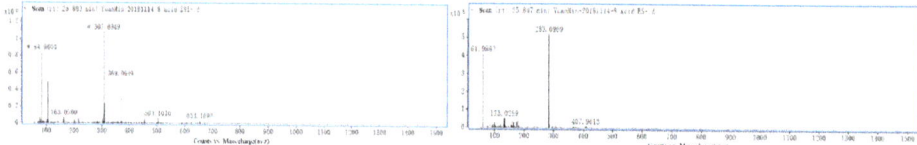

Figure 2. *Cont.*

Artepillin C

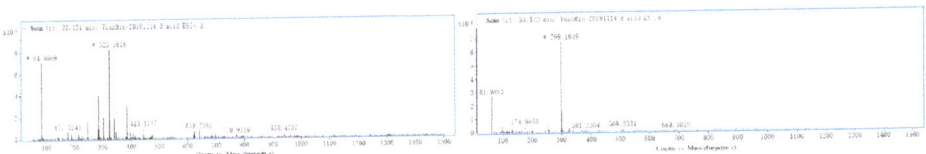

Figure 2. The primary mass spectrum for each of the seven phenolic acids in both positive and negative ESI modes: Chlorogenic acid (1) with (M + Na)$^+$ at m/z 377 and (M − H)$^-$ at m/z 353, whereas caffeic acid (2) with (M + Na)$^+$ at m/z 203 and (M − H)$^-$ at m/z 179, isochlorogenic acid B (3) with (M + Na)$^+$ at m/z 539 and (M − H)$^-$ at m/z 515, isochlorogenic acid A (4) with (M + Na)$^+$ at m/z 539 and (M − H)$^-$ at m/z 515, isochlorogenic acid C (5) with (M + Na)$^+$ at m/z 539 and (M − H)$^-$ at m/z 549, caffeic acid phenethyl ester (6) with (M + Na)$^+$ at m/z 307 and (M − H)$^-$ at m/z 283, and artepillin C (7) with (M + Na)$^+$ at m/z 323 and (M − H)$^-$ at m/z 299.

Table 1. The identification of seven phenolic acids from Brazilian propolis samples in both positive and negative ESI modes.

No.	t_R/min	Positive Ion Mode			Negative Ion Mode			Compound
		Molecular Ion (m/z)	Molecular Formula	Error (ppm)	Molecular Ion (m/z)	Molecular Formula	Error (ppm)	
1	2.391	[M + Na]$^+$ 377.0855	$C_{16}H_{18}O_9$	1.591	[M − H]$^-$ 353.0879	$C_{16}H_{18}O_9$	1.699	Chlorogenic acid
2	5.159	[M + Na]$^+$ 203.0021	$C_9H_8O_4$	−6.206	[M − H]$^-$ 179.0430	$C_9H_8O_4$	4.934	Caffeic acid
3	7.526	[M + Na]$^+$ 539.1169	$C_{25}H_{24}O_{12}$	−0.557	[M − H]$^-$ 515.1195	$C_{25}H_{24}O_{12}$	0.971	Isochlorogenic acid B
4	7.806	[M + Na]$^+$ 539.1169	$C_{25}H_{24}O_{12}$	0.742	[M − H]$^-$ 515.1198	$C_{25}H_{24}O_{12}$	1.553	Isochlorogenic acid A
5	9.820	[M + Na]$^+$ 539.1169	$C_{25}H_{24}O_{12}$	−0.371	[M − H]$^-$ 515.1197	$C_{25}H_{24}O_{12}$	1.359	Isochlorogenic acid C
6	25.948	[M + Na]$^+$ 307.9490	$C_{17}H_{16}O_4$	0.977	[M − H]$^-$ 283.0969	$C_{17}H_{16}O_4$	−0.353	caffeic acid phenethyl ester
7	33.078	[M + Na]$^+$ 323.1618	$C_{19}H_{24}O_3$	−1.547	[M − H]$^-$ 299.1649	$C_{19}H_{24}O_3$	0.669	Artepillin C

Brazilian green propolis has become a popular health supplement due to its many biological properties. Characteristically, it has an herbal odor and a unique, irritating taste. Previous work provided the first evidence that artepillin C was the main, pungent ingredient in the ethanol extract of Brazilian green propolis (EEBP). Moreover, that artepillin C potently activated human transient receptor potential ankyrin 1 (TRPA1) channels [23].

In this study, artepillin C was successfully identified and was the same compound that has previously been shown to have a variety of beneficial, biological activities. Notably, three isomers of chlorogenic acid were identified by the UPLC-ESI-QTOF-MS, which has rarely been reported. Thus, these results indicate that this method is useful for identification of the constituents of Brazilian green propolis. It should be noted that Brazilian green propolis contains predominantly phenolic compounds, including flavonoids and phenolic acid as well as its derivatives [24]. There were many unidentified flavonoids in the total ion chromatogram; moreover, the TIC of the methanol extracts obtained from Brazilian green propolis (Figure 1) did not include analysis of its water extracts. In subsequent studies, we will need to further identify these characteristic compounds obtained from Brazilian green propolis.

2.2. Determination of Phenolic Acids in Brazilian Green Propolis

After the seven phenolic acids obtained from the Brazilian green propolis were identified from the total ion chromatogram, we further quantified them using HPLC. According to the study carried out by Cuiping Zhang et al., nine phenolic compounds were quantified using HPLC by comparing them with standard substances [22]. The polyphenol fraction in propolis was quantitatively characterized by HPLC-ESI-MS/MS [25]. Using aqueous ethanol along with the addition of the internal standard veratraldehyde, an RP-HPLC procedure for phenolic compounds was developed and 10 compounds were subsequently quantified [26].

Similarly, and as presented here, the main, characteristic peaks were identified by their chromatographic behavior and UV spectra relative to those reference compounds in the HPLC chromatogram (Figure 3). The seven phenolic compounds were separated using the chromatographic conditions indicated in the experimental section of this paper. The content of each phenolic acid component as obtained from the Brazilian green propolis was based on a linear regression equation of the phenolic acid component standard. Each component's content ratio was calculated based on the relationship between the peak area of the phenolic acid component in the sample and the injection amount. We also conducted a methodological verification to evaluate the scientific nature of our HPLC-mediated, determination method for different phenolic acid compounds found in Brazilian green propolis.

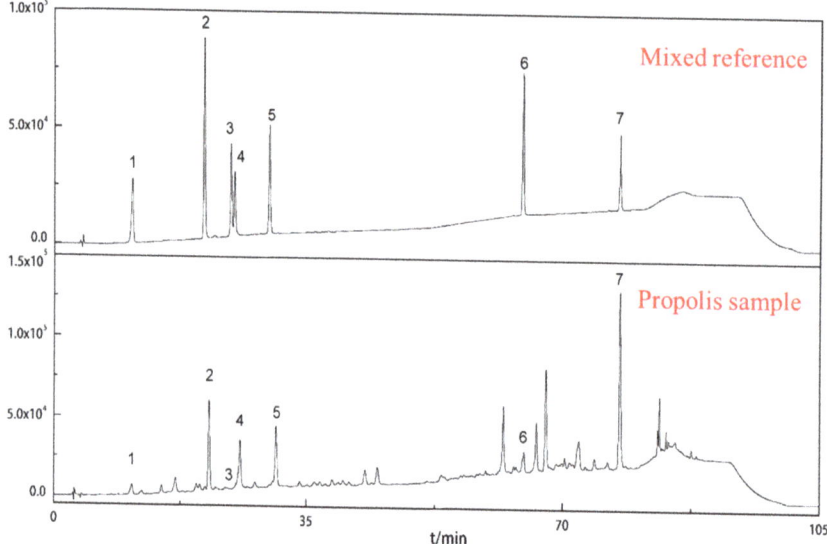

Figure 3. Comparison of chromatograms obtained at 310 nm of chlorogenic acid (1), caffeic acid (2), isochlorogenic acid B (3), isochlorogenic acid A (4), isochlorogenic acid C (5), caffeic acid phenethyl ester (6), and artepillin C (7) mix of standards and Brazilian green propolis sample.

2.3. Method Validation

Methodological verification was performed according to International Council for Harmonization (ICH) guidelines [27] and included measurements for: Linearity estimation, system precision and repeatability, and accuracy and stability.

2.3.1. Linearity

The linearity of the method used to identify the aforementioned compounds was determined by analyzing the standards used. Equations for the calibration curves were determined by plotting the relationship between the corrected peak areas (peak area/migration time), ratio of the analysis and the internal standard and the concentration (µg/mL). The concentrations of all compounds obtained from the Brazilian green propolis samples were calculated based on the peak area ratio and data are shown in Table 2. As indicated, all R^2 values obtained using linear regression analysis were > 0.99.

Linear regression equations for the identified compounds are also presented in Table 2, where y is the peak area and x is the concentration.

Table 2. Linearity, sensitivity, system precision and accuracy ($n = 6$).

Phenolic Acids	Equation	R^2	Range (μg/mL)	Average Recovery (Mean ± SD)
[b] Chlorogenic acid	[a] $Y = 1.25 \times 10^6 X - 5405.19$	0.9997	3.75–22.50	100.5% ± 3.80%
Caffeic acid	$Y = 4.00 \times 10^6 X - 8763.30$	0.9997	2.70–21.60	96.7% ± 1.39%
Isochlorogenic acid B	$Y = 3.09 \times 10^6 X - 5324.83$	0.9999	0.95–5.70	97.8% ± 2.31%
Isochlorogenic acid A	$Y = 2.25 \times 10^6 X + 18885.5$	0.9999	0.90–11.25	100.4% ± 2.81%
Isochlorogenic acid C	$Y = 2.53 \times 10^6 X - 55085.10$	0.9999	8.50–51.00	99.7% ± 2.51%
caffeic acid phenethyl ester	$Y = 2.36 \times 10^6 X - 9337.66$	0.9996	12.00–72.00	98.5% ± 1.66%
Artepillin C	$Y = 3.14 \times 10^6 X + 63207.59$	0.9987	12.30–98.30	99.5% ± 1.32%

[a] Response y, is the peak area ratio (area/migration time) of the analytes versus that of standard compound.
[b] Detection was carried out at 310 nm (Chlorogenic acid, Caffeic acid, Isochlorogenic acid B, Isochlorogenic acid A, Isochlorogenic acid C, caffeic acid phenethyl ester, Artepillin C).

The UPLC method enables higher efficiency and higher precision detection. In a previous study, the propolis analysis was conducted using HPLC. In general, and in the case of simple, sensitive, and specific reversed-phase high performance liquid chromatography (RP-HPLC), a rapid determination method of salicin was developed and verified to distinguish poplar gum and propolis [28].

2.3.2. System Precision and Repeatability

System accuracy was assessed by repeated injections ($n = 6$) of the standard mixture. The relative standard deviation (RSD)% values of each compound as well as the chromatogram similarity are calculated; all results indicated that instrument variability was sufficiently low at low concentrations. These results showed that the RSD% of each phenolic acid in peak area is less than 2% and similarity of the chromatogram of each standard mixture sample was more than 98%. Collectively, these results indicated that the precision of the instrument met testing requirements.

The repeatability was obtained as the RSD% by analysis of six same green propolis samples of the standard components and instrumental variability, by taking into account the chromatographic peak similarity: such as peak areas and compound retention. The results were considered satisfactory, since the RSD% ($n = 6$) of seven phenolic acids content is less than 2%. Moreover, the similarity of chromatograms from six propolis samples were more than 98%, indicating sound repeatability of our HPLC analysis.

2.3.3. Accuracy

Accuracy was estimated using recovery experiments performed on random Brazilian green propolis. Regarding accuracy and recovery studies, each of the phenolic acids standards was added to the same Brazilian green propolis. Approximately 20% of the analysis used native content obtained before the extraction process. These results are shown in Table 2. The average recovery rate was more than 95%; the acceptable RSD% for all obtained results was less than 5%. It is worth emphasizing that accuracy studies were undertaken for seven phenolic acid compounds. Moreover, the results were considered to be satisfactory for the purposes of our method.

2.3.4. Stability

Regarding the stability of this approach, sample size, pH of the mobile phase, and different solvent brands were mandatory in order to standardize our results. The stability study was implemented by following a "time-by-time" approach, in which the injection time of a sample of the same Brazilian green propolis sample was altered (0, 4, 8, 12 and 24 h) when conducting HPLC. The chromatographic peak similarity at different time points and the RSD% of the seven standards compounds were greater than 98% and less than 2.0%, respectively. Therefore, the developed method was considered to be stable, recognizing its use in different laboratories.

In summary, the validation parameters evaluated in the present study indicated that the HPLC method met the requirements for quality control of our Brazilian green propolis analysis [26].

2.4. Data Analysis

The seven identified phenolic acids obtained from Brazilian green propolis were quantified using a validated HPLC method. The contents of each of these phenolic acid compounds are reported in Table 3. Although Brazilian green propolis comes from different parts of Brazil, there was no significant difference in the content of a given phenolic acid across different kinds of Brazilian green propolis samples. This is likely due to these samples coming from the same plant resin sources. Specifically, isochlorogenic acid B had the lowest content (0.08 ± 0.04), while the artepillin C had the highest (2.48 ± 0.94). Artepillin C has been shown to be the main pungent ingredient in Brazilian green propolis [29]; its content as determined here varied from 0–11%, depending on the geographical origin.

Table 3. Determination of seven phenolic acids compounds obtained from fourteen Brazilian green propolis samples.

No.	Compounds (%)							Total Content (%)
	C1	C2	C3	C4	C5	C6	C7	
BP01	0.484	0.095	0.115	1.238	2.662	0.669	2.906	8.17
BP02	0.221	0.111	0.037	0.220	0.588	0.706	1.087	2.97
BP03	0.405	0.095	0.104	0.953	1.525	0.471	3.509	7.06
BP04	0.408	0.181	0.067	0.644	0.917	0.288	1.728	4.23
BP05	0.360	0.055	0.073	0.785	1.117	0.375	1.901	4.67
BP06	0.442	0.070	0.099	1.069	1.899	0.429	2.628	6.64
BP07	0.478	0.093	0.066	0.971	1.901	0.598	3.993	8.10
BP08	0.347	0.080	0.109	0.902	1.501	0.392	2.891	6.22
BP09	0.753	0.178	0.141	0.749	1.370	0.263	1.504	4.96
BP10	0.502	0.097	0.117	1.242	2.780	0.755	3.824	9.32
BP11	0.540	0.094	0.113	1.313	2.232	0.621	3.273	8.19
BP12	0.092	0.017	0.005	0.171	0.494	0.037	1.327	2.14
BP13	0.183	0.024	0.009	0.275	0.797	0.288	2.069	3.65
BP14	0.246	0.060	0.069	0.575	1.110	0.601	2.097	4.76
Mean ± SD	0.39 ± 0.17	0.09 ± 0.05	0.08 ± 0.04	0.79 ± 0.38	1.49 ± 0.72	0.47 ± 0.21	2.48 ± 0.94	5.79 ± 2.2

The data obtained here were analyzed using a one-way analysis of variance (ANOVA), followed by Tukey's honestly significant difference (HSD) test. Tukey's multiple comparisons test was performed for different phenolic acids groups, with results showing that artepillin C had an extremely significant difference in terms of its content in Brazilian green propolis when compared with other compounds ($p < 0.01$; Figure 4). Regarding the isochlorogenic acid C group, a one-way ANOVA also detected an extremely significant difference between its content in Brazilian green propolis and other tested compounds ($p < 0.01$). The data for the different phenolic acids for each group were normally distributed (Figure 4), a requirement necessary to conduct a one-way ANOVA. Using our validated HPLC method, these results suggest that artepillin C quantification can be used as an important factor for determining Brazilian green propolis quality. Moreover, it has potential for use as a chemical marker for the future development of better quality control measures for Brazilian green propolis.

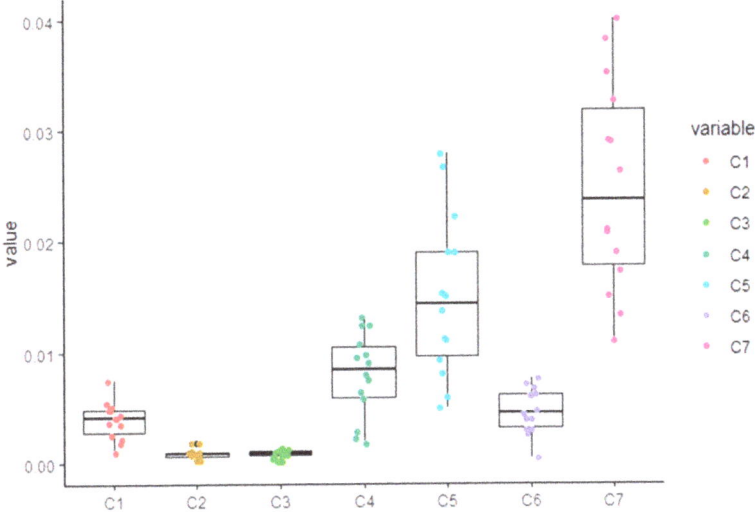

Figure 4. Statistical analysis using one-way (ANOVA) followed by Tukey's honestly significant difference (HSD) test. C1–C7 are represented with Chlorogenic acid, caffeic acid, isochlorogenic acid B, isochlorogenic acid A, isochlorogenic acid C, caffeic acid phenethyl ester, Artepillin C, respectively. $p < 0.01$ indicates a significant difference between the test groups.

3. Experimental Section

3.1. Reagents and Chemicals

Chlorogenic acid, caffeic acid, isochlorogenic acid A, isochlorogenic acid B, isochlorogenic acid C, caffeic acid phenethyl ester (all used as standard) were from Chengdu Alfa Biotechnology Co., Ltd. (Chengdu, Sichuan, China). Artepillin C (used as standard) was purchased from Richmond, VA (USA). Methanol (HPLC grade) and ethanol (95%) were from Merck Chemicals. Formic acid (95%) was from Sigma-Aldrich (Milan, Italy).

3.2. Sample Preparation

All Brazilian green propolis samples were collected in summer 2017 from different manufacturers (Figure 5) and stored at −25 °C until analysis [30]. Three samples were randomly selected from 14 samples of green propolis tested, and only 0.1 g of each was weighed into a 10 mL volumetric flask and well mixed. After adding methanol to the propolis sample and diluting to volume (10 mg/mL), it was ultrasonically extracted (360 W, 25 KHz) for 30 min, and then the supernatant was prepared. Resulting supernatants were then filtered using a 0.45 μm filter from VWR (Radnor, PA, USA) prior to detection by UPLC-ESI-QTOF-MS (Agilent Technologies, Waldbronn, Germany).

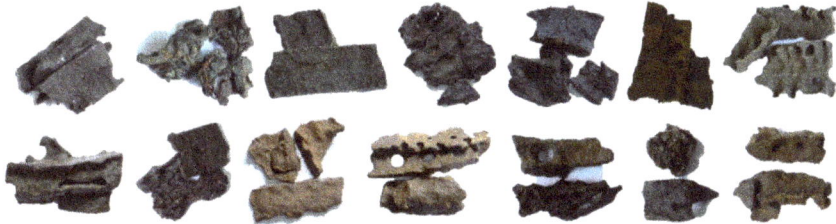

Figure 5. Fourteen Brazilian green propolis obtained from commercial suppliers.

The standard Chlorogenic acid, caffeic acid, isochlorogenic acid A, isochlorogenic acid B, isochlorogenic acid C, caffeic acid phenethyl ester, Artepillin C (5 mg of each) were placed in a 5 mL volumetric flask and dissolved in methanol. The standard was identified after the analysis of UPLC-ESI-QTOF-MS. The standard solution was stored at 4 °C until later use. The three mL of 95% ethanol was added to 100 mg of each Brazilian green propolis sample. The sample was then extracted using ultrasound (360 W, 25 KHz) for 1 h, after which it was centrifuged at 3000 r/min for 10 min. Finally, the 0.1 mL supernatant was obtained and adjusted to 1 mL with ethanol, after which it was filtered using a 0.45 µm filter. The resulting solution was then used for HPLC.

3.3. UPLC-ESI-QTOF-MS

Brazilian green propolis was identified using an Agilent 1290 ESI-QTOF-MS spectrometer and an Agilent 6545 Series UPLC system (Agilent Technologies, Waldbronn, Germany). The instrument was equipped with an electrospray ionization (ESI) source (Dual AJS ESI) and a proprietary Agilent jet stream dual nebulizer. In the UPLC analysis, chromatographic separations of Brazilian green propolis were conducted using a C18 Agilent SB column (Waldbronn, Germany) (RP-18,100 mm × 2.1 mm, 1.8 µm particle size) at a flow rate of 0.3 mL/min with 0.1% formic acid (A) and methanol (B) as solvents (99.9%, HPLC grade; Merck, Darmstadt, Germany). Starting with 25% B, to reach 45% B at 11 min, 55% B at 22 min, 70% B at 29 min, 95% B at 40 min, and then it became isocratic for 4 min. The injection volume was 2 µL for each sample.

The mass spectrometer was operated in the positive and negative electrospray ionization modes using Agilent technology. The optimized ESI operating conditions were as follows: Capillary voltage of 3500 V and drying and sheath gas temperature of 320 °C and 350 °C, respectively. The drying and sheath gas flows were set at 8 L/min and 11 L/min, respectively. The range for mass spectrometry detection was: MS: 100–1700 (m/z) and MS/MS: 50–1000 (m/z). The ion source temperature was 150 °C. Finally, the nebulizer pressure was 35 psi [31].

3.4. HPLC

Quantification of Brazilian green propolis was achieved using different instruments; specifically, a Shimadzu HPLC-20AT (Shimadzu, Japanese) using a Kromasil C18 (AKZONOBEL, Sweden) column (RP-18, 250 mm × 4.6 mm, 5 µm particle size) at a flow rate of 1.0 mL/min. The HPLC system consisted of a binary pump, an auto sampler, and photodiode-array detector, which was software-controlled. The mobile phase used was water/formic acid (999:1, v/v) (solvent A) and HPLC grade methanol (solvent B) (99.9%, HPLC grade). Elution was performed with a gradient starting with 75% B to reach 30% B at 22 min, 45% B at 45 min, 30% B at 58 min, 20% B at 75 min, 5% B at 80 min, 75% B at 95 min, and then it became isocratic for 10 min. The injection volume for both the sample and the standard was 2 µL. Finally, all chromatograms were measured at 310 nm [32].

3.5. Method Validation

In total, 14 samples of Brazilian green propolis were analyzed using HPLC. To verify the rationality of the HPLC method, we conducted a method validation test, which assessed the system's suitability, linearity, system precision, accuracy, and stability.

3.5.1. Linearity (Calibration Curve)

The calibration curves were constructed using five concentrations—including the Lower Limit of Quantitation (LLOQ)—that ranged from 0.5 to 100 µg/mL. The linear regression equation was determined by taking the sample injection amount as the abscissa and the peak area as the ordinate. The peak area of each standard was considered for the purpose of plotting the linearity graph. Linearity was evaluated using linear regression analysis, which was calculated by the least square regression method.

3.5.2. System Precision

System precision was assessed by repeated injections ($n = 6$) of a standard mixture of the analytes (concentration ≥ Limit of Quantity (LOQ) values). The RSD% values of peak area as well as the similarity of chromatograms were then determined. The acceptance criterion was ±2% for the RSD.

3.5.3. Repeatability

Repeatability was assessed by repeated injection ($n = 6$) of the same Brazilian green propolis sample, weighing approximately 0.25 g. The RSD% values of the seven phenolic acids as well as the similarity of the chromatograms of the six green propolis samples were then determined. The acceptance criterion was ±2% for the RSD.

3.5.4. Accuracy

Accuracy was conducted by a recovery experiment performed on a representative sample ($n = 6$) of Brazilian green propolis. More specifically, equal amounts of standard solution were added to each of the Brazilian green propolis samples and the average recovery rate of the Brazilian green propolis was then calculated. The accuracy method was also evaluated on the basis of RSD.

3.5.5. Stability

The stability of the solution was determined using the green propolis samples for short-term stability by keeping at room temperature for 12 h prior to analysis. Representative propolis samples were then injected at 0, 4, 8, 12 and 24 h. The stability of the instrument detection was judged by the chromatogram similarity at different time points as well as the RSD of the peak area.

3.6. Statistical Analysis

The validation experiment as well as the analysis of the quantified sample solution of the Brazilian green propolis extract were performed in six replicates. Experimental data are represented as means ± SD and $p < 0.05$ was considered to be statistically significant. Multiple comparisons were implemented using Tukey's honestly significant difference (HSD) test. To control for relevant confounding factors, one-way analysis of variance (ANOVA) was used. A p-value of < 0.01 indicated extreme statistical significance.

4. Conclusions

We present here a simple identification and determination method that was optimized and validated for the analysis of seven phenolic acids. This approach was then applied to the quantitative analysis of 14 Brazilian green propolis samples. When compared with other methods cited in the literature, this approach offers a number of additional advantages, including the use of fewer reagents and reducing the cost of analysis. Given these improvements, one quality control laboratory could analyze more samples per day in addition to saving time and money. And compared with previous publications, the combination of UPLC-ESI-QTOF-MS and HPLC system was the first application in Brazilian green propolis study. The advancement and practicality of the method greatly improved the research of analytical performances. Our results showed that there were some significant differences in phenolic acid content across different Brazilian green propolis samples. Notably, artepillin C has been found only in Brazilian green propolis, indicating promising development for this particular propolis. We report for the first time three different isomers of isochlorogenic acid, indicating the precision and accuracy of our UPLC-ESI-QTOF-MS method. In the present study, we focused on the identification and quantification of different phenolic acids in Brazilian green propolis. Our results suggest that this method could be considered new and effective method that could provide a valuable reference for the future quality control of Brazilian green propolis.

Author Contributions: S.S., M.L. and J.H. conceived and designed the experiments; K.L. performed the sampling and carried out the sample preparation; G.Y. and K.L. analysed the data; S.S. wrote the paper; X.Z. revised the manuscript; all authors read and approved the final manuscript to be submitted to Molecules.

Funding: This work was supported Guangdong Pharmaceutical University.

Acknowledgments: We really appreciate that the supplier provides all Brazilian green propolis samples for us.

Conflicts of Interest: All authors had full access to study data and had final responsibility to submit the manuscript for publication. The authors had declared that there is no conflict of interest.

References

1. Cao, Y.H.; Wang, Y.; Yuan, Q. Analysis of Flavonoids and Phenolic Acid in Propolis by Capillary Electrophoresis. *Chromatographia* **2004**, *59*, 135–140. [CrossRef]
2. Dobrowolski, J.W.; Vohora, S.B.; Sharma, K.; Shah, S.A.; Naqvi, S.A.; Dandiya, P.C. Antibacterial, antifungal, antiamoebic, antiinflammatory and antipyretic studies on propolis bee products. *J. Ethnopharmacol.* **1991**, *35*, 77. [CrossRef]
3. Marcucci, M.; Rodriguez, J.; Ferreres, F.; Bankova, V.; Groto, R.; Popov, S. Chemical composition of Brazilian propolis from São Paulo state. *Z. Naturforsch. C* **1998**, *53*, 117–119. [CrossRef]
4. Yong, K., Park; Alencar, S.M.; Aguiar, C.L. Botanical origin and chemical composition of Brazilian propolis. *J. Agri. Food Chem.* **2002**, *50*, 2502. [CrossRef]
5. De Castro, S.L. Propolis: Biological and pharmacological activies. Therapeutic uses of this bee-product. *Ann. Rev. Biol. Sci.* **2001**, *3*, 49–83. [CrossRef]
6. Afd, P.A.P.; Trugo, L.C.; Frd, N. Distribution of quinic acid derivatives and other phenolic compounds in Brazilian propolis. *Z. Naturforsch. C* **2003**, *58*, 590–593. [CrossRef]
7. Bankova, V.S.; de Castro, S.L.; Marcucci, M.C. Propolis: Recent advances in chemistry and plant origin. *Apidologie* **2000**, *31*, 3–15. [CrossRef]
8. de Barros, M.P.; Sousa, J.P.B.; Bastos, J.K.; de Andrade, S.F. Effect of Brazilian green propolis on experimental gastric ulcers in rats. *J. Ethnopharmacol.* **2007**, *110*, 567–571. [CrossRef] [PubMed]
9. De-Funari, C.; De-Oliveira-Ferro, V. Mb, Analysis of propolis from Baccharis dracunculifolia DC. (Compositae) and its effects on mouse fibroblasts. *J. Ethnopharmacol.* **2007**, *111*, 206–212. [CrossRef]
10. Falcão, S.I.; Vilas-Boas, M.; Estevinho, L.M.; Barros, C.; Domingues, M.R.; Cardoso, S.M. Phenolic characterization of Northeast Portuguese propolis: Usual and unusual compounds. *Anal. Bioanal. Chem.* **2010**, *396*, 887–897. [CrossRef]
11. Gardana, C.; Scaglianti, M.; Pietta, P.; Simonetti, P. Analysis of the polyphenolic fraction of propolis from different sources by liquid chromatography–tandem mass spectrometry. *J. Pharm. Biomed. Anal.* **2007**, *45*, 390–399. [CrossRef]
12. Pellati, F.; Orlandini, G.; Pinetti, D.; Benvenuti, S. HPLC-DAD and HPLC-ESI-MS/MS methods for metabolite profiling of propolis extracts. *J. Pharm. Biomed. Anal.* **2011**, *55*, 934–948. [CrossRef] [PubMed]
13. Volpi, N.; Bergonzini, G. Analysis of flavonoids from propolis by on-line HPLC–electrospray mass spectrometry. *J. Pharm. Biomed. Anal.* **2006**, *42*, 354–361. [CrossRef]
14. Cuyckens, F.; Claeys, M. Mass spectrometry in the structural analysis of flavonoids. *J. Mass Spectr.* **2004**, *39*, 1–15. [CrossRef]
15. Falcão, S.I.; Vale, N.; Gomes, P.; Domingues, M.R.; Freire, C.; Cardoso, S.M.; Vilas-Boas, M. Phenolic profiling of Portuguese propolis by LC–MS spectrometry: Uncommon propolis rich in flavonoid glycosides. *Phytochem. Anal.* **2013**, *24*, 309–318. [CrossRef]
16. Zhou, S.-D.; Xu, X.; Lin, Y.-F.; Xia, H.-Y.; Huang, L.; Dong, M.-S. On-line screening and identification of free radical scavenging compounds in Angelica dahurica fermented with Eurotium cristatum using an HPLC-PDA-Triple-TOF-MS/MS-ABTS system. *Food Chem.* **2019**, *272*, 670–678. [CrossRef] [PubMed]
17. Midorikawa, K.; Banskota, A.H.; Tezuka, Y.; Nagaoka, T.; Matsushige, K.; Message, D.; Huertas, A.A.; Kadota, S. Liquid chromatography–mass spectrometry analysis of propolis. *Phytochem. Anal. Int. J. Plant Chem. Biochem. Tech.* **2001**, *12*, 366–373. [CrossRef] [PubMed]
18. Sawaya, A.C.; Tomazela, D.M.; Cunha, I.B.; Bankova, V.S.; Marcucci, M.C.; Custodio, A.R.; Eberlin, M.N. Electrospray ionization mass spectrometry fingerprinting of propolis. *Analyst* **2004**, *129*, 739–744. [CrossRef]

19. Banskota, A.H.; Tezuka, Y.; Midorikawa, K.; Matsushige, K.; Kadota, S. Two novel cytotoxic benzofuran derivatives from Brazilian propolis. *J. Nat. Prod.* **2000**, *63*, 1277–1279. [CrossRef] [PubMed]
20. Basnet, P.; Matsushige, K.; Hase, K.; Kadota, S.; Namba, T. Four di-O-caffeoyl quinic acid derivatives from propolis. Potent hepatoprotective activity in experimental liver injury models. *Biol. Pharm. Bull.* **1996**, *19*, 1479–1484. [CrossRef]
21. Castro, C.; Mura, F.; Valenzuela, G.; Figueroa, C.; Salinas, R.; Zuñiga, M.C.; Torres, J.L.; Fuguet, E.; Delporte, C. Identification of phenolic compounds by HPLC-ESI-MS/MS and antioxidant activity from Chilean propolis. *Food Res. Int.* **2014**, *64*, 873–879. [CrossRef]
22. Zhang, C.; Shen, X.; Chen, J.; Jiang, X.; Hu, F. Identification of free radical scavengers from Brazilian green propolis using off-line HPLC-DPPH assay and LC-MS. *J. Food Sci.* **2017**, *82*, 1602–1607. [CrossRef]
23. Hata, T.; Tazawa, S.; Ohta, S.; Rhyu, M.-R.; Misaka, T.; Ichihara, K. Artepillin C, a major ingredient of Brazilian propolis, induces a pungent taste by activating TRPA1 channels. *PLoS ONE* **2012**, *7*, e48072. [CrossRef] [PubMed]
24. Teixeira, É.W.; Negri, G.; Meira, R.M.; Salatino, A. Plant origin of green propolis: Bee behavior, plant anatomy and chemistry. *Evi. Based Compl. Altern. Med.* **2005**, *2*, 85–92. [CrossRef]
25. Medana, C.; Carbone, F.; Aigotti, R.; Appendino, G.; Baiocchi, C. Selective analysis of phenolic compounds in propolis by HPLC-MS/MS. *Phytochem. Anal. Int. J. Plant Chem. Biochem. Tech.* **2008**, *19*, 32–39. [CrossRef] [PubMed]
26. de Sousa, J.P.; Bueno, P.C.; Gregório, L.E.; da Silva Filho, A.A.; Furtado, N.A.; de Sousa, M.L.; Bastos, J.K. A reliable quantitative method for the analysis of phenolic compounds in Brazilian propolis by reverse phase high performance liquid chromatography. *J. Sep. Sci.* **2007**, *30*, 2656–2665. [CrossRef] [PubMed]
27. Guideline, I.H.T. Validation of Analytical Procedures: Text and Methodology Q2 (R1). In Proceedings of the International Conference on Harmonization; 2005; pp. 11–12.
28. Zhang, C.-p.; Zheng, H.-q.; Liu, G.; Hu, F.-l. Development and validation of HPLC method for determination of salicin in poplar buds: Application for screening of counterfeit propolis. *Food Chem.* **2011**, *127*, 345–350. [CrossRef]
29. Matsuda, A.H.; de Almeida-Muradian, L.B. Validated method for the quantification of artepillin-C in Brazilian propolis. *Phytochem. Anal. Int. J. Plant Chem. Biochem. Tech.* **2008**, *19*, 179–183. [CrossRef] [PubMed]
30. Chasset, T.; Häbe, T.T.; Ristivojevic, P.; Morlock, G.E. Profiling and classification of French propolis by combined multivariate data analysis of planar chromatograms and scanning direct analysis in real time mass spectra. *J. Chromatogr. A* **2016**, *1465*, 197–204. [CrossRef]
31. Tan, G.H.; Wong, R.C. Determination of aflatoxins in food using liquid chromatography coupled with electrospray ionization quadrupole time of flight mass spectrometry (LC-ESI-QTOF-MS/MS). *Food Control* **2013**, *31*, 35–44. [CrossRef]
32. Truchado, P.; Ferreres, F.; Tomas-Barberan, F.A. Liquid chromatography–tandem mass spectrometry reveals the widespread occurrence of flavonoid glycosides in honey, and their potential as floral origin markers. *J. Chromatogr. A* **2009**, *1216*, 7241–7248. [CrossRef]

Sample Availability: Samples of the compounds **1–7** in this paper and **14** Brazilian green propolis are available from the authors.

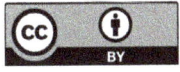

© 2019 by the authors. Licensee MDPI, Basel, Switzerland. This article is an open access article distributed under the terms and conditions of the Creative Commons Attribution (CC BY) license (http://creativecommons.org/licenses/by/4.0/).

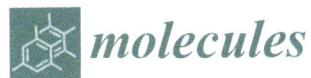

Article

Simultaneous Determination and Pharmacokinetic Characterization of Glycyrrhizin, Isoliquiritigenin, Liquiritigenin, and Liquiritin in Rat Plasma Following Oral Administration of Glycyrrhizae Radix Extract

You Jin Han [1], Bitna Kang [2], Eun-Ju Yang [1], Min-Koo Choi [2,*] and Im-Sook Song [1,*]

1. College of Pharmacy and Research Institute of Pharmaceutical Sciences, Kyungpook National University, Daegu 41566, Korea; gksdbwls2@nate.com (Y.J.H.); ejy125@gmail.com (E.-J.Y.)
2. College of Pharmacy, Dankook University, Cheon-an 31116, Korea; qlcska8520@naver.com
* Correspondence: isssong@knu.ac.kr (I.-S.S.); minkoochoi@dankook.ac.kr (M.-K.C.); Tel.: +82-53-950-8575 (I.-S.S.); +82-41-550-1432 (M.-K.C.)

Academic Editors: In-Soo Yoon and Hyun-Jong Cho
Received: 12 April 2019; Accepted: 9 May 2019; Published: 10 May 2019

Abstract: Glycyrrhizae Radix is widely used as herbal medicine and is effective against inflammation, various cancers, and digestive disorders. We aimed to develop a sensitive and simultaneous analytical method for detecting glycyrrhizin, isoliquiritigenin, liquiritigenin, and liquiritin, the four marker components of Glycyrrhizae Radix extract (GRE), in rat plasma using liquid chromatography-tandem mass spectrometry and to apply this analytical method to pharmacokinetic studies. Retention times for glycyrrhizin, isoliquiritigenin, liquiritigenin, and liquiritin were 7.8 min, 4.1 min, 3.1 min, and 2.0 min, respectively, suggesting that the four analytes were well separated without any interfering peaks around the peak elution time. The lower limit of quantitation was 2 ng/mL for glycyrrhizin and 0.2 ng/mL for isoliquiritigenin, liquiritigenin, and liquiritin; the inter- and intra-day accuracy, precision, and stability were less than 15%. Plasma concentrations of glycyrrhizin, isoliquiritigenin, liquiritigenin, and liquiritin were quantified for 24 h after a single oral administration of 1 g/kg GRE to four rats. Among the four components, plasma concentration of glycyrrhizin was the highest and exhibited a long half-life (23.1 ± 15.5 h). Interestingly, plasma concentrations of isoliquiritigenin and liquiritigenin were restored to the initial concentration at 4–10 h after the GRE administration, as evidenced by liquiritin biotransformation into isoliquiritigenin and liquiritigenin, catalyzed by fecal lysate and gut wall enzymes. In conclusion, our analytical method developed for detecting glycyrrhizin, isoliquiritigenin, liquiritigenin, and liquiritin could be successfully applied to investigate their pharmacokinetic properties in rats and would be useful for conducting further studies on the efficacy, toxicity, and biopharmaceutics of GREs and their marker components.

Keywords: Glycyrrhizae Radix extract; glycyrrhizin; isoliquiritigenin; liquiritigenin; liquiritin; LC–MS/MS analysis; pharmacokinetics

1. Introduction

Glycyrrhizae Radix (licorice root) has been used as a herbal medicine because of a variety of pharmacological activities, including anti-oxidative, anti-cancer, and anti-diabetic activities as well as memory enhancing and inflammation reducing effects [1]. In addition, it has been used as a flavoring agent in food products [2] and also as an adjuvant to increase the therapeutic efficacy of other drugs. For example, Glycyrrhizae Radix lowers the risk of aphthous ulcers caused by aspirin intake and the side effect of spironolactone. It also increased the efficacy of corticosteroids and improved the elimination of nitrofurantoin [3]. Recently, our group prepared an ethanol extract of Glycyrrhizae Radix and investigated the efficacy of Glycyrrhizae Radix extract (GRE) in relation to the modulation of reactive splenic T cells. The oral administration of GRE (0.1–0.5 g/kg) for 9 days could effectively ameliorate interferon-γ-related autoimmune responses in a mouse model of experimental autoimmune encephalomyelitis [1]. For understanding the relationship between the response elicited by GRE and its pharmacokinetics, it was important to carry out the bioanalysis of the predominant or pharmacological components of GRE in biological samples following herbal extract administration and to understand their pharmacokinetics.

Glycyrrhizae Radix contains many bioactive saponins and flavonoids along with glycyrrhizin, a major and marker component of Glycyrrhizae Radix [2,4–6]. It has recently been reported that glycyrrhizin exerts strong neuroprotective effects on a mouse model of experimental autoimmune encephalomyelitis [1,7]. In addition, glycyrrhizin is commonly used owing to its therapeutic effects against arthritis, hepatotoxicity, leukemia, allergies, stomach ulcers, and inflammation. Moreover, the major active flavonoids of Glycyrrhizae Radix, such as isoliquiritigenin, liquiritin, and liquiritigenin [8], are often used as anti-depressants or as anticancer, cardio-protective, anti-microbial, and neuroprotective agents [9–14]. Based on the literature search, glycyrrhizin, isoliquiritigenin, liquiritin, and liquiritigenin were selected as predominant or pharmacological components of GRE. An analytical method for simultaneously detecting these four components from a traditional Chinese herbal formulation Sijunzi decoction or from Glycyrrhizae Radix, using high-performance liquid chromatography (HPLC) with a detection limit of >300 ng/mL has been previously reported [15,16]. The previous analytical methods and pharmacokinetic studies on bioactive saponins and flavonoids following GRE administration mainly focused on pharmacokinetic drug–drug interaction between the Jiegeng and Gancao or the co-extract of Shaoyao Gancao decoction [17–19]. Moreover, their pharmacokinetic application has been carried out at a high dose of the extract. Plasma concentrations of the 10 active constituents including glycyrrhizin, isoliquiritigenin, liquiritin, and liquiritigenin were determined following a single oral administration of 9.5 g/kg Shaoyao–Gancao decoction extract [17]. Mao et al. determined the plasma concentrations of glycyrrhizin, glycyrrhetinic acid, isoliquiritigenin, liquiritigenin, isoliquiritin, and liquiritin after administering a single oral dose of 20 g/kg of GRE [18]. Shan et al. determined the pharmacokinetics of nine active components including these four components on repeated oral administration of Zushima–Gancao extract (2.7 g/kg) for 20 days [19]. A high dose of GRE might be administered owing to the lower concentration of active components. Even the concentration of glycyrrhizin, which was the highest in GRE, was <2% and that of other flavones was <1% [2,4–6].

Therefore, the purpose of this study was to establish simultaneous and sensitive assays to quantify the major and pharmacologically active components in GRE, such as glycyrrhizin, isoliquiritigenin, liquiritin, and liquiritigenin, and to implement the developed method in the pharmacokinetic studies of these four components following a single oral administration of RGE (1 g/kg) in rats. The method was developed using triple quadrupole liquid chromatography–tandem mass spectrometry (LC–MS/MS) and to validate this bioanalytical method in terms of linearity, selectivity, accuracy, precision, recovery, stability, and matrix effects according to the U.S. Food and Drug Administration Guideline for Bioanalytical Method [20].

2. Results

2.1. LC–MS/MS Analysis

2.1.1. MS/MS Analysis

In order to optimize ESI conditions for four components, each compound was injected directly into the mass spectrometer ionization source. Glycyrrhizin showed optimal ionization in positive mode and isoliquiritigenin, liquiritigenin, and liquiritin showed optimal ionization in negative mode. Figure 1 shows the mass spectra and chemical structure of glycyrrhizin, isoliquiritigenin, liquiritigenin, and liquiritin. The selection of berberine as an internal standard (IS) was based on its simultaneous determination with glycyrrhizin, which was present at the highest concentration in GRE, in a positive ionization mode [21,22]. In addition, berberine eluted in the middle of glycyrrhizin and the three flavones and it showed a stable extraction recovery with low coefficient of variation (CV). The optimized analytical conditions including mass transition from the precursor to product ion (m/z) for glycyrrhizin, isoliquiritigenin, liquiritigenin, liquiritin, and berberine (IS) are listed in Table 1.

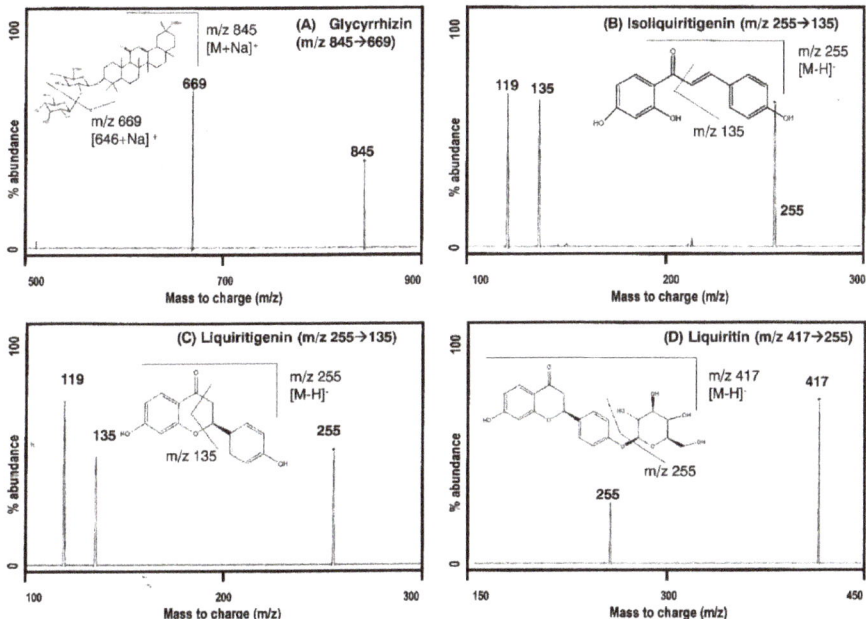

Figure 1. Structure and product ion mass spectra of (**A**) glycyrrhizin, (**B**) isoliquiritigenin, (**C**) liquiritigenin, and (**D**) liquiritin.

Table 1. MS/MS parameters for the detection of the analytes and IS.

Compounds	MRM Transitions (m/z)		Ionization Mode	Collision Energy (eV)
	Precursor Ion	Product Ion		
Glycyrrhizin	845	669	Positive	35
Isoliquiritigenin	255	135	Negative	15
Liquiritigenin	255	135	Negative	15
Liquiritin	417	255	Negative	20
Berberine (IS)	336	320	Positive	30

2.1.2. Specificity

Representative multiple reaction monitoring (MRM) chromatograms of glycyrrhizin, isoliquiritigenin, liquiritigenin, and liquiritin, and IS (Figure 2) showed that the four analytes and berberine (IS) peaks were well-separated with no interfering peaks at their respective retention times corresponding to the concentration of the lower limit of quantification (LLOQ). The retention times of glycyrrhizin, isoliquiritigenin, liquiritigenin, and liquiritin, and IS were 7.8 min, 4.1 min, 3.1 min, 2.0 min, and 4.8 min, respectively, and the total run time was 10.0 min. The selectivity of the analytes was confirmed from six different blank rat plasma and plasma samples obtained from rats at 2 h after oral administration of GRE (1 g/kg) (Figure 3).

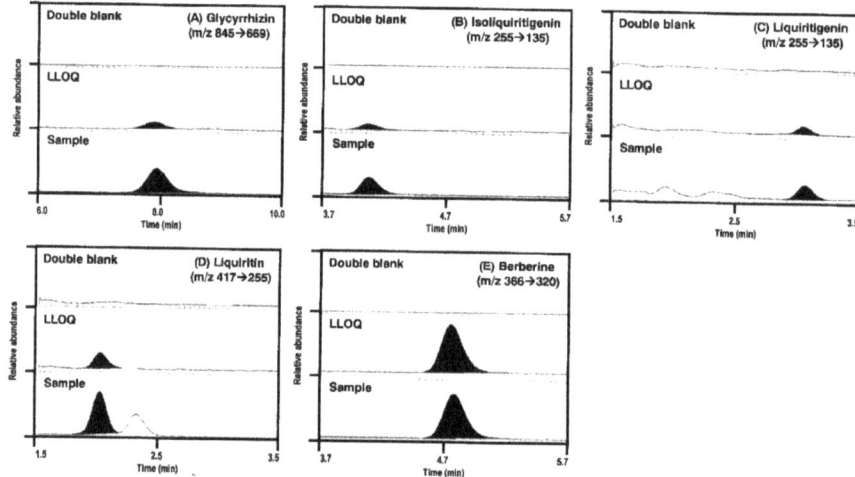

Figure 2. Representative multiple reaction monitoring (MRM) chromatograms of (**A**) glycyrrhizin, (**B**) isoliquiritigenin, (**C**) liquiritigenin, (**D**) liquiritin, and (**E**) berberine (IS) in rat double blank plasma (upper), rat blank plasma spiked with standard solution at lower limit of quantification (LLOQ) (center), and rat plasma samples at 2 h following single oral administration of Glycyrrhizae Radix extract (GRE) (1 g/kg) (lower).

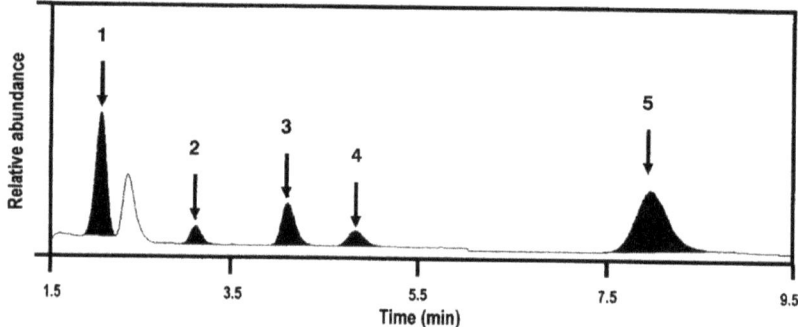

Figure 3. Representative MRM chromatograms of glycyrrhizin (**5**), isoliquiritigenin (**3**), liquiritigenin (**2**), liquiritin (**1**), and berberine (**4**) in rat plasma samples at 2 h following single oral administration of GRE (1 g/kg).

2.1.3. Linearity and LLOQs

To access linearity, the calibration curve consisting of seven different concentrations of glycyrrhizin, isoliquiritigenin, liquiritigenin, and liquiritin was analyzed, and the calibration curves and equations for each component have been shown in Figure 4 and Table 2. The LLOQs for glycyrrhizin, isoliquiritigenin, liquiritigenin, and liquiritin in our analytical system was defined by a signal-to-noise ratio of >5, the precision was ≤15%, and the accuracy was 80–120%; these results have been listed in Table 2.

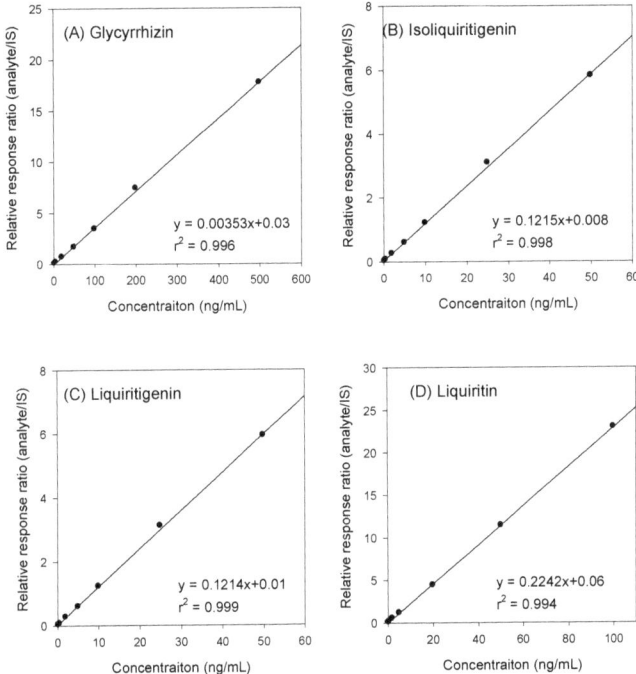

Figure 4. Representative calibration curves of (**A**) glycyrrhizin, (**B**) isoliquiritigenin, (**C**) liquiritigenin, and (**D**) liquiritin in rat plasma.

Table 2. Linearity and LLOQs of glycyrrhizin, isoliquiritigenin, liquiritin and liquiritigenin.

Analytes	Representative Regression Equation	r^2	Linear Range (ng/mL)	LLOQ (ng/mL)
Glycyrrhizin	y = 0.0035x + 0.03	0.996	2–500	2
Isoliquiritigenin	y = 0.1215x + 0.008	0.998	0.2–50	0.2
Liquiritigenin	y = 0.1214x + 0.01	0.999	0.2–50	0.2
Liquiritin	y = 0.2242x + 0.06	0.994	0.2–100	0.2

2.1.4. Accuracy and Precision

The inter- and intra-day accuracy and precision were assessed using three concentrations of quality control (QC) samples consisting of the mixture of four analytes (Table 3). The results showed that inter- and intra-day precision for glycyrrhizin, isoliquiritigenin, liquiritin, and liquiritigenin was below 13.6%. The inter- and intra-day accuracy for glycyrrhizin, isoliquiritigenin, liquiritin, and liquiritigenin ranged from 87.4% to 112.2% (Table 3).

Table 3. Intra- and inter-day precision and accuracy of glycyrrhizin, isoliquiritigenin, liquiritin and liquiritigenin.

Analytes	Nominal Concentration (ng/mL)	Intra-day			Inter-day		
		Measured Concentration (ng/mL)	Precision (%)	Accuracy (%)	Measured Concentration (ng/mL)	Precision (%)	Accuracy (%)
Glycyrrhizin	6	5.8	13.3	96.1	5.2	6.3	87.4
	75	70.1	13.6	93.5	77.5	6.8	103.3
	400	416.8	13.3	104.2	410.1	7.4	102.5

Table 3. Cont.

Analytes	Nominal Concentration (ng/mL)	Intra-day			Inter-day		
		Measured Concentration (ng/mL)	Precision (%)	Accuracy (%)	Measured Concentration (ng/mL)	Precision (%)	Accuracy (%)
Isoliquiritigenin	0.6	0.7	4.9	108.6	0.6	8.9	101.8
	7.5	7.9	10.8	105.6	7.7	4.7	102.1
	30	32.8	7.9	109.2	33.3	7.0	111.0
Liquiritigenin	0.6	0.6	4.0	98.6	0.6	7.6	97.7
	7.5	7.7	3.7	103.0	7.5	5.8	100.5
	30	32.6	3.7	108.6	33.6	5.6	112.0
Liquiritin	0.6	0.6	9.8	99.2	0.6	8.8	103.3
	10	9.9	10.0	99.2	10.0	5.5	99.9
	75	74.2	8.9	98.9	84.1	3.8	112.2

Data represented as mean ± SD from six independent experiments.

2.1.5. Matrix Effect and Recovery

The extraction recoveries of glycyrrhizin, isoliquiritigenin, liquiritin, and liquiritigenin in the low, medium, high QC samples ranged from 70.3% to 99.1% with CV of <14.0%. The matrix effects ranged from 76.2 to 114.2% with CV of <14.8%. These results indicate that no significant interference occurred during the ionization and methanol precipitation process. The extraction recovery and matrix effect of the IS at 0.1 ng/mL were 86.2% and 108.2%, respectively (Table 4).

Table 4. Extraction recoveries and matric effects for the determination of liquiritin, liquiritigenin, isoliquiritigenin, glycyrrhizin and of IS.

Analyte		Concentration (ng/mL)	Extraction Recovery (%)	CV (%)	Matrix Effects (%)	CV (%)
Glycyrrhizin	Low QC	6	89.06 ± 7.38	8.29	98.80 ± 5.89	5.96
	Medium QC	75	77.2 ± 7.7	9.9	92.1 ± 3.6	3.9
	High QC	400	75.0 ± 4.9	6.6	96.4 ± 4.6	4.8
Isoliquiritigenin	Low QC	0.6	80.2 ± 10.8	13.6	78.9 ± 3.0	3.8
	Medium QC	7.5	74.6 ± 8.1	10.8	88.3 ± 4.9	5.5
	High QC	30	70.3 ± 4.9	7.1	93.6 ± 5.3	5.6
Liquiritigenin	Low QC	0.6	99.1 ± 7.9	8.0	76.2 ± 3.1	4.1
	Medium QC	7.5	88.9 ± 9.5	10.7	96.6 ± 8.1	8.4
	High QC	30	83.5 ± 6.4	7.7	104.9 ± 8.2	7.8
Liquiritin	Low QC	0.6	79.2 ± 11.1	14.0	114.2 ± 10.4	9.1
	Medium QC	10	83.2 ± 11.3	13.6	97.2 ± 14.4	14.8
	High QC	75	90.7 ± 6.4	7.1	101.8 ± 7.7	7.6
IS		0.1	86.2 ± 2.7	3.1	108.2 ± 1.8	1.7

Data represented as mean ± SD from six independent experiments.

2.1.6. Stability

It was found that the precision and accuracy of QC samples consisting of a mixture of the four analytes were within 12.9% for short-term stability, below 6.4% for post-preparative stability, and below 11.1% for three freeze–thaw cycle stability (Table 5). Therefore, glycyrrhizin, isoliquiritigenin, liquiritin, and liquiritigenin in plasma samples were found to exhibit no problems in these three stability tests during the bioanalytical procedure.

Table 5. Stability of glycyrrhizin, isoliquiritigenin, liquiritin and liquiritigenin.

Storage Conditions	Analytes	Concentration (ng/mL)		Precision %	Accuracy %
		Spiked	Measured		
Short-term stability	Glycyrrhizin	6	5.6	6.8	94.0
		400	390.8	9.5	97.7
	Isoliquiritigenin	0.6	0.6	12.9	101.8
		30	30.1	7.5	100.3
	Liquiritigenin	0.6	0.6	3.3	93.6
		30	28.8	8.9	102.7
	Liquiritin	0.6	0.6	9.1	92.8
		75	71.3	10.1	99.5
Post-preparative stability	Glycyrrhizin	6	5.8	4.9	96.2
		400	390.8	3.7	97.7
	Isoliquiritigenin	0.6	0.6	4.1	92.4
		30	32.2	3.6	107.3
	Liquiritigenin	0.6	0.6	6.4	93.0
		30	32.8	4.8	109.5
	Liquiritin	0.6	0.6	3.7	97.3
		75	76.4	2.5	101.9
Three freeze-thaw cycle stability	Glycyrrhizin	6	6.8	0.8	113.9
		400	394.1	10.3	98.5
	Isoliquiritigenin	0.6	0.5	5.8	90.9
		30	30.0	7.1	99.9
	Liquiritigenin	0.6	0.5	5.1	90.0
		30	29.2	8.2	97.2
	Liquiritin	0.6	0.5	4.3	87.3
		75	72.6	11.1	96.7

Data represented as mean ± SD from six independent experiments.

2.2. Contents of Glycyrrhizin, Liquiritin, Isoliquiritigenin, and Liquiritigenin in GRE

The concentration of glycyrrhizin, isoliquiritigenin, liquiritigenin, and liquiritin in GRE are summarized in Table 6. The concentration of glycyrrhizin was the highest (1.3%), consistent with the findings of previous studies [2,4–6]. Isoliquiritigenin, liquiritigenin, and liquiritin were present at lower concentrations (0.014%, 0.027%, and 0.38%, respectively) in GRE.

Table 6. The mean contents of four compounds in GRE.

Compounds	Content (%)
Glycyrrhizin	1.3 ± 0.2
Isoliquiritigenin	0.014 ± 0.004
Liquiritigenin	0.027 ± 0.010
Liquiritin	0.38 ± 0.07

Data represented as mean ± SD from six independent experiments.

2.3. Plasma Concentration of Glycyrrhizin, Liquiritin, Isoliquiritigenin, and Liquiritigenin

Next, we investigated the plasma concentrations of glycyrrhizin, isoliquiritigenin, liquiritigenin, and liquiritin following a single oral GRE administration at a dose of 1 g/kg. Plasma concentrations of glycyrrhizin, isoliquiritigenin, liquiritigenin, and liquiritin over time and their PK parameters are shown in Figure 5 and Table 7, respectively. Among the four major components present in rat plasma, glycyrrhizin was found to be maintained at the highest concentration for a period of 24 h. In contrast, the plasma concentration of liquiritin gradually reduced at an elimination half-life ($T_{1/2}$) of 3.7 ± 2.2 h. Concentrations of isoliquiritigenin and liquiritigenin were similar and increased up to 8 h and then gradually reduced; therefore, T_{max} and MRT values of both these compounds were very similar. The area under the plasma concentration–time curve (AUC) of isoliquiritigenin and liquiritigenin were comparable but higher than that of liquiritin, despite their concentration (0.014% and 0.027%, respectively) in GRE being lower than that of liquiritin (0.38%). Collectively, these results suggested that isoliquiritigenin and liquiritigenin were transformed during the intestinal absorption process.

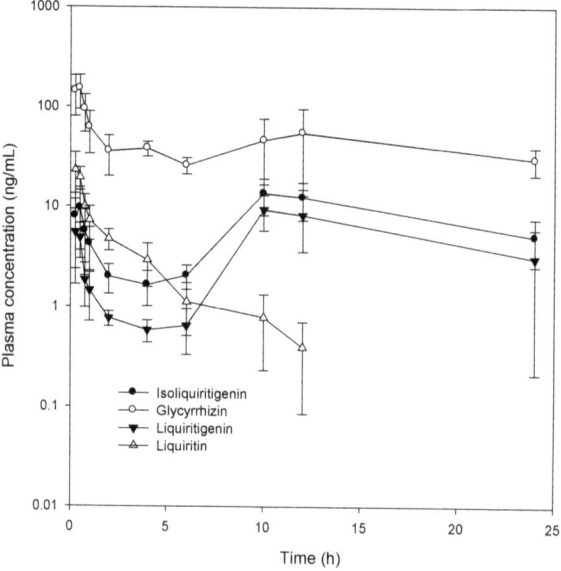

Figure 5. Plasma concentration–time profiles of glycyrrhizin, isoliquiritigenin, liquiritigenin, and liquiritin and after oral administration of GRE to rats. Data were expressed as mean ± SD from four rats per group.

Table 7. Pharmacokinetic parameters of glycyrrhizin, isoliquiritigenin, liquiritin, liquiritigenin after oral administration of GRE (1 g/kg) to rats.

Parameters	Glycyrrhizin	Isoliquiritigenin	Liquiritigenin	Liquiritin
C_{max} (ng/mL)	164.4 ± 62.0	16.6 ± 2.7	10.8 ± 3.6	26.8 ± 8.5
AUC_{last} (ng·h/mL)	1051.0 ± 487.5	179.2 ± 46.3	112.5 ± 36.4	39.5 ± 7.8
T_{max} (h)	0.4 ± 0.1	8.1 ± 5.2	8.1 ± 5.3	0.4 ± 0.1
$T_{1/2}$ (h)	23.1 ± 15.5	-	-	3.7 ± 2.2
MRT_{last} (h)	10.7 ± 0.7	12.5 ± 1.3	12.8 ± 1.8	3.3 ± 1.3

Data were expressed as mean ± SD from four rats; C_{max}: maximum plasma concentration; AUC_{last}: Area under plasma concentration-time curve from zero to last time; T_{max}, time to reach C_{max}; $T_{1/2}$: elimination half-life; MRT: mean residence time.

2.4. Biotransformation in the Rat Intestine

We investigated whether the biotransformation of isoliquiritigenin and liquiritigenin from liquiritin could occur in the rat intestine. Because the plasma concentration of isoliquiritigenin and liquiritigenin was increased at 4–10 h after oral GRE administration, we measured biotransformation in the rat ileum segment. After a 2 h incubation of a single component of GRE such as isoliquiritigenin, liquiritigenin, and liquiritin with rat ileum segments and intestinal contents, liquiritin was found to transform into isoliquiritigenin and liquiritigenin and the formation rate of both these compounds were similar to each other (Figure 6A–C). Moreover, although isoliquiritigenin and liquiritigenin were interchangeable, they did not transform into liquiritin (Figure 6D).

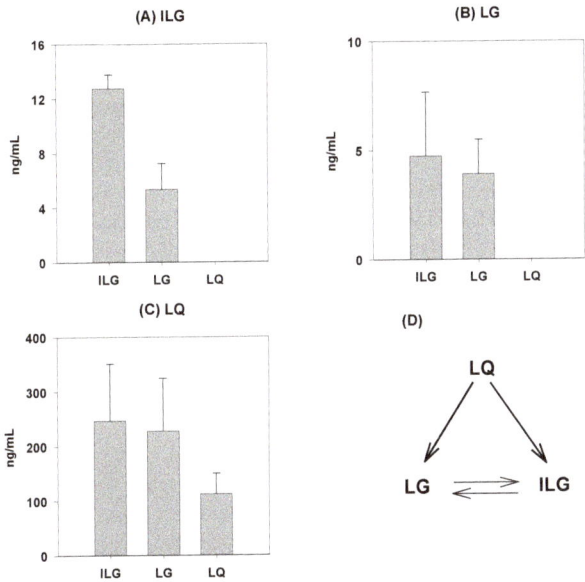

Figure 6. Formation of isoliquiritigenin (ILG), liquiritigenin (LG), and liquiritin (LQ) 2 h incubation after the addition of (**A**) isoliquiritigenin (ILG), (**B**) liquiritigenin (LG), and (**C**) liquiritin (LQ) in rat ileum. (**D**) Proposed biotransformation scheme among LQ, LG, and ILG in rat intestine. Data were expressed as mean ± SD from six independent experiments per group.

3. Discussion

In this study, the newly developed analytical method for glycyrrhizin, isoliquiritigenin, liquiritigenin, and liquiritin using an LC–MS/MS system showed relatively higher sensitivity (i.e., LLOQ 2 ng/mL for glycyrrhizin and 0.2 ng/mL for isoliquiritigenin, liquiritigenin, and liquiritin) despite using lower plasma sample volume (50 µL). For example, Wang et al. implemented a protein-precipitation method and sample preparations via evaporation and reconstitution for detecting 10 active constituents in Shaoyao–Gancao decoction. The LLOQs for glycyrrhizin and three flavone compounds were 5 and 0.5 ng/mL, respectively [17]. Mao et al. applied analytical methods for glycyrrhizin, glycyrrhetinic acid, isoliquiritigenin, liquiritigenin, isoliquiritin, and liquiritin using an LC–MS/MS system with 10 and 0.4 ng/mL of LLOQ for glycyrrhizin and three flavones, respectively [18]. Additionally, previously established methods by Shan et al. applied liquid–liquid extraction which requires acidification with HCl for the extraction of glycyrrhizin and glycyrrhetinic acid and a larger plasma sample volume (100 µL) and the LLOQs for glycyrrhizin and three flavones were 1 and 0.34–0.5 ng/mL, respectively [19]. Herein, we used a protein-precipitation method with methanol containing IS rather than a previously described liquid–liquid extraction method or sample preparation via evaporation and reconstitution method [8,17,19], and then directly injected an aliquot of the supernatant after centrifugation of protein-precipitated plasma samples.

We further validated our simple, sensitive, and simultaneous analytical method by performing a pharmacokinetic study after orally administering rats with 1 g/kg of GRE. We successfully measured the plasma concentrations of glycyrrhizin, isoliquiritigenin, liquiritin, and liquiritigenin for 24 h. However, we should take into account the fact that the pharmacological efficacy was investigated following repeated oral administration for 9 days at a dose range of 0.1–0.5 g/kg. Thus, the pharmacokinetic study involving repeated administration of GRE at a lower dose range of 0.1–0.5 g/kg needs to be performed to understand the pharmacokinetic–pharmacodynamic correlation of GRE.

The pharmacokinetic features of glycyrrhizin, including its long half-life, were consistent with those reported in previous studies [23,24]. The plasma concentrations of isoliquiritigenin and liquiritigenin were similar and showed fast elimination up to 4 h but rebounded to the initial plasma concentration over 10 h. As demonstrated in this study (Figure 6), liquiritin was hydrolyzed to isoliquiritigenin and liquiritigenin, and both isoliquiritigenin and liquiritigenin were interchangeable. The results suggested that liquiritin in GRE could be a precursor for isoliquiritigenin and liquiritigenin and is a more potent pharmacological component [25]; therefore, the hydrolysis of liquiritin could be attributed to an increased plasma concentration of isoliquiritigenin and liquiritigenin during the absorption period (from 4 to 10 h in this study). The results were consistent with the previous report that isoliquiritigenin and liquiritigenin, which were generated from liquiritin, were absorbed from the jejunum to colon with the help of gut wall enzymes and intestinal flora [26].

Mao et al. reported that the metabolism of some active components of Gancao, including glycyrrhizin and liquiritigenin, in rat fecal lysate was changed after co-administration with Jiegeng; consequently, this could be an important factor for alterations in the pharmacokinetic profiles of glycyrrhizin and liquiritigenin [18]. According to their results, not only Jiegeng but also Gancao changed the hydrolysis of liquiritigenin [18], which is similar to this study and could be a factor responsible for higher plasma concentration of liquiritigenin after GRE administration. In addition to this biotransformation, liquiritin permeability was much greater when added as a part of GRE as compared with the addition of an equal amount of liquiritin alone [18]. These results should also be clarified by performing a pharmacokinetic comparison between GRE administration and the administration of an equal amount of a single component as well as a comparison between intestinal absorption and metabolism; these topics are currently being investigated by our research group.

4. Materials and Methods

4.1. Materials

Glycyrrhizin (Dipotassium Glycyrrhizinate, purity > 75.0%, for High Performance Liquid Chromatography grade) was purchased from Santa Cruz Biotechnology, Inc. (Dallas, TX, USA). Berberine chloride (internal standard, purity ≥ 98.0%), isoliquiritigenin (purity > 99.0%), liquiritin (purity > 98.0%), and liquiritigenin (purity > 97.0%) were gained from Sigma-Aldrich (St. Louis, MO, USA). Water, methanol, and other solvents were obtained from J.T. Baker Korea (Seoul, Korea) and TEDIA (Fairfield, OH, USA). All other chemicals and solvents are of reagent and analytical grade.

Glycyrrhizae Radix extract (GRE; #KNUNPM GR-2015-001, deposited at the laboratory of Natural Products Medicine in Kyungpook National University) was used [1]. Briefly, dried Glycyrrhizae Radix, imported from China to Republic of Korea in 2015, was extracted with 94% ethanol for 3 h. The extracted solution was filtrated and concentrated by a rotary evaporator to obtain the GRE.

4.2. Animals

Male Sprague–Dawley rats (7 weeks of age, 249 ± 6 g), obtained from Samtako Bio Korea (Osan, Kyunggido, Korea) were used for pharmacokinetic experiments. All animal procedures were approved by the Animal Care and Use Committee of Kyungpook National University (approval No. KNU-2017-0126) and conducted in accordance with the National Institutes of Health guidance for the care and the use of laboratory animals. Rats were maintained in an animal facility at the College of Pharmacy, Kyungpook National University at a temperature of 21–27 °C with 13 h light (08:00–21:00) and a relative humidity of 60 ± 5%.

4.3. Preparation of Calibration Curve and Quality Control Samples

Calibration curve samples containing glycyrrhizin (2 to 500 ng/mL), liquiritin (0.2 to 100 ng/mL), isoliquiritigenin (0.2 to 50 ng/mL), and liquiritigenin (0.2 to 50 ng/mL) were prepared using an internal standard method. Briefly, aliquots of calibration curve samples (50 µL) was added to 300 µL of methanol containing 0.1 ng/mL berberine, vortex-mixed for 10 min, and centrifuged at $10,000\times g$ for 10 min at 4 °C. An aliquot (10 µL) of the supernatant was injected into the LC–MS/MS system.

4.4. LC–MS/MS Analysis of Glycyrrhizin, Liquiritin, Isoliquiritigenin, and Liquiritigenin

4.4.1. LC–MS/MS Condition

The LC–MS/MS system connected to Agilent 6470 triple-quadrupole mass spectrometer (Agilent, Wilmington, DE, USA) via electrospray ionization (ESI) interface. The mobile phase consisted of methanol: water (65:35, v:v) with 0.1% formic acid. The analytical column of a Synergi Polar-RP (4 µm particle size, 150 × 2 mm, Phenomenex, Torrance, CA, USA) equipped with an guard column (4 × 2 mm, Phenomenex) was used. The sample injection volume, dwell time, and flow rate were 10 µL, 10 min, and 0.3 mL/min, respectively.

4.4.2. Specificity

Six individual blank plasma samples from rats were used and specificity was defined as no interfering signal at the peak region of each analyte (glycyrrhizin, isoliquiritigenin, liquiritigenin, and liquiritin) and internal standard from background and endogenous signal.

4.4.3. Linearity

The linearity of the method was evaluated by analyzing a series of calibration samples consisting glycyrrhizin (from 2 to 500 ng/mL), liquiritin (from 0.2 to 100 ng/mL), isoliquiritigenin and liquiritigenin (from 0.2 to 50 ng/mL). Least square linear regression equation of the peak area ratios of each analyte to IS against the corresponding concentrations was obtained with a weighting factor of $1/x^2$.

4.4.4. Accuracy and Precision

The accuracy and precision of intra-day and inter-day were analyzed by six replicate QC samples on the same day and six consecutive days, respectively.

Accuracy is described in relative percentage of measured concentration compared to the spiked concentration and precision are determined by relative standard deviation compared to the average concentration of QC samples.

4.4.5. Extraction Recovery and Matrix Effect

Extraction recovery was calculated by comparing the peak areas of each analytes in QC samples through the extraction process with those in blank plasma extracts spiked with corresponding concentrations [27]. Matrix effects were monitored by dividing the peak areas in blank plasma extracts spiked with QC concentrations by those in neat solutions of corresponding concentrations [27].

4.4.6. Stability

The stability of four analytes in the rat plasma was tested from QC samples exposed to three different conditions [28]. Short-term stability was calculated by comparing QC samples that were stored for 5 h at 25 °C before sample preparation with the untreated QC samples. The three freeze–thaw cycle stability was analyzed by comparing QC samples that underwent three freeze–thaw cycles (−80 °C to 25 °C and standing for 3 h at 25 °C defined as one cycle) with the untreated QC samples. Post-preparative stability was evaluated by comparing the post-preparative QC samples maintained in the autosampler at 4 °C for 12 h with the untreated QC samples [28].

4.5. Determination of Glycyrrhizin, Isoliquiritigenin, Liquiritigenin, and Liquiritin in GRE

One hundred mg of GRE was diluted 50 times with methanol, and the diluted samples (50 µL) were added to 300 µL of methanol containing berberine (0.1 ng/mL), vortex-mixed for 10 min, and centrifuged at 10,000 × g for 10 min at 4 °C. An aliquot (10 µL) of the supernatant was injected into the LC–MS/MS system.

4.6. Pharmacokinetic Study

Rats were fasted for at least 12 h with water ad libitum before pharmacokinetic experiments and femoral arteries of rats were cannulated with polyethylene tube (PE50, Jungdo, Seoul, Korea) under anesthesia with isoflurane (30 mmol/kg).

GRE (1 g/kg, 2 mL/kg suspended in distilled water) was administered orally to rats by oral gavage. Blood samples (about 250 µL) were taken via the femoral artery at 0, 0.25, 0.5, 0.75, 1, 2, 4, 6, 8, 10 and 12 h and centrifuged at 10,000× g for 10 min at 4 °C. Obtained plasma (50 µL) were stored at −80 °C until analysis.

Glycyrrhizin, isoliquiritigenin, liquiritigenin, and liquiritin concentrations in plasma samples were analyzed using the developed LC–MS/MS method. Plasma samples (50 µL) were added to 300 µL of methanol containing berberine (0.1 ng/mL), vortex-mixed for 10 min, and centrifuged at 10,000× g for 10 min at 4 °C. An aliquot (10 µL) of the supernatant was injected into the LC–MS/MS system.

Pharmacokinetic parameters of glycyrrhizin, isoliquiritigenin, liquiritigenin, and liquiritin were calculated from the plasma concentration vs. time profile using the WinNonlin software (version 5.0, Certara Inc., Princeton, NJ, USA).

4.7. Biotransformation of Isoliquiritigenin and Liquiritigenin from Liquiritin

Rats were fasted for at least 12 h with water ad libitum before performing dissection of the rat ileum. The ileal segment (approximately 20 cm) was excised after the rats were euthanized by cervical dislocation. The dissected ileal segments were washed using a 10 mL syringe filled with 30 mL pre-warmed Hank's balanced salt solution (HBSS, pH 7.4; Sigma, St. Louis, MO, USA); the eluent was vortexed for 1 min followed by centrifugation at 1000× g for 5 min at 4 °C. The supernatant was used for incubation with isoliquiritigenin, liquiritigenin, and liquiritin. The ileal segments were mounted onto the Ussing chambers (Navicyte, Holliston, MA, USA) and were acclimatized with HBSS for 30 min.

To mimic the intestinal situation that occurred when GRE was administered to rats via the oral route, the concentrations of isoliquiritigenin, liquiritigenin, and liquiritin were determined based on the oral dose of GRE, their content in GRE, and fluid volume of the small intestine. For example, 1 g of GRE suspended in 2 mL water was administered at a dose of 1 g/kg to rats having stomach fluid volumes of 3.2–7.8 mL [29], which resulted in a 5–10-fold dilution. Therefore, 14 µg/mL of isoliquiritigenin, 27 µg/mL of liquiritigenin, or 380 µg/mL of liquiritin was present in the intestinal diluent.

The experiments began by changing HBSS with pre-warmed intestinal eluent (1 mL) containing 14 µg/mL of isoliquiritigenin, 27 µg/mL of liquiritigenin, or 380 µg/mL of liquiritin to the apical side of the ileal segment, followed by 2 h of incubation. Carbogen gas (5% CO_2/ 95% O_2) was bubbled into the Ussing chambers at a rate of 150 drops/min during the experiment. Aliquots (50 µL) of the samples were mixed with 300 µL of methanol containing berberine (0.1 ng/mL), vortex-mixed for 10 min, and centrifuged at 10,000× g for 10 min at 4 °C. An aliquot (10 µL) of the supernatant was injected into the LC–MS/MS system.

5. Conclusions

A sensitive and simultaneous LC–MS/MS method for the determination of the four marker components of Glycyrrhizae Radix, namely glycyrrhizin, isoliquiritigenin, liquiritin, and liquiritigenin, has been developed and validated in rat plasma; this analytical method was successfully applied to investigate the pharmacokinetic profiles of glycyrrhizin, isoliquiritigenin, liquiritin, and liquiritigenin in rats following a single oral administration of GRE (1 g/kg) for 24 h.

This method can easily be applied in the bioanalysis and pharmacokinetic studies of GRE, including its administration at multiple therapeutic doses, or for making pharmacokinetic comparisons among individual components in small experimental animals. Moreover, following an appropriate validation, the present method can be extended to determine routine drug monitoring of glycyrrhizin, isoliquiritigenin, liquiritin, and liquiritigenin in plasma samples as well as in other biological samples, and thus, can be applied to in vivo pharmacokinetic–pharmacodynamic correlation studies.

Author Contributions: Conceptualization, M.-K.C. and I.-S.S.; methodology, investigation, and data interpretation, Y.J.H., B.K., E.-J.Y., M.-K.C., and I.-S.S.; writing—original draft preparation, Y.J.H.; writing—review and editing and supervision, M.-K.C. and I.-S.S.

Funding: This research received no external funding.

Conflicts of Interest: The authors declare no conflict of interest.

References

1. Wang, T.; Ding, L.; Jin, H.; Shi, R.; Li, Y.; Wu, J.; Li, Y.; Zhu, L.; Ma, Y. Simultaneous quantification of catechin, epicatechin, liquiritin, isoliquiritin, liquiritigenin, isoliquiritigenin, piperine and glycyrrhetinic acid in rat plasma by hplc-ms/ms: Application to a pharmacokinetic study of longhu rendan pills. *Biomed. Chromatogr.* **2016**, *30*, 1166–1174. [CrossRef]
2. Xie, J.; Zhang, Y.; Wang, W.; Hou, J. Identification and simultaneous determination of glycyrrhizin, formononetin, glycyrrhetinic acid, liquiritin, isoliquiritigenin, and licochalcone a in licorice by lc-ms/ms. *Acta Chromatogr.* **2014**, *26*, 507–516. [CrossRef]
3. Qiao, X.; Ji, S.; Yu, S.W.; Lin, X.H.; Jin, H.W.; Duan, Y.K.; Zhang, L.R.; Guo, D.A.; Ye, M. Identification of key licorice constituents which interact with cytochrome p450: Evaluation by lc/ms/ms cocktail assay and metabolic profiling. *AAPS J.* **2014**, *16*, 101–113. [CrossRef]
4. Kobayashi, S.; Miyamoto, T.; Kimura, I.; Kimura, M. Inhibitory effect of isoliquiritin, a compound in licorice root, on angiogenesis in vivo and tube formation in vitro. *Biol. Pharm. Bull.* **1995**, *18*, 1382–1386. [CrossRef] [PubMed]
5. Wang, Y.; Yao, Y.; An, R.; You, L.; Wang, X. Simultaneous determination of puerarin, daidzein, baicalin, wogonoside and liquiritin of gegenqinlian decoction in rat plasma by ultra-performance liquid chromatography-mass spectrometry. *J. Chromatogr. B Analyt. Technol. Biomed. Life Sci.* **2009**, *877*, 1820–1826. [CrossRef] [PubMed]
6. Lin, Z.J.; Qiu, S.-X.; Wufuer, A.; Shum, L. Simultaneous determination of glycyrrhizin, a marker component in radix glycyrrhizae, and its major metabolite glycyrrhetic acid in human plasma by lc–ms/ms. *J. Chromatogr. B* **2005**, *814*, 201–207. [CrossRef]
7. Hu, F.W.; Yu, C.C.; Hsieh, P.L.; Liao, Y.W.; Lu, M.Y.; Chu, P.M. Targeting oral cancer stemness and chemoresistance by isoliquiritigenin-mediated grp78 regulation. *Oncotarget* **2017**, *8*, 93912–93923. [CrossRef]
8. Liao, M.; Zhao, Y.; Huang, L.; Cheng, B.; Huang, K. Isoliquiritigenin and liquiritin from glycyrrhiza uralensis inhibit α-synuclein amyloid formation, rcs advances, 2016. *RCS Adv.* **2016**, *6*, 86640–86649.
9. Peng, F.; Du, Q.; Peng, C.; Wang, N.; Tang, H.; Xie, X.; Shen, J.; Chen, J. A review: The pharmacology of isoliquiritigenin. *Phytother. Res.* **2015**, *29*, 969–977. [CrossRef] [PubMed]
10. Maggiolini, M.; Statti, G.; Vivacqua, A.; Gabriele, S.; Rago, V.; Loizzo, M.; Menichini, F.; Amdò, S. Estrogenic and antiproliferative activities of isoliquiritigenin in mcf7 breast cancer cells. *J. Steroid. Biochem.* **2002**, *82*, 315–322. [CrossRef]
11. Cuendet, M.; Guo, J.; Luo, Y.; Chen, S.; Oteham, C.P.; Moon, R.C.; Van Breemen, R.B.; Marler, L.E.; Pezzuto, J.M. Cancer chemopreventive activity and metabolism of isoliquiritigenin, a compound found in licorice. *Cancer Prev. Res.* **2010**, *3*, 221–232. [CrossRef]
12. Cuendet, M.; Oteham, C.P.; Moon, R.C.; Pezzuto, J.M. Quinone reductase induction as a biomarker for cancer chemoprevention. *J. Nat. Prod.* **2006**, *69*, 460–463. [CrossRef]
13. Jang, D.S.; Park, E.J.; Hawthorne, M.E.; Vigo, J.S.; Graham, J.G.; Cabieses, F.; Santarsiero, B.D.; Mesecar, A.D.; Fong, H.H.; Mehta, R.G. Potential cancer chemopreventive constituents of the seeds of dipteryx o dorata (tonka bean). *J. Nat. Prod.* **2003**, *66*, 583–587. [CrossRef]

14. Zhang, X.; Qiao, H.; Zhang, T.; Shi, Y.; Ni, J. Enhancement of gastrointestinal absorption of isoliquiritigenin by nanostructured lipid carrier. *Adv. Powder Technol.* **2014**, *25*, 1060–1068. [CrossRef]
15. Liu, Y.; Yang, J.-S. Determination of liquiritigenin, liquiritin, isoliquiritigenin and isoliquiritin in extract of traditional chinese medicine sijunzi decoction by high-performance liquid chromatography. *J. Chinese Pharma. Sci.* **2005**, *14*, 227.
16. Zhang, Y.; Cao, J.; Wang, Y.; Xiao, S. Simultaneous determination of glycyrrhizin and 15 flavonoids in licorice and blood by high performance liquid chromatography with ultraviolet detector. *ISRN Anal. Chem.* **2013**, *10*, 1–7. [CrossRef]
17. Wang, Y.; Xu, C.; Wang, P.; Lin, X.; Yang, Y.; Li, D.; Li, H.; Wu, X.; Liu, H. Pharmacokinetic comparisons of different combinations of shaoyao-gancao-decoction in rats: Simultaneous determination of ten active constituents by hplc–ms/ms. *J. Chromatogr. B* **2013**, *932*, 76–87. [CrossRef]
18. Mao, Y.; Peng, L.; Kang, A.; Xie, T.; Xu, J.; Shen, C.; Ji, J.; Di, L.; Wu, H.; Shan, J. Influence of jiegeng on pharmacokinetic properties of flavonoids and saponins in gancao. *Molecules* **2017**, *22*, 1587. [CrossRef]
19. Shan, J.; Qian, W.; Peng, L.; Chen, L.; Kang, A.; Xie, T.; Di, L. A comparative pharmacokinetic study by uhplc-ms/ms of main active compounds after oral administration of zushima-gancao extract in normal and adjuvant-induced arthritis rats. *Molecules* **2018**, *23*, 227. [CrossRef]
20. Zimmer, D. New us fda draft guidance on bioanalytical method validation versus current fda and ema guidelines: Chromatographic methods and isr. *Bioanalysis* **2014**, *6*, 13–19. [CrossRef]
21. Lin, S.J.; Tseng, H.H.; Wen, K.C.; Suen, T.T. Determination of gentiopicroside, mangiferin, palmatine, berberine, baicalin, wogonin and glycyrrhizin in the traditional chinese medicinal preparation sann-joong-kuey-jian-tang by high-performance liquid chromatography. *J. Chromatogr. A* **1996**, *730*, 17–23. [CrossRef]
22. Okamura, N.; Miki, H.; Ishida, S.; Ono, H.; Yano, A.; Tanaka, T.; Ono, Y.; Yagi, A. Simultaneous determination of baicalin, wogonoside, baicalein, wogonin, berberine, coptisine, palmatine, jateorrhizine and glycyrrhizin in kampo medicines by ion-pair high-performance liquid chromatography. *Biol. Pharm. Bull.* **1999**, *22*, 1015–1021. [CrossRef]
23. Cantelli-Forti, G.; Maffei, F.; Hrelia, P.; Bugamelli, F.; Bernardi, M.; D'Intino, P.; Maranesi, M.; Raggi, M. Interaction of licorice on glycyrrhizin pharmacokinetics. *Environ. Health Perspect.* **1994**, *102*, 65. [CrossRef]
24. ISHIDA, S.; SAKIYA, Y.; ICHIKAWA, T.; TAIRA, Z. Dose-dependent pharmacokinetics of glycyrrhizin in rats. *Chem. Pharm. Bull.* **1992**, *40*, 1917–1920. [CrossRef] [PubMed]
25. Zhou, Y.; Ho, W.S. Combination of liquiritin, isoliquiritin and isoliquirigenin induce apoptotic cell death through upregulating p53 and p21 in the a549 non-small cell lung cancer cells. *Oncol Rep.* **2014**, *31*, 298–304. [CrossRef]
26. Zhang, L.; Zhao, H.; Liu, Y.; Dong, H.; Lv, B.; Fang, M.; Zhao, H. Metabolic routes along digestive system of licorice: Multicomponent sequential metabolism method in rat. *Biomed. Chromatogr.* **2016**, *30*, 902–912. [CrossRef]
27. Huang, P.; Zhang, L.; Chai, C.; Qian, X.C.; Li, W.; Li, J.S.; Di, L.Q.; Cai, B.C. Effects of food and gender on the pharmacokinetics of ginkgolides a, b, c and bilobalide in rats after oral dosing with ginkgo terpene lactones extract. *J. Pharm. Biomed. Anal.* **2014**, *100*, 138–144. [CrossRef]
28. Guo, P.; Dong, L.; Yan, W.; Wei, J.; Wang, C.; Zhang, Z. Simultaneous determination of linarin, naringenin and formononetin in rat plasma by lc-ms/ms and its application to a pharmacokinetic study after oral administration of bushen guchi pill. *Biomed. Chromatogr.* **2015**, *29*, 246–253. [CrossRef]
29. McConnell, E.L.; Basit, A.W.; Murdan, S. Measurements of rat and mouse gastrointestinal ph, fluid and lymphoid tissue, and implications for in-vivo experiments. *J. Pharm. Pharmacol.* **2008**, *60*, 63–70. [CrossRef] [PubMed]

Sample Availability: Samples of Glycyrrhizae Radix extract (#KNUNPM GR-2015-001) are available from the authors.

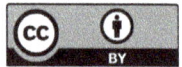

© 2019 by the authors. Licensee MDPI, Basel, Switzerland. This article is an open access article distributed under the terms and conditions of the Creative Commons Attribution (CC BY) license (http://creativecommons.org/licenses/by/4.0/).

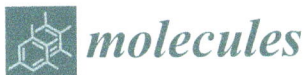

Article

Liquid Chromatography-Tandem Mass Spectrometry of Desoxo-Narchinol a and Its Pharmacokinetics and Oral Bioavailability in Rats and Mice

Subindra Kazi Thapa [1,†], Mahesh Upadhyay [1,†], Tae Hwan Kim [2], Soyoung Shin [1], Sung-Joo Park [3,4] and Beom Soo Shin [5,*]

[1] Department of Pharmacy, College of Pharmacy, Wonkwang University, Iksan, Jeonbuk 54538, Korea; thapasubindra@gmail.com (S.K.T.); maheshupadhyay@gmail.com (M.U.); shins@wku.ac.kr (S.S.)
[2] College of Pharmacy, Daegu Catholic University, Gyeongsan, Gyeongbuk 38430, Korea; thkim@cu.ac.kr
[3] Department of Herbology, School of Korean Medicine, Wonkwang University, Iksan, Jeonbuk 54538, Korea; parksj08@wku.ac.kr
[4] Hanbang Cardio-Renal Syndrome Research Center, Wonkwang University, Iksan, Jeonbuk 54538, Korea
[5] School of Pharmacy, Sungkyunkwan University, Suwon, Gyeonggi 16419, Korea
* Correspondence: bsshin@skku.edu; Tel.: +82-31-290-7705
† Subindra Kazi Thapa and Mahesh Upadhyay contributed equally to this work.

Academic Editors: In-Soo Yoon and Hyun-Jong Cho
Received: 11 May 2019; Accepted: 27 May 2019; Published: 28 May 2019

Abstract: Desoxo-narchinol A is one of the major active constituents from *Nardostachys jatamansi*, which has been reported to possess various pharmacological activities, including anti-inflammatory, antioxidant, and anticonvulsant activity. A simple and sensitive liquid chromatography-tandem mass spectrometry (LC-MS/MS) method was developed and validated for the quantification of desoxo-narchinol A in two different biological matrices, i.e., rat plasma and mouse plasma, using sildenafil as an internal standard (IS). The method involved simple protein precipitation with acetonitrile and the analyte was separated by gradient elution using 100% acetonitrile and 0.1% formic acid in water as a mobile phase. The MS detection was performed with a turbo electrospray in positive ion mode. The lower limit of quantification was 10 ng/mL in both rat and mouse plasma. Intra- and inter-day accuracies were in the ranges of 97.23–104.54% in the rat plasma and 95.90–110.11% in the mouse plasma. The precisions were within 8.65% and 6.46% in the rat and mouse plasma, respectively. The method was applied to examine the pharmacokinetics of desoxo-narchinol A, and the oral bioavailability of desoxo-narchinol A was 18.1% in rats and 28.4% in mice. The present results may be useful for further preclinical and clinical studies of desoxo-narchinol A.

Keywords: desoxo-narchinol A; Nardostachys jatamansi; LC-MS/MS; pharmacokinetics; bioavailability

1. Introduction

Nardostachys jatamansi is a pharmacologically versatile herb found in alpine Himalayas [1]. Traditionally, the roots of *Nardostachys jatamansi* have been used as an aromatic, bitter tonic, antispasmodic, stimulant, antiseptic, diuretic, and emmenagogue [2,3]. The pharmacological activities of *Nardostachys jatamansi* have been well demonstrated in experimental animals. For example, studies have reported that *Nardostachys jatamansi* possesses hepato-protective [1], gamma-aminobutyric acid (GABA) enhancing [4], anti-parkinsonian [5], and anticonvulsant [6] activities in rats. Various activities of *Nardostachys jatamansi*, including antidepressant [7], improvement of learning and memory [8], antidiabetic [9], and anti-inflammatory [10], have also been demonstrated in mice. Recently, in-vitro-derived plants of *Nardostachys jatamansi* have also shown an anti-cholinesterases, anti-hyperglycemic, anti-inflammatory, anti-hypertensive, and anti-tyrosinase potential [11].

The pharmacological activities of *Nardostachys jatamansi* might be attributed to the various compounds present in *Nardostachys jatamansi*, including sesquiterpenes, lignans, and neolignans, terpinic coumarins, phenols, flavonoids, and alkaloids [3,12]. Desoxo-narchinol A is a nardosinone-type sesquiterpenoid found in the rhizomes and roots of *Nardostachys jatamansi*. Desoxo-narchinol A has shown protective effects against lipopolysaccharide (LPS)-induced inflammation through p38 deactivation [13]. Inhibitory activity of desoxo-narchinol A against LPS-induced nitric-oxide (NO) production has been reported as well [14]. Recently, it has also been reported that desoxo-narchinol A inhibited the excessive production of pro-inflammatory mediators and cytokines in LPS-stimulated BV2 and primary microglial cells [15,16]. Therefore, desoxo-narchinol A may be useful as a potential therapeutic agent for the treatment of inflammation or prevention of neurodegenerative diseases.

Despite extensive research on its pharmacological activities, there has been limited information regarding the pharmacokinetics of *Nardostachys jatamansi* or its active ingredient, desoxo-narchinol A. To better understand the biological actions and the therapeutic effects for further development as a therapeutic agent, comprehensive pharmacokinetic studies based on robust analytical methods are essential. To date, a liquid chromatography-tandem mass spectrometry (LC-MS/MS) of nardosinone, another active ingredient of *Nardostachys jatamansi*, has been developed and applied to characterize its pharmacokinetics following intravenous injection in rats [17]. For desoxo-narchinol A, there is only one recent pharmacokinetic study after oral administrations of desoxo-narchinol A and extracts of *Nardostachys jatamansi* in rats by applying an LC-MS/MS method [18]. However, the LC-MS/MS utilized solid-phase extraction, which requires long sample preparation time and cost. Moreover, the pharmacokinetics were only determined following oral administration in rats [18]. Its oral bioavailability and comprehensive pharmacokinetic characteristics are still unknown. The potential differences in pharmacokinetics in different animal species that have been utilized for the pharmacological studies need to be elucidated as well.

Therefore, the aim of the present study was to develop and validate a simple, rapid, and sensitive LC-MS/MS analysis for the quantification of desoxo-narchinol A in the biological fluids. The method was successfully applied to determine the oral bioavailability and pharmacokinetics of desoxo-narchinol A in two animal species, i.e., rats and mice, following intravenous and oral administration. To our knowledge, this is the first study investigating the comprehensive pharmacokinetics of desoxo-narchinol A in rats as well as in mice.

2. Results and Discussion

2.1. Optimization of Sample Preparation

Sample pretreatment procedure was needed to remove protein and potential interferences before LC-MS/MS analysis. Various sample extraction techniques have been applied to extract analytes from biological samples, including protein precipitation, liquid–liquid extraction, and solid–phase extraction. Since the protein precipitation provides a simple and rapid method to extract analytes from the biological matrices [19,20], we applied protein precipitation to prepare samples in the present study. Different organic solvents, namely methanol and acetonitrile, were investigated as protein precipitation solvents to achieve good resolution and high recovery of analytes from spiked biological matrices. Finally, a direct protein precipitation method using acetonitrile was found to be optimal and was selected for biological sample preparation. The main advantages of the present method include the simplicity and low cost of the single-step protein precipitation over other extraction methods. Although solid-phase extraction has been effectively used to extract desoxo-narchinol A and nardosinonediol from plasma [18], it involves greater complexity, lengthy sample preparation time, and higher cost.

2.2. Chromatography

The observed multiple reaction monitoring (MRM) transitions and assay parameters for desoxo-narchinol A and sildenafil (internal standard, IS) are summarized in Table 1. The representative chromatograms in the rat and mouse plasma are shown in Figures 1 and 2, respectively. Desoxo-narchinol A and IS were eluted for 2.74 min and 2.54 min, respectively, in the rat plasma. Similarly, the retention time of desoxo-narchinol A was 2.73 min and that of IS was 2.53 min in the mouse plasma. The complete chromatographic run took 7 min.

Specificity is the ability to determine accurately and specifically the analyte in the presence of other components that may be expected to be present in the matrix. Specificity was assessed by comparing the chromatograms of the blank rat and mouse plasma with the blank matrix spiked with the analyte and IS. Examination of blank, zero sample, and other calibrators showed no interfering peaks at the retention times corresponding to desoxo-narchinol A or IS.

Table 1. Observed MRM transitions and mass spectrometry settings.

Compounds	MRM Transition (*m/z*)	Retention Time (min)		DP (V)	FP (V)	CE (eV)	CXP (V)
		Rat Plasma	Mouse Plasma				
Desoxo-narchinol A	192.94 → 99.00	2.74	2.73	56	310	19	2
IS	474.76 → 58.10	2.54	2.53	96	370	67	0

Note: DP, declustering potential; FP, focusing potential; CE, collision energy; CXP, collision cell exit potential.

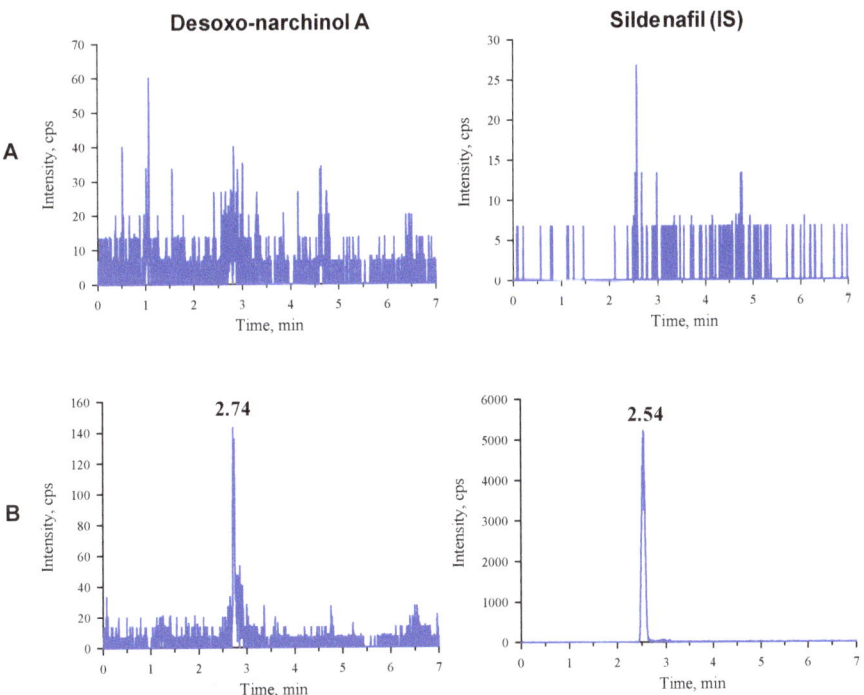

Figure 1. Representative chromatograms of desoxo-narchinol A (left) and the internal standard (right) in the (**A**) blank rat plasma and (**B**) blank rat plasma spiked with desoxo-narchinol A (LLOQ) and IS.

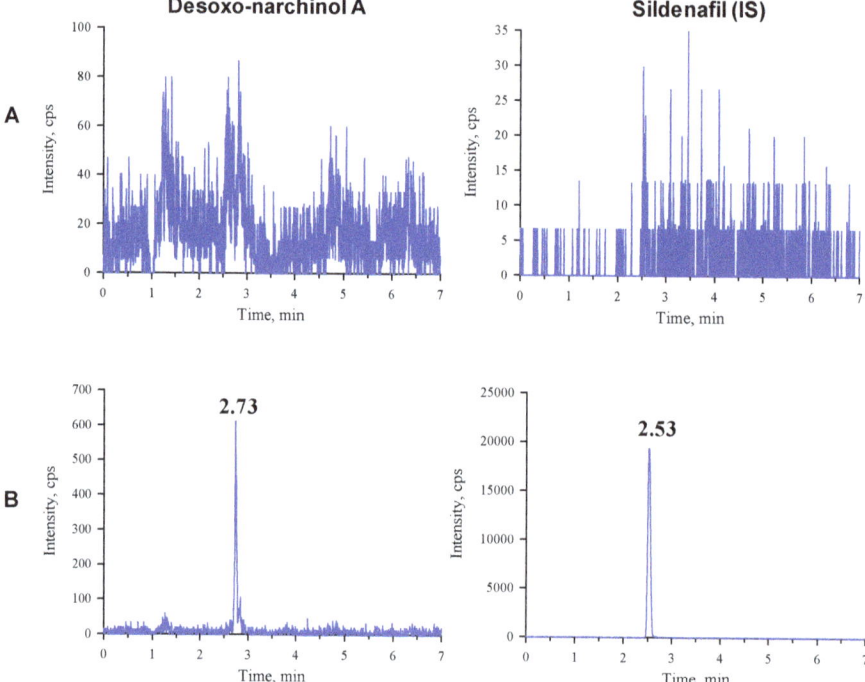

Figure 2. Representative chromatograms of desoxo-narchinol A (left) and the internal standard (right) in the (**A**) blank mouse plasma and (**B**) blank mouse plasma spiked with desoxo-narchinol A (LLOQ) and IS.

2.3. Linearity and Sensitivity

Linearity refers to the ability to obtain test results that are proportional to analyte concentration within a given range. The calibration curves for desoxo-narchinol A in both rat and mouse plasma were linear in the concentration range of 10–1000 ng/mL with correlation coefficients (r^2) > 0.999. The calibration curves had a reliable reproducibility over the standard concentrations of the analyte across the calibration range. The lower limit of quantification (LLOQ) was defined as the lowest standard concentration on the calibration curve with an accuracy of 80–120% and a precision less than 20% [21]. The LLOQ of desoxo-narchinol A was 10 ng/mL for both rat and mouse plasma, which provided sufficient sensitivity to characterize its pharmacokinetics following intravenous and oral administration.

2.4. Accuracy, Precision, and Recovery

The accuracy indicates the closeness between the measurement and the true or theoretical value, and precision is the closeness among a series of measurements. Assessment of accuracy and precision of the analytical method is essential to determine whether the method is ready for validation [21]. The present method was validated in two different biological matrices, i.e., rat and mouse plasma, by using matrix matched quality control (QC) samples to demonstrate its accuracy and precision. The intra- and inter-day accuracy and precision were assessed by analyzing five replicates of LLOQ (10 ng/mL), and QC samples at three different concentrations (25, 125, and 800 ng/mL) in the blank rat and mouse plasma each day for five days. According to the FDA guidance [21], the mean accuracy should not deviate by ±15 %, except for LLOQ, where it can be ±20% of the nominal concentration. Similarly, the deviation at each concentration level from the nominal concentration was expected to be within ± 15%, except LLOQ, for which it should not be more than ± 20% [21].

The determined intra- and inter-day accuracy and precision are summarized in Table 2. The intra- and inter-day accuracies were 97.23–104.54% and the precisions were within 8.65% in the rat plasma. In the mouse plasma, the intra- and inter-day accuracies were 95.90–110.11% and the precisions were within 6.46%. The intra- and inter-day accuracy and precision of the present assay satisfied the criteria of the FDA guidance on bioanalytical methods validation [21] and indicated that the established method was accurate and reliable.

Table 2. Intra- and inter-day accuracy and precision of desoxo-narchinol A assay in rat and mouse plasma.

Matrix	Concentration (ng/mL)	Intra-Day ($n = 5$)		Inter-Day ($n = 5$)	
		Accuracy (%)	Precision (%)	Accuracy (%)	Precision (%)
Rat plasma	10	97.23	8.65	104.54	8.30
	25	99.80	3.90	100.81	1.97
	125	102.24	5.26	99.54	1.66
	800	102.64	1.10	98.28	3.23
Mouse plasma	10	98.41	1.59	110.11	6.46
	25	97.81	0.67	104.20	3.64
	125	97.31	0.78	100.85	2.13
	800	95.90	0.46	99.93	2.93

The total recovery of desoxo-narchinol A that was determined by comparing the peak responses of the drug free plasma or Milli-Q water spiked with desoxo-narchinol A is summarized in Table 3. Although recovery does not need to be 100%, it has been recommended that the extent of recovery of an analyte and IS should be consistent and reproducible [21]. The average recovery for desoxo-narchinol A was 95.15–99.10% in the rat plasma and 95.53–100.07% in the mouse plasma, indicating that the extraction of desoxo-narchinol A via a single-step protein precipitation was efficient and reproducible.

Table 3. Total recovery (%) for desoxo-narchinol A and IS in rat and mouse plasma ($n = 5$).

	Concentration (ng/mL)	Rat Plasma (%)	Mouse Plasma (%)
Desoxo-narchinol A	10	98.77 ± 3.18	99.37 ± 0.65
	25	99.10 ± 2.00	100.07 ± 0.88
	125	95.15 ± 1.63	95.53 ± 1.33
	800	96.10 ± 1.56	96.22 ± 1.29
IS	200	103.90 ± 2.32	100.12 ± 3.48

2.5. Stability

Analyte stability in a given matrix should be determined during sample collection, processing, and storage of the analysis to ensure that the analytical method generates reliable data. The stability was evaluated by comparing the peak responses of the QC samples of desoxo-narchinol A at two different concentrations (25 and 800 ng/mL) in the rat or mouse plasma that were stored in four different conditions against those of freshly prepared QC samples. Results of autosampler stability, freeze-thaw stability, short-term stability, and long-term stability are shown in Table 4. As shown in Table 4, the stability QC samples displayed average 96.62–104.98% recoveries in the rat plasma and 97.43–106.11% in the mouse plasma. Any significant deviations were not observed compared to the freshly prepared samples, indicating that there was no significant degradation of desoxo-narchinol A under the tested conditions.

Table 4. Stability of desoxo-narchinol A in blank rat and mouse plasma ($n = 5$).

Matrix	Conc (ng/mL)	Percentage over Theoretical Concentration (%)			
		Autosampler Stability (24 h, 4 °C)	Freeze-Thaw Stability (3 cycles, −20 °C)	Short-Term Stability (4 h, 20 °C)	Long-Term Stability (2 wk, −20 °C)
Rat plasma	25	102.34 ± 1.75	96.62 ± 0.89	98.23 ± 1.63	104.98 ± 1.05
	800	99.06 ± 1.76	98.45 ± 1.15	99.68 ± 1.49	102.86 ± 1.66
Mouse plasma	25	104.24 ± 0.50	106.11 ± 0.70	105.23 ± 0.49	98.61 ± 0.84
	800	99.59 ± 0.43	103.46 ± 0.80	100.00 ± 0.56	97.43 ± 1.07

2.6. Pharmacokinetics of Desoxo-Narchinol A in Rats

The developed method was successfully applied to pharmacokinetic studies of desoxo-narchinol A following intravenous and oral administration in two animal species.

The average plasma concentration-time profiles of desoxo-narchinol A after intravenous and oral administration in rats are shown in Figure 3. The corresponding pharmacokinetic parameters of desoxo-narchinol A calculated via non-compartmental analysis are shown in Table 5.

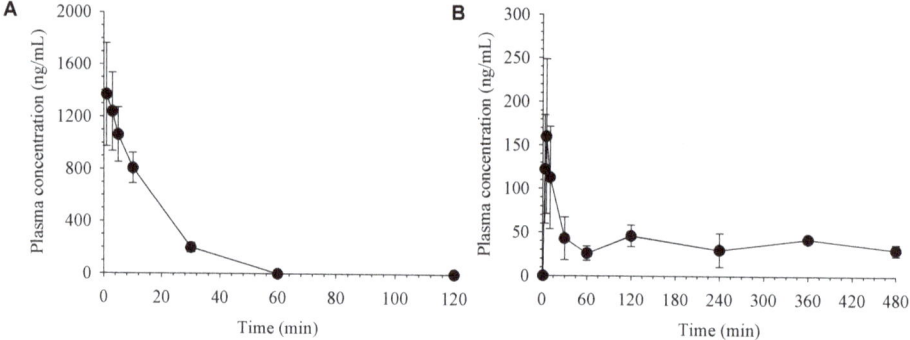

Figure 3. Average plasma concentration vs. time profiles of desoxo-narchinol A after (A) intravenous administration at a dose of 5 mg/kg ($n = 4$) and (B) oral administration at a dose of 50 mg/kg ($n = 4$) in rats. Data represent the mean ± SD.

Table 5. Non-compartmental pharmacokinetic parameters of desoxo-narchinol A following intravenous injection (IV) or oral administration (PO) in rats and mice.

Pharmacokinetic Parameters	Rat		Mouse	
	IV (5 mg/kg, $n = 4$)	PO (50 mg/kg, $n = 4$)	IV (2 mg/kg, $n = 6$)	PO (50 mg/kg, $n = 5$)
$t_{1/2}$ (min)	10.2 ± 0.7	516.9 ± 99.4 [a]	7.4 ± 5.0	9.8 ± 2.3
T_{max} (min)	-	5.0 ± 0.0	-	10.0 ± 0.0
C_0 or C_{max} (ng/mL)	1442.5 ± 463.6	159.8 ± 88.8	624.9 ± 434.8	1978.5 ± 1114.4
AUC_{all} (ng·h/mL)	399.8 ± 73.0	317.9 ± 46.6	80 ± 25.8	688.9 ± 279.5
AUC_{inf} (ng·h/mL)	400.8 ± 73.1	725.1 ± 213.3 [a]	102.2 ± 27.2	726.6 ± 303.4
CL or CL/F (mL/min/kg)	213.8 ± 39.3	950.1 ± 574.0 [a]	343.9 ± 83.1	1302.5 ± 505.3
V_{ss} (L/kg)	2.9 ± 0.6	-	3.6 ± 2.7	-
Bioavailability (F)	-	18.1%	-	28.4%

Note: [a], $n = 3$; $t_{1/2}$, terminal half-life; T_{max}, time to reach C_{max}; C_0 or C_{max}, maximum plasma concentration after i.v. or oral administration, respectively; AUC_{all}, area under the plasma concentration-time curve from time zero to the last observation time point; AUC_{inf}, AUC to infinity; CL or CL/F, systemic clearance or apparent clearance; V_{ss}, volume of distribution at steady state.

In rats, following intravenous injection, plasma concentrations of desoxo-narchinol A were declined with the elimination half-life ($t_{1/2}$) of 10.2 ± 0.7 min and not detected after 60 min. Following oral administration, desoxo-narchinol A was rapidly absorbed, reached the maximum plasma concentration (C_{max}) at 5 min. Then, the plasma concentration of desoxo-narchinol A showed a multi-exponential decline with an extended terminal phase, resulting in the prolonged terminal $t_{1/2}$ compared to that after intravenous injection. Multiple peaks were observed in most of the individual plasma concentration-time profiles. Due to the presence of secondary peaks in the plasma concentration-time profiles, terminal phase could not be easily defined and $t_{1/2}$, area under the plasma concentration-time curve (AUC_{inf}), and apparent clearance (CL/F) were estimated from the limited number of animals. The rapid absorption and prolonged terminal $t_{1/2}$ after oral absorption is consistent with the recent literature report, which reported the T_{max} and $t_{1/2}$ of desoxo-narchinol A of 7.5 ± 2.7 min and 248.8 ± 135.2 min, respectively, following oral administration in rats [18]. The extended terminal phases of desoxo-narchinol A was also observed following oral administration of extracts from *Nardostachys jatamansi* [18]. Finally, the oral bioavailability of desoxo-narchinol A was estimated at 18.1% in rats.

Extensive enterohepatic recirculation typically leads to multiple peaks or shoulders in the plasma concentration-time profiles and a prolonged terminal half-life [22,23]. Alternatively, complex absorption processes, including the presence of different absorption sites in the gastrointestinal tract, may also be associated with the double peak phenomenon [24]. Although multiple peaks and prolonged terminal half-lives were observed only after oral administration, further studies are required to elucidate its mechanisms including enterohepatic recirculation, which may have a pronounced impact on the systemic exposure, and thus on the pharmacological effects of desoxo-narchinol-A.

2.7. Pharmacokinetics of Desoxo-Narchinol A in Mice

Figure 4 depicts the average plasma concentration-time profiles of desoxo-narchinol A after intravenous and oral administration in mice. The non-compartmental pharmacokinetic parameters of desoxo-narchinol A in mice are summarized in Table 5. Similar to the pharmacokinetics in rats, desoxo-narchinol A was rapidly disappeared from the plasma with $t_{1/2}$ of 7.4 ± 5.0 min and not detected after 45 min following intravenous injection in mice. Following oral administration, desoxo-narchinol A was rapidly absorbed to reach C_{max} within 10 min and decreased with the elimination $t_{1/2}$ of 9.8 ± 2.3 min. The extended terminal $t_{1/2}$ and multiple peaks were not observed in mice either after intravenous or oral administration. The species differences in the pharmacokinetic disposition may be worthy of further studies. The oral bioavailability of desoxo-narchinol A was 30.9% in mice, which was higher than that in rats. To best of our knowledge, this is the first report of oral bioavailability of desoxo-narchinol A in animals.

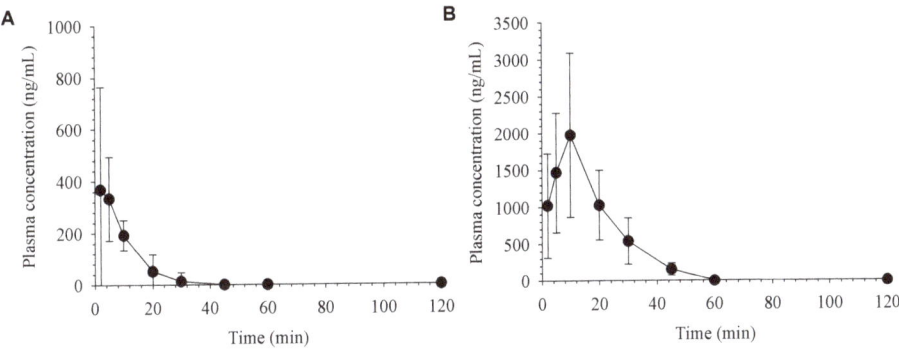

Figure 4. Average plasma concentration vs. time profiles of desoxo-narchinol A after (A) intravenous administration at a dose of 2 mg/kg (n = 6) and (B) oral administration at a dose of 50 mg/kg (n = 5) in mice. Data represent the mean ± SD.

3. Materials and Methods

3.1. Materials

Desoxo-narchinol A was supplied by the School of Oriental Medicine, Wonkwang University (Iksan, South Korea) and stored at −20 °C. Sildenafil (IS), dimethyl sulfoxide (DMSO), and formic acid were purchased from Sigma-Aldrich, Inc. (St. Louis, MO, USA). Acetonitrile and methanol were the products of Burdick and Jackson (Muskegon, MI, USA). All other reagents were high-performance liquid chromatography (HPLC) grades. Water used during the entire study was purified using a Milli-Q water purification system.

3.2. Animal Study

The animal studies were approved by the Institutional Animal Care and Use Committee (IACUC) at Wonkwang University (WKU17-02) and conducted following the Guidelines for the Care and Use of Animals. Male Sprague-Dawley (SD) rats (7 weeks old) and ICR (CD-1) mice (7 weeks old) were purchased from Hanil sirhamdongmul center (Wanju, South Korea). Animals were kept in plastic cages with free access to standard diet and water. The animals were maintained at a temperature of 22–24 °C with a 12 h light-dark cycle and relative humidity of 50 ± 10%.

3.2.1. Rat Study

Rats were anesthetized with intraperitoneal injection of 20 mg/kg Zoletil 50® (tiletamine HCl 125 mg/5 mL + zolazepam HCl 125 mg/5 mL) and cannulated with a polyethylene tubing (0.58 mm i.d., 0.96 mm o.d., Natsume, Tokyo, Japan) in the right jugular vein. After 24 h of recovery, the rats were examined for their physical condition and the experiment was carried out only if the animal was found to be stable. After overnight fasting, desoxo-narchinol A dissolved in 10% DMSO was administered to rats by intravenous (IV, 5 mg/kg, $n = 4$) injection or oral (PO, 50 mg/kg, $n = 4$) administration. Blood samples (200 µL) were collected from the jugular vein before and at 1, 3, 5, 10, 30 min, 1, and 2 h after IV injection, and at 1, 3, 5, 10, 30 min, 1, 2, 4, 6, and 8 h after oral administration. Plasma samples were harvested by centrifugation of the blood samples at 4,000× g for 10 min and stored at −20 °C until analysis.

3.2.2. Mice Study

Mice were administered with desoxo-narchinol A by IV injection into the caudal vein (2 mg/kg, $n = 6$) or oral administration (50 mg/kg, $n = 5$). Blood samples (approximately 40 µL) were collected from the retro-orbital sinus before and at 2, 5, 10, 20, 30, 45 min, 1, and 2 h after drug administration. By centrifugation of the blood samples at 4,000 × g for 10 min, plasma samples were stored at −20 °C until analysis.

3.2.3. Noncompartmental Analysis

The pharmacokinetic parameters of desoxo-narchinol A were determined by noncompartmental analysis using the Phoenix® WinNonlin® (Certara, L.P., Princeton, NJ, USA). The apparent terminal half-life ($t_{1/2}$) was calculated as $0.693/\lambda_z$, where λ_z is the terminal slope. The area under the plasma concentration-time curve from time zero to the last observation time point (AUC_{all}) was calculated using the trapezoidal method and AUC to infinity (AUC_{inf}) was obtained by adding C_{last}/λ_z to AUC_{all}. The systemic clearance (CL) and apparent clearance (CL/F) were estimated by Dose/AUC_{inf}. Volume of distribution at steady state (V_{ss}) was calculated as CL·MRT, where MRT is the mean residence time. Maximum plasma concentration (C_{max}) and time to reach C_{max} (T_{max}) were obtained directly from the observed data. The oral bioavailability (F) was calculated as $F = (AUC_{inf, oral} \cdot Dose_{iv})/(AUC_{inf, iv} \cdot Dose_{oral})$.

3.3. Calibration Standards and Quality Control Samples

The standard stock solutions of desoxo-narchinol A and IS were prepared in methanol at the concentration of 1.0 mg/mL. The working standard solutions of desoxo-narchinol A were prepared by serial dilution of the stock solution with acetonitrile, yielding concentrations of 10, 50, 100, 250, 500, and 1000 ng/mL. The IS working solution 200 ng/mL was prepared by dilution of the stock solution with acetonitrile.

To prepare calibration standard samples, blank rat or mouse plasma were diluted 10-fold with water. Then, 50 μL of the diluted plasma were spiked with 50 μL of the IS working solution and 50 μL of the desoxo-narchinol A standard working solution. Acetonitrile 100 μL was added to the mixture as a protein precipitation solvent. The mixture was mixed on a vortex mixer for 1 min followed by centrifugation at 16,000× g for 20 min at 4 °C. The supernatant 10 μL was injected onto the LC-MS/MS.

The matrix-matched QC samples were prepared by spiking the desoxo-narchinol A working solutions to the freshly harvested blank rat or mouse plasma to provide LLOQ (10 ng/mL), low concentration QC (25 ng/mL), medium concentration QC (125 ng/mL), and high concentration QC (800 ng/mL). The QC samples were stored at −20 °C until analysis.

To prepare plasma samples, the obtained plasma samples were diluted 10-fold with water and 50 μL of the diluted plasma samples were mixed with 150 μL of acetonitrile and 50 μL of the IS solution (200 ng/mL) on a vortex mixer. After the mixture was centrifuged at 16,000× g for 20 min at 4 °C, the supernatant was collected and 10 μL was injected onto the LC-MS/MS.

3.4. LC-MS/MS Conditions

LC-MS/MS system consisted of API 2000 triple quadrupole mass spectrometer (AB Sciex, Concord, ON, Canada) coupled with a Nanospace, Shiseido HPLC system (Shiseido, Yokohama, Japan). Plasma samples were separated on a Kinetex C_{18} column (100 × 2.10 mm i.d., 5 μm). The composition of mobile phase was a mixture of 0.1% of formic acid in water (mobile phase A) and acetonitrile (mobile phase B) with gradient elution program set as: 10% B (0 → 0.5 min), 10% → 90% B (0.5 → 1 min), 90% B (1 → 4.5 min), 90% → 10% B (4.5 → 5 min), and 10% B (5 → 7 min). The flow rate was 0.2 mL/min and the temperature of the autosampler and column were set to be 4 °C and 40 °C, respectively.

The electrospray ionization (ESI) source was operated in positive mode with the curtain and turbo-gas (all nitrogen) set at 30 and 6 psi, respectively. The turbo-gas temperature and the ion spray needle voltage were set at 400 °C and 4500 V, respectively. The mass spectrometer was operated in the MRM mode with a dwell time of 150 ms per MRM channel. The selected precursor/product ion pairs were m/z 192.94 → 99.00 for desoxo-narchinol A and m/z 474.76 → 58.1 for IS. The collision energy was set at 19 and 67 eV for desoxo-narchinol A and IS, respectively. Table 1 summarizes the observed MRM transitions and mass spectrometry settings for desoxo-narchinol A and IS. Data acquisition was performed with Analyst 1.4 software (AB Sciex).

3.5. Assay Validation

3.5.1. Specificity, linearity, and Sensitivity

Specificity was evaluated by analyzing the blank matrix and the blank matrix spiked with the analyte and IS. The linearity was assessed over the concentration ranges of 10–1000 ng/mL in both rat and mouse plasma. The calibration curves were constructed by the weighted regression method (1/x) of peak area ratios of desoxo-narchinol A to IS compared to the actual concentration. The determination of $r^2 > 0.999$ was considered desirable for the calibration curve. The lowest standard concentration on the calibration curve was accepted as the LLOQ. The analyte peak of LLOQ sample should be identifiable, discrete, and reproducible with accuracy within ±20% and precision ≤20%. The deviation of standards of other than LLOQ from the nominal concentration should be within ±15%.

3.5.2. Accuracy and Precision

The accuracy, precision, and recovery were assessed by using the matrix-matched LLOQ and QC samples. Intra- and inter-day accuracies and precisions were expressed as a percent of deviation from the respective nominal values. The intra-day accuracy and precision of QC samples were determined within one day. The inter-day accuracy and precision of the QC samples were determined on five different days.

3.5.3. Recovery

The total recovery of the analyte at LLOQ and three QC samples were determined by analyzing samples prepared by spiking desoxo-narchinol A in drug-free plasma and Milli-Q water separately, and that spiked in Milli-Q water served as un-extracted QC samples. The recovery of desoxo-narchinol A and IS were determined by using five replicates and were processed as usual and analyzed along with five replicates of un-extracted QC samples. The extraction recovery of analyte was determined by measuring the peak area ratios of the analyte after extraction of plasma samples to those of un-extracted QC samples.

3.5.4. Stability

The stability of desoxo-narchinol A was examined under four different conditions using five replicates of low (25 ng/mL) and high (800 ng/mL) matrix-matched QC samples. To assess the stability of desoxo-narchinol A in the rat and mouse plasma at room and storage temperature, low and high QC samples were left at 20 °C for 4 h and at −20 °C for 2 weeks, respectively, and desoxo-narchinol A concentrations were determined. The autosampler storage stability was determined by storing the QC samples in the autosampler at 4 °C for 24 h before being analyzed. The freeze-thaw stability was assessed by determining the remaining concentrations after low and high QC samples were subjected to three freeze-thaw cycles. The results were expressed as the percentage of the mean calculated over theoretical concentrations

4. Conclusions

In this study, a simple and rapid LC-MS/MS method for the analysis of desoxo-narchinol A was developed and validated in two biological matrices—rat plasma, and mouse plasma. The assay involves small sample volumes and single-step protein precipitation resulting in simple and sensitive analysis of desoxo-narchinol A with the LLOQ of 10 ng/mL in both rat and mouse plasma. The developed method was fully validated to demonstrate its reproducibility, as well as specificity, sensitivity, accuracy, precision, recovery, and stability. By applying the LC-MS/MS method, the pharmacokinetics and oral bioavailability of desoxo-narchinol A were determined after intravenous and oral administration in two animal species. The LC-MS/MS assay and the pharmacokinetic information of desoxo-narchinol A in rats and mice may provide useful information for further preclinical and clinical studies of desoxo-narchinol A.

Author Contributions: Conceptualization, S.S., T.H.K., S.-J.P., and B.S.S.; methodology, S.S., T.H.K., and B.S.S.; formal analysis, S.K.T., M.U., and B.S.S.; investigation, S.K.T., M.U., and B.S.S.; writing—original draft preparation, S.K.T., M.U., and B.S.S.; writing—review and editing, S.S., T.H.K., S.-J.P., and B.S.S.; funding acquisition, S.-J.P.

Funding: This research was funded by the National Research Foundation of Korea, grant number NRF-2015R1A2A1A15055913.

Conflicts of Interest: The authors declare no conflict of interest.

References

1. Ali, S.; Ansari, K.A.; Jafry, M.; Kabeer, H.; Diwakar, G. Nardostachys jatamansi protects against liver damage induced by thioacetamide in rats. *J. Ethnopharmacol.* **2000**, *71*, 359–363. [CrossRef]

2. Bagchi, A.; Oshima, Y.; Hikino, H. Neolignans and lignans of nardostachys jatamansi roots1. *Planta Medica.* **1991**, *57*, 96–97. [CrossRef]
3. Chaudhary, S.; Chandrashekar, K.S.; Pai, K.S.R.; Setty, M.M.; Devkar, R.A.; Reddy, N.D.; Shoja, M.H. Evaluation of antioxidant and anticancer activity of extract and fractions of nardostachys jatamansi dc in breast carcinoma. *Bmc Complementary Altern. Med.* **2015**, *15*, 50. [CrossRef] [PubMed]
4. Salim, S.; Ahmad, M.; Zafar, K.S.; Ahmad, A.S.; Islam, F. Protective effect of nardostachys jatamansi in rat cerebral ischemia. *Pharmacol. Biochem. Behav.* **2003**, *74*, 481–486. [CrossRef]
5. Ahmad, M.; Yousuf, S.; Khan, M.B.; Hoda, M.N.; Ahmad, A.S.; Ansari, M.A.; Ishrat, T.; Agrawal, A.K.; Islam, F. Attenuation by nardostachys jatamansi of 6-hydroxydopamine-induced parkinsonism in rats: Behavioral, neurochemical, and immunohistochemical studies. *Pharmacol. Biochem. Behav.* **2006**, *83*, 150–160. [CrossRef] [PubMed]
6. Rao, V.S.; Rao, A.; Karanth, K.S. Anticonvulsant and neurotoxicity profile of nardostachys jatamansi in rats. *J. Ethnopharmacol.* **2005**, *102*, 351–356. [CrossRef]
7. Dhingra, D.; Goyal, P.K. Inhibition of mao and gaba: Probable mechanisms for antidepressant-like activity of nardostachys jatamansi dc. In mice. *Indian J. Exp. Biol.* **2008**, *46*, 212–218.
8. Joshi, H.; Parle, M. Nardostachys jatamansi improves learning and memory in mice. *J. Med. Food* **2006**, *9*, 113–118. [CrossRef]
9. Song, M.Y.; Bae, U.J.; Lee, B.H.; Kwon, K.B.; Seo, E.A.; Park, S.J.; Kim, M.S.; Song, H.J.; Kwon, K.S.; Park, J.W.; et al. Nardostachys jatamansi extract protects against cytokine-induced beta-cell damage and streptozotocin-induced diabetes. *World J. Gastroenterol.* **2010**, *16*, 3249–3257. [CrossRef]
10. Bae, G.-S.; Heo, K.-H.; Choi, S.B.; Jo, I.-J.; Kim, D.-G.; Shin, J.-Y.; Seo, S.-H.; Park, K.-C.; Lee, D.-S.; Oh, H. Beneficial effects of fractions of nardostachys jatamansi on lipopolysaccharide-induced inflammatory response. *Evid. Based Complementary Altern. Med.* **2014**, *2014*. [CrossRef] [PubMed]
11. Bose, B.; Tripathy, D.; Chatterjee, A.; Tandon, P.; Kumaria, S. Secondary metabolite profiling, cytotoxicity, anti-inflammatory potential and in vitro inhibitory activities of nardostachys jatamansi on key enzymes linked to hyperglycemia, hypertension and cognitive disorders. *Phytomedicine: Int. J. Phytother. Phytopharm.* **2018**, *55*, 58–69. [CrossRef]
12. Bae, G.S.; Park, K.C.; Koo, B.S.; Jo, I.J.; Choi, S.B.; Song, H.J.; Park, S.J. Nardostachys jatamansi inhibits severe acute pancreatitis via mitogen-activated protein kinases. *Exp. Med.* **2012**, *4*, 533–537. [CrossRef]
13. Shin, J.Y.; Bae, G.S.; Choi, S.B.; Jo, I.J.; Kim, D.G.; Lee, D.S.; An, R.B.; Oh, H.; Kim, Y.C.; Shin, Y.K.; et al. Anti-inflammatory effect of desoxo-narchinol-a isolated from nardostachys jatamansi against lipopolysaccharide. *Int. Immunopharmacol.* **2015**, *29*, 730–738. [CrossRef]
14. Hwang, J.S.; Lee, S.A.; Hong, S.S.; Han, X.H.; Lee, C.; Lee, D.; Lee, C.-K.; Hong, J.T.; Kim, Y.; Lee, M.K. Inhibitory constituents of nardostachys chinensis on nitric oxide production in raw 264.7 macrophages. *Bioorganic Med. Chem. Lett.* **2012**, *22*, 706–708. [CrossRef]
15. Yoon, C.S.; Kim, K.W.; Lee, S.C.; Kim, Y.C.; Oh, H. Anti-neuroinflammatory effects of sesquiterpenoids isolated from nardostachys jatamansi. *Bioorg. Med. Chem. Lett.* **2018**, *28*, 140–144. [CrossRef]
16. Kim, K.W.; Yoon, C.S.; Kim, Y.C.; Oh, H. Desoxo-narchinol a and narchinol b isolated from nardostachys jatamansi exert anti-neuroinflammatory effects by up-regulating of nuclear transcription factor erythroid-2-related factor 2/heme oxygenase-1 signaling. *Neurotox. Res.* **2019**, *35*, 230–243. [CrossRef]
17. Lu, Z.; Zhou, P.; Zhan, Y.; Su, J.; Yi, D. Quantification of nardosinone in rat plasma using liquid chromatography–tandem mass spectrometry and its pharmacokinetics application. *J. Chromatogr. Sci.* **2015**, *53*, 1725–1729. [CrossRef]
18. Le, V.N.H.; Zhao, Y.; Cho, C.W.; Na, M.; Quan, K.T.; Kim, J.H.; Hwang, S.Y.; Kim, S.W.; Kim, K.T.; Kang, J.S. Pharmacokinetic study comparing pure desoxo-narchinol a and nardosinonediol with extracts from nardostachys jatamansi. *J. Chromatogr. B Anal. Technol. Biomed. Life Sci.* **2018**, *1102–1103*, 152–158. [CrossRef]
19. Shin, S.; Jeong, H.M.; Chung, S.E.; Kim, T.H.; Thapa, S.K.; Lee, D.Y.; Song, C.H.; Lim, J.Y.; Cho, S.M.; Nam, K.Y.; et al. Simultaneous analysis of acetylcarnitine, proline, hydroxyproline, citrulline, and arginine as potential plasma biomarkers to evaluate nsaids-induced gastric injury by liquid chromatography-tandem mass spectrometry. *J. Pharm. Biomed. Anal.* **2019**, *165*, 101–111. [CrossRef]

20. Thapa, S.K.; Weon, K.Y.; Jeong, S.W.; Kim, T.H.; Upadhyay, M.; Han, Y.H.; Jin, J.S.; Hong, S.H.; Youn, Y.S.; Shin, B.; et al. Simple and rapid liquid chromatography-tandem mass spectrometry analysis of arctigenin and its application to a pharmacokinetic study. *Mass Spectrom. Lett.* **2017**, *8*, 23–28.
21. U.S. FDA. *Guidance for industry: Bioanalytical method validation. Center for Drug Evaluation and Research (CDER)*; U.S. FDA: Rockville, MD, USA, 2018.
22. Roberts, M.S.; Magnusson, B.M.; Burczynski, F.J.; Weiss, M. Enterohepatic circulation: Physiological, pharmacokinetic and clinical implications. *Clin. Pharm.* **2002**, *41*, 751–790. [CrossRef]
23. Kim, T.H.; Shin, S.; Landersdorfer, C.B.; Chi, Y.H.; Paik, S.H.; Myung, J.; Yadav, R.; Horkovics-Kovats, S.; Bulitta, J.B.; Shin, B.S. Population pharmacokinetic modeling of the enterohepatic recirculation of fimasartan in rats, dogs, and humans. *Aaps. J.* **2015**, *17*, 1210–1223. [CrossRef]
24. Kim, T.H.; Shin, S.; Bulitta, J.B.; Youn, Y.S.; Yoo, S.D.; Shin, B.S. Development of a physiologically relevant population pharmacokinetic in vitro-in vivo correlation approach for designing extended-release oral dosage formulation. *Mol. Pharm.* **2017**, *14*, 53–65. [CrossRef]

Sample Availability: Samples of the compounds are not available from the authors.

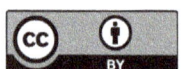 © 2019 by the authors. Licensee MDPI, Basel, Switzerland. This article is an open access article distributed under the terms and conditions of the Creative Commons Attribution (CC BY) license (http://creativecommons.org/licenses/by/4.0/).

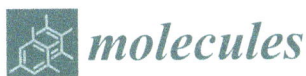

Communication

A Simple HPLC Method for the Quantitative Determination of Silybin in Rat Plasma: Application to a Comparative Pharmacokinetic Study on Commercial Silymarin Products

Eun-Sol Ha [†], Dong-Gyun Han [†], Seong-Wook Seo, Ji-Min Kim, Seon-Kwang Lee, Woo-Yong Sim, In-Soo Yoon * and Min-Soo Kim *

Department of Manufacturing Pharmacy, College of Pharmacy, Pusan National University, Busan 46241, Korea; edel@pusan.ac.kr (E.-S.H.); hann9607@pusan.ac.kr (D.-G.H.); sswook@pusan.ac.kr (S.-W.S.); jiminkim@pusan.ac.kr (J.-M.K.); lsk7079@pusan.ac.kr (S.-K.L.); popo923@pusan.ac.kr (W.-Y.S.)
* Correspondence: insoo.yoon@pusan.ac.kr (I.-S.Y.); minsookim@pusan.ac.kr (M.-S.K.);
 Tel.: +82-51-510-2806 (I.-S.Y.); +82-51-510-2813 (M.-S.K.)
† These authors contributed equally to this work.

Received: 13 May 2019; Accepted: 6 June 2019; Published: 10 June 2019

Abstract: Silybin (SBN) is a major active constituent of silymarin, a mixture of flavonoids found in fruits and seeds of milk thistle. The aim of this study was to describe a simple bioanalytical method for quantifying SBN in rat plasma. A simple protein deproteinization procedure with acetonitrile (ACN) was employed for plasma sample preparation. A reversed column and gradient elution of a mobile phase (mixture of phosphate buffer (pH 5.0) and ACN) were used for chromatographic separation. The selectivity, linearity (50–5000 ng/mL), precision, accuracy, recovery, matrix effect, and stability for this method were validated as per the current Food and Drug Administration (FDA) guidelines. Our method for SBN was applied to a comparative pharmacokinetic study on four different commercial silymarin products. This in vivo rat study demonstrated that product #4 significantly enhanced the relative oral bioavailability of SBN, as compared to product #1–3. Therefore, the bioanalytical method proposed herein could serve as a promising alternative for preclinical pharmacokinetic studies on silymarin products and, by extension, clinical use after partial modification and validation.

Keywords: silybin; HPLC; silymarin product; rat; comparative pharmacokinetics

1. Introduction

Milk thistle (*Silybum marianum* L.) is a well-recognized medicinal plant widely used to prevent and treat various acute and chronic liver disorders [1]. Silymarin is a mixture of flavonoids found in fruits and seeds of milk thistle [2,3]. It is known as a clinically effective hepatoprotectant against alcoholic liver disease, toxin-/drug-induced hepatitis, viral hepatitis, and cirrhosis [4]. Silybin (SBN; Figure 1), a flavone, is the major and most active constituent of silymarin, constituting approximately 60%–70% [5]. It possesses antioxidant, anti-inflammatory, antifibrotic, hepatoprotective, and anticancer activities [6]. However, the oral bioavailability of SBN is very poor (0.73% in rats) due to its low aqueous solubility and permeability, limiting its wide clinical application [5,7]. Thus, the determination of relevant plasma pharmacokinetic parameters (including AUC, C_{max}, and bioavailability) would be essential in developing new silymarin formulations to enhance the oral absorption of SBN, the major active compound of silymarin [4,8,9].

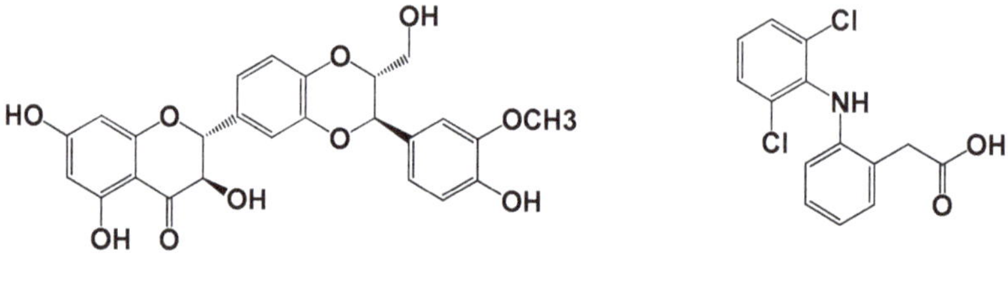

Silybin **Diclofenac**

Figure 1. Chemical structures of silybin (SBN) and diclofenac (internal standard, IS).

So far, several bioanalytical methods using high-performance liquid chromatography (HPLC) combined with ultraviolet/visible (UV) [5,10–12] and mass [13] detectors have been reported for the quantitative determination of SBN in human and rat plasma samples. However, these methods have some limitations and need for improvements on such aspects of insufficient sensitivity with a lower limit of quantification (LLOQ) of 0.5 μg/mL [5,10], time-consuming procedures of sample preparation with liquid–liquid extraction [11,12], and relatively expensive instrumentation for mass spectrometry [13]. Thus, there is a need to develop an alternative bioanalytical method with simpler sample preparation procedure and sufficient sensitivity for pharmacokinetic research and development.

Here, we developed and fully validated a simple and efficient HPLC method for quantifying SBN in rat plasma. The linearity, sensitivity, precision, accuracy, recovery, matrix effect, and stability of this HPLC method were assessed [14,15]. Next, the developed bioanalytical method was applied to investigate the comparative pharmacokinetics of SBN following the oral administration of commercially available functional food products of silymarin that were manufactured by four different pharmaceutical companies located in South Korea.

2. Results and Discussion

2.1. Method Development

Several conditions relevant to chromatographic analysis were assessed for acceptable sensitivity and good separation of the analytes from the endogenous matrix substances and metabolites within a suitable run time. Several trials were performed to select a suitable stationary phase, internal standard (IS), and sample preparation procedures.

To choose a stationary phase, several types of HPLC columns including Kinetex® C8 and C18 columns (250 × 4.6 mm, 5 μm, 100 Å; Phenomenex) and Luna® HILIC column (150 × 3 mm, 5 μm, 200 Å; Phenomenex) were evaluated. Our test revealed that Kinetex® C18 column exhibited better resolution and intensity of peaks compared to other columns (data not shown). Thus, Kinetex® C18 column was chosen as the stationary phase for SBN.

Several compounds such as celecoxib, repaglinide, ketoconazole, and quinidine were tested as potential IS that could compensate for possible analytical errors. However, these were found to be unsuitable owing to poor separation from SBN and endogenous plasma components. We finally settled for diclofenac (Figure 1) as it exhibited good separation; additionally, it displayed acceptable peak resolution, retention time, and UV absorbance intensity at the same wavelength as SBN.

Rat plasma samples were pretreated by solvent precipitation-reconstitution technique, a simpler and more efficient sample preparation method, compared to the solid phase or liquid–liquid extraction method. To optimize sample preparation procedures, various organic solvents for protein precipitation including acetone, methanol, acetonitrile (ACN), trichloroacetic acid, and their combinations, were examined. Among these, ACN yielded the lowest matrix effect and highest recovery for SBN and DIC with a centrifugation speed of 15,000g for an acceptable precipitation period of 5 min.

2.2. Method Validation

As shown in Figure 2, SBN peaks were well separated from the peaks of IS and endogenous substances in the blank plasma. These results imply that the bioanalytical method developed herein may provide acceptable selectivity without endogenous interferences occurring at the appearance of SBN and IS peaks. The calibration curves (SBN-to-IS peak area ratio versus SBN-to-IS concentration ratio) for SBN were observed to be linear from 50 to 5000 ng/mL. A representative equation for the calibration curves is as follows: $y = 0.2224 \times x + 0.0001$, where y indicates the ratio of SBN peak area to that of IS, and x indicates the ratio of nominal concentration of SBN to that of IS. The correlation coefficients (r^2) were more than 0.999, indicating an acceptable linearity of our method. The intra- and inter-day accuracy and precision were determined for SBN at the LLOQ (50 ng/mL) and three quality control (QC) levels (3000 ng/mL (high; HQC), 600 ng/mL (middle; MQC), 150 ng/mL (low; LQC)), as shown in Table 1. The precision of the method was determined to be 8.8% or less, and its accuracy ranged from 96.6% to 111.2%. These values are within the acceptable range, indicating that the present method is reproducible, accurate, and precise. Notably, our present method with a simple protein deproteinization procedure achieved an equivalent LLOQ (50 ng/mL) in a previous study involving liquid–liquid extraction [4].

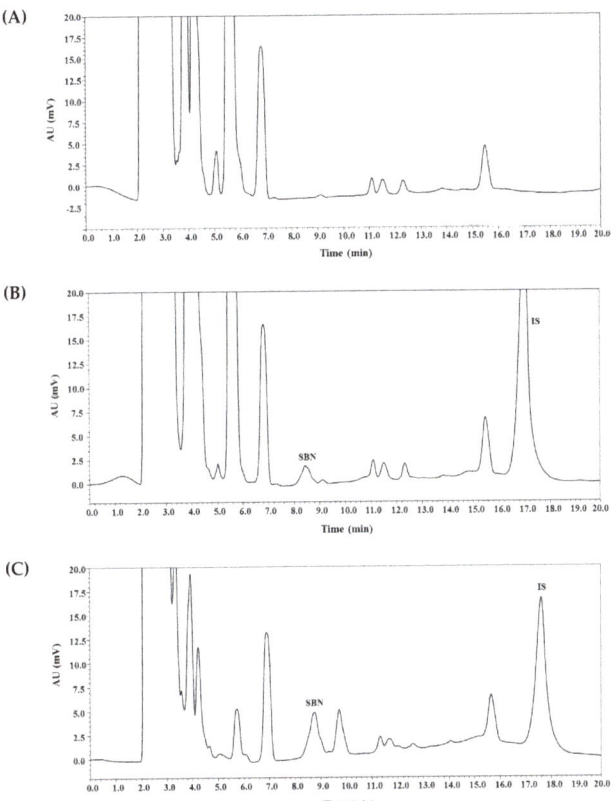

Figure 2. Typical chromatograms of SBN and IS in rat plasma: blank rat plasma (**A**); blank rat plasma spiked with analytes (600 ng/mL, middle quality control (MQC)) and IS (**B**); plasma sample collected at 30 min after oral administration of commercial silymarin product #4 (200 mg/kg as silybin) in rats, where calculated concentrations of SBN was 1055 ng/mL, respectively (**C**).

Table 1. Intra- and inter-day precision and accuracy of SBN in rat plasma (n = 5).

Nominal Concentration (ng/mL)	Precision (%)		Accuracy (%)	
	Intra-Day	Inter-Day	Intra-Day	Inter-Day
LLOQ (50)	4.3	4.3	106.7	103.2
LQC (150)	1.4	7.1	104.1	100.6
MQC (600)	2.3	8.8	107.4	96.6
HQC (3000)	3.1	8.5	111.2	99.3

The recovery and matrix effects were determined for SBN at the QC levels and for IS at 1000 ng/mL (Table 2). The recovery of SBN was 92.3%–100.1% with CV values of <4.4%. The mean matrix effect was 91.4%–98.8% with CV values of <5.4%. The SBN stability was measured under various conditions relevant to the present method. The bench-top, freeze-thaw, autosampler, and long-term stabilities were measured for SBN at the levels tested. We observed the bias in the concentration to be within ±15% of the corresponding nominal value; the remaining fraction of SBN was 88.6%–113.3% with CV values of <5.0% (Table 3). Our results show that the sample preparation procedures used herein could offer acceptable matrix effect with good extraction recovery, and that SBN remains stable under various storage and handling conditions relevant to this bioanalytical method.

Table 2. Recovery and matrix effect of SBN and IS in rat plasma (n = 5).

Nominal Concentration (ng/mL)	Recovery (%)	Matrix Effect (%)
LLOQ (50)	100.1 ± 4.5	95.0 ± 5.1
LQC (150)	98.6 ± 2.1	92.9 ± 4.6
MQC (600)	93.6 ± 1.5	91.4 ± 1.8
HQC (3000)	92.3 ± 3.9	98.0 ± 1.4
IS (Diclofenac, 1000)	93.3 ± 3.1	98.8 ± 1.6

Table 3. Stability (%) of SBN in rat plasma (n = 5).

Nominal Concentration (ng/mL)	Bench–Top [a]	Autosampler [b]	Freeze–Thaw [c]	Long–Term [d]
LLOQ (50)	103.7 ± 5.2	91.8 ± 3.5	95.1 ± 1.7	92.3 ± 4.4
LQC (150)	100.3 ± 3.6	88.6 ± 1.6	98.4 ± 3.2	93.6 ± 3.4
MQC (600)	101.5 ± 2.3	107.1 ± 3.7	94.7 ± 1.6	100.5 ± 2.0
HQC (3000)	100.7 ± 0.9	98.1 ± 3.1	113.3 ± 1.6	98.6 ± 0.3

[a] Room temperature during 3 h. [b] 25 °C during 24 h in the autosampler. [c] Three freezing and thawing cycles. [d] −20 °C during 14 days.

2.3. Application to a Comparative Pharmacokinetic Study in Rats

Rats were administered oral silymarin products at 200 mg/kg as SBN. Following this, plasma concentrations versus time profiles of SBN were assessed (Figure 3). Their relevant pharmacokinetic parameters are listed in Table 4. The oral SBN dose was selected based on previous preclinical pharmacokinetic studies on SBN [4,5,8,9]. We identified linear terminal phases of plasma concentration profiles obtained from oral studies. After the oral administration of the four silymarin products, plasma SBN levels reached respective peaks (C_{max}) at 2–30 min, which was rather consistent with previously reported rat data (11 ± 1.8 min) [5]. As shown in Table 4, the C_{max}, AUC_{inf}, and AUC_{last} of SBN after oral administration of commercial product #4 were significantly higher than those after administration of the other commercial silymarin products #1–3 as follows: the AUC_{inf} after administration of product #4 was 6.3-, 8.3-, and 4.4-fold higher; the AUC_{last} after administration of product #4 was 8.9-, 11.8-, and 6.2-fold higher; and the C_{max} after administration of product #4 was 12.5-, 6.9-, and 4.2-fold higher than those after administration of products #1–3, respectively. These results clearly indicated that the commercial silymarin products exhibited fast oral absorption of SBN and that the bioavailability of SBN was higher with product #4 than with the other three products.

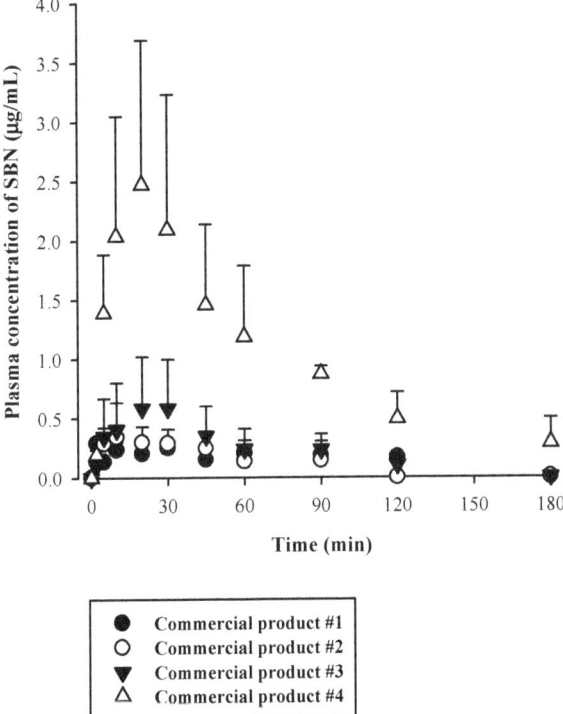

Figure 3. Plasma concentration versus time profiles of SBN following oral administration of four different commercial silymarin products in rats (n = 5).

Table 4. Pharmacokinetic parameters of SBN following oral administration of four different commercial silymarin products in rats (n = 5).

Parameter	AUC_{inf} (µg·min/mL)	AUC_{last} (µg·min/mL)	C_{max} (µg/mL)	T_{max} (min)
Commercial product #1	35.6 ± 16.2	23.2 ± 13.6	0.250 ± 0.056	30 (2–30)
Commercial product #2	26.9 ± 11.2	17.6 ± 11.0	0.455 ± 0.277	10 (5–30)
Commercial product #3	50.6 ± 24.9	33.2 ± 18.6	0.744 ± 0.331	10 (5–20)
Commercial product #4	224.5 ± 37.4 *	207.0 ± 28.0 *	3.13 ± 0.49 *	20 (10–20)

* Significantly different from the other groups ($p < 0.05$).

3. Materials and Methods

3.1. Materials

SBN (purity ≥95.0%), potassium phosphate monobasic/dibasic, and dimethyl sulfoxide (DMSO) were obtained from Sigma-Aldrich Co. (St. Louis, MO, USA). Diclofenac (purity ≥98.0%) was obtained from Tokyo Chemical Industry Co. (Tokyo, Japan). HPLC-grade acetonitrile (ACN) was obtained from Honeywell, Inc. (Muskegon, MA, USA). The silymarin products from four different manufacturers, indicated as 'Commercial product #1–4', were evaluated. The names of the manufacturers were not disclosed for privacy reasons.

3.2. Calibration Standards and QC Samples

Stocks of SBN and IS were prepared in DMSO at 1 mg/mL. The stock solution of SBN was diluted serially using methanol to make working solutions with concentrations 5–500 µg/mL. The working solution of IS (100 µg/mL) was prepared in ACN. The calibration standard samples were made by spiking the blank rat plasma with each corresponding working solution, thereby yielding final concentrations of 50, 100, 200, 500, 1000, 2000, and 5000 ng/mL. The QC samples were prepared with new stock solutions of SBN using the same procedure adopted in preparing calibration standards.

3.3. Chromatographic Conditions

A Shimadzu HPLC-UV system with a pump (LC-20AT), an autosampler (SIL-20AC), a column oven (CTO-20A), and an ultraviolet detector (SPD-20A) was used in this study (Shimadzu Co., Kyoto, Japan). A Kinetex C18 column (250 × 4.6 mm, 5 µm, 100 Å; Phenomenex, Torrance, CA, USA) protected by a C18 guard column (SecurityGuard HPLC Cartridge System, Phenomenex) was used for chromatographic separation at 40 °C. The mobile phase for the HPLC system consisted of phosphate buffer (pH 5.0; 10 mM) (solvent A) and ACN (solvent B) at a flow rate of 1 mL/min. The gradient elution protocol was as follows (solvent A/solvent B (v/v)): ramped from 71:29 (v/v) to 59:41 (v/v) during 10 min; back to 71:29 (v/v) for 10 min. The wavelength for SBN and IS was set as 220 nm. The total run time and injection volume were 20 min and 20 µL, respectively. All solvents used for sample preparation and HPLC analysis were degassed by sonication under vacuum and in-line electronic vacuum degasser modules.

3.4. Method Validation

The bioanalytical method for determining SBN in biological samples was validated as per the US FDA guidelines [16]. The selectivity, linearity, precision, accuracy, recovery, matrix effect, bench–top, freeze–thaw, post–preparative (autosampler), and long-term stabilities were evaluated as previously described [17,18].

3.5. Pharmacokinetic Study in Rats

Male, 9-week-old Sprague–Dawley rats (approximately 300 g) were purchased from Samtako Bio Korea Co. (Gyeonggi-do, South Korea). Animal study protocols used in this study were approved by the Pusan National University-Institutional Animal Care and Use Committee (approval number: PNU-2018-1848). Rats were fasted during 12 h and anesthetized by intramuscular injection of zoletil at 20 mg/kg. Their femoral arteries were cannulated with a polyethylene tube (Clay Adams) 4 h before drug administration. The rats were randomly divided into four treatment groups (n = 5 per group) receiving four different commercial silymarin products. All the products tested are currently marketed in soft gelatin capsules. Their undiluted liquid contents, with no further formulation, were administered orally to rats at a single dose of 200 mg/kg as silybin. Approximately 300 µL blood was collected through the femoral artery at 0, 2, 5, 10, 20, 30, 45, 60, 90, 120, and 180 min after the oral dosing. Following centrifugation of the blood sample at 2000g at 4 °C for 10 min, a 120 µL aliquot of the plasma was stored at −20 °C until HPLC analysis.

3.6. Sample Pretreatment

A plasma sample (120 µL) was deproteinized with 400 µL of ice-cold ACN (IS dissolved at 1000 ng/mL). After vortexing during 5 min and centrifugation for 5 min at 15,000g, 400 µL supernatant was transferred to a 1.7 mL microcentrifuge tube and dried under a gentle nitrogen gas stream. The resultant residue was reconstituted with 40 µL mobile phase, and a 20 µL aliquot was analyzed by the HPLC system.

3.7. Data Analysis

The analytical data acquisition and processing were conducted using the LC Solution Software (Version 1.25; Shimadzu Co.). All chromatograms were analyzed using the IS. Peak area ratios of SBN to IS were used for calculations (least squares regression, weighting factor of $1/x$, x = concentration). For pharmacokinetic analysis, non-compartmental analysis (WinNonlin, version 3.1, NCA200 and 201; Certara USA Inc., Princeton, NJ, USA) was used to estimate the following pharmacokinetic parameters: total area under the plasma concentration versus time curve from time zero to the last sampling time (AUC_{last}) and to time infinity (AUC_{inf}). The peak plasma concentration (C_{max}) and time to reach C_{max} (T_{max}) were directly read from observed data.

3.8. Statistical Analysis

Statistical analysis was conducted using *t*-test for comparing unpaired two means or Tukey's honestly significant difference (HSD) test with posteriori analysis of variance (ANOVA) for comparing unpaired three means. A p-value < 0.05 indicated statistical significance. Unless indicated otherwise, all data are expressed as mean ± standard deviation and rounded to one decimal place, except T_{max} values expressed as median (range) and as an integer number.

4. Conclusions

A simple and efficient HPLC–UV method was successfully developed and validated for the quantitative determination of SBN in rat plasma. The developed method offers several advantages including simplicity of sample preparation procedures, good recovery, negligible matrix effect, and acceptable sensitivity comparable to the previously reported HPLC method which employs more complex sample pretreatment procedure. The comparative pharmacokinetic study on commercial silymarin products revealed that product #4 significantly enhanced the relative oral bioavailability of SBN compared to product #1–3. Therefore, the bioanalytical method proposed herein could serve as a promising alternative for preclinical pharmacokinetic studies on silymarin products and, by extension, clinical use after partial modification and validation.

Author Contributions: Conceptualization, E.-S.H. and D.-G.H.; methodology, S.-W.S.; software, J.-M.K. and S-K.L.; validation, S.-W.S. and W.-Y.S.; formal analysis, E.-S.H., D.-G.H., and S.-W.S.; investigation, J.-M.K.; resources, W.-Y.S.; data curation, S.-W.S. and J.-M.K.; writing—original draft preparation, E.-S.H. and D.-G.H.; writing—review and editing, I.-S.Y. and M.-S.K.; supervision, I.-S.Y. and M.-S.K.

Funding: This research was supported by Basic Science Research Program through the National Research Foundation of Korea (NRF) funded by the Ministry of Science, ICT & Future Planning (NRF-2017R1C1B1006483) and the Ministry of Education (NRF-2017R1D1A3B03030252).

Conflicts of Interest: The authors declare no conflict of interest. The funders had no role in the design of the study; in the collection, analyses, or interpretation of data; in the writing of the manuscript, or in the decision to publish the results.

References

1. Federico, A.; Dallio, M.; Di Fabio, G.; Zarrelli, A.; Zappavigna, S.; Stiuso, P.; Tuccillo, C.; Caraglia, M.; Loguercio, C. Silybin-Phosphatidylcholine Complex Protects Human Gastric and Liver Cells from Oxidative Stress. *In Vivo* **2015**, *29*, 569–575. [PubMed]
2. Lee, J.I.; Narayan, M.; Barrett, J.S. Analysis and comparison of active constituents in commercial standardized silymarin extracts by liquid chromatography-electrospray ionization mass spectrometry. *J. Chromatogr. B* **2007**, *845*, 95–103. [CrossRef] [PubMed]
3. Byeon, J.C.; Ahn, J.B.; Jang, W.S.; Lee, S.-E.; Choi, J.-S.; Park, J.-S. Recent formulation approaches to oral delivery of herbal medicines. *J. Pharm. Investig.* **2019**, *49*, 17–26. [CrossRef]
4. Wei, Y.; Ye, X.; Shang, X.; Peng, X.; Bao, Q.; Liu, M.; Guo, M.; Li, F. Enhanced oral bioavailability of silybin by a supersaturatable self-emulsifying drug delivery system (S-SEDDS). *Colloid. Surf. A* **2012**, *396*, 22–28. [CrossRef]

5. Wu, J.W.; Lin, L.C.; Hung, S.C.; Chi, C.W.; Tsai, T.H. Analysis of silibinin in rat plasma and bile for hepatobiliary excretion and oral bioavailability application. *J. Pharm. Biomed. Anal.* **2007**, *45*, 635–641. [CrossRef] [PubMed]
6. Ma, Y.; He, H.; Xia, F.; Li, Y.; Lu, Y.; Chen, D.; Qi, J.; Lu, Y.; Zhang, W.; Wu, W. In vivo fate of lipid-silybin conjugate nanoparticles: Implications on enhanced oral bioavailability. *Nanomedicine* **2017**, *13*, 2643–2654. [CrossRef] [PubMed]
7. Ershadi, S.; Jouyban, A.; Molavi, O.; Shayanfar, A. Development of a Terbium-Sensitized Fluorescence Method for Analysis of Silibinin. *J. AOAC Int.* **2017**, *100*, 686–691. [CrossRef] [PubMed]
8. Yi, T.; Liu, C.; Zhang, J.; Wang, F.; Wang, J.; Zhang, J. A new drug nanocrystal self-stabilized Pickering emulsion for oral delivery of silybin. *Eur. J. Pharm. Sci.* **2017**, *96*, 420–427. [CrossRef] [PubMed]
9. Wu, W.; Wang, Y.; Que, L. Enhanced bioavailability of silymarin by self-microemulsifying drug delivery system. *Eur. J. Pharm. Biopharm.* **2006**, *63*, 288–294. [CrossRef] [PubMed]
10. Wu, J.W.; Lin, L.C.; Hung, S.C.; Lin, C.H.; Chi, C.W.; Tsai, T.H. Hepatobiliary excretion of silibinin in normal and liver cirrhotic rats. *Drug Metab. Dispos.* **2008**, *36*, 589–596. [CrossRef] [PubMed]
11. Kim, Y.C.; Kim, E.J.; Lee, E.D.; Kim, J.H.; Jang, S.W.; Kim, Y.G.; Kwon, J.W.; Kim, W.B.; Lee, M.G. Comparative bioavailability of silibinin in healthy male volunteers. *Int. J. Clin. Pharmacol. Ther.* **2003**, *41*, 593–596. [CrossRef] [PubMed]
12. Rickling, B.; Hans, B.; Kramarczyk, R.; Krumbiegel, G.; Weyhenmeyer, R. Two high-performance liquid chromatographic assays for the determination of free and total silibinin diastereomers in plasma using column switching with electrochemical detection and reversed-phase chromatography with ultraviolet detection. *J. Chromatogr. B* **1995**, *670*, 267–277. [CrossRef]
13. Zhu, H.J.; Brinda, B.J.; Chavin, K.D.; Bernstein, H.J.; Patrick, K.S.; Markowitz, J.S. An assessment of pharmacokinetics and antioxidant activity of free silymarin flavonolignans in healthy volunteers: A dose escalation study. *Drug Metab. Dispos.* **2013**, *41*, 1679–1685. [CrossRef] [PubMed]
14. Shim, J.H.; Chae, J.I.; Cho, S.S. Identification and extraction optimization of active constituents in *Citrus junos* Seib ex TANAKA peel and its biological evaluation. *Molecules* **2019**, *24*, 680. [CrossRef] [PubMed]
15. Thakur, D.; Jain, A.; Ghoshal, G.; Shivhare, U.; Katare, O. RP-HPLC method development using analytical QbD approach for estimation of cyanidin-3-O-glucoside in natural biopolymer based microcapsules and tablet dosage form. *J. Pharm. Investig.* **2017**, *47*, 413–427. [CrossRef]
16. US Food and Drug Administration (FDA). Bioanalytical Method Validation Guidance for Industry. 2018. Available online: https://www.fda.gov/regulatory-information/search-fda-guidance-documents/bioanalytical-method-validation-guidance-industry (accessed on 4 June 2019).
17. Kim, K.T.; Lee, J.Y.; Park, J.H.; Kim, M.H.; Kim, J.S.; Shin, H.J.; Kang, N.; Cho, H.J.; Yoon, I.S.; Kim, D.D. Development of HPLC Method for the Determination of Buspirone in Rat Plasma Using Fluorescence Detection and Its Application to a Pharmacokinetic Study. *Chem. Pharm. Bull.* **2016**, *64*, 1582–1588. [CrossRef] [PubMed]
18. Kim, S.B.; Kim, K.T.; Joo, J.; Seo, K.A.; Hwang, H.; Kim, S.H.; Song, M.; Lee, S.; Jahn, A.; Cho, H.J.; et al. Assessment of pharmacokinetics, bioavailability and protein binding of anacetrapib in rats by a simple high-performance liquid chromatography-tandem mass spectrometry method. *Biomed. Chromatogr.* **2017**, *31*, e3791. [CrossRef] [PubMed]

Sample Availability: Samples of the compounds are not available from the authors.

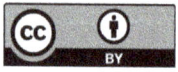

© 2019 by the authors. Licensee MDPI, Basel, Switzerland. This article is an open access article distributed under the terms and conditions of the Creative Commons Attribution (CC BY) license (http://creativecommons.org/licenses/by/4.0/).

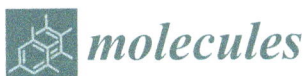

Article

Detection of 13 Ginsenosides (Rb1, Rb2, Rc, Rd, Re, Rf, Rg1, Rg3, Rh2, F1, Compound K, 20(*S*)-Protopanaxadiol, and 20(*S*)-Protopanaxatriol) in Human Plasma and Application of the Analytical Method to Human Pharmacokinetic Studies Following Two Week-Repeated Administration of Red Ginseng Extract

Sojeong Jin [1], Ji-Hyeon Jeon [2], Sowon Lee [2], Woo Youl Kang [3,4], Sook Jin Seong [3,4], Young-Ran Yoon [3,4], Min-Koo Choi [1,*] and Im-Sook Song [2,*]

1. College of Pharmacy, Dankook University, Cheon-an 31116, Korea
2. College of Pharmacy and Research Institute of Pharmaceutical Sciences, Kyungpook National University, Daegu 41566, Korea
3. Clinical Trial Center, Kyungpook National University Hospital, Daegu 41944, Korea
4. Department of Biomedical Science, BK21 Plus KNU Bio-Medical Convergence Program for Creative Talent, College of Medicine, Kyungpook National University, Daegu 41944, Korea
* Correspondence: minkoochoi@dankook.ac.kr (M.-K.C.); isssong@knu.ac.kr (I.-S.S.); Tel.: +82-41-550-1438 (M.-K.C.); +82-53-950-8575 (I.-S.S.)

Academic Editors: In-Soo Yoon and Hyun-Jong Cho
Received: 19 June 2019; Accepted: 17 July 2019; Published: 18 July 2019

Abstract: We aimed to develop a sensitive method for detecting 13 ginsenosides using liquid chromatography–tandem mass spectrometry and to apply this method to pharmacokinetic studies in human following repeated oral administration of red ginseng extract. The chromatograms of Rb1, Rb2, Rc, Rd, Re, Rf, Rg1, Rg3, Rh2, F1, compound K (CK), protopanaxadiol (PPD), and protopanaxatriol (PPT) in human plasma were well separated. The calibration curve range for 13 ginsenosides was 0.5–200 ng/mL and the lower limit of quantitation was 0.5 ng/mL for all ginsenosides. The inter- and intra-day accuracy, precision, and stability were less than 15%. Among the 13 ginsenosides tested, nine ginsenosides (Rb1, Rb2, Rc, Rd, Rg3, CK, Rh2, PPD, and PPT) were detected in the human plasma samples. The plasma concentrations of Rb1, Rb2, Rc, Rd, and Rg3 were correlated with the content in red ginseng extract; however, CK, Rh2, PPD, and PPT were detected although they are not present in red ginseng extract, suggesting the formation of these ginsenosides through the human metabolism. In conclusion, our analytical method could be effectively used to evaluate pharmacokinetic properties of ginsenosides, which would be useful for establishing the pharmacokinetic–pharmacodymic relationship of ginsenosides as well as ginsenoside metabolism in humans.

Keywords: ginsenosides; red ginseng extract; pharmacokinetics; human

1. Introduction

Ginsenosides are classified into two types according to their hydroxylation position on the core triterpene saponin structure: 20(*S*)-protopanaxadiol (PPD) and 20(*S*)-protopanaxatriol (PPT) [1]. These ginsenosides are considered to be the major active pharmacological constituents of ginseng [2,3]. Several studies have described the immunological, antioxidant, anticoagulant, anti-neoplastic, neuroprotective, and hepatoprotective effects of ginseng and its associated ginsenosides [3–8]. The content and types of ginsenosides vary depending on the preparation method of ginseng product such as steaming times, temperature, and the extraction method [9,10]. For example, ginsenosides Rg1 and Re decreased, but ginsenosides Rb1, Rb2, Rc, Rd, and Rg3 increased after several hours of steaming and extraction. As results, the ratio of PPD-type to PPT-type ginsenoside of Korean red ginseng extract was higher than that of Korean ginseng [10]. Ginsenosides generally have low intestinal permeability in Caco-2 cells and low oral bioavailability in rats [1]. For example, the oral bioavailability of Rb1 and Rh2 is around 1.18–4.35 % and 4.0–6.4%, respectively. Other ginsenosides such as Rg1, Rd, Rh1, and Re have a low oral bioavailability, of less than 10% [1]. Owing to the low oral bioavailability of these ginsenosides, their plasma concentration is also low. The maximum plasma concentration of Rb1, Rb2, Rc, and Rd, major ginsenosides found in rat plasma, was lower than 10 ng/mL in rats following oral administration of red ginseng extract at a dose of 1.5 g/kg [8,11]

Because of the low plasma concentration of ginsenosides, the analysis of ginsenosides in human plasma following oral administration of ginseng product has been limited to the selected ginsenoside. Moreover, analytical methods have also been limited to liquid chromatography–tandem mass spectrometry (LC-MS/MS) rather than high-performance liquid chromatography (HPLC) with UV or fluorescence detection [12]. In human study, there are some reports on the analysis of ginsenosides but they used large volume of plasma or provided limited concentrations on ginsenosides because of the high lower limit of quantitation (LLOQ). For example, the plasma concentration of Rb1 and CK following single oral administration of 10 g of American ginseng powder was investigated. In this study, Rb1 and CK in 0.7 mL of plasma samples were extracted using a solid-phase extraction procedure and detected by time-of-flight mass spectrometry coupled with ultra-high pressure liquid chromatography [13]. Another study developed a simultaneous analysis method for Rb1 and Rg1 in human plasma by LC-MS/MS. In this study, for the analysis of Rb1 and Rg1, 100 µL of human plasma was subjected to protein precipitation and analyzed with a calibration curve range of 10–1000 ng/mL [14]. The ginsenoside Rb1 was detected but Rg1 was not detected. This could be attributed to the low plasma concentration of Rg1 after oral administration of the ginseng product (1.5 g/day) [14].

Recently, more sensitive analytical methods have been developed. Choi et al. reported the plasma concentrations of Rb1 and CK in human plasma following single oral administration of 3 g of fermented red ginseng extract with a calibration curve range of 1–1000 ng/mL [15]. In another study, ginsenoside PPD was analyzed after a single oral administration of a PPD 25 mg capsule with a calibration curve range of 0.1–100 ng/mL [16]. Ginsenoside Re was analyzed after a single oral administration of a Re 200 mg tablet with a calibration curve range of 0.5–200 ng/mL. The metabolite peaks of Rg1, Rg2, F1, Rh1, and PPT in human plasma and urine were also monitored following oral administration of Re tablet (200 mg) without quantification [12]. Our group simultaneously determined the plasma concentrations of the ginsenosides Rb1, Rb2, Rc, Rd, and CK in human subjects following single and 2-week repeated administration of three pouches of red ginseng product with a calibration curve range of 0.5–200 ng/mL [17].

However, minor ginsenosides or metabolites of ginsenosides may also have beneficial pharmacological effects and, therefore, the pharmacokinetic properties of minor components and metabolites should also be measured. In rats, following single or repeated oral administration of high doses of ginseng extract (2–8 g/kg), various ginsenosides such as Ra3, Rb1, Rd, CK, Re, and Rg1 could be detected in the plasma of rats by LC-MS/MS with calibration curves ranging from 1.37 or 12.3 ng/mL to 3000 ng/mL [18]. These results suggest that sensitive analytical methods could be useful for the detection of various ginsenosides in human plasma.

Therefore, the objective of this study was to develop an analytical method for the detection of various ginsenosides in human plasma and to apply this validated method to pharmacokinetic studies after multiple administration of red ginseng extract (three pouches/day for two weeks) in human subjects. We analyzed 13 ginsenosides (Rb1, Rb2, Rc, Rd, Re, Rf, Rg1, Rg3, Rh2, F1, CK, PPD, and PPT), which are ginsenosdies found in red ginseng extract and their biological metabolites that could be transformed by intestinal microbiota (Figure 1).

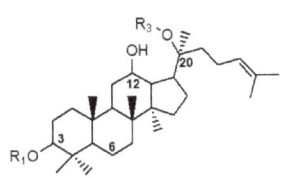
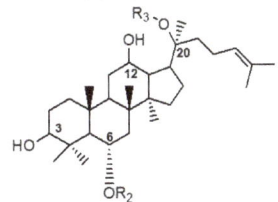
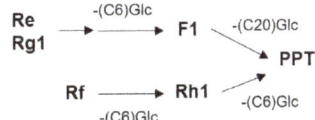

Figure 1. Structure and metabolic pathway of 20(S)-protopanaxadiol (PPD) and 20(S)-protopanaxatriol (PPT) type ginsenosides. Metabolic pathway represents deglycosylation at C3, C6, or C20 position by β-glucosidase from intestinal microbiota. Glc: glucose; Arap: arabinopyranose; Araf: arabinofuranose; Rha: rhamnose; Xyl: xylose.

2. Results

2.1. MS/MS Analysis

The mass spectrometer was operated with electrospray ionization (ESI) in the positive ionization mode. Table 1 shows the selected precursor and product ions of analytes and respective mass spectrometric conditions in the MS/MS stage of the ginsenosides, which were optimized based on the fragmentation patterns of precursor and product ions of target ginsenoside, the specificity of target ginsenoside compared to the other ginsenosides, and the consistency with the previously published findings [11,19]. Since ginsenosides Rb2 and Rc resulted in the same m/z values of precursor and product ion, these ginsenosides should be separated each other during the elution. Retention times were 5.7 min for Rb2 and 4.8 min for Rc (Table 1 and Figure 2B).

2.2. Sample Praperations

For sample preparation, both protein precipitation and liquid–liquid extraction (LLE) methods should be applied depend on the number of glycosylation of ginsenosides. For example, we used the protein precipitation method for ginsenosides glycosylated with more than two glucose units (i.e., Rb1, Rb2, Rc, Rd, Re, Rf, Rg1, Rg3, and F2; hydrophilic ginsenosides) and the LLE method for monoglycosylated ginsenosides and their aglycones (i.e., Rh1, Rh2, CK, PPD, and PPT; lipophilic ginsenosides) based on the extraction recovery after sample preparation and the interference of endogenous peaks in human blank plasma (the plasma withdrawn from human subjects who did not take ginseng or ginsenosides). The monoglycosylated ginsenoside F1 could be extracted with both the protein precipitation and LLE method; however, the detection sensitivity of analyte was better for precipitation samples than for LLE samples. Therefore, F1 were extracted with the protein precipitation method. Methyl tert-butyl ether (MTBE) was chosen as an extraction solvent based on the extraction efficiency and reproducibility of the ginsenosides Rh1, Rh2, CK, PPD, and PPT and based on previous findings [15].

The ginsenosides F2 and Rh1 were excluded in the validation process because their peaks could not be completely separated from the endogenous peaks that detected at the same m/z as F2 and Rh1 in human blank plasma, and the peak response of F2 and Rh1 at LLOQ was less than five times the response of a blank sample [20,21].

2.3. Analytical Method Validation

The method was fully validated according to the FDA Guidance for Industry: Bioanalytical Method Validation (May 2018) [21] for its specificity, accuracy, precision, matrix effect and extraction recovery, and stability.

Table 1. Mass spectrometry (MS/MS) parameters for the detection of the ginsenosides and internal standard (IS).

Sample Preparation Method	Compound	Precursor Ion (m/z)	Product Ion (m/z)	Retention Time (min)	Fragmentor Voltage (V) [a]	Collision Energy (V)
Protein precipitation	Rb1	1131.6	365.1	4.6	165	65
	Rb2	1101.6	335.1	5.7	185	60
	Rc	1101.6	335.1	4.8	185	60
	Rd	969.9	789.5	6.8	170	50
	Re	969.9	789.5	2.1	170	50
	Rf	823.5	365.1	3.3	135	55
	Rg1	824.0	643.6	2.2	135	40
	Rg3	807.5	365.2	9.3	165	60
	F1	661.5	203.1	4.6	185	40
	F2	807.5	627.5	9.4	135	40
	Berberine (IS)	336.1	320.0	4.5	135	30
LLE	Rh1	603.4	423.4	2.9	135	10
	Rh2	587.4	407.4	4.5	135	15
	CK	645.5	203.1	6.4	160	35
	PPD	425.3	109.1	11.0	125	25
	PPT	441.3	109.1	4.0	130	30
	13C-caffeine (IS)	198	140	2.9	120	20

[a] Fragmentor voltage (V) is the voltage difference between capillary and skimmer.

2.3.1. Specificity

Representative multiple reaction-monitoring (MRM) chromatograms of the ginsenosides Rb1, Rb2, Rc, Rd, Re, Rf, Rg1, Rg3, Rh2, F1, F2, CK, PPD, and PPT (Figure 2) showed that all the ginsenoside peaks obtained using the protein precipitation or LLE method were well separated with no interfering peaks at their respective retention times. The retention times of the 13 ginsenosides are shown in Table 1. The specificity of the analytes was confirmed using six different human blank plasma samples and test plasma samples obtained from human subjects at 1 h after the last oral administration of red ginseng extract (Figure 2).

2.3.2. Linearity and LLOQ

To assess linearity, the standard calibration curve of eight different concentrations of 13 ginsenosides was analyzed, and the standard calibration curve and equation for each component are shown in Table 2. The LLOQ was defined as a signal-to-noise ratio of > 5.0 with a precision rate of ≤ 15% and an accuracy rate of 80–120%. The LLOQ for the ginsenosides in our analytical system was set at 0.5 ng/mL in all cases.

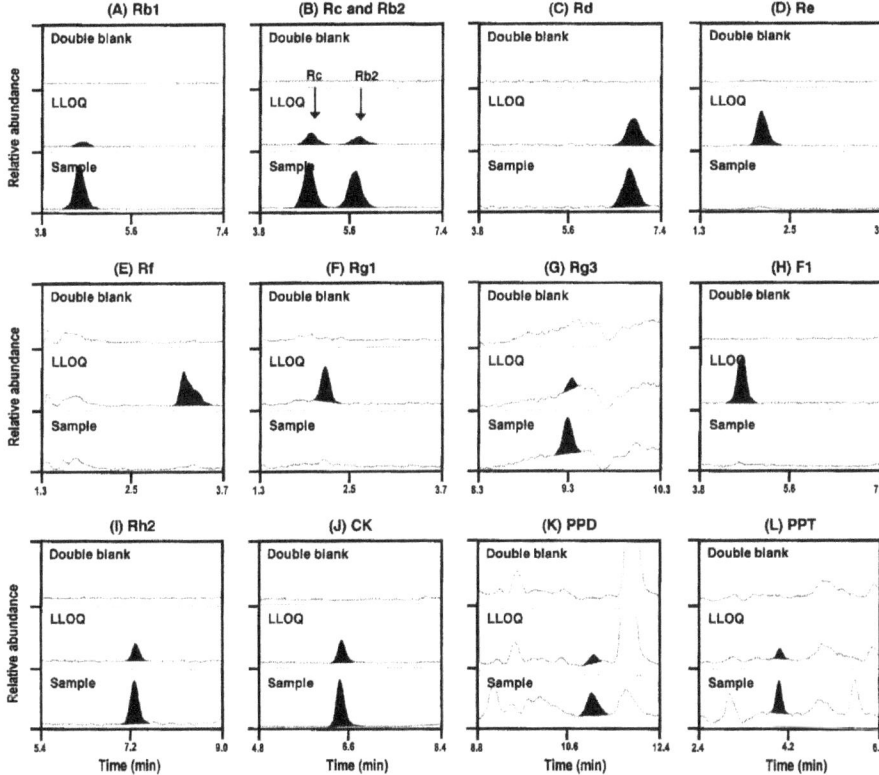

Figure 2. Representative multiple reaction-monitoring (MRM) chromatograms of the ginsenosides (**A**) Rb1, (**B**) Rc and Rb2, (**C**) Rd, (**D**) Re, (**E**) Rf, (**F**) Rg1, (**G**) Rg3, (**H**) F1, (**I**) Rh2, (**J**) CK, (**K**) PPD, and (**L**) PPT in human double blank plasma (**upper**), human blank plasma spiked with standard samples with a lower limit of quantification (LLOQ) (**center**), and human plasma at 1 h following 2 weeks of repeated oral administration of red ginseng extract (**lower**).

Table 2. Linear range, slope and intercept of regression equation, and correlation coefficient of 13 ginsenosides.

Analyte	Linear Range (ng/mL)	Slope ± SD [a]	Intercept ± SD [a]	Correlation Coefficient [a]
Rb1	0.5–200	0.0485 ± 0.0205	0.0007 ± 0.0019	0.997
Rb2	0.5–200	0.1069 ± 0.0394	−0.0003 ± 0.0041	0.997
Rc	0.5–200	0.1408 ± 0.0393	0.0003 ± 0.0047	0.997
Rd	0.5–200	0.2597 ± 0.0536	−0.0388 ± 0.0903	0.996
Re	0.5–200	0.2509 ± 0.0290	−0.0048 ± 0.0095	0.997
Rf	0.5–200	0.1980 ± 0.0308	−0.0056 ± 0.0095	0.995
Rg1	0.5–200	0.0648 ± 0.0081	−0.0010 ± 0.0071	0.994
Rg3	0.5–200	0.0687 ± 0.0092	0.0008 ± 0.0069	0.987
F1	0.5–200	0.8728 ± 0.2221	−0.0337 ± 0.0437	0.995
Rh2	0.5–200	0.0146 ± 0.0035	−0.0006 ± 0.0009	0.996
CK	0.5–200	0.0860 ± 0.0442	−0.0071 ± 0.0076	0.990
PPD	0.5–200	0.0476 ± 0.0120	0.0004 ± 0.0024	0.995
PPT	0.5–200	0.0221 ± 0.0022	−0.0019 ± 0.0037	0.996

[a] Average of six determinations.

2.3.3. Precision and Accuracy

The inter-day and intra-day precision and accuracy were assessed using three different concentrations (1.5, 15, and 150 ng/mL) of quality control (QC) samples consisting of a specific ginsenoside mixture (Rb1, Rb2, Rc, Rd, Re, Rf, Rg1, Rg3, and F1 for protein precipitation; Rh2, CK, PPD, and PPT for LLE) (Table 3). The results showed that inter-day and intra-day precision (CV in Table 3) for the 13 ginsenosides was below 13.0%, and the inter-day and intra-day accuracy (RE in Table 3) for the 13 ginsenosides was below 15.0% (Table 3).

Table 3. Intra- and inter-day precision and accuracy of 13 ginsenosides.

Analyte	QC (ng/mL)	Inter-day (n = 5)				Intra-day (n = 6)			
		Measured (ng/mL)	SD	CV (%)	RE (%)	Measured (ng/mL)	SD	CV (%)	RE (%)
Rb1	1.5	1.5	0.1	6.1	0.9	1.5	0.1	7.7	1.9
	15	15.1	0.7	4.5	0.5	15.0	0.3	1.9	0.2
	150	150.3	8.8	5.9	0.2	154.8	5.8	3.7	3.2
Rb2	1.5	1.5	0.1	4.7	2.5	1.5	0.1	5.2	1.4
	15	15.0	0.6	4.2	−0.1	15.2	0.3	2.2	1.4
	150	154.5	10.3	6.6	3.0	162.6	6.6	4.1	8.4
Rc	1.5	1.5	0.1	4.4	−0.8	1.5	0.1	5.0	0.3
	15	14.9	0.8	5.0	−0.4	14.8	0.5	3.2	−1.3
	150	154.1	11.9	7.7	2.7	160.2	7.6	4.7	6.8
Rd	1.5	1.5	0.1	6.4	2.0	1.6	0.1	5.8	6.3
	15	14.9	0.7	5.0	−0.8	15.2	0.3	2.1	1.2
	150	155.8	10.7	6.9	3.9	164.4	6.4	3.9	9.6
Re	1.5	1.5	0.1	3.7	−0.7	1.6	0.1	3.9	6.1
	15	15.1	0.6	4.2	0.5	15.4	0.5	3.1	2.8
	150	150.1	9.8	6.5	0.1	158.6	6.0	3.8	5.7
Rf	1.5	1.5	0.1	6.0	0.4	1.6	0.1	5.2	4.4
	15	15.0	0.6	3.7	−0.3	15.3	0.9	5.6	2.2
	150	156.7	11.4	7.3	4.5	166.3	7.9	4.8	10.8
Rg1	1.5	1.6	0.1	6.1	3.9	1.6	0.1	5.9	6.2
	15	15.2	0.9	5.8	1.5	15.8	0.5	2.9	5.1
	150	151.1	7.7	5.1	0.7	155.5	5.6	3.6	3.7
Rg3	1.5	1.4	0.2	10.3	−5.9	1.6	0.1	5.9	8.5
	15	15.8	1.6	10.2	5.2	15.9	1.2	7.5	5.9
	150	159.2	16.0	10.1	6.1	166.4	11.7	7.0	11.0
F1	1.5	1.5	0.1	6.5	−3.3	1.5	0.1	3.7	−0.3
	15	14.9	0.8	5.5	−1.0	14.9	0.3	2.2	−0.7
	150	154.8	10.9	7.1	3.2	160.8	7.4	4.6	7.2
Rh2	1.5	1.4	0.1	8.2	−4.9	1.3	0.1	9.5	−11.8
	15	15.2	0.4	2.6	1.5	13.6	1.2	8.6	−9.2
	150	151.5	7.5	5.0	1.0	151.2	16.9	11.2	0.8
CK	1.5	1.4	0.2	10.6	−4.9	1.5	0.1	6.5	−3.4
	15	14.5	1.9	13.0	−3.5	12.8	1.4	10.8	−15.0
	150	163.2	12.0	7.3	8.8	141.1	10.0	7.1	−6.0
PPD	1.5	1.5	0.2	11.7	−1.1	1.5	0.1	5.1	3.0
	15	14.9	0.5	3.5	−0.5	15.0	0.5	3.2	−0.1
	150	166.4	17.2	10.3	10.9	155.4	6.3	4.1	3.6
PPT	1.5	1.5	0.1	5.0	2.4	1.5	0.1	4.2	1.4
	15	14.8	0.4	2.8	−1.5	15.7	0.4	2.4	4.6
	150	153.8	2.0	1.3	2.5	156.8	2.3	1.5	4.5

Data represented as mean ± SD from five or six independent experiments.

2.3.4. Extraction Recovery and Matrix Effect

The extraction recovery of the ginsenosides Rb1, Rb2, Rc, Rd, Re, Rf, Rg1, Rg3, and F1, which were prepared with the protein precipitation method using three different concentrations (1.5, 15, and 150 ng/mL) of QC samples, ranged from 85.5% to 99.2% with a CV of < 14.9%. In the case of the LLE method, the extraction recovery of the ginsenosides Rh2, CK, PPD, and PPT ranged from 56.3% to 81.9% with a CV of < 14.9% (Table 4).

Table 4. Extraction recoveries and matrix effects for 13 ginsenosides.

Analyte	QC (ng/mL)	Recovery (%)		Matrix Effect (%)		Analyte	QC (ng/mL)	Recovery (%)		Matrix Effect (%)	
		Recovery	CV	Matrix Effect	CV			Recovery	CV	Matrix Effect	CV
Rb1	1.5	93.5	8.5	74.5	13.6	Rg3	1.5	91.9	14.9	92.2	12.2
	15	85.5	8.1	78.3	7.0		15	90.3	6.4	70.3	6.8
	150	89.3	4.0	75.8	5.8		150	94.2	10.2	67.9	4.2
Rb2	1.5	96.0	6.5	79.4	8.5	F1	1.5	96.9	7.2	56.6	4.0
	15	86.0	5.9	82.1	6.1		15	90.1	6.5	57.9	3.2
	150	89.3	2.9	78.5	6.3		150	93.1	3.3	57.1	3.2
Rc	1.5	93.8	6.7	69.8	12.5	Rh2	1.5	64.9	11.8	99.7	3.2
	15	87.7	6.4	70.4	8.9		15	64.9	3.7	95.6	2.4
	150	91.3	4.3	67.8	8.4		150	65.4	3.6	98.5	2.6
Rd	1.5	96.4	7.3	73.9	8.0	CK	1.5	60.0	14.9	88.6	7.3
	15	88.7	5.2	75.5	8.4		15	64.0	14.4	93.1	6.6
	150	90.8	3.8	72.4	6.8		150	56.3	12.4	77.0	5.1
Re	1.5	99.2	13.1	9.5	7.4	PPD	1.5	79.9	5.0	98.4	14.9
	15	93.5	5.8	7.0	5.5		15	70.7	5.4	96.7	4.1
	150	95.5	3.1	7.9	6.6		150	71.6	5.2	100.1	5.7
Rf	1.5	93.0	4.2	19.5	13.6	PPT	1.5	81.7	7.2	77.8	11.8
	15	88.1	6.7	16.4	9.9		15	77.5	4.3	77.3	5.3
	150	94.0	7.1	18.2	10.9		150	81.9	6.8	76.6	5.4
Rg1	1.5	97.5	13.4	9.9	5.8						
	15	97.6	8.5	7.2	3.4						
	150	96.2	5.5	7.7	4.2						

Data represented as mean ± SD from six independent experiments.

The matrix effects for the ginsenosides Rh2, CK, PPD, and PPT ranged from 77.0% to 100.1%. The matrix effects for the protein-precipitated ginsenosides (Rb1, Rb2, Rc, Rd, Re, Rf, Rg1, Rg3, and F1) ranged from 7.0% to 92.9%. The matrix effect of ginsenosides Re, Rf, and Rg1 was in the range of 7.0%–19.5%, suggesting that Re, Rf, and Rg1 showed significant signal suppression during the ionization and protein precipitation process; however, the values of CV of Re, Rf, and Rg1 was less than 15% and the matrix effect of Re, Rf, and Rg1 was similar for the three different QC levels with an acceptable CV, and 10 other ginsenosides showed no significant interference during ionization and sample preparation. According to the EMA guideline [22], we concluded our analytical method was acceptable even though Re, Rf, and Rg1 had significant ion suppression.

2.3.5. Stability

The precision (CV) and accuracy (RE) of three different concentrations of QC samples consisting of a mixture of the ginsenosides Rb1, Rb2, Rc, Rd, Re, Rf, Rg1, Rg3, and F1, which were prepared using the protein precipitation method, were within 13.5% for short-term stability, below 14.9% for post-preparative stability, and below 12.9% for three freeze–thaw cycle stability (Table 5). The precision (CV) and accuracy (RE) of three different concentrations of QC samples consisting of a mixture of the ginsenosides Rh2, CK, PPD, and PPT, which were prepared using the LLE method, were within 10.6% for short-term stability, below 12.4% for post-preparative stability, and below 14.7% for three freeze–thaw cycle stability (Table 5). Therefore, the 13 ginsenosides in human plasma samples had no stability issues during the storage in the freezer, sample preparation process, and analysis time after the samples were processed, as demonstrated by the three stability tests.

Table 5. Stability of 13 ginsenosides.

Analyte	Short-Term Stability (6 h, 25 °C)				Analyte	Short-Term Stability (6 h, 25 °C)			
	QC (ng/mL)	Measured (ng/mL)	CV (%)	RE (%)		QC (ng/mL)	Measured (ng/mL)	CV (%)	RE (%)
Rb1	1.5	1.6	5.3	3.9	Rg3	1.5	1.4	13.5	−7.9
	15	13.5	3.3	−9.9		15	13.7	4.7	−8.7
	150	137.0	6.8	−8.7		150	133.7	4.2	−10.8
Rb2	1.5	1.5	1.6	−2.9	F1	1.5	1.5	2.3	−2.9
	15	13.3	4.7	−11.5		15	13.3	4.5	−11.1
	150	137.5	8.7	−8.3		150	138.9	6.4	−7.4
Rc	1.5	1.4	2.8	−4.3	Rh2	1.5	1.5	5.1	0.2
	15	13.4	3.4	−10.6		15	14.9	2.9	−0.8
	150	138.5	8.2	−7.6		150	149.7	4.3	−0.2
Rd	1.5	1.5	4.0	−3.5	CK	1.5	1.4	4.7	−6.5
	15	13.2	4.2	−12.2		15	13.4	1.5	−10.6
	150	139.7	8.0	−6.9		150	143.7	7.9	−4.2
Re	1.5	1.5	1.8	−1.3	PPD	1.5	1.6	5.0	5.4
	15	14.1	2.0	−5.8		15	15.3	2.2	2.0
	150	143.4	3.7	−4.4		150	146.2	5.6	−2.5
Rf	1.5	1.4	3.0	−7.6	PPT	1.5	1.5	3.0	1.0
	15	13.6	3.4	−9.1		15	15.0	2.0	−0.3
	150	150.3	9.2	0.2		150	146.0	5.0	−2.7
Rg1	1.5	1.5	5.6	2.0					
	15	14.0	3.1	−6.9					
	150	144.9	4.7	−3.4					

Analyte	Post-Preparative Stability (24 h, 8 °C)				Analyte	Post-Preparative Stability (24 h, 8 °C)			
	QC (ng/mL)	Measured (ng/mL)	CV (%)	RE (%)		QC (ng/mL)	Measured (ng/mL)	CV (%)	RE (%)
Rb1	1.5	1.5	14.9	−0.3	Rg3	1.5	1.4	9.7	−8.7
	15	13.9	5.3	−7.5		15	14.3	5.3	−4.5
	150	133.3	2.9	−11.1		150	131.2	3.1	−12.5
Rb2	1.5	1.4	10.1	−9.3	F1	1.5	1.3	4.9	−12.4
	15	13.6	7.7	−9.5		15	13.5	6.7	−10.1
	150	135.3	3.4	−9.8		150	134.9	1.8	−10.1
Rc	1.5	1.4	9.7	−5.5	Rh2	1.5	1.5	5.2	2.0
	15	13.6	6.1	−9.7		15	15.6	2.5	3.7
	150	135.4	2.8	−9.8		150	164.8	3.1	9.9
Rd	1.5	1.3	5.4	−11.3	CK	1.5	1.4	12.4	−5.9
	15	13.4	7.0	−10.7		15	13.7	4.9	−8.8
	150	136.2	3.0	−9.2		150	160.7	3.3	7.2
Re	1.5	1.5	5.1	−2.6	PPD	1.5	1.6	2.0	5.0
	15	14.2	4.8	−5.4		15	15.5	3.0	3.1
	150	141.7	0.6	−5.5		150	156.9	1.8	4.6
Rf	1.5	1.7	1.9	14.6	PPT	1.5	1.7	4.5	10.8
	15	14.8	2.7	−1.2		15	15.7	2.7	4.5
	150	154.2	7.3	2.8		150	158.2	2.7	5.5
Rg1	1.5	1.4	2.5	−4.0					
	15	14.2	9.7	−5.3					
	150	142.8	3.3	−4.8					

Table 5. Cont.

Analyte	Freeze-Thaw Stability (3 Cycles)				Analyte	Freeze-Thaw Stability (3 Cycles)			
	QC (ng/mL)	Measured (ng/mL)	CV (%)	RE (%)		QC (ng/mL)	Measured (ng/mL)	CV (%)	RE (%)
Rb1	1.5	1.5	2.3	−2.6	Rg3	1.5	1.6	2.7	9.2
	15	13.6	3.2	−9.5		15	13.6	1.4	−9.2
	150	143.6	5.4	−4.3		150	140.1	4.7	−6.6
Rb2	1.5	1.4	4.3	−4.7	F1	1.5	1.5	3.1	−0.7
	15	13.3	2.2	−11.1		15	13.4	1.4	−10.4
	150	145.2	5.4	−3.2		150	145.8	5.0	−2.8
Rc	1.5	1.5	1.7	−0.3	Rh2	1.5	1.5	4.0	0.4
	15	13.5	2.1	−10.3		15	15.6	4.7	3.7
	150	147.8	5.8	−1.5		150	152.3	2.1	1.5
Rd	1.5	1.4	2.0	−5.7	CK	1.5	1.5	7.8	−3.3
	15	13.1	2.3	−12.9		15	13.1	14.7	−12.4
	150	144.7	5.4	−3.6		150	167.3	4.7	11.5
Re	1.5	1.5	2.4	0.4	PPD	1.5	1.6	6.0	6.6
	15	13.9	2.4	−7.1		15	15.7	3.7	4.5
	150	144.5	5.8	−3.7		150	160.4	2.2	7.0
Rf	1.5	1.4	1.3	−5.5	PPT	1.5	1.4	5.6	−3.5
	15	14.0	2.9	−6.8		15	15.4	1.6	2.8
	150	156.8	7.7	4.5		150	158.7	1.7	5.8
Rg1	1.5	1.5	3.1	−2.5					
	15	14.1	4.6	−6.3					
	150	147.3	3.1	−1.8					

Data represented as mean ± SD from six independent experiments.

2.4. Contents of Ginsenosides in Red Ginseng Extract

The ginsenoside content of the red ginseng extract provided to participants daily for 14 days (three pouches of Hongsamjung All Day^{TM}/day) is summarized in Table 6. The most abundant ginsenoside was Rb1 (18.8–23.6 mg/day), followed by Rb2, Rc, Rd, and Rg3 (12.9–5.9 mg/day). The abundance of Re, Rh1, and Rg1 was 1.6–6.6 mg/day. The daily intake of PPT-type ginsenosides was lower than that of PPD-type ginsenosides. The values of daily intake of PPD-type ginsenosides are ranged between 50.2–64.7 mg/day and those of PPT-type ginsenoside are ranged between 11.2–14.9 mg/day.

Table 6. Daily intake amount of ginsenoside from red ginseng extract.

Ginsenoside		mg/day	Ginsenoside		mg/day
PPD-type	Rb1	21.9 ± 2.1	PPT-type	Re	6.6 ± 1.3
	Rb2	10.4 ± 1.2		Rg1	5.2 ± 0.6
	Rc	12.9 ± 1.5		F1	0.0 ± 0.0
	Rd	5.9 ± 0.7		PPT	0.0 ± 0.0
	Rh2	0.0 ± 0.0			
	Rg3	7.9 ± 2.3			
	CK	0.0 ± 0.0			
	PPD	0.0 ± 0.0			

Data represented as mean ± SD from four independent experiments.

The oral administration of three pouches of red ginseng for two weeks was well tolerated and did not produce any unexpected or serious adverse events, as previously reported [17].

2.5. Pharmacokinetics of Rb1, Rb2, Rc, Rd, Rg3, Rh2, CK, PPD, and PPT Following 2 Weeks-Repeated Administration of Red Ginseng Extract

Of the 13 ginsenosides examined, nine ginsenosides (Rb1, Rb2, Rc, Rd, Rg3, CK, Rh2, PPD, and PPT) were detected in the human plasma samples; the plasma concentrations of these ginsenosides are shown in Figure 3. The ginsenosides Rb1, Rb2, Rc, Rd, and Rg3, which were detected in the plasma samples, are all PPD-type ginsenosides and present at a relatively high content in red ginseng extract. In contrast, the PPT-type ginsenosides Re and Rh1 were not detected in the human plasma samples despite their high content in red ginseng extract. CK, Rh2, and PPD, which are metabolites from Rb1, Rb2, and Rc, were also detected even though they are not present in red ginseng extract, suggesting that these PPD-type metabolites could be formed in the human intestine during the intestinal absorption stage (Figure 1) [11,23,24]. Among the reported PPT-type metabolites, only PPT was detected in the human plasma.

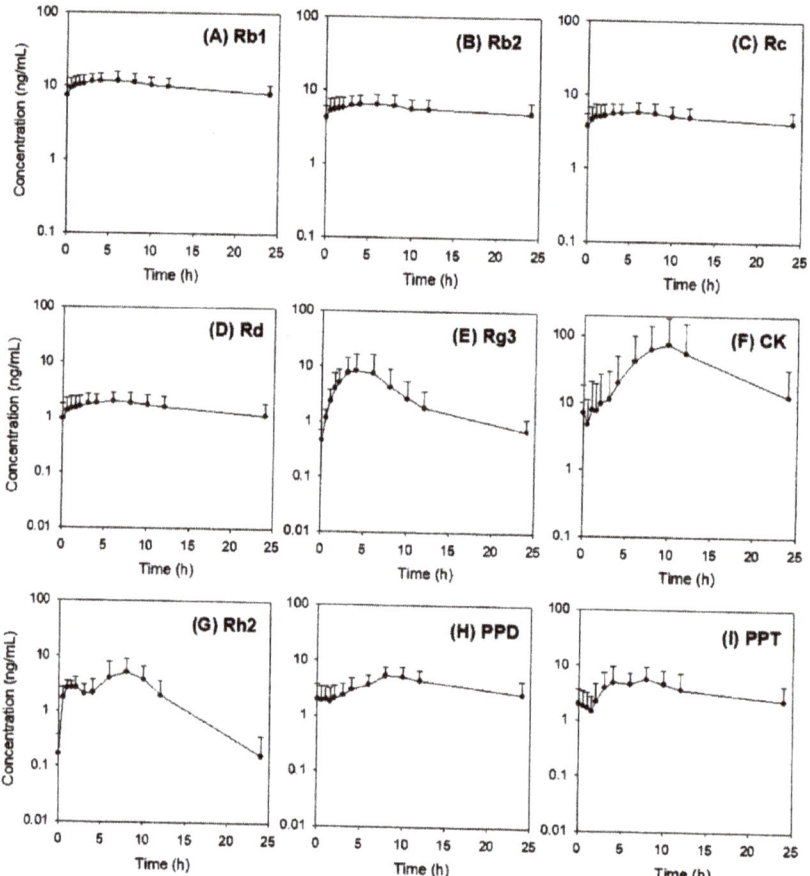

Figure 3. Plasma concentration-time profiles of ginsenosides (**A**) Rb1, (**B**) Rb2, (**C**) Rc, (**D**) Rd, (**E**) Rg3, (**F**) CK, (**G**) Rh2, (**H**) PPD, and (**I**) PPT in human plasma after two-weeks repeated administrations of red ginseng extract. Data represented as mean ± SD from eleven subjects.

The pharmacokinetic parameters from the plasma concentration-time profiles of these ginsenosides are shown in Table 7. The plasma Rb1, Rb2, Rc, and Rd concentrations were constant over time, and they had a long terminal half-life. The AUC and C_{max} values of Rb1, Rb2, Rc, and Rd were correlated with the content of red ginseng extract. In contrast to the plasma concentrations of Rb1, Rb2, Rc, and Rd, the plasma concentrations of Rg3, Rh2, and CK showed a bell-shaped profile (Figure 3); this may be attributed to further metabolism to PPD. The T_{max} of Rg3 (3.6 h) was smaller than that of Rh2 and CK (5.6–9.1 h), which may be associated with the high content of Rg3 that the absorption of Rg3 could occur following oral administration of red ginseng extract and absence of Rh2 and CK in the red ginseng extract that the absorption of Rh1 and CK could occur after they were transformed from Rb1, Rb2, Rc, and Rd.

Table 7. Pharmacokinetic parameters of ginsenosides in human plasma after two-weeks repeated administrations of red ginseng extract.

Ginsenosides	PK Parameters				
	AUC (ng·h/mL)	C_{max} (ng/mL)	T_{max} (h)	MRT (h)	$T_{1/2}$ (h)
Rb1	227.6 ± 73.5	12.7 ± 3.6	4.5 ± 1.8	10.7 ± 1.5	42.9 ± 20.8
Rb2	137.0 ± 48.8	6.9 ± 2.3	4.5 ± 2.3	11.8 ± 1.5	51.2 ± 22.8
Rc	123.0 ± 46.1	6.2 ± 2.1	4.3 ± 3.2	11.7 ± 1.5	34.5 ± 12.9
Rd	35.1 ± 19.5	2.2 ± 0.9	6.2 ± 2.1	10.4 ± 1.5	24.6 ± 8.0
Re	ND	ND	ND	ND	ND
Rf	ND	ND	ND	ND	ND
Rg1	ND	ND	ND	ND	ND
Rg3	68.0 ± 60.5	8.7 ± 8.9	3.6 ± 0.9	8.2 ± 1.4	9.4 ± 3.9
F1	ND	ND	ND	ND	ND
Rh2	49.9 ± 27.8	6.1 ± 3.5	6.0 ± 3.3	7.7 ± 1.5	3.1 ± 1.3
CK	873.0 ± 1236.0	81.6 ± 112.5	9.5 ± 1.6	10.6 ± 1.2	5.2 ± 1.1
PPD	85.1 ± 39.5	6.1 ± 2.3	8.7 ± 1.6	11.3 ± 1.9	12.6 ± 8.2
PPT	86.5 ± 49.8	7.9 ± 4.6	8.3 ± 6.2	11.2 ± 3.0	10.6 ± 8.4

AUC: area under the plasma concentration-time curve from 0 to last sampling time. C_{max}: maximum plasma concentration; T_{max}: time to reach C_{max}; MRT: mean residence time. $T_{1/2}$: half-life; ND: not detected. Data represented as mean ± SD from eleven subjects

The plasma concentration profiles of PPD and PPT were similar but flatter compared with those of Rg3, Rh2, and CK. Since PPD was derived from Rg3, Rh2, and CK and could undergo further metabolism [11,23,24], the plasma profile of PPD and PPT could be attributed to the faster elimination in human body rather than intestinal formation via intestinal microbiota. Lin et al. reported that 40 metabolites of PPD were identified in human plasma and urine and the major metabolites of PPD was the hydroxylated form in human body through phase I hepatic metabolism [19].

To explain time-dependent metabolism and absorption of ginsenosides, the plasma concentrations of ginsenosides at absorption phase (from 4 to 10 h) depend on the deglycosylation states was shown in Figure 4. The plasma concentrations of Rb1, Rb2, Rc, and Rd, tri- and tetraglycosylated ginsenosides, were stable for 4–10 h of post dose (Figure 4A), suggesting the stable absorption and slow elimination process. The plasma concentrations of Rg3 was decreased along with increasing time (4–10 h) but the monoglycosylated ginsenosides Rh2 and CK, metabolites from Rg3 and F2, increased over time (Figure 4B,C), suggesting the gut metabolism from Rg3 to Rh2 during the absorption stage. The delayed absorption of Rh2, CK, and PPD indicated that formation and absorption of Rh2, CK, and PPD might occur in the lower part of intestine. On the other hand, the formation and absorption of PPT was faster than PPD (Figure 4D), suggesting the rapid metabolism of PPT-type ginsenosides in human intestine and it partly attributed to the absence of Re and Rg1 in human plasma despite of the higher content in Korean red ginseng extract.

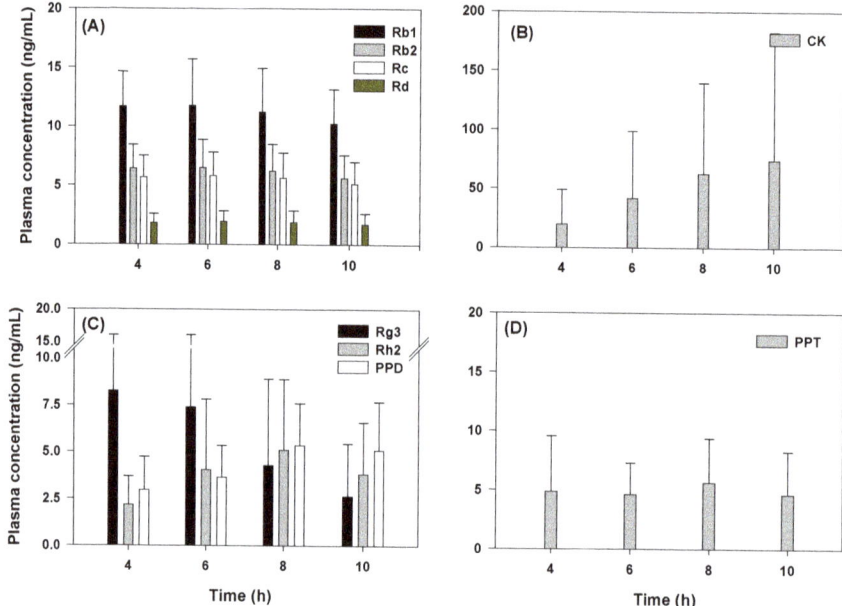

Figure 4. Plasma concentration of ginsenosides (**A**) Rb1, Rb2, Rc, and Rd, (**B**) CK, (**C**) Rg3, Rh2, and PPD, and (**D**) PPT at 4, 6, 8, and 10 h after two-weeks repeated administrations of red ginseng extract. Data represented as mean ± SD from eleven subjects.

3. Discussion

Despite the therapeutic benefits of various ginsenosides, which include anti-cancer, anti-diabetic, anti-oxidative, and immune-stimulating effects [3–8], the plasma concentration of these ginsenosides and their pharmacokinetic-pharmacodynamic relationship need to be further investigated. As its first step, analytical methods for various ginsenosides and pharmacokinetic profile of these ginsenosides are critical. We developed an analytical method for 13 ginsenosides (Rb1, Rb2, Rc, Rd, Re, Rf, Rg1, Rg3, and F1, Rh2, CK, PPD, and PPT) using a LC-MS/MS system, which had high sensitivity (i.e., the LLOQ of all ginsenosides was 0.5 ng/mL) and required a small plasma sample volume (100 μL). The glycosylation number of the ginsenosides was different: tetraglycosylated ginsenosides for Rb1, Rb2, and Rc; triglycosylated ginsenosides for Rd, Re, and Rg1; diglycosylated ginsenosides for F2, Rg3, and Rf; monoglycosylated ginsenosides for Rh2, CK, Rh1, and F1; aglycones for PPD and PPT (Figure 1). Because of different extraction efficiencies, di-, tri-, and tetraglycosylated ginsenosides were extracted by protein precipitation, and aglycones were extracted by LLE. Monoglycosylated ginsenosides could be extracted using both methods; however, CK and Rh2 were extracted by LLE, and F1 was extracted by protein precipitation based on the extraction recovery and matrix effect.

We further validated our sensitive analytical method by performing a pharmacokinetic study after the oral administration of red ginseng extract (three pouches of red ginseng extract), which has demonstrated tolerability for two weeks of repeated administration [17]. We successfully measured the plasma concentration of Rb1, Rb2, Rc, Rd, Rg3, Rh2, CK, PPD, and PPT. Except for PPT, detectable ginsenosides were all PPD-type ginsenosides and their deglycosylated metabolites. Interestingly, the plasma AUC values of three glycosylated ginsenosides (Rb1, Rb2, and Rc) were correlated with the content of red ginseng extract and showed similar T_{max} values, suggesting the similar intestinal absorption kinetics of these ginsenosides despite of the different structures and glycosidation patterns, which is consistent with the previous report [17]. The long terminal half-life suggested that the intestinal metabolism (to other PPD-type metabolites) and excretion of Rb1, Rb2, and Rc may be a slow process. The T_{max} values of Rd, Rh2, CK, and PPD were increased according to the deglycosylated status, suggesting that deglycosylation mediated by β-glucosidase in the intestinal microbiome could occur sequentially and steadily [11,23,24], and Rh2, CK, and PPD could be detected in human plasma even though they are not present in red ginseng extract.

In the case of Rg3, its T_{max} was smaller compared with that of Rh2 and CK because of its high content in red ginseng extract. Re and Rg1 (PPT-type ginsenosides) were not detected even though they are present in red ginseng extract; however, PPT was detected. It is possible that Re and Rg1 are metabolized to PPT by intestinal microbiota before the absorption occur [11,23,24] and biotransformation of PPT could be faster than the formation rate of PPD. However, we should note that the time-dependent gut metabolism of ginsenosides in human intestine has never been investigated, therefore we speculated time-dependent gut metabolism of ginsenoside from the plasma concentration and T_{max} of ginsenosides and their deglycosylated metabolites. Particularly, for CK concentration, large inter-subject variation was shown in Figure 4B and previous publication [17]. This variability could be attributed to inter-subject variable metabolism related to the intestinal microbiota [25] and further studies should focus on the characterization of microorganisms that produce it and the potential beneficial effects of this metabolite.

4. Materials and Methods

4.1. Materials

Red ginseng extract (Hongsamjung All Day™; lot no. 731902) was purchased from the Punggi Ginseng Cooperative Association (Youngjoo, Kyungpook, Republic of Korea). The ginsenosides Rb1, Rb2, Rc, Rd, Re, Rf, Rg1, Rg3, Rh1, Rh2, F1, F2, CK, PPD, and PPT were purchased from the Ambo Institute (Daejeon, Republic of Korea). Berberine and 13C-caffeine, used as internal standards (IS), were purchased from Sigma-Aldrich Chemical Co. (St. Louis, MO, USA). All other chemicals and solvents were of reagent or analytical grade.

4.2. LC-MS/MS Analysis

4.2.1. Instrument

The LC-MS/MS system consisted of an Agilent 1260 Infinity HPLC system (Agilent Technologies, Wilmington, DE, USA) and Agilent 6470 Triple Quadrupole MS system (Agilent Technologies, Wilmington, DE, USA). The system was operated using Mass Hunter Acquisition Software (Version B.08.00; Agilent Technologies, Wilmington, DE, USA). The pressure of drying gas was set at 35 psi and the gas temperature was kept at 300 °C. The ion spray voltage was set at 4000 V in the positive mode.

4.2.2. HPLC Condition

Chromatographic separation was performed using a Phenomenex Polar RP analytical column (150 × 2.0 mm i.d., 4.0 μm particle size) for protein precipitation samples and a Phenomenex Luna C18 analytical column (150 × 2.0 mm i.d., 3.0 μm particle size) for liquid–liquid extraction (LLE) samples. The HPLC mobile phase for protein precipitation samples consisted of 0.1% formic acid in water (phase A) and 0.1% formic acid in methanol (phase B), and the following gradient elution was used: 69% of phase B for 0–2.0 min, 69–85% of phase B for 2.0–4.0 min, 85–69% of phase B for 6.0–6.5 min. The flow rate was 0.27 mL/min, and the injection sample volume was 10 μL. The HPLC mobile phase for LLE samples was isocratic, consisting of 0.1% formic acid in water (8%) and 0.1% formic acid in methanol (92%) at a flow rate of 0.15 mL/min. The sample injection volume was 10 μL.

4.2.3. Preparation of Stock, Working, and Quality Control (QC) Solutions

Ginsenosides and their metabolites (Rb1, Rb2, Rc, Rd, Re, Rf, Rg1, Rg3, Rh2, F1, CK, PPD, and PPT) were accurately weighed and dissolved in methanol to obtain a concentration of 1000 μg/mL each.

The above stock solutions were divided and mixed according to the sample preparation method (i.e., protein precipitation and LLE). The ginsenosides for protein precipitation method (Rb1, Rb2, Rc, Rd, Re, Rf, Rg1, Rg3, and F1) were mixed and diluted with methanol to a concentration of 2000 ng/mL. The ginsenosides for LLE (Rh2, CK, PPD, and PPT) were mixed and diluted with methanol to a concentration of 2000 ng/mL. Working solutions were then serially diluted with methanol to obtain calibration working solutions of 5, 10, 20, 50, 200, 500, 1000, and 2000 ng/mL. Quality control (QC) working solutions were prepared at 15, 150, and 1500 ng/mL with each ginsenoside.

4.2.4. Preparation of Calibration Curve and QC Samples

Calibration curve samples were prepared by spiking 10 μL of working solution into 90 μL of human blank plasma at final concentrations of 0.5, 1, 2, 5, 20, 50, 100, and 200 ng/mL. QC samples were prepared by spiking 10 μL of QC working solution into 90 μL of human blank plasma at final concentrations of 1.5, 15, and 150 ng/mL of QC samples.

For protein precipitation, 600 μL of an IS (0.05 ng/mL berberine in methanol) was added to 100 μL of calibration curve samples and QC samples. Then, the mixture was vortexed for 15 min and centrifuged at 16,100× g for 5 min. After centrifugation, 500 μL of the supernatant was transferred to a clean tube and evaporated to dryness under a nitrogen stream at 40 °C. The residue was reconstituted with 150 μL of 70% methanol consisting of 0.1% formic acid.

For LLE, 50 μL of an IS (20 ng/mL 13C-caffeine in water) and 800 μL of MTBE was added to 100 μL of calibration curve samples and QC samples. The mixture was vortexed for 10 min and centrifuged at 16,100× g for 5 min. After centrifugation, the samples were frozen at −80 °C for 4 h. The upper layer was transferred to a clean tube and evaporated to dryness under a nitrogen stream. The residue was reconfigured with 150 μL of 80% methanol consisting of 0.1% formic acid.

4.3. Method Validation

4.3.1. Specificity

The specificity of the method was assessed by comparing chromatogram responses of six lots of human blank plasma with lower limit of quantification (LLOQ) sample.

4.3.2. Linearity

The linearity of the method was assessed using six calibration curves analyzed on six different days. The calibration curve was obtained by plotting the peak area ratio against the concentration of each drug at eight-point levels with a weighting factor of $1/x^2$.

4.3.3. Precision and Accuracy

The intra-day ($n = 5$) and inter-day ($n = 6$) precision and accuracy were evaluated using three different QC samples for each analyte. The precision and accuracy at each concentration level were evaluated in terms of the coefficient of variance (CV, %) and relative error (RE, %).

4.3.4. Extraction Recovery and Matrix Effect

The extraction recovery and matrix effect were assessed for three different QC samples using six different blank plasma samples. The extraction recoveries were evaluated by comparing the peak areas of the extracted samples (spiked before extraction) with those of the unextracted samples (spiked after blank extraction) [26]. The matrix factor for the analyte and IS was calculated in each lot by comparing the peak responses of the post-extraction samples (spiked after blank extraction) against neat solutions, which have the same amount of analyte as the extracted sample [26].

4.3.5. Stability

Short-term stability was evaluated to determine whether the sample was stable during treatment. All analytes and IS of the spiked plasma samples were left for at least 6 h at 25 °C. The spiked plasma samples were also subjected to a freeze (−80 °C) and thaw cycle (25 °C and stand for 2 h) three times. After the samples were processed, it was confirmed that they were stable at 8 °C for 24 h. The stability test was conducted using three different concentrations of QC samples.

4.4. Pharmacokinetic Study

The study was approved by the Institutional Review Board of Kyungpook National University Hospital (KNUH, Daegu, Republic of Korea) and was conducted at the KNUH Clinical Trial Center in accordance with the applicable Good Clinical Practice guidelines (IRB approval no. KNUH 2018-04-028-002). All subjects provided written informed consent before study enrollment and underwent clinical evaluation including physical examination, serology tests, 12-lead electrocardiography, and clinical history assessment. A total of 11 healthy Korean male subjects aged ≥ 19 years and with a body weight of ≥ 50 kg were enrolled in this study.

The volunteers took 3 pouches of red ginseng extract per day at 9 AM for 2 weeks. On the 14th day, after taking the last dose of the red ginseng extract, blood samples (5 mL) were collected in a heparinized tube at 0.25, 0.5, 1, 2, 3, 4, 6, 8, 10, 12, and 24 h post-dose via a saline-locked angiocatheter. The plasma was collected by centrifugation for 10 min at 3000 × g and stored at −80 °C until analysis.

To analyze the ginsenosides Rb1, Rb2, Rc, Rd, Re, Rf, Rg1, Rg3, and F1, 600 µL of an IS (0.05 ng/mL berberine in methanol) was added to 100 µL of plasma samples. Then, the mixture was vortexed for 15 min and centrifuged at 16,100× g for 5 min. After centrifugation, 500 µL of the supernatant was transferred to a clean tube and evaporated to dryness under a nitrogen stream at 40 °C. The residue was reconstituted with 150 µL of 70% methanol consisting of 0.1% formic acid, and a 10 µL aliquot was injected into the LC-MS/MS system.

To analyze the ginsenosides Rh2, CK, PPD, and PPT, 50 µL of an IS (20 ng/mL 13C-caffeine in water) and 800 µL of MTBE were added to 100 µL of plasma samples. The mixture was vortexed for 10 min and centrifuged at 16,100× g for 5 min. After centrifugation, the samples were frozen at −80 °C for 4 h. The upper layer was transferred to a clean tube and evaporated to dryness under a nitrogen stream. The residue was reconfigured with 150 µL of 80% methanol consisting of 0.1% formic acid, and a 10 µL aliquot was injected into the LC-MS/MS system.

Similarly, the ginsenoside content in the red ginseng extract was quantified. The red ginseng extract (100 mg) was diluted 50-fold with methanol, and 100 µL of the diluted sample was prepared using the method described previously. Aliquots (10 µL) of the supernatant were directly injected into the LC-MS/MS system.

4.5. Data Analysis

Pharmacokinetic parameters were estimated using non-compartmental methods (WinNonlin version 2.0; Pharsight Co., Certara, NJ, USA). All pharmacokinetic parameters are presented as the mean ± standard deviation (SD).

5. Conclusions

A sensitive LC–MS/MS method for the detection of 13 ginsenosides (Rb1, Rb2, Rc, Rd, Re, Rf, Rg1, Rg3, and F1, Rh2, CK, PPD, and PPT) in human plasma with a LLOQ of 0.5 ng/mL was developed and validated. This method can be used in the bioanalysis and pharmacokinetic studies of ginseng products administered at multiple therapeutic doses. Following repeated oral administration of red ginseng extract for two weeks, the plasma concentrations of Rb1, Rb2, Rc, Rd, Rg3, Rh2, CK, PPD, and PPT were detected. The findings can provide valuable information on ginsenoside metabolism in the human body and contribute to in vivo pharmacokinetic-pharmacodynamic correlation studies.

Author Contributions: Conceptualization, M.-K.C. and I.-S.S.; methodology and validation, S.J., M.-K.C., and I.-S.S.; investigation, S.J., J.-H.J., S.L., W.Y.K., S.J.S., Y.-R.Y., M.-K.C., and I.-S.S.; resources, W.Y.K., S.J.S., Y.-R.Y.; writing—original draft preparation, S.J. and I.-S.S.; supervision, M.-K.C. and I.-S.S.; writing—review and editing, M.-K.C. and I.-S.S.; funding acquisition, I.-S.S.

Funding: This work was supported by the Korea Institute of Planning and Evaluation for Technology in Food, Agriculture, Forestry and Fisheries (IPET) through Export Promotion Technology Development Program, funded by Ministry of Agriculture, Food and Rural Affairs (MAFRA) [No 316017-3], Republic of Korea.

Conflicts of Interest: The authors declare no conflict of interest.

References

1. Won, H.J.; Kim, H.I.; Park, T.; Kim, H.; Jo, K.; Jeon, H.; Ha, S.J.; Hyun, J.M.; Jung, A.; Kim, J.S.; et al. Non-clinical pharmacokinetic behavior of ginsenosides. *J. Ginseng Res.* **2018**, *43*, 354–360. [CrossRef] [PubMed]
2. Ru, W.; Wang, D.; Xu, Y.; He, X.; Sun, Y.E.; Qian, L.; Zhou, X.; Qin, Y. Chemical constituents and bioactivities of Panax ginseng (C. A. Mey.). *Drug Dis. Ther.* **2015**, *9*, 23–32. [CrossRef] [PubMed]
3. Kim, J.H.; Yi, Y.S.; Kim, M.Y.; Cho, J.Y. Role of ginsenosides, the main active components of Panax ginseng, in inflammatory responses and diseases. *J. Ginseng Res.* **2017**, *41*, 435–443. [CrossRef] [PubMed]
4. Choi, K.T. Botanical characteristics, pharmacological effects and medicinal components of Korean Panax ginseng C A Meyer. *Acta Pharmacol. Sin.* **2008**, *29*, 1109–1118. [CrossRef] [PubMed]
5. Yun, T.K.; Choi, S.Y.; Yun, H.Y. Epidemiological study on cancer prevention by ginseng: Are all kinds of cancers preventable by ginseng? *J. Korean Med. Sci.* **2001**, *16*, S19–S27. [CrossRef]
6. Gui, Q.F.; Xu, Z.R.; Xu, K.Y.; Yang, Y.M. The efficacy of ginseng-related therapies in type 2 Diabetes mellitus: An updated systematic review and meta-analysis. *Medicine (Baltimore)* **2016**, *95*, e2584. [CrossRef]
7. Park, T.Y.; Hong, M.; Sung, H.; Kim, S.; Suk, K.T. Effect of Korean Red Ginseng in chronic liver disease. *J. Ginseng Res.* **2017**, *41*, 450–455. [CrossRef]
8. Lee, S.; Kwon, M.; Choi, M.K.; Song, I.S. Effects of red ginseng extract on the pharmacokinetics and elimination of methotrexate via Mrp2 regulation. *Molecules* **2018**, *23*. [CrossRef]
9. Seong, S.J.; Kang, W.Y.; Heo, J.K.; Jo, J.; Choi, W.G.; Liu, K.H.; Lee, S.; Choi, M.K.; Han, Y.H.; Lee, H.S.; et al. A comprehensive in vivo and in vitro assessment of the drug interaction potential of red ginseng. *Clin. Ther.* **2018**, *40*, 1322–1337. [CrossRef]
10. Lee, S.M.; Bae, B.S.; Park, H.W.; Ahn, N.G.; Cho, B.G.; Cho, Y.L.; Kwak, Y.S. Characterization of Korean Red Ginseng (Panax ginseng Meyer): History, preparation method, and chemical composition. *J. Ginseng Res.* **2015**, *39*, 384–391. [CrossRef]
11. Jin, S.; Lee, S.; Jeon, J.H.; Kim, H.; Choi, M.K.; Song, I.S. Enhanced Intestinal permeability and plasma concentration of metformin in rats by the repeated administration of Red Ginseng extract. *Pharmaceutics* **2019**, *11*. [CrossRef] [PubMed]
12. Liu, L.; Huang, J.; Hu, X.; Li, K.; Sun, C. Simultaneous determination of ginsenoside (G-Re, G-Rg1, G-Rg2, G-F1, G-Rh1) and protopanaxatriol in human plasma and urine by LC-MS/MS and its application in a pharmacokinetics study of G-Re in volunteers. *J. Chromatogr. B Analyt. Technol. Biomed. Life Sci.* **2011**, *879*, 2011–2017. [CrossRef] [PubMed]
13. Wang, C.Z.; Kim, K.E.; Du, G.J.; Qi, L.W.; Wen, X.D.; Li, P.; Bauer, B.A.; Bissonnette, M.B.; Musch, M.W.; Chang, E.B.; et al. Ultra-performance liquid chromatography and time-of-flight mass spectrometry analysis of ginsenoside metabolites in human plasma. *Am. J. Chin. Med.* **2011**, *39*, 1161–1171. [CrossRef] [PubMed]
14. Ji, H.Y.; Lee, H.W.; Kim, H.K.; Kim, H.H.; Chang, S.G.; Sohn, D.H.; Kim, J.; Lee, H.S. Simultaneous determination of ginsenoside Rb1 and Rg1 in human plasma by liquid chromatography–mass spectrometry. *J. Pharm. Biomed. Anal.* **2004**, *35*, 207–212. [CrossRef] [PubMed]
15. Choi, I.D.; Ryu, J.H.; Lee, D.E.; Lee, M.H.; Shim, J.J.; Ahn, Y.T.; Sim, J.H.; Huh, C.S.; Shim, W.S.; Yim, S.V.; et al. Enhanced absorption study of ginsenoside compound K (20-O-beta-(D-Glucopyranosyl)-20(S)-protopanaxadiol) after oral administration of fermented red ginseng extract (HYFRG) in healthy Korean volunteers and rats. *Evid. Based Complement. Alternat. Med.* **2016**, *2016*, 3908142. [CrossRef] [PubMed]
16. Zhang, D.; Wang, Y.; Han, J.; Yu, W.; Deng, L.; Fawcett, J.P.; Liu, Z.; Gu, J. Rapid and sensitive LC-MS/MS assay for the quantitation of 20(S)-protopanaxadiol in human plasma. *J. Chromatogr. B Analyt. Technol. Biomed. Life Sci.* **2009**, *877*, 581–585. [CrossRef] [PubMed]

17. Choi, M.K.; Jin, S.J.; Jeon, J.H.; Kang, W.Y.; Seong, S.J.; Yoon, Y.R.; Han, Y.H.; Song, I.S. Tolerability and pharmacokinetics of ginsenosides Rb1, Rb2, Rc, Rd, and compound K after single or multiple administration of red ginseng extract in human beings. *J. Ginseng Res.* **2018**. [CrossRef]
18. Liu, H.; Yang, J.; Du, F.; Gao, X.; Ma, X.; Huang, Y.; Xu, F.; Niu, W.; Wang, F.; Mao, Y.; et al. Absorption and disposition of ginsenosides after oral administration of Panax notoginseng extract to rats. *Drug Metab. Dispos.* **2009**, *37*, 2290–2298. [CrossRef] [PubMed]
19. Ling, J.; Yu, Y.; Long, J.; Li, Y.; Jiang, J.; Wang, L.; Xu, C.; Duan, G. Tentative identification of 20(S)-protopanaxadiol metabolites in human plasma and urine using ultra-performance liquid chromatography coupled with triple quadrupole time-of-flight mass spectrometry. *J. Ginseng Res.* **2018**. [CrossRef]
20. Kadian, N.; Raju, K.S.; Rashid, M.; Malik, M.Y.; Taneja, I.; Wahajuddin, M. Comparative assessment of bioanalytical method validation guidelines for pharmaceutical industry. *J. Pharm. Biomed. Anal.* **2016**, *126*, 83–97. [CrossRef]
21. FDA. FDA guidance for industry: Bioanalytical method validation. 2018. Available online: https://www.gmp-compliance.org/guidelines/gmp-guideline/fda-guidance-for-industry-bioanalytical-method-validation (accessed on 17 July 2019).
22. EMA. EMA Guideline on bioanalytical method validation. 2011. Available online: https://www.therqa.com/forum/good-laboratory-practice-discussion-forum/thread/3049/ (accessed on 17 July 2019).
23. Park, S.E.; Na, C.S.; Yoo, S.A.; Seo, S.H.; Son, H.S. Biotransformation of major ginsenosides in ginsenoside model culture by lactic acid bacteria. *J. Ginseng Res.* **2017**, *41*, 36–42. [CrossRef] [PubMed]
24. Yang, X.D.; Yang, Y.Y.; Ouyang, D.S.; Yang, G.P. A review of biotransformation and pharmacology of ginsenoside compound K. *Fitoterapia* **2015**, *100*, 208–220. [CrossRef] [PubMed]
25. Kim, D.H. Gut microbiota-mediated pharmacokinetics of ginseng saponins. *J. Ginseng. Res.* **2018**, *42*, 255–263. [CrossRef] [PubMed]
26. Matuszewski, B.K.; Constanzer, M.L.; Chavez-Eng, C.M. Strategies for the assessment of matrix effect in quantitative bioanalytical methods based on HPLC-MS/MS. *Anal. Chem.* **2003**, *75*, 3019–3030. [CrossRef] [PubMed]

Sample Availability: Samples of the ginsenoside Rc and Rg3 are available from the authors.

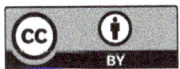

© 2019 by the authors. Licensee MDPI, Basel, Switzerland. This article is an open access article distributed under the terms and conditions of the Creative Commons Attribution (CC BY) license (http://creativecommons.org/licenses/by/4.0/).

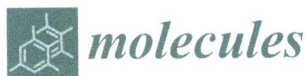

Article

Simultaneous Quantification of Four Phenylethanoid Glycosides in Rat Plasma by UPLC-MS/MS and Its Application to a Pharmacokinetic Study of Acanthus Ilicifolius Herb

Mengqi Zhang [1,2,†], Xia Ren [1,2,†], Shijun Yue [1,2], Qing Zhao [1,2], Changlun Shao [1,2,*] and Changyun Wang [1,2,*]

1   Key Laboratory of Marine Drugs, The Ministry of Education of China, School of Medicine and Pharmacy, Ocean University of China, Qingdao 266003, China
2   Laboratory for Marine Drugs and Bioproducts, Qingdao National Laboratory for Marine Science and Technology, Qingdao 266237, China
*   Correspondence: shaochanglun@ouc.edu.cn (C.S.); changyun@ouc.edu.cn (C.W.);
    Tel.: +86-532-8203-1381 (C.S.); +86-532-8203-1536 (C.W.); Fax: +86-532-8203-1536 (C.S. & C.W.)
†   Contributed equally.

Academic Editors: In-Soo Yoon and Hyun-Jong Cho
Received: 29 June 2019; Accepted: 19 August 2019; Published: 28 August 2019

Abstract: Acanthus ilicifolius herb (AIH), the dry plant of *Acanthus ilicifolius* L., has long been used as a folk medicine for treating acute and chronic hepatitis. Phenylethanoid glycosides (PhGs) are one family of the main components in AIH with hepatoprotective, antioxidant, and anti-inflammatory activities. In this study, the pharmacokinetics of AIH was investigated preliminarily by ultra-performance liquid chromatography coupled with triple quadrupole mass spectrometry (UPLC-MS/MS). A simultaneously quantitative determination method for four PhGs (acteoside, isoacteoside, martynoside, and crenatoside) in rat plasma was first established by UPLC-MS/MS. These four PhGs were separated with an ACQUITY UPLC BEH C_{18} column (2.1 × 50 mm, 1.7 μm) by gradient elution (mobile phase: MeCN and 0.1% formic acid in water, 0.4 mL/min). The mass spectrometry detection was performed using negative electrospray ionization (ESI^-) in multiple reaction monitoring (MRM) mode. By the established method, the preliminary pharmacokinetics of AIH was elucidated using the kinetic parameters of the four PhGs in rat plasma after intragastric administration of AIH ethanol extract. All four PhGs showed double peaks on concentration-time curves, approximately at 0.5 h and 6 h, respectively. Their elimination half-lives ($t_{1/2}$) were different, ranging from 3.42 h to 8.99 h, although they shared similar molecular structures. This work may provide a basis for the elucidation of the pharmacokinetic characteristics of bioactive components from AIH.

Keywords: acanthus ilicifolius herb; phenylethanoid glycosides; pharmacokinetics; UPLC-MS/MS

1. Introduction

Acanthus ilicifolius L. is a mangrove shrub belonging to the *Acanthus* genus in the Acanthaceae family which grows in tropical and subtropical intertidal habitats. Acanthus ilicifolius herb (AIH, "laoshule" in Chinese), the dry plant of *A. ilicifolius* L., is a folk medicine to treat acute and chronic hepatitis, lymphatic intumescence, spleen enlargement, paralysis, and rheumatism [1–6]. Modern pharmaceutical studies have demonstrated that the extracts of AIH possess hepatoprotective, antioxidant, anti-inflammatory, anticarcinogenic, and antibacterial activities [6–10]. Numerous chemical constituents have been isolated from AIH, including phenylethanoid glycosides (PhGs), alkaloids, flavones, lignans, triterpenoid saponins, and sterols [11–17]. Among them, PhGs were reported as one family of the main components from AIH, such as acteoside, isoacteoside, martynoside, and crenatoside with potential pharmacological effects [18–23]. The pharmacologic actions of AIH extracts, as well as these four PhGs, have been reported, whereas no pharmacokinetics have been studied till now.

During our ongoing research of pharmacodynamic material basis of medical plants, we found that AIH and its efficient components, PhGs, exhibited potent hepatoprotective, antiviral, and antioxidant activities. Specifically, PhGs were found to be abundant in AIH, of which acteoside and isoacteoside were the main components, while martynoside and crenatoside were in relatively lower contents. In the present study, the pharmacokinetics of AIH were investigated with these four PhGs as representatives in rat plasma after intragastric administration of AIH extract. To achieve this purpose, a simple, sensitive and rapid ultra-performance liquid chromatography coupled with triple quadrupole mass spectrometry (UPLC-MS/MS) method was established, first, for the simultaneous and quantitative determination of the four PhGs in rat plasma. Herein, we report the establishment and optimization of UPLC-MS/MS method, the validation of the established method, and the pharmacokinetic study of AIH.

2. Results and Discussion

2.1. Establishment and Optimization of the UPLC-MS/MS Method

The UPLC-MS/MS method was established and optimized to determine the four PhGs (acteoside, isoacteoside, martynoside, and crenatoside) simultaneously and quantitatively. In preliminary experiments, the two isomer analytes, acteoside and isoacteoside, were found to have the same MS fragmentation characteristics. Therefore, it was required to separate these two analytes from each other by UPLC because of their influence on each other. In our study, different mobile phase compositions were screened, including methanol and water, methanol and 0.1% formic acid in water, MeCN and water, MeCN and 0.1% formic acid in water, and MeCN and 0.5% formic acid in water. It was found that the mobile phase consisting of MeCN and 0.1% formic acid in water significantly improved the peak shapes and achieved the baseline separation of acteoside and isoacteoside (Figure 1). Moreover, in comparison with isocratic elution, the gradient elution with MeCN and 0.1% formic acid shortened analysis duration and increased separation efficiency.

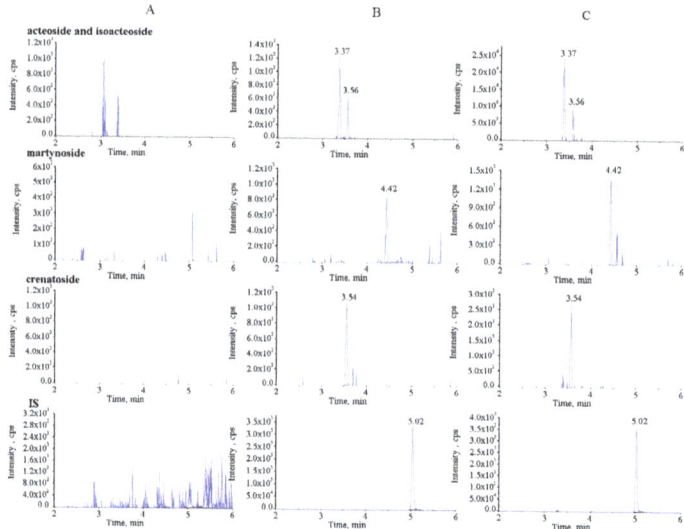

Figure 1. The multiple reaction monitoring (MRM) chromatograms for the four phenylethanoid glycosides (PhGs) and genistein (IS) in (**A**) blank plasma, (**B**) blank plasma spiked with the four PhGs at the lowest limit of quantification (LLOQ) and IS (1000 ng/mL), and (**C**) test plasma collected at 30 min after intragastric administration.

The mass conditions were modified to find the optimum precursor-to-product ion pairs for MRM detection by the production scan procedure. Both positive and negative ionization ESI modes were tested for the four PhGs and genistein (IS). It was observed that the negative mode (ESI⁻) of the four PhGs achieved better sensitivity as compared with the positive mode. Among them, acteoside, isoacteoside, and crenatoside displayed the same characteristic MS fragments of m/z 161.02 in the mass spectra due to their similar molecular structures (Figure 2 and Table 1).

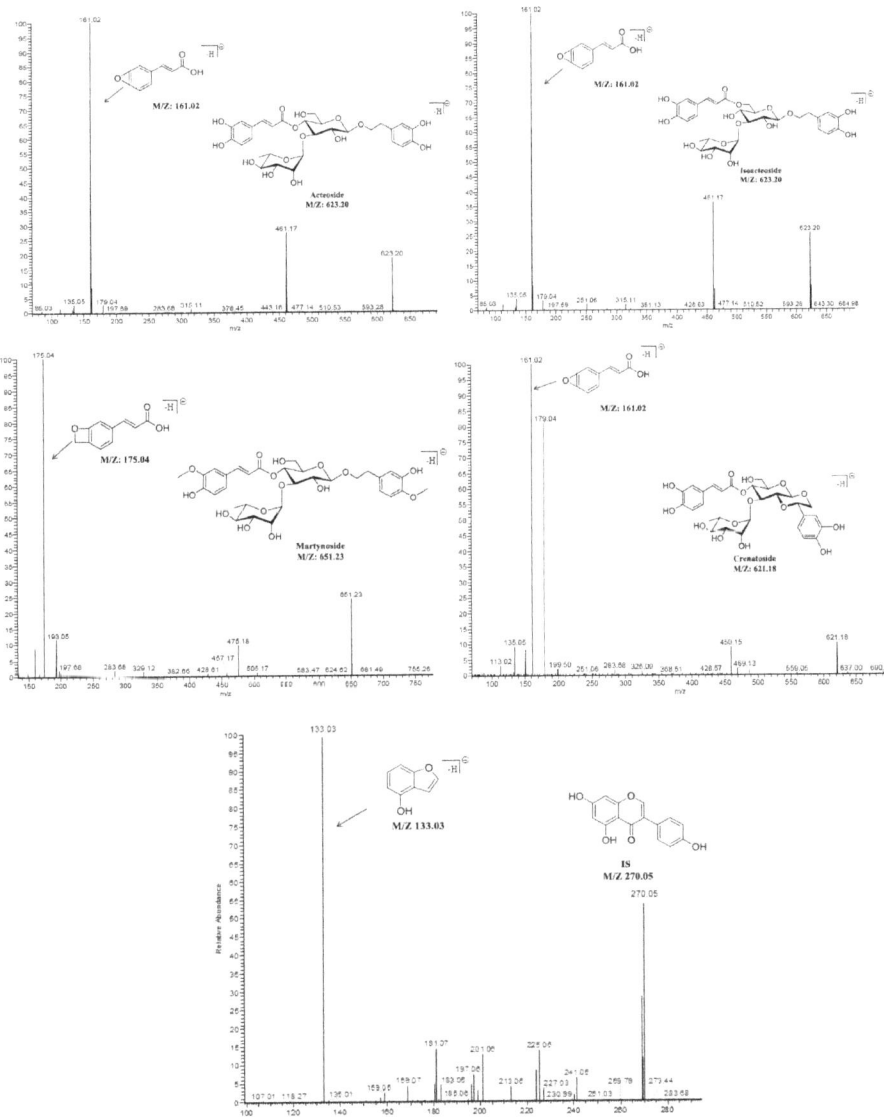

Figure 2. The structures, conjectural fragments, and MS/MS spectra of PhGs and IS at 30 V collision energy.

Table 1. The optimized mass spectrometry parameters of the PhGs and IS.

Components	Retention Time (min)	MRM Transitions (precursor→product)	Collision Energy (v)	Cone Voltage (v)
Acteoside	3.37	623.2→161.0	50	76
Isoacteoside	3.56	623.2→161.0	50	76
Martynoside	4.42	651.2→175.0	36	78
Crenatoside	3.54	621.2→161.0	44	72
Genistein (IS)	5.02	270.0→133.0	34	78

It should be pointed that genistein was selected as the IS because it displayed a strong MS response under negative ion mode (ESI$^-$) and presented satisfactory chromatographic behavior (Figure 2 and Table 1).

2.2. Contents of the Four PhGs in AIH

The contents of the four PhGs were analyzed by UPLC-MS/MS utilizing the same chromatography method as described in Section 3.6. The contents of acteoside, isoacteoside, martynoside, and crenatoside in AIH ranged from 0.02 to 6.24 mg/g (Table 2).

Table 2. Contents of the four PhGs in AIH (means ± SD).

Components	Contents (mg/g)
Acteoside	6.245 ± 0.723
Isoacteoside	0.822 ± 0.102
Martynoside	0.071 ± 0.023
Crenatoside	0.023 ± 0.008

2.3. Method Validation

The established UPLC-MS/MS method was validated for its selectivity, linearity, accuracy, precision, extraction recovery, matrix effect, and stability according to the FDA Guidance for Industry on Bioanalytical Method Validation [24].

2.3.1. Selectivity

Representative chromatograms of the blank plasma sample, blank plasma sample added with PhGs at the lowest limit of quantification (LLOQ) and IS, and treated plasma samples are shown in Figure 1. The results suggest that no significant endogenous interference was found around the retention time of the PhGs and IS.

2.3.2. Linearity and LLOQ

The concentrations of PhGs in test samples were calculated by the calibration curves, which showed good linearities with $r^2 > 0.993$. The LLOQ of the four PhGs were determined ranging from 0.2 to 2.0 ng/mL in accordance with the signal-to-noise ratios (S:N) > 10 (Table 3). These results indicated that the linearity and LLOQ were feasible for quantificational detection of the four PhGs in rat plasma.

Table 3. Regression equation and LLOQ for the four PhGs.

Components	Linear Regression Equation	r^2	Range (ng/mL)	LLOQ (ng/mL)
Acteoside	y = 0.000655 x − 0.001804	0.9979	2.0–1000	2.0
Isoacteoside	y = 0.000917 x − 0.000488	0.9935	0.2–100	0.2
Martynoside	y = 0.005864 x − 0.001393	0.9990	0.4–200	0.4
Crenatoside	y = 0.000592 x − 0.000034	0.9949	0.4–200	0.4

2.3.3. Accuracy and Precision

Our results showed that the intra- and inter-day accuracies of the four PhGs ranged from −8.92% to 9.88%, while the precisions ranged from 1.47% to 13.08% (Table 4), indicating that the method had satisfactory accuracy and precision.

Table 4. Accuracy and precision of the four PhGs in rat plasma ($n = 6$).

Components	Concentration (ng/mL)	Accuracy (RE%)		Precision (RSD%)	
		Intra-day	Inter-day	Intra-day	Inter-day
Acteoside	2.0	4.36	5.53	7.24	6.17
	5.0	−5.26	−3.81	2.17	3.60
	50.0	−7.25	−4.89	7.32	2.37
	800.0	4.70	4.27	7.04	5.90
Isoacteoside	0.2	9.88	−4.86	6.42	3.80
	0.5	2.98	−0.98	5.53	8.46
	5.0	4.24	−4.38	8.35	11.90
	80.0	9.26	7.27	8.27	9.47
Martynoside	0.4	−7.24	4.18	5.54	10.00
	1.0	2.04	3.41	9.09	10.49
	10.0	−1.02	1.54	2.70	1.80
	160.0	1.44	−2.71	1.47	3.39
Crenatoside	0.4	9.43	6.63	9.72	6.42
	1.0	−8.53	−5.12	12.37	13.08
	10.0	−5.32	−8.92	2.08	8.10
	160.0	−2.95	−5.22	6.39	4.35

2.3.4. Extraction Recovery and Matrix Effect

It was found that the extraction recoveries of the four PhGs ranged from 70.56% to 104.54% at three concentration levels (Table 5). It should be noted that there were large variations of extraction recovery for acteoside and isoacteoside. The reason may be that the extraction recoveries of acteoside and isoacteoside suffered from low to moderate suppression due to matrix effects, which would not limit the use of this method, given the satisfactory precision and reproducibility obtained.

Table 5. The extraction recovery and matrix effects of the four PhGs in rat plasma ($n = 6$).

Components	Concentration (ng/mL)	Extraction Recovery		Absolute Matrix Effect		Relative Matrix Effect	IS Normalized MF	
		Mean (%)	RSD (%)	Mean (%)	RSD (%)	RSD (%)	Mean ± SD	RSD (%)
Acteoside	5.0	75.51	8.03	99.00	12.97	9.41	0.95 ± 0.06	7.62
	50.0	88.51	9.75	85.03	4.40	3.22	0.93 ± 0.03	3.11
	800.0	97.14	3.43	86.70	6.21	8.97	0.92 ± 0.02	6.23
Isoacteoside	0.5	98.50	11.47	95.66	9.83	10.11	1.00 ± 0.10	7.96
	5.0	70.56	1.48	89.52	6.38	3.98	1.02 ± 0.09	12.14
	80.0	71.01	2.76	88.11	5.34	2.32	1.04 ± 0.11	2.35
Martynoside	1.0	104.54	12.41	89.27	12.66	4.78	0.96 ± 0.05	9.76
	10.0	92.81	9.64	101.02	7.78	6.33	0.98 ± 0.09	4.12
	160.0	98.19	4.14	96.23	3.42	5.22	0.99 ± 0.08	10.35
Crenatoside	1.0	82.96	11.42	85.31	2.34	10.90	1.00 ± 0.08	8.62
	10.0	90.11	9.57	89.72	10.64	3.51	0.97 ± 0.04	10.69
	160.0	80.38	5.33	106.66	4.47	2.96	0.90 ± 0.03	7.62

The absolute matrix effects of these PhGs were from 85.03% to 106.66% (Table 5). And the relative standard deviation (RSD) values of relative matrix effects were less than 10.90%. The IS normalized matrix factors were 0.90–1.04. The above results indicated that the extraction recoveries of these PhGs were reliable, and there was almost no significant matrix effect in this experiment.

2.3.5. Stability

The stability results of the four PhGs at three concentrations under four conditions are summarized in Table 6. These four PhGs were observed to be stable under a variety of storage and process conditions with the RSD values less than 12.48% and the RE values from −11.62% to 4.70%.

Table 6. The stability of the four PhGs in rat plasma ($n = 6$).

Components	Concentration (ng/mL)	Freeze and Thaw		Short-Term		Long-Term		Post-Preparative	
		RSD (%)	RE (%)	RSD (%)	RE (%)	RSD (%)	RE (%)	RSD (%)	RE (%)
Acteoside	5.0	2.92	−1.58	2.17	−5.26	2.51	−2.45	4.68	−2.72
	50.0	4.60	−5.42	7.32	−7.25	8.01	−8.44	11.78	1.40
	800.0	6.32	1.50	7.04	4.70	6.49	−0.01	2.27	−2.16
Isoacteoside	0.5	6.59	0.61	7.53	2.98	7.43	−1.42	9.61	−2.70
	5.0	9.90	−1.65	11.69	4.24	10.32	2.20	10.68	1.88
	80.0	1.99	0.61	6.28	2.98	6.06	−1.42	7.32	−2.70
Martynoside	1.0	9.46	3.03	9.09	2.04	8.74	1.27	7.47	2.27
	10.0	3.13	−0.19	2.70	−1.02	2.82	−0.79	1.82	−0.66
	160.0	1.13	−2.71	1.47	1.44	1.69	−0.91	2.47	−0.60
Crenatoside	1.0	6.42	2.46	12.37	−8.53	6.36	0.71	9.38	−3.03
	10.0	10.87	−8.98	10.42	−5.32	9.94	−11.6	12.48	−10.95
	160.0	5.27	−3.37	6.39	−2.95	3.80	−4.97	6.02	−1.40

2.4. Pharmacokinetic Study

The established and validated UPLC-MS/MS method was used to investigate the pharmacokinetics of AIH represented by the four PhGs in rat plasma after intragastric administration of AIH ethanol extract.

We found that all of the four PhGs could be detected from plasma at 5 min after intragastric administration of AIH ethanol extract (Figure 3). All of the PhGs showed double peaks on concentration-time curves. The first concentration peaks of all the PhGs appeared at about 0.5 h, and then, reached the second peaks at approximately 6 h in rat plasma. Interestingly, a literature survey indicated that the concentration-time curve features of acteoside and isoacteoside have been reported as double peaks within 1 h in rat plasma after intragastric administration of individual components [25,26], whereas, they have been reported as single peaks [27,28] or double peaks [26,29] within 2 h when administrated medicinal plant extracts. In our study, the relatively distant double peaks of the PhGs might attribute to multiple reasons, such as the influences of complex compositions in AIH, enterohepatic circulation, multiple absorption sites, and gastric emptying process.

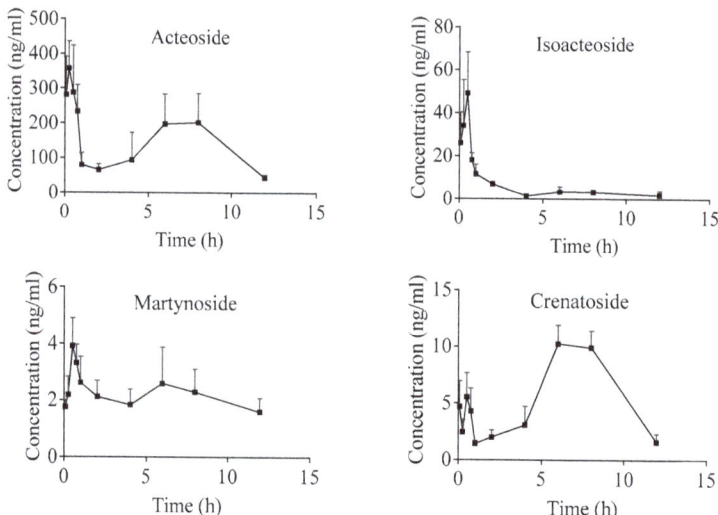

Figure 3. Mean plasma concentration-time curves of the four PhGs in rat plasma ($n = 6$).

Among the four PhGs, the concentration of the second peak of crenatoside was higher than that of the first peak, but the concentration of the second peaks of the other three analytes were lower than those of their first peaks. The peak times (t_{max}) of acteoside and isoacteoside were at 0.3 ± 0.1 h and 0.4 ± 0.2 h (Table 7), respectively, which were consistent with previous studies [26,28–30]. The t_{max} of martynoside and crenatoside were at 3.1 ± 3.6 h and 6.8 ± 1.1 h, respectively, which were longer than those of acteoside and isoacteoside.

Table 7. Pharmacokinetic parameters for the four PhGs in rat plasma after intragastric administration (means ± SD, $n = 6$).

Parameter	Acteoside	Isoacteoside	Martynoside	Crenatoside
$AUC_{0-t}/(\mu g/L \times h)$	1826.3 ± 680.2	70.9 ± 26.9	23.6 ± 6.9	64.7 ± 14.5
$AUC_{0-\infty}/(\mu g/L \times h)$	2243.1 ± 894.6	87.0 ± 40.0	39.5 ± 15.5	76.0 ± 30.0
$t_{1/2}/(h)$	5.6 ± 3.4	4.6 ± 3.1	9.0 ± 2.7	3.4 ± 3.1
$t_{max}/(h)$	0.3 ± 0.1	0.4 ± 0.2	3.1 ± 3.6	6.8 ± 1.1
$C_{max}/(\mu g/L)$	356.9 ± 64.2	58.2 ± 15.0	4.0 ± 0.9	10.9 ± 0.9

The areas under the curves (AUC_{0-t}) of the four PhGs were consistent with their contents in AIH, for example, acteoside exhibited the highest AUC_{0-t} as 1826.3 ± 680.2 μg/L × h and the highest content up to 6.24 mg/g. The four PhGs displayed different elimination half-lives ($t_{1/2}$), ranging from 3.4 h to 9.0 h, although they have similar molecular structures.

3. Materials and Methods

3.1. Chemicals and Reagents

The authentic phenylethanoid glycoside compounds were purchased as follows: acteoside (purity 98.0%) from Dalian Meilun Biological Technology Co., Ltd. (Dalian, China); isoacteoside (purity 98.0%) from Chengdu Push Bio-Technology Co., Ltd. (Chengdu, China); and genistein (internal standard, IS) from Shanghai Aladdin Biochemical Technology Co., Ltd. (Shanghai, China). Martynoside and crenatoside (>98.0% purity) were isolated from AIH in our laboratory and identified by combination of NMR, HPLC, and MS. HPLC-grade acetonitrile (MeCN) and methanol were purchased from Fisher Scientific Co., Ltd. (St. Louis, MO, USA). HPLC-grade formic acid was obtained from Shanghai Macklin Biochemical Co., Ltd. (Shanghai, China), and experimental water was purified by a Milli-Q Reagent Water System (Millipore, Burlington, MA, USA).

3.2. Preparation of AIH Extracts

The plant *A. ilicifolius* L. was collected from Jiangmen, Guangdong Province, China and authenticated by Professor Feng-Qin Zhou, Shandong University of Traditional Chinese Medicine. Voucher specimen number for *A. ilicifolius* L. is 2018060805. Voucher specimen of the plant is deposited at the Key Laboratory of Marine Drugs, the Ministry of Education of China, Ocean University of China, Qingdao, China.

The whole plant was dried in the shade and ground into crude powder. The crude powder (200 g) was immersed in 95% ethanol (v/w, 10:1) for 1 h, and then heated to reflux at 80 °C for 2 h. The extraction solution was filtered, and the residue was refluxed again in 95% ethanol (v/w, 8:1) at 80 °C for 2 h. The filtrate was pooled together and concentrated by a rotary evaporator to dryness at 45 °C. Finally, the product was dissolved in distilled water to acquire the AIH extract for testing with the concentration of 5.0 g crude herb/mL. This extract sample was stored at 4 °C until use.

3.3. Animals

Ten male Sprague-Dawley (250–280 g) rats were purchased from Jinan Pengyue Experimental Animal Center (SCXK (Lu) 20140007). The animal experiments were approved by the Animal Ethics

Committee of Marine Biomedical Research Institute of Qingdao (MBRI-2018-0606), and the guidelines of the institute were strictly followed. All rats had free access to water and food, and were maintained in an environmentally controlled breeding room under the following conditions: 20 ± 2 °C temperature, 60–70% relative humidity, and 12 h light/dark for 1 week before the experiment operated. After fasted for 12 h with free access to water, blank plasma was obtained from four rats after intragastric administration of 2.0 mL/kg water for the UPLC-MS/MS method validation, and the other six rats which were administrated with AIH extract were used for the pharmacokinetic study as in Section 2.4.

3.4. Preparation of Stock Solutions, Calibration Samples, and Quality Control Samples

The stock solutions of four PhGs, acteoside, isoacteoside, martynoside, and crenatoside, were prepared with methanol as a solvent. A stock solution of the PhGs mixture was prepared by combining these four PhGs to attain the final concentrations of 10,000 ng/mL acteoside, 1000 ng/mL isoacteoside, 2000 ng/mL martynoside, and 2000 ng/mL crenatoside. The working solutions were obtained from the stock solution by sequential dilution with methanol at the concentrations of 20.0–10,000 ng/mL acteoside, 2.0–1000 ng/mL isoacteoside, 4.0–2000 ng/mL martynoside, and 4.0–2000 ng/mL crenatoside. Calibration samples were prepared by adding 5 µL working solutions to 45 µL blank plasmas in 1.5 mL Eppendorf tubes. Therefore, the final calibration samples contained 2.0–1000 ng/mL acteoside, 0.2–100 ng/mL isoacteoside, 0.4–200 ng/mL martynoside, and 0.4–200 ng/mL crenatoside. The quality control (QC) samples were prepared in the same way as calibration samples, with the final dilutions of 5.0, 50, and 800 ng/mL acteoside, 0.5, 5, and 80 ng/mL isoacteoside, 1.0, 10, and 160 ng/mL martynoside, and 1.0, 10, and 160 ng/mL crenatoside. The stock solution of the internal standard (IS), geistein, was prepared in methanol at the concentration of 1.0 mg/mL. The IS working solution of 1000 ng/mL was obtained by diluting the stock solution with methanol.

3.5. Pretreatment of Calibration Samples and QC Samples

The 10 µL IS working solution and 140 µL methanol were added to each calibration sample (50 µL) and QC sample (50 µL). The mixture was vortexed for 60 s and centrifuged at 15,000× g for 15 min to separate the precipitated protein. Then, 2 µL of supernatant of the mixture was used for the UPLC-MS/MS analysis.

3.6. Instrumentation and Chromatographic Conditions

A Waters ACQUITY™ UPLC system (Waters Corp., Milford, MA, USA) was interfaced with a Waters Xevo™ TQ/MS (Waters, USA) equipped with an electrospray ionization (ESI) source. Separation of the PhGs was performed on an ACQUITY UPLC BEH C_{18} column (2.1 × 50 mm, 1.7 µm), and the column temperature was maintained at 40 °C during the analysis. The mobile phase consisted of MeCN (solvent A) and 0.1% formic acid in water (solvent B) at a flow rate of 0.4 mL/min. The gradient elution conditions were as follows: 0–1 min, 2–2% A; 1–1.5 min, 2–10% A; 1.5–7 min, 10–43% A; 7–8 min, 43–95% A; 8–9 min, 95% A; 9–10 min, 95–2% A. The injection volume was 2 µL. The detection wavelength was at 330 nm.

The PhGs were detected and quantified by multiple reaction monitoring (MRM) in negative ionization mode (ESI$^-$). The MS parameters of the ionization source were as follows: source temperature, 150 °C; capillary voltage, 3.15 kV; desolvation gas temperature, 400 °C; desolvation gas flow rate, 800 L/h; and cone gas flow rate, 150 L/h. Other optimized parameters, collision energies, and cone voltages are shown in Table 1. All raw data were processed using MassLynx V4.1 workstation (Waters Corp., Milford, MA, USA).

3.7. Method Validation

The selectivity of the method was assessed by chromatograms of blank plasma, blank plasma spiked with working solution of the four PhGs at the lowest limit of quantification (LLOQ) together with working solution of IS, and test plasma acquired at 30 min after intragastric administration of AIH extract. The samples were prepared and pretreated in the same approaches as in Sections 3.4 and 3.5.

Various concentrations of calibration standards (2.0, 5.0, 10, 25, 50, 100, 200, 400, 800, and 1000 ng/mL acteoside; 0.2, 0.5, 1.0, 2.5, 5.0, 10, 20, 40, 80, and 100 ng/mL isoacteoside; and 0.4, 1.0, 2.0, 5.0, 10, 20, 40, 80, 160, and 200 ng/mL martynoside and crenatoside) were processed according to the above procedures for sample preparation. The calibration curve was constructed by plotting analyte-to-IS peak area ratio (y) versus the concentration (x, ng/mL) of analyte and fitted to linear regression (y = ax + b) using 1/x as the weighting factor. The calibration curves were acceptable only if their correlation coefficients (r^2) represented linearity of 0.99 or greater. The calibration curve was established daily throughout the method development and pharmacokinetic analysis. The LLOQ was determined by testing the lowest analytical concentration of the calibration curve.

The accuracy and precision of the method were evaluated by analyzing QC samples at three concentrations prepared as in Section 3.4 with six replicates. To determine the intra- and inter-day accuracy and precision, six replicates at each concentration level were analyzed for five consecutive days. Accuracy was expressed as relative error (RE, %) values within ±15%, and precision was described as relative standard deviation (RSD, %) values less than 15%.

The extraction recoveries at different QC levels were investigated by comparing the mean peak areas of the PhGs pipetted into blank plasma before and after protein precipitation, respectively. The absolute matrix effect expressed as matrix factor (MF) was evaluated by comparing the peak areas of the PhGs pipetted into rat plasma after protein precipitation with those dissolved in the initial mobile phase solution. The relative matrix effect was assessed based on the peak areas of the PhGs pipetted into six different individual sources of rat plasma. The IS normalized MF was determined by the absolute MF of analyte over that of the IS.

The stabilities of the four PhGs were determined by using QC samples in different conditions. Freeze-thaw stability was assessed after three freeze-thaw cycles (from −80 °C to room temperature). Short-term stability was determined after exposure of the QC samples at room temperature (25 °C) for 10 h. Long-term stability was assessed by exposing the samples at −20 °C for 20 days. The samples stored in the autosampler at 4 °C for 24 h were used to evaluate the post-preparative stability. Each QC concentration level was prepared in six replicate samples.

3.8. Pharmacokinetic Study

AIH extract was given to the six rats at a dose of 10.0 g crude herb/kg body weight by intragastric administration. Blood samples (200 μL) were collected from the fossa orbitalis vein before dosing and at the time points of 5, 15, 30, and 45 min and 1, 2, 4, 6, 8, and 12 h after administration and transformed into heparinized Eppendorf tubes. Then, the blood samples were centrifuged at 12,000 × g, 4 °C, for 10 min. Each rat plasma sample (50 μL) was prepared in the same approaches as in Section 3.5.

3.9. Data Analysis

Drug and Statistics (DAS) 3.2.8 software (Shanghai University of Traditional Chinese Medicine, Shanghai, China) was applied to calculate the pharmacokinetic parameters ($t_{1/2}$, t_{max}, C_{max}, AUC_{0-t}, and $AUC_{0-\infty}$) of the four PhGs. All data were shown as mean ± standard deviation (SD).

4. Conclusions

In this study, an accurate and sensitive UPLC-MS/MS method was established and validated for the simultaneously quantitative determination of four PhGs (acteoside, isoacteoside, martynoside, and crenatoside) in rat plasma. This method which was specific to PhGs had good linearity, high accuracy and precision, and no significant matrix effect. By the established method, the preliminary pharmacokinetic features were firstly elucidated for AIH represented by the four PhGs in rats after intragastric administration of AIH extract. It was concluded that these four PhGs manifested relatively distant double peaks on the concentration-time curves and different elimination half-lives although they shared similar molecular structures. The achieved pharmacokinetic parameters may provide primary data and a scientific basis for the further research on the pharmacokinetics of AIH.

Author Contributions: Conceptualization, M.Z. and S.Y.; methodology, M.Z. and X.R.; software, S.Y.; validation, M.Z., X.R., and S.Y.; formal analysis, M.Z. and X.R.; investigation, M.Z.; resources, X.R.; data curation, M.Z. and X.R.; writing—original draft preparation, M.Z. and X.R.; writing—review and editing, M.Z., X.R., Q.Z., and C.W.; visualization, C.W. and C.S.; supervision, C.W. and C.S.; project administration, C.W. and C.S.; and funding acquisition, C.W. and C.S.

Funding: This work was financially supported by the National Natural Science Fund of China (Nos. 41806191 and U1606403), the National High Technology Research and Development Program of China (863 Program) (No. 2013AA093001), the project supported by the Marine S&T Fund of the Shandong Province for Pilot National Laboratory for Marine Science and Technology (Qingdao) (No. 2018SDKJ0406-5), the Natural Science Foundation of Shandong Province (No. ZR2019BD049), and the Taishan Scholars Program, China.

Acknowledgments: We wish to acknowledge Dan Yan, the Capital Medical University, and Juan Liu, master student at the Capital Medical University for their kindness and help in the technical support.

Conflicts of Interest: The authors declare no conflict of interest.

References

1. Nanjing University of Chinese Medicine. *Dictionary of Chinese Herbal Medicine*; Shanghai Science and Technology Press: Shanghai, China, 1977; pp. 844–845.
2. Guan, H.S.; Wang, S.G. *Chinese Marine Materia Medica*; Shanghai Scientific and Technical Publishers: Shanghai, China, 2009; Volume 2, pp. 371–372.
3. Guan, H.S.; Wang, S.G. *Selection of Chinese Marine Materia Medica*; Shanghai Scientific and Technical Publishers: Shanghai, China, 2013; pp. 96–98.
4. Guan, H.S.; Wang, S.G. *Illustrated Handbook of Chinese Marine Materia Medica*; Shanghai Scientific and Technical Publishers: Shanghai, China, 2015; Volume 1, pp. 228–231.
5. Fu, X.M.; Zhang, M.Q.; Shao, C.L.; Li, G.Q.; Bai, H.; Dai, G.L.; Chen, Q.W.; Kong, W.; Fu, X.J.; Wang, C.Y. Chinese Marine Materia Medica Resources: Status and Potential. *Mar. Drugs* **2016**, *14*, 46. [CrossRef] [PubMed]
6. Babu, B.H.; Shylesh, B.S.; Padikkala, J. Antioxidant and hepatoprotective effect of *Acanthus ilicifolius*. *Fitoterapia* **2001**, *72*, 272–277. [CrossRef]
7. Babu, B.H.; Shylesh, B.S.; Padikkala, J. Tumour reducing and anticarcinogenic. activity of *Acanthus ilicifolius* in mice. *J. Ethnopharmacol.* **2002**, *79*, 27–33. [CrossRef]
8. Kumar, K.T.M.S.; Gorain, B.; Roy, D.K.; Samanta, S.K.; Pal, M.; Biswas, P.; Roy, A.; Adhikari, D.; Karmakar, S.; Sen, T. Anti-inflammatory activity of *Acanthus ilicifolius*. *J. Ethnopharmacol.* **2008**, *120*, 7–12. [CrossRef] [PubMed]
9. Kalaskar, P.S.; Karande, V.V.; Bannalikar, A.S.; Gatne, M.M. Antifungal activity of leaves of mangroves plant *Acanthus ilicifolius* against *Aspergillus fumigatus*. *Indian J. Pharm. Sci.* **2012**, *74*, 575–579. [CrossRef]
10. Firdaus, M.; Prihanto, A.A.; Nurdiani, R. Antioxidant and cytotoxic activity of *Acanthus ilicifolius* flower. *Asian Pac. J. Trop. Biomed.* **2013**, *3*, 17–21. [CrossRef]
11. Wahidulla, S.; Bhattacharjee, J.J. Benzoxazinoids from *Acanthus ilicifolius*. *J. Indian Inst. Sci.* **2001**, *81*, 485–490.
12. Kanchanapoom, T.; Kamel, M.S.; Kasai, R.; Yamasaki, K.; Picheansoonthon, C.; Hiraga, Y. Benzoxazinoid glucosides from *Acanthus ilicifolius*. *Phytochemistry* **2001**, *58*, 637–640. [CrossRef]
13. Kanchanapoom, T.; Kamel, M.S.; Kasai, R.; Yamasaki, K.; Picheansoonthon, C.; Hiraga, Y. Lignan glucosides from *Acanthus ilicifolius*. *Phytochemistry* **2001**, *56*, 369–372. [CrossRef]
14. Kanchanapoom, T.; Kasai, R.; Yamasaki, K. Flavonoid glycosides from *Acanthus ilicifolius* L. *Nat. Med.* **2002**, *56*, 122.
15. Wu, J.; Zhang, S.; Huang, J.; Xiao, Q.; Li, Q.; Long, L. Phenylethanoid and aliphatic alcohol glycosides from *Acanthus ilicifolius*. *Phytochemistry* **2003**, *63*, 491–495. [CrossRef]
16. Wu, J.; Huang, J.S.; Xiao, Q.; Zhang, S.; Xiao, Z.H.; Li, Q.X.; Long, L.J.; Huang, L.M. Complete assignments of ^{1}H and ^{13}C NMR data for 10 phenylethanoid glycosides. *Magn. Reson. Chem.* **2004**, *42*, 659–662. [CrossRef] [PubMed]

17. Van, K.P.; Quang, T.H.; Huong, T.T.; Nhung le, L.T.; Cuong, N.X.; Van, M.C. Chemical constituents of *Acanthus ilicifolius* L. and effect on osteoblastic MC3T3E1 cells. *Arch. Pharm. Res.* **2008**, *31*, 823–829.
18. Morikawa, T.; Pan, Y.; Ninomiya, K.; Imura, K.; Matsuda, H.; Yoshikawa, M.; Yuan, D.; Muraoka, O. Acylated phenylethanoid oligoglycosides with hepatoprotective activity from the desert plant *Cistanche tubulosa*. *Bioorg. Med. Chem.* **2010**, *18*, 1882–1890. [CrossRef] [PubMed]
19. Pan, Y.N.; Morikawa, T.; Ninomiya, K.; Imura, K.; Yuan, D.; Yoshikawa, M.; Muraoka, O. Bioactive constituents from Chinese nature medicines: Four new acylated phenylethanoid oligoglycosides, kankanosides J1, J2, K1 and K2 from stems of *Cistanche tubulosa*. *Chem. Pharm. Bull.* **2010**, *58*, 575–578. [CrossRef] [PubMed]
20. Li, Y.X.; Chen, Z.; Feng, Z.M.; Yang, Y.N.; Jiang, J.S.; Zhang, P.C. Hepatoprotective glycosides from *Leonurus japonicus* Houtt. *Carbohydr. Res.* **2012**, *348*, 42–46. [CrossRef] [PubMed]
21. Ma, Q.G.; Guo, Y.M.; Luo, B.M.; Liu, W.M.; Wei, R.R.; Yang, C.X.; Ding, C.H.; Xu, X.F.; He, M.H. Hepatoprotective phenylethanoid glycosides from *Cirsium setosum*. *Nat. Prod. Res.* **2016**, *30*, 1824–1829. [CrossRef]
22. Shen, T.; Li, X.Q.; Hu, W.C.; Zhang, L.J.; Xu, X.D.; Wu, H.F.; Ji, L.L. Hepatoprotective effect of phenylethanoid glycosides from *Incarvillea compacta* against CCl$_4$-induced cytotoxicity in HepG2 cells. *J. Korean Soc. Appl. Biol. Chem.* **2015**, *58*, 617–625. [CrossRef]
23. Xue, Z.Z.; Yang, B. Phenylethanoid glycosides: Research advances in their phytochemistry, pharmacological activity and pharmacokinetics. *Molecules* **2016**, *21*, 991. [CrossRef]
24. U.S. Food and Drug Administration. (FDA) Guidance for Industry: Bioanalytical Method Validation. 2018. Available online: https://www.fda.gov/ucm/groups/fdagov-public/@fdagovdrugs-gen/documents/document/ucm070107.pdf (accessed on 24 May 2018).
25. Gan, P.; Huo, S.X.; Bai, P.; Li, G.; Peng, X.M.; He, Y.; Yan, M. Pharmacokinetics and tissue distribution of acteoside in rats. *Chin. Pharm. Bull.* **2014**, *30*, 417–420.
26. Feng, B.W.; Song, Y.G.; Xu, Q.M.; Xu, P.F.; Zeng, Q.; Shan, B.X.; Liu, K.Y.; Su, D. Simultaneous determination of savaside A, acteoside, and isoacteoside in rat plasma by UHPLC-MS/MS: Comparative pharmacokinetic and bioavailability characteristics of *Monochasma savatieri* via different routes of administration. *J. Sep. Sci.* **2018**, *41*, 4408–4418. [CrossRef] [PubMed]
27. Zheng, D.K.; Chen, W.K.; Ma, S.C.; Shao, J.; Wang, J.; Luo, Y.H. Simultaneous determination of three phenolic glycosides in *Callicarpa nudiflora* by UHPLC-MS methods and analysis of their pharmacokinetics in plasma of rats. *Chin. Tradit. Herb. Drugs* **2015**, *46*, 3533–3538. [CrossRef]
28. Zhao, M.; Qian, D.W.; Liu, P.; Shang, E.X.; Jiang, S.; Guo, J.M.; Su, S.L.; Duan, J.A.; Du, L.Y.; Tao, J.H. Comparative pharmacokinetics of catalpol and acteoside in normal and chronic kidney disease rats after oral administration of *Rehmannia glutinosa* extract. *Biomed. Chromatogr.* **2015**, *29*, 1842–1848. [CrossRef] [PubMed]
29. Li, Y.J.; Gan, L.; Li, G.Q.; Deng, L.; Zhang, X.S.; Deng, Y.L. Pharmacokinetics of plantamajoside and acteoside from *Plantago asiatica* in rats by liquid chromatography-mass spectrometry. *J. Pharm. Biomed. Ana.* **2014**, *89*, 251–256. [CrossRef] [PubMed]
30. Wen, Y.; Huo, S.; Zhang, W.; Xing, H.; Qi, L.; Zhao, D.; Li, N.; Xu, J.; Yan, M.; Chen, X. Pharmacokinetics, biodistribution, excretion and plasma protein binding studies of acteoside in rats. *Drug Res.* **2016**, *66*, 148–153. [CrossRef] [PubMed]

Sample Availability: Not available.

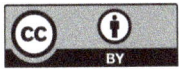

© 2019 by the authors. Licensee MDPI, Basel, Switzerland. This article is an open access article distributed under the terms and conditions of the Creative Commons Attribution (CC BY) license (http://creativecommons.org/licenses/by/4.0/).

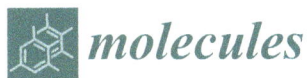

Communication

Tyrosinase Inhibition Antioxidant Effect and Cytotoxicity Studies of the Extracts of *Cudrania tricuspidata* Fruit Standardized in Chlorogenic Acid

Ha-Na Oh [1,†], Dae-Hun Park [2,†], Ji-Yeon Park [1], Seung-Yub Song [1], Sung-Ho Lee [1], Goo Yoon [1], Hong-Seop Moon [1], Deuk-Sil Oh [3], Sang-Hoon Rhee [4], Eun-Ok Im [5], In-Soo Yoon [5], Jung-Hyun Shim [1,*] and Seung-Sik Cho [1,*]

[1] College of Pharmacy, Mokpo National University, Muan-gun, Jeonnam 58554, Korea;
543ab@naver.com (H.-N.O.); 2162162@naver.com (J.-Y.P.); tgb1007@naver.com (S.-Y.S.);
tjdgh0730@naver.com (S.-H.L.); gyoon@mokpo.ac.kr (G.Y.); hbsmoon@mokpo.ac.kr (H.-S.M.)
[2] Department of Nursing, Dongshin University, Naju-si, Jeonnam 58245, Korea; dhj1221@hanmail.net
[3] Jeollanam-do Forest Resource Research Institute, Naju, Jeonnam 58213, Korea; ohye@korea.kr
[4] Department of Biological Sciences, Oakland University, Rochester, MI 48309, USA; srhee@oakland.edu
[5] Department of Pharmacy, College of Pharmacy, Pusan National University, Busan 46241, Korea;
eoim@pusan.ac.kr (E.-O.I.); insoo.yoon@pusan.ac.kr (I.-S.Y.)
* Correspondence: s1004jh@gmail.com (J.-H.S.); sscho@mokpo.ac.kr (S.-S.C.);
Tel.: +82-614502684 (J.-H.S.); +82-614502687 (S.-S.C.)
† These authors contributed equally to this work.

Received: 21 August 2019; Accepted: 6 September 2019; Published: 7 September 2019

Abstract: In the present study, various extracts of *C. tricuspidata* fruit were prepared with varying ethanol contents and evaluated for their biomarker and biological properties. The 80% ethanolic extract showed the best tyrosinase inhibitory activity, while the 100% ethanolic extract showed the best total phenolics and flavonoids contents. The HPLC method was applied to analyze the chlorogenic acid in *C. tricuspidata* fruit extracts. The results suggest that the observed antioxidant and tyrosinase inhibitory activity of *C. tricuspidata* fruit extract could partially be attributed to the presence of marker compounds in the extract. In this study, we present an analytical method for standardization and optimization of *C. tricuspidata* fruit preparations. Further investigations are warranted to confirm the in vivo pharmacological activity of *C. tricuspidata* fruit extract and its active constituents and assess the safe use of the plant for the potential development of the extract as a skin depigmentation agent.

Keywords: *C.tricuspidata* Bureau; HPLC; tyrosinase

1. Introduction

Cudrania tricuspidata (Moraceae) is used as traditional medicine for inflammation, gastritis, cancer, and liver injury [1]. In the previous reports, active constituents from roots and leaves of *Cudrania tricuspidata* contain pharmaceutically active substances such as neuroprotective [2], anti-inflammatory [3,4], pancreatic lipase inhibitory [5], monoamine oxidase inhibitory [6], and anti-obesity effects [7]. Additively, prenylated isoflavonoids, benzylated flavonoids, xanthones from the fruits displayed potential antioxidant, anti-inflammatory, and neuroprotective activities [8–10].

The efficacy of extracts and purified bioactive substances prepared using *C. tricuspidata* as a medical source has been studied broadly to date. The content of a single compound present in fruits was insufficient for use as biomarkers for pharmaceutical/cosmetic application. Moreover, preparations involving the fruit could be beneficial for productivity purpose as *C. tricuspidata* is a perennial plant (Table 1).

Table 1. Chemical constituents and biological activities of *C. tricuspidata* fruit reported in previous literatures.

Constituent	Activity	Contents	Effective Dose (mg/kg/day)(route/animal)	Ref.
6,8-diprenylgenistein	Anti-obesity	Single compound	30 (oral/mouse)	[7]
Cudraisoflavones etc	Neuroprotective	*N.D	N.D	[2]
Genistein etc	Lipase inhibition	N.D	N.D	[5]
5,7,3′,4′-Tetrahydroxy-6,8-diprenylisoflavone	Antiallergy	N.D	N.D	[11]
Water extract	Dermatitis	Rutin was identified	60 (oral/mouse)	[3]
Gancaonin A etc	Monoamine oxidase inhibition	N.D	N.D	[6]
Water and etnaolic extract	Tyrosinase inhibition	Chlorogenic acid	N.D	This study
Scandenolone	Anti-cancer	Single compound	5 and 7.5 (intravenous/mouse)	[12]

*ND; not decribed.

Few studies have been conducted on the fruits of *C. tricuspidata* and the contents of bioactive substances were observed to be insufficient for use as key compounds for pharmaceutical industrialization. Considerable effort has been focused on developing *C. tricuspidata* as materials, but no positive results have been achieved.

The aim of this study was to evaluate the fruit extract of *C. tricuspudata* for tyrosinase inhibitory activity, as well as to characterize the chromatographic profile of its optimized extract to identify the compounds responsible for antioxidant and tyrosinase inhibition. Validation of a High Performance Liquid Chromatography (HPLC) method was preformed for standardize of chlorogenic acid.

In the preliminary study, we purified and identified the main substance, chlorogenic acid with antioxidant and tyrosinase inhibitory activity from fruits of *C. tricuspidata*. Previous reports have demonstrated that chlorogenic acid plays important roles in melanogenesis of B16 melanoma cells. Although chlorogenic acid did not exhibit strong tyrosinase inhibitory effect, its metabolic product(s) showed suppression of melanogenesis in B16 melanoma cells by inhibiting tyrosinase activity [13]. Consequently, we set chlorogenic acid as a biomarker for the extract of *C. tricuspidata* fruit.

Cytotoxicity test was assessed in cell lines to test the cell viability in the presence of the extract of *C. tricuspudata* fruit with an aim to incorporate the extract in topical form as a skin whitening agent. This is the first study that assess tyrosinase inhibition and quantifythe presence of biomarkers such as chlorogenic acid in *C. tricuspudata* fruit.

Previously, we had investigated the biological properties of extracts and their biomarkers obtained from *C. tricuspidata* leaves for the development of medicinal/food sources. In this study, fruit components of *C. tricuspidata* were screened for cosmetic application. Extracts of *C. tricuspidata* fruit were prepared for the assessment of chemical composition and biological properties.

2. Results and Discussion

2.1. Chromatographic Conditions for Extract of C. tricuspidata Fruit

The HPLC conditions were established as follows. A gradient program was used to separate the chlorogenic acid (Table 6). Detection wavelengths were set as 330 nm. As shown in Figure 1, chlorogenic acid was identified as the main component in the extract from *C. tricuspidata*.

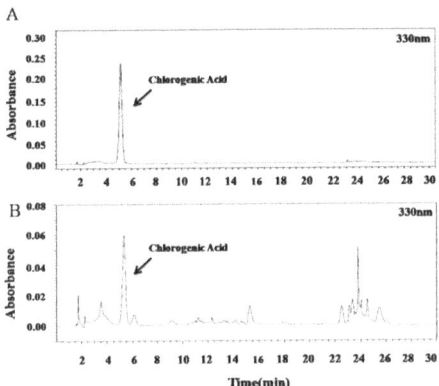

Figure 1. Analysis of *C. tricuspidata* fruit extracts by High Performance Liquid Chromatography (HPLC) method. (**A**) standard; (**B**) sample extract (fruit).

Lee et al. reported that the extraction yield of water extract of *C. tricuspidata* fruit was 12.7% and extract contained rutin [3]. However, the content of rutin in the water extract was not described. In the present study, rutin was not found in the extract of *C. tricuspidata* fruit.

Jiang et al. purified and identified anticancer compound named scandenolone from *C. tricuspidata* fruit [12]. Jiang described the detailed purification process in the reported study. However, the study lacked a description of the content of active compound in the fruits of *C. tricuspidata*. Although it has been reported that scandenolone plays an important role in mediating anticancer activity, the potential of the compound to prevent cancer cannot be guaranteed by just consuming *C. tricuspidata* fruits. In addition, there exists no data on permissible levels of consumption for human. Therefore, scandenolone can be considered as one of the trace components of fruits of *C. tricuspidata*.

Jo et al. reported about anti-obesity efficacy of 6,8-Diprenylgenisteinusing 70% ethanol extract of *C. tricuspidata* fruit in their study [7]. The daily intake was set as 10–15 g of fruit. In the present study, 6,8-Diprenylgenistein was analyzed using HPLC, but it was difficult to confirm its presence in the extract of *C. tricuspidata* fruit. As the species, harvesting time of *C. tricuspidata* fruit, and the places of cultivation are different, we presumed that the presence of 6,8-Diprenylgenisteinmight also be different.

2.2. Method Validation

2.2.1. Linearity, Limit of Detection (LOD), and Limit of Quantification (LOQ)

In the present study, calibration curves, limit of detection, and quantification were conducted. Calibration curves were set in the range of 3.125–50 μg/mL for chlorogenic acid and exhibited good linear regressions (r^2 = 0.998). The LOD was found to be 0.7 μg/mL for chlorogenic acid. The LOQ value for chlorogenic acid was found to be 2.1 μg/mL (Table 2).

Table 2. HPLC data for the calibration graphs and limit of quantification of the active compound.

Analyte	Retention Time (min)	R^2	Linear Range (μg/mL)	LOQ (μg/mL)	LOD (μg/mL)
Chlorogenic acid	4.7	0.998	3.125–50	2.11	0.7

2.2.2. Precision and Accuracy

The results of the intraday and interday precision experiments are shown in Table 3. The overall recovery percentages were in the range of 104.04–107.78% for chlorogenic acid. These results demonstrate that the developed method is reproducible with a good accuracy (Table 3).

Table 3. Analytical results of intra-day and inter-day precision and accuracy.

Analyte	Conc (µg/mL)	Intra-Day (n = 3)		Inter-Day (n = 3)	
		RSD (%) [a]	Accuracy (%)	RSD (%)	Accuracy (%)
Chlorogenic acid	6.25	2.65	105.29	2.74	104.04
	12.5	7.86	105.32	5.94	107.78
	25	2.59	104.50	3.17	105.91

[a] RSD: relative standard deviation.

2.2.3. Repeatability

The results of the repeatability are shown in Table 4. RSD values were below 2.0%. Thus, HPLC method is suitable for analysis of *C. tricuspidata* fruit.

Table 4. Analytical data of recovery (n = 6).

Analyte	Added (µg/mL)	Recovery (%) (Mean ± SD)	RSD (%) [a]
Cholorogenic acid	6.25	103.39 ± 0.35	0.4
	12.5	96.79 ± 0.96	1.08
	25	98.59 ± 1.20	1.26

[a] RSD: relative standard deviation.

2.3. Contents of Marker Compounds from C. tricuspidata Fruit Extracts

Plant samples were extracted with various solvent compositions to select the best extraction solvent conditions: hot water, 20–100% ethanol (v/v). The validated HPLC method was applied to analyze the samples. The contents (%wt.) of chlorogenic acid is presented in Figure 2. The contents of the chlorogenic acid in the 80% ethanolic extract were greater compared to other ethanolic extracts. Based on these results, the 80% ethanol was selected as the most effective extraction solvent (0.34 ± 0.01%, w/w).

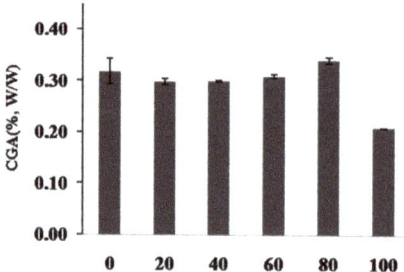

Figure 2. Content of chlorogenic acid (CGA) in hot water and ethanolic extracts from *C. tricuspidata* fruit. 0 (hot water ex); 20 (20% ethantol ex); 40 (40% ethanol ex); 60 (60% ethanol ex); 80 (80% ethanol ex); 100 (100% ethanol ex). Each value was the mean ± SD (n = 3).

2.4. Cell Viability and Tyrosinase Inhibition of C. tricuspidata Fruit Extracts

Cytotoxicity of various extracts of *C. tricuspidata* was determined by MTT (3-(4,5-dimethylthiazol-2-yl)-2,5-diphenyltetrazolium bromide) assay [14]. Cytotoxicity was assessed after treatment of B16F10 cells with a various sample concentration of 100 µg/mL for 24 h. For further study, 100 µg/mL or less should be considered as optimal for conducting experiments on unraveling the mechanism of action of *C. tricuspidata* extract (Figure 3).

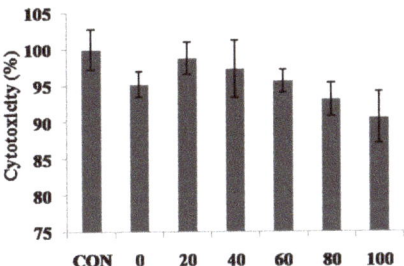

Figure 3. Cell viability of water and ethanolic extracts from *C. tricuspidata* fruit. 0–100 represent 0–100% ethanolic extract (100 μg/mL). Each value was the mean ± SD ($n = 3$).

The tyrosinase inhibition of various extracts of *C. tricuspidata* was determined by the tyrosinase inhibitory assays. The measured tyrosinase inhibitory activity is shown in Figure 4. The tyrosinase inhibition decreased in the following order: 80% ethanol extract (68.3 ± 7.3%) > 100% ethanol extract (64.1 ± 5.2%) > 60% ethanol extract (51.2 ± 1.3%) > 40% ethanol extract (24.5 ± 6.8%) > 20% ethanol extract (10.68 ± 0.4%) > hot water extract (5.22 ± 0.5%).

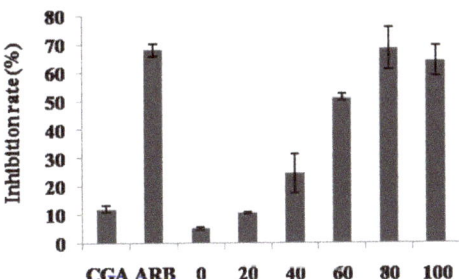

Figure 4. Tyrosinate inhibition in hot water and ethanolic extracts from *C. tricuspidata* fruit. CGA: chlorogenic acid (8 μg/mL); ARB (150 μg/mL): arbutin. 0–100 represent 0–100% ethanolic extract (100 μg/mL). Each value was the mean ± SD ($n = 3$).

In the present study, we identified chlorogenic acid as one of the tyrosinase inhibitory (anti-whitening related) efficacy factors. Content of chlorogenic acid and the extent of tyrosinase inhibition were the highest in 80% *C. tricuspidata* fruit extract. In the previous report, chlorogenic acid was reported to affect melanogenesis through tyrosinase inhibition when converted into metabolites in cells [11]. Therefore, we established chlorogenic acid as the biomarker of *C. tricuspidata* fruit. HPLC chromatograms revealed chlorogenic acid as the major component of *C. tricuspidata* fruit.

In the present study, total phenolic and total flavonoids content of *C. tricuspidata* fruit extracts were compared. Total phenolic and flavonoids were the highest in 100% ethanolic extracts. Extracts containing phenolic compounds have been reported to exhibit tyrosinase inhibition [15–17].

Tyrosinase inhibition was the highest in 80% ethanolic extract. Besides, total phenolic and total flavonoid levels were highest in 100% ethanolic extract, thus indicating that the 80% ethanolic extract contains unknown tyrosinase inhibitors. It is hypothesized that through further studies, unknown tyrosinase inhibitors in 80% ethanolic extracts can be identified (Table 5).

Table 5. Antioxidant activity and total phenolic contents of C. tricuspidata fruit extracts.

Extract	Total Flavonoid (Ascorbic Acid eq. µg/100 µg Extract)	Total Phenolic Content (Gallic Acid eq. mg/g)
Hot water	7.9	31.9 ± 1.4
20% EtOH Ex	14.0	36.0 ± 3.0
40% EtOH Ex	10.8	29.9 ± 1.8
60% EtOH Ex	11.2	33.9 ± 2.1
80% EtOH Ex	19.5	35.9 ± 2.2
100% EtOH Ex	26.0	40.6 ± 2.7

3. Experimental Section

3.1. Plant Material and Preparation of the Extract

C. tricuspidata fruit was collected in May 2017 near Naju, Jeonnam Province, Korea. A voucher specimen (MNUCSS-CTF-01) was deposited in the College of Pharmacy, Mokpo National University. Fruits were dried and used for extract preparation. The air-dried and powdered *C. tricuspidata* fruits (10 g) were subjected to extraction twice with 20–100% ethanol (100 mL) at room temperature for three days. The 0% extract was prepared using hot water extraction (100 °C, 4 h). After filtration, the resultant ethanol solution was evaporated, freeze-dried, and stored at -50 °C. The crude extract was resuspended in ethanol and filtered using a 0.4 µm membrane. All samples were used for the optimization of the extraction process and in vitro experiments.

3.2. Instrumentation and Chromatographic Conditions

The HPLC conditions were established as shown in Table 6.

Table 6. Analytical HPLC conditions for *C. tricuspidata* fruit extracts.

Parameters	Conditions		
Instruments and Column	Alliance 2695 HPLC system (Waters, Millford, MA, USA) Zorbax extended-C18 (C18, 4.6 mm × 150 mm, 5 µm)		
Flow rate	0.8 mL/min		
Injection volumn	10 µL		
UV detection	330 nm		
Run time	30 min		
	Time (min)	A (%)	B (%)
	0	10	90
	7	10	90
	8	20	80
Gradient	20	25	75
	21	100	0
	25	10	90
	30	10	90

3.3. Preparation of Standards and Sample Solutions

Accurately weighed appropriate amounts of chlorogenic acid was mixed and dissolved in methanol in a 50 mL volumetric flask, to obtain a stock solution of 50 µg/mL. Solutions were subsequently 2-fold serially diluted to 3.125 µg/mL.

Samples (0.5 g) were dissolved in methanol (10 mL). Subsequently, 1 mL was diluted with 9 mL of mobile phase A to obtain a final solution with a known concentration of 25 mg/mL [18].

3.4. Method Validation

The analytical method usedfor the quantification of chlorogenic acid in the various extract of C. tricuspidata fruit was validated in terms of specificity, linearity, sensitivity, accuracy, precision, and recovery. Experiments were performed as previously described [16].

3.5. Analysis of the Extract from C. tricuspidata Fruit

The HPLC method developed herein was used to quantitatively determinate of the amounts of chlorogenic acid in 6 extracts from C. tricuspidata fruit.

3.6. Cell Viability

Human melanoma cells (B16F10) were purchased from the American Tissue Culture Collection (Manassas, VA, USA). Cells were seeded in 96-well plates and treated with 100 µg/mL of sample for 24 h. MTT was added and plates were incubated at 37 °C for 2 h. After dissolving the formazan crystals in 100 µL of DMSO, the absorbance was measured at 490 nm using an Enspire Multimode Plate reader (Perkin-Elmer, Akron, OH) [19].

3.7. Tyrosinase Inhibitory Assay

Tyrosinase inhibition assay was performed following a previously described method with some modification [20]. Briefly, reaction mixtures (total volume of 150 µL) with 49.5 µL of phosphate buffer (pH 6.8, 100 mM), 45 µL of distilled water, and 5 µL of sample dissolved in DMSO (100 µg/mL) were prepared. This was followed by the addition of 0.5 µL of mushroom tyrosinase (10 units) and 50 µL of the substrate, mixed well, and incubated for 10 min at 37 °C. Absorbance was measured at 475nm.

The percent inhibition of the enzyme reaction was calculated as follows:

$$\text{Inhibition rate (\%)} = (B - S)/B \times 100 \qquad (1)$$

where B and S are the absorbance values for the blank and sample, respectively.

3.8. Determination of Total Phenolic Content

The total phenolic content was determined using Folin-Ciocalteu assay [18]. A 1 mL of sample solution (5 mg/mL) was mixed with 1 mL of 2% (w/v) Na_2CO_3 solution and 1 mL of 10% Folin-Ciocalteu phenol reagent. After 10 min, the absorbance was measured at 750 nm using a microplate reader (Perkin Elmer, Waltham, MA, USA). The phenolic content was calculated from calibration curve of gallic acid. The results were expressed as mg of gallic acid equivalents per g of sample.

3.9. Determination of Total Flavonoids

The total flavonoid content was determined based on a previously reported colorimetric method [18]. Briefly, a 0.5 mL aliquot of the sample solution was mixed with distilled water (2 mL) and subsequently with 5% $NaNO_2$ solution (0.15 mL). After incubation for 5 min, a 0.15 mL aliquot of 10% $AlCl_3$ solution was added to the mixture and after 5 min, 4% NaOH solution (2 mL) was added to the mixture. Water was added to the sample to bring the final volume to 5 mL, and the mixture was thoroughly mixed and allowed to stand for 15 min. The absorbance of the resultant mixture was measured at 415 nm. Then, the total flavonoid content was calculated as quercetin equivalents (mg quercetin/g extract) by reference to a standard curve ($r^2 = 0.999$).

4. Conclusions

In our preliminary study, we identified chlorogenic acid in the fruits of C. tricuspidata as antioxidant compound using bioassay-guided purification. The validated HPLC method was developed and applied to confirm the presence of chlorogenic acid in C. tricuspidata fruit extracts. Various ethanolic extracts of *C. tricuspidata* fruit were prepared, and 80% ethanolic extract was found to exhibit the highest tyrosinase inhibitory activity. Besides, 100% ethanolic extract possessed the highest content of total phenolics and flavonoids. Based on the results, it is evident that the 80% ethanolic extract contains unknown tyrosinase inhibitors. Further studies are necessitated to identify the unknown tyrosinase inhibitors in 80% ethanolic extracts. The results suggest that the observed antioxidant and tyrosinase inhibitory activity of *C. tricuspidata* fruit extract could partially be attributed to the presence of marker compounds in the extract. We report ananalytical method for standardization and extraction optimization of *C. tricuspidata* fruit for the first time. Further investigations are needed to confirm the biological effect of *C. tricuspidata* fruit extract for the potential development of the extract as a cosmetic source.

Author Contributions: Conceptualization, H.-A.O., D.-H.P., J.-H.S., and S.-S.C.; methodology, H.-N.O., D.-H.P., S.-H.L., G.Y., H.-S.M., D.-S.O., S.-H.R., E.-O.I., I.-S.Y., J.-H.S., and S.-S.C.; software, H.-N.O., D.-H.P., S.-H.L., G.Y., H.-S.M., D.-S.O., S.-H.R., E.-O.I., I.-S.Y., J.-H.S., and S.-S.C.; validation, H.-N.O., D.-H.P., J.-Y.P., S.-Y.S., J.-H.S., and S.-S.C.; formal analysis, H.-N.O., D.-H.P., J.-Y.P., S.-Y.S., J.-H.S., and S.-S.C.; investigation, H.-N.O., D.-H.P., J.-Y.P., S.-Y.S., S.-H.L., G.Y., H.-S.M., D.-S.O., S.-H.R., E.-O.I., I.-S.Y., J.-H.S., and S.-S.C.; resources, J.-H.S. and S.-S.C.; data curation, H.-N.O., D.-H.P., J.-Y.P., and S.-Y.S.,; writing—original draft preparation, H.-N.O. and D.-H.P.; writing—review and editing, D.-H.P. S.-H.L., G.Y., H.-S.M., D.-S.O., S.-H.R., E.-O.I., I.-S.Y., J.-H.S., and S.-S.C.; supervision, J.-H.S. and S.-S.C.

Funding: Korea Institute of Planning and Evaluation for Technology in Food, Agriculture, Forestry and Fisheries: MAFRA 316007-5, Mokpo National University: MNU Innovative Programs for National University in 2019.

Acknowledgments: This work was supported by Korea Institute of Planning and Evaluation for Technology in Food, Agriculture, Forestry and Fisheries (IPET) through Agri-Bio industry Technology Development Program, funded by Ministry of Agriculture, Food and Rural Affairs (MAFRA)(316007-5), and this research was supported by the funds of the MNU Innovative Programs for National University in 2019.

Conflicts of Interest: The authors declare no conflict of interest.

References

1. Chang, S.H.; Jung, E.J.; Lim, D.G.; Oyungerel, B.; Lim, K.I.; Her, E.; Choi, W.S.; Jun, M.H.; Choi, K.D.; Han, D.J. Anti-inflammatory action of *Cudrania tricuspidata* on spleen cell and T lymphocyte proliferation. *J. Pharm. Pharmacol.* **2008**, *60*, 1221–1226. [CrossRef] [PubMed]
2. Hiep, N.T.; Kwon, J.; Kim, D.-W.; Hwang, B.Y.; Lee, H.-J.; Mar, W.; Lee, D. Isoflavones with neuroprotective activities from fruits of *Cudrania tricuspidata*. *Phytochemistry* **2015**, *111*, 141–148. [CrossRef] [PubMed]
3. Lee, H.; Ha, H.; Lee, J.K.; Seo, C.s.; Lee, N.h.; Jung, D.Y.; Park, S.J.; Shin, H.K. The fruits of *Cudrania tricuspidata* suppress development of atopic dermatitis in NC/Nga mice. *Phytother. Res.* **2012**, *26*, 594–599. [CrossRef] [PubMed]
4. Han, X.H.; Hong, S.S.; Jin, Q.; Li, D.; Kim, H.-K.; Lee, J.; Kwon, S.H.; Lee, D.; Lee, C.-K.; Lee, M.K. Prenylated and benzylated flavonoids from the fruits of *Cudrania tricuspidata*. *J. Nat. Prod.* **2008**, *72*, 164–167. [CrossRef] [PubMed]
5. Jo, Y.H.; Kim, S.B.; Liu, Q.; Do, S.-G.; Hwang, B.Y.; Lee, M.K. Comparison of pancreatic lipase inhibitory isoflavonoids from unripe and ripe fruits of *Cudrania tricuspidata*. *PLoS ONE* **2017**, *12*, e0172069. [CrossRef] [PubMed]
6. Han, X.H.; Hong, S.S.; Hwang, J.S.; Jeong, S.H.; Hwang, J.H.; Lee, M.H.; Lee, M.K.; Lee, D.; Ro, J.S.; Hwang, B.Y. Monoamine oxidase inhibitory constituents from the fruits of *Cudrania tricuspidata*. *Arch. Pharm. Res.* **2005**, *28*, 1324–1327. [CrossRef] [PubMed]
7. Jo, Y.H.; Choi, K.-M.; Liu, Q.; Kim, S.B.; Ji, H.-J.; Kim, M.; Shin, S.-K.; Do, S.-G.; Shin, E.; Jung, G. Anti-obesity effect of 6,8-diprenylgenistein, an isoflavonoid of *Cudrania tricuspidata* fruits in high-fat diet-induced obese mice. *Nutrients* **2015**, *7*, 10480–10490. [CrossRef] [PubMed]
8. Xin, L.-T.; Yue, S.-J.; Fan, Y.-C.; Wu, J.-S.; Yan, D.; Guan, H.-S.; Wang, C.-Y. *Cudrania tricuspidata*: An updated review on ethnomedicine, phytochemistry and pharmacology. *RSC Adv.* **2017**, *7*, 31807–31832. [CrossRef]
9. Lee, B.; Lee, J.; Lee, S.-T.; Suk, T.; Lee, W.; Jeong, T.-S.; Hun Park, K. Antioxidant and Cytotoxic Activities of Xanthones from *Cudrania tricuspidata*. *Bioorg. Med. Chem. Lett.* **2005**, *15*, 5548–5552. [CrossRef] [PubMed]

10. Jeong, C.-H.; Nam Choi, G.; Hye Kim, J.; Hyun Kwak, J.; Rok Jeong, H.; Kim, D.-O.; Heo, h.j. Protective Effects of Aqueous Extract from *Cudrania tricuspidata* on Oxidative Stress-induced Neurotoxicity. *Food Sci. Biotechnol.* **2010**, *19*, 1113–1117. [CrossRef]
11. Lee, T.; Kwon, J.; Lee, D.; Mar, W. Effects of Cudrania tricuspidata Fruit Extract and Its Active Compound, 5, 7, 3′, 4′-Tetrahydroxy-6, 8-diprenylisoflavone, on the High-Affinity IgE Receptor-Mediated Activation of Syk in Mast Cells. *J. Agric. Food Chem.* **2015**, *63*, 5459–5467. [CrossRef] [PubMed]
12. Jiang, X.; Cao, C.; Sun, W.; Chen, Z.; Li, X.; Nahar, L.; Sarker, S.D.; Georgiev, M.I.; Bai, W. Scandenolone from *Cudrania tricuspidata* fruit extract suppresses the viability of breast cancer cells (MCF-7) in vitro and in vivo. *Food. Chem. Toxicol.* **2019**, *126*, 56–66. [CrossRef] [PubMed]
13. Li, H.-R.; Habasi, M.; Xie, L.-Z.; Akber Aisa, H. Effect of Chlorogenic Acid on Melanogenesis of B16 Melanoma Cells. *Molecules* **2014**, *19*, 12940–12948. [CrossRef] [PubMed]
14. Stockert, J.C.; Horobin, R.W.; Colombo, L.L.; Blazquez-Castro, A. Tetrazolium salts and formazan products in Cell Biology: Viability assessment, fluorescence imaging, and labeling perspectives. *Acta Histochem.* **2018**, *120*, 159–167. [CrossRef] [PubMed]
15. Di Petrillo, A.; Gonzalez-Paramas, A.M.; Era, B.; Medda, R.; Pintus, F.; Santos-Buelga, C.; Fais, A. Tyrosinase inhibition and antioxidant properties of *Asphodelus microcarpus* extracts. *BMC Complement. Altern. Med.* **2016**, *16*, 453. [CrossRef] [PubMed]
16. Karim, A.A.; Azlan, A.; Ismail, A.; Hashim, P.; Abd Gani, S.S.; Zainudin, B.H.; Abdullah, N.A. Phenolic composition, antioxidant, anti-wrinkles and tyrosinase inhibitory activities of cocoa pod extract. *BMC Complement. Altern. Med.* **2014**, *14*, 381.
17. Kim, S.B.; Jo, Y.H.; Liu, Q.; Ahn, J.H.; Hong, I.P.; Han, S.M.; Hwang, B.Y.; Lee, M.K. Optimization of Extraction Condition of Bee Pollen Using Response Surface Methodology: Correlation between Anti-Melanogenesis, Antioxidant Activity, and Phenolic Content. *Molecules* **2015**, *20*, 19764–19774. [CrossRef] [PubMed]
18. Choi, H.J.; Park, D.H.; Song, S.H.; Yoon, I.S.; Cho, S.S. Development and Validation of a HPLC-UV Method for Extraction Optimization and Biological Evaluation of Hot-Water and Ethanolic Extracts of *Dendropanax morbifera* Leaves. *Molecules* **2018**, *23*, 650. [CrossRef] [PubMed]
19. Oh, H.N.; Seo, J.H.; Lee, M.H.; Kim, C.; Kim, E.; Yoon, G.; Cho, S.S.; Cho, Y.S.; Choi, H.W.; Shim, J.H.; et al. Licochalcone C induced apoptosis in human oral squamous cell carcinoma cells by regulation of the JAK2/STAT3 signaling pathway. *J. Cell. Biochem.* **2018**, *119*, 10118–10130. [CrossRef] [PubMed]
20. Mirmortazavi, S.S.; Farvandi, M.; Ghafouri, H.; Mohammadi, A.; Shourian, M. Evaluation of novel pyrimidine derivatives as a new class of mushroom tyrosinase inhibitor. *Drug. Des. Dev. Ther.* **2019**, *13*, 2169–2178. [CrossRef] [PubMed]

Sample Availability: Samples of the compounds are not available from the authors.

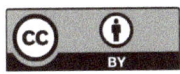

© 2019 by the authors. Licensee MDPI, Basel, Switzerland. This article is an open access article distributed under the terms and conditions of the Creative Commons Attribution (CC BY) license (http://creativecommons.org/licenses/by/4.0/).

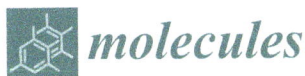

Communication

Validation of a Cell Proliferation Assay to Assess the Potency of a Dialyzable Leukocyte Extract Intended for Batch Release

Gregorio Carballo-Uicab [1], José E. Linares-Trejo [1], Gabriela Mellado-Sánchez [1], Carlos A. López-Morales [1], Marco Velasco-Velázquez [2], Lenin Pavón [3], Sergio Estrada-Parra [4], Sonia Mayra Pérez-Tapia [1,4,5,*] and Emilio Medina-Rivero [1,*]

1. Unidad de Desarrollo e Investigación en Bioprocesos (UDIBI), Escuela Nacional de Ciencias Biológicas, Instituto Politécnico Nacional, Ciudad de Mexico 11340, Mexico; gjcarballo@ipn.mx (G.C.-U.); jelt92@gmail.com (J.E.L.-T.); gmellados@ipn.mx (G.M.-S.); carlos.lopez@udibi.com.mx (C.A.L.-M.)
2. Departamento de Farmacología y Unidad Periférica de Investigación en Biomedicina Traslacional (CMN 20 de noviembre, ISSSTE), Facultad de Medicina, Universidad Nacional Autónoma de México, Ciudad Universitaria, Ciudad de Mexico 04510, Mexico; marcovelasco@unam.mx
3. Laboratorio de Psicoinmunología, Dirección de Investigaciones en Neurociencias del Instituto Nacional de Psiquiatría Ramón de la Fuente, Cuida de Mexico 14370, Mexico; lkuriaki@imp.edu.mx
4. Departamento de Inmunología, Escuela Nacional de Ciencias Biológicas, Instituto Politécnico Nacional, Ciudad de Mexico 11340, Mexico; sestradap07@hotmail.com
5. Laboratorio Nacional para Servicios Especializados de Investigación, Desarrollo e Innovación (I+D+i) para Farmacoquímicos y Biotecnológicos, LANSEIDI-FarBiotec-CONACyT, Ciudad de Mexico 11340, Mexico
* Correspondence: sperezt@ipn.mx (S.M.P.-T.); emilio.medina@udibi.com.mx (E.M.-R.); Tel.: +52-1-5729-6000 (ext. 62543) (S.M.P.-T. & E.M.-R.)

Academic Editors: In-Soo Yoon and Hyun-Jong Cho
Received: 28 August 2019; Accepted: 8 September 2019; Published: 20 September 2019

Abstract: Transferon® is a blood product with immunomodulatory properties constituted by a complex mixture of peptides obtained from a human dialyzable leukocyte extract (DLE). Due to its complex nature, it is necessary to demonstrate batch consistency in its biological activity. Potency is the quantitative measure of biological activity and is also a quality attribute of drugs. Here we developed and validated a proliferation assay using Jurkat cells exposed to azathioprine, which is intended to determine the potency of Transferon® according to international guidelines for pharmaceuticals. The assay showed a linear response (2.5 to 40 µg/mL), coefficients of variation from 0.7 to 13.6% demonstrated that the method is precise, while $r^2 = 0.97$ between the nominal and measured values obtained from dilutional linearity showed that the method is accurate. We also demonstrated that the cell proliferation response was specific for Transferon® and was not induced by its vehicle nor by other peptide complex mixtures (glatiramer acetate or hydrolyzed collagen). The bioassay validated here was used to assess the relative potency of eight released batches of Transferon® with respect to a reference standard, showing consistent results. The collective information from the validation and the assessment of several batches indicate that the bioassay is suitable for the release of Transferon®.

Keywords: dialyzable leukocyte extract; Transferon®; complex mixture of peptides; quality specifications; biological potency; development and validation

1. Introduction

Dialyzable leukocyte extracts (DLEs) are blood products obtained from healthy human donors. These extracts are composed of complex mixtures of peptides that induce immunomodulatory activity [1–3].

Several DLEs have been used worldwide as food supplements but only a few are considered drug products after establishing several controls in the process and in the quality of the finished product. Among the controls, the consistency of batches is essential to ensure the efficacy and safety of a drug product. Consistency is demonstrated through the compliance of the criteria established in quality specifications using suitable analytical methods to assess identity, purity, heterogeneity, and potency [3,4].

The development of analytical methods to be included in the specifications is key to guaranteeing the robustness of the results. Therefore, these methodologies must be validated to demonstrate that the system is suitable for its intended use under a quality control environment [5,6]. However, the development of the methods employed to determine the quality attributes of a drug product containing a complex mixture of peptides is challenging due to its intrinsic heterogeneity [7]. Potency assays are critical for determining batch-to-batch biological activity. In general, in vitro potency methods require cell lines that express specific receptors that recognize the analyte and the measurement of the response elicited by the drug (for example, proliferation, death, cytokines, or growth factors expression) [6,8].

The properties of Transferon®, such as polydispersity of low-molecular-weight peptides, confirm that it is a complex drug [9]. In most of the complex drugs, the mechanism of action is not well understood; however, their therapeutic effect has been well determined for some diseases. Transferon®, a drug product made of DLEs, has been tested in several models. Whereas the in vitro assays allow for obtaining basic knowledge [2,10], the in vivo animal models allow for the evaluation of its effects on pathologies such as viral diseases and neoplasia [1,11]. In humans, it has been specifically proved to be effective as a coadjuvant to conventional therapies of certain diseases involving immunological dysregulation, such as major depressive disorders [12], hypersensitivities (allergic rhinitis, atopic dermatitis, allergic asthma) [13], and some infectious diseases such as herpes zoster and sepsis [14,15].

So far, the batch release tests of Transferon® include an in vivo assay, which evaluates the effect of Transferon® on the survival of mice infected with herpes simplex virus 1 [11], and an in vitro assay, which analyzes the ability of Transferon® to induce interferon-γ expression in Jurkat cells [3]. Although the two methods are convenient alternatives used to determine the biological activity of Transferon®, both also present some disadvantages. For instance, the in vivo assay is affected by multiple variables, and implies complex logistics, high costs, and bioethical issues. Despite the issues involved with the in vitro assay, it is a more feasible alternative since it does not exhibit a dose–response curve because it is a limit test. Thus, new bioassays for the evaluation of DLEs potency are still required.

Recently, the capacity of DLEs to induce Jurkat cell proliferation exposed to azathioprine has been reported without describing the mechanism of action involved for this biological effect, additionally the assay lacks potency estimation with respect to a reference standard and system suitability for a linear response [16], which are required as a routine batch release assay in a quality control environment. In this work, we report the validation of a Jurkat-cells-based assay according to the recommendations for the development, validation, and analysis of bioassays of the United States Pharmacopeia (USP), the European Pharmacopoeia (Ph. Eur.), and the International Council for Harmonization of Technical Requirements for Pharmaceuticals for Human Use (ICH) [5,8,17–19]. Once validated, this bioassay was used to evaluate the biological potency of eight batches of Transferon®, as rendered in the demonstration of the consistency of this attribute.

2. Results and Discussion

2.1. Method Development

Proliferation inhibition of Jurkat clone E6.1 T leukemia cells is induced by a purine analogue, azathioprine, which interferes with the DNA replication [20]. Conversely, the treatment of the cells with both Transferon® and azathioprine avoided this effect in a concentration range from 1 to 180 µg/mL. The obtained dose–response curve exhibited a sigmoidal behavior with a half-maximal effective concentration (EC_{50}) of 13.07 µg/mL, which fitted into the four-parameters logistic model

($r^2 = 0.95$) (Figure 1A). Based on these results we defined a concentration range of Transferon® from 2.5 to 40 µg/mL to obtain a linear response ($r^2 = 0.94$) (Figure 1B). Transferon® did not modify the proliferation of Jurkat cells, unlike the inhibition observed in cells exposed to azathioprine. Additionally, the effect of Transferon® was also evaluated in Daudi cells exposed to azathioprine, showing a similar dose-dependent response (data not shown). These results are evidence of a favorable effect of Transferon® on cell proliferation (Figure 1). Due to the complex composition of the product, it was difficult to elucidate its mechanism of action; however, the biological responses evidenced a modulation of cytokine production, such as interleukine 6, and the ability to promote early differentiation of CD11c$^+$ NK cells [2,10,11]. It allowed for the development and validation of in vitro models to contribute toward biological characterization of the product.

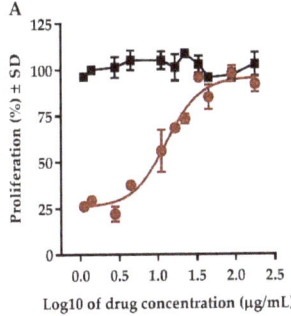
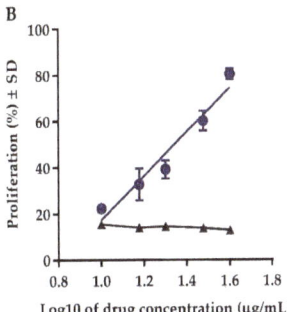

Figure 1. Effect of Transferon® on the proliferation of Jurkat cells. (**A**) Comparison of the Transferon® dose–response curve (1–180 µg/mL) using cells exposed (red circles) and not exposed to azathioprine (black squares). (**B**) Dose–response curve exhibiting a linear behavior in a concentration range from 2.5 to 40 µg/mL Transferon® (blue circles) compared to the response of cells exposed to azathioprine and treated with a vehicle (grey triangles).

In our study, we confirmed that Transferon® was capable of inducing the proliferation of Jurkat cells exposed to azathioprine in a specific concentration range. This was unlike the previous study, which evaluated the batch to batch consistency in biological activity using a single concentration of the product [16]. Usually, the assays for the evaluation of biologics exhibit a non-linear behavior, mainly sigmoidal. We observed this behavior; however, we established the linear range to determine the potency through parallel line analysis (PLA) [17,18,21] in order to evaluate the potency as a critical quality attribute of Transferon®. In this sense, the bioassay validation according to international pharmaceutical guidelines, such as ICH, USP, and Ph. Eur., is mandatory in biological potency tests as a quality specification for biologics and complex drugs [5–8,17].

2.2. Method Validation

The characteristics chosen to demonstrate that the bioassay is suitable for its intended purpose include: concentration range, precision, accuracy, specificity, and system suitability. The parameters and acceptance criteria were defined according to guidelines for pharmaceuticals and previous studies [5,8,17,21,22].

2.2.1. Precision

Repeatability results from three independent samples for each analytic run showed percentage coefficient of variation (%CV) values lower than 25% at each concentration level of the dose–response curve. The intermediate precision (IP) values (inter-analyst, inter-instrument, and inter-assay CV) remained within the established acceptance criterion (≤25%) (Table 1). All the curves employed for the evaluation of precision showed an $r^2 \geq 0.82$ with no significant differences between the slopes or the intercepts obtained for each IP analysis (Table 1, Figure S1).

Table 1. Evaluation of repeatability and intermediate precision.

	Repeatability			Intermediate Precision			Equality Analysis	
	r^2	CV (%)	n	r^2	CV (%)	n	Slopes	Intercepts
Analyst 1	0.85	3.6–13.6	3	0.90	3.9–10.5	6	$F_{(1, 26)} = 0.4851$	$F_{(1, 27)} = 0.3962$
Analyst 2	0.95	0.7–8.9	3				$p = 0.4923$	$p = 0.5344$
Microplate Reader 1	0.95	0.7–8.9	3	0.96	2.4–7.6	6	$F_{(1, 26)} = 0.1471$	$F_{(1, 27)} = 0.2936$
Microplate reader 2	0.96	1.9–7.5	3				$p = 0.7040$	$p = 0.5923$
Run 1	0.82	7.3–22.6	3	0.83	8.4–16.6	6	$F_{(1, 26)} = 0.3208$	$F_{(1, 27)} = 0.4033$
Run 2	0.85	0.6–12.6	3				$p = 0.5760$	$p = 0.5308$

2.2.2. Accuracy

The results obtained from the dilutional linearity showed an upper shift in the vertical distance at 130 and 140% levels, while 60 and 70% levels showed a lower shift in the vertical distance with respect to the 100% linearity level (Figure 2A). All the curves obtained at each level of the dilutional linearity were demonstrated to be parallels using PLA analysis. All curves showed $r^2 \geq 0.85$ during the linear regression analysis and $r^2 = 0.97$ between the nominal and the measured potency (Figure 2B).

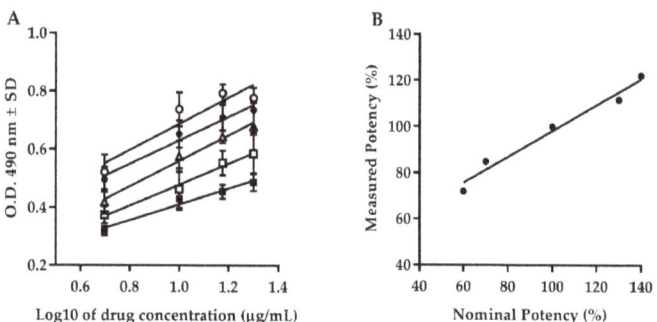

Figure 2. Accuracy. (**A**) Behavior of dilutional linearity at dilution levels of 60% (black squares), 70% (white squares), 100% (white triangles), 130% (black circles), and 140% (white circles) of Transferon®. (**B**) Relationship between nominal and measured potency at dilution levels from 60 to 140% ($r^2 = 0.97$). O.D.: Optical Density; SD: Standard Deviation.

2.2.3. Specificity

After comparing the responses exhibited by Transferon®, Colagenart®, and Copaxone®, and the vehicle control, it was observed that only Transferon® induced proliferation activity in cells exposed to azathioprine.

In the slope comparison analysis, Colagenart® ($F_{(1, 2)} = 3.086$, $p = 0.2210$), Copaxone® ($F_{(1, 2)} = 0.023$, $p = 0.8934$), and the vehicle control ($F_{(1, 2)} = 2.836$, $p = 0.2342$) did not show significant differences with respect to zero during the F-test. The response obtained with Transferon® ($F_{(1, 2)} = 69.06$, $p = 0.0142$) remained within the acceptance criterion for this attribute (Figure 3). The results demonstrated that this method is specific for the evaluation of the biological activity of Transferon®.

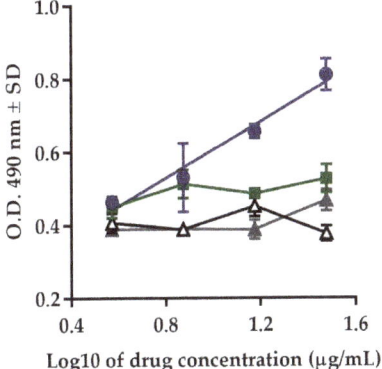

Figure 3. Specificity. Comparison of the response of Transferon® (blue circles) with Colagenart® (green squares), Copaxone® (white triangles), and the vehicle control (grey triangles).

2.2.4. System Suitability

The system suitability was established during the development and validation of the bioassay. All the established parameters were defined as pre-requisites to assess the potency of Transferon® by demonstrating linearity of response, parallelism, and evident biological response (Table 2).

Table 2. Results of the parameters determined during the evaluation of eight batches of Transferon® for system suitability.

Batch	Potency (80–125%)	C.I. 95% (74–136%)	Δ Response (≥2)	r^2 (≥0.8)	CV (≤25%)
	Results	Results	Results	Results	Results
18E13	100.0	100–100	2.9	0.96	0.7–8.9
18E14	112.8	104–121	3.5	0.94	14–22
18C08	110.5	102–118	3.5	0.92	3.0–16
18D10	97.8	90–105	2.9	0.96	3.7–14
18D09	87.0	79–94	2.5	0.95	3.3–13
18D11	98.2	94–102	3.0	0.98	4.5–9.1
18D12	95.5	91–99	2.9	0.98	1.2–7.9
18B06	102.3	98–106	3.2	0.97	0.5–2.7
18C07	103.9	99–108	3.1	0.98	0.7–4.7

A linear response was observed in a concentration range (from 5 to 30 μg/mL) for all the evaluated batches ($r^2 \geq 0.92$) with curves constructed with five data points. The %CV was established between 0.5 to 22. All the evaluated batches showed a response ratio ≥ 2.5 compared to the control containing cells treated only with azathioprine. This means that Transferon® doubled the proliferation response (optical density, O.D.) of Jurkat cells despite the presence of a cell proliferation inhibitor (azathioprine).

2.2.5. Batch Consistency

The F-test ($F_{(4, 15)} = 0.7519$, $p = 0.5721$) showed equality of slopes in all the evaluated batches, demonstrating the parallelism among curves. The consistency of relative potency among batches was observed between 87 and 113%, while the C.I. 95% range was from 79 to 121% for the eight evaluated batches, complying with the acceptance criteria for this attribute (Figure 4 and Table 2).

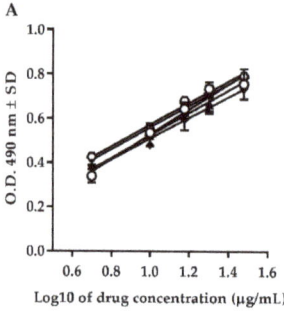 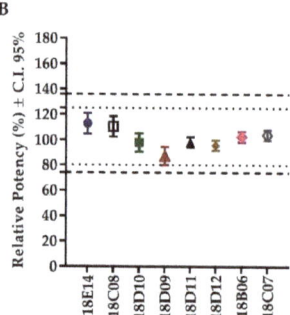

Figure 4. Consistency of the potency among batches of Transferon®. (**A**) Dose–response curves of different batches of Transferon®. (**B**) Relative potency of eight batches of Transferon® with confidence intervals (C.I.) at 95% ($n = 3$).

The results obtained during the validation exercise showed that the bioassay was linear, precise, accurate, specific, and suitable to evaluate the biological potency of Transferon®. Our results demonstrated consistency in the biological potency of the product and supported our proposal of using this bioassay as an additional suitable method for batch release. Currently, the analytical methods indicated within the Transferon® specification included protein content, endotoxin, sterility, identity, and biological activity [3,11]. All batches used in this work met the acceptance criteria for release using an in vivo method and the in vitro assay validated in this work.

3. Materials and Methods

3.1. Materials

We employed Jurkat E6.1 cells (American Type Culture Collection, ATCC, Manassas, VA, USA), Roswell Park Memorial Institute (RPMI) medium (ATCC, Manassas, VA, USA), fetal bovine serum (FBS) (Gibco, Thermo Scientific, Waltham, MA, USA), cell proliferation assay kit ([3-(4,5-dimethylthiazol-2-yl)-5-(3-carboxymethoxyphenyl)-2-(4-sulfophenyl)-2H-tetrazolium, inner salt; MTS) (Promega Corporation, Madison, WI, USA), and azathioprine (Sigma-Aldrich, St. Louis, MO, USA).

Two products containing a complex mixture of peptides were used as controls, glatiramer acetate (Copaxone®) acquired from Teva Pharmaceutical Industries (Central District, Israel) and hydrolyzed collagen (Colagenart®) acquired from LEMAR S.A.P.I. de C.V. (Mexico City, Mexico).

The development and validation of the bioassay were performed using nine commercial batches of human DLEs (Transferon®) (18B06, 18C07, 18C08, 18D09, 18D10, 18D11, 18D12, 18E13, and 18E14) provided by Pharma-FT (Mexico City, Mexico). Batch 18E13 was used as a reference standard.

3.2. Cell Culture and In Vitro Cell-Based Assay

Jurkat E6.1 cells were grown in RPMI-1640 medium with 10% FBS and placed at 37 °C in 5% CO_2 at maximum concentration of 1×10^6 cells/mL. Prior to the assay, the cells were maintained in RPMI-1640 medium without FBS for 12–18 h. Afterwards, the cells were plated at 2×10^4 cells/well in a sterile 96-well plate and co-treated with azathioprine (6.25 µg/mL) and different concentrations of Transferon® (2.5–40 µg/mL) in a final volume of 200 µL/well with RPMI medium supplemented with 10% FBS. Cultures were incubated at 37 °C, 5% CO_2 for 72 h. Azathioprine-untreated cells and vehicle (water for injection) plus azathioprine were used as negative controls. After the incubation, MTS was added to every well of the plate and incubated for 4 h at 37 °C in 5% CO_2. The O.D. was measured at 490 nm using a microplate reader (SpectraMax® M3, Molecular Devices, San Jose, CA, USA, and EPOCH spectrophotometer for IP determination, BioTek, Winooski, VT, USA).

3.3. International Pharmaceutical Guidelines

All the work in this paper was executed following the recommendations of Chapters 1032 [8], 1033 [19], and 1034 [18] of the USP for the development, validation, and analysis of bioassays, respectively, as well as Chapter 5.3 of the Ph. Eur. [17], and Validation of analytical procedures: text and methodology Q2 (R1) from ICH [5].

3.4. Method Development

The aims of the development was, first, to evaluate whether Transferon® was capable of inducing the proliferation of Jurkat cells exposed to azathioprine, and second, to establish the experimental conditions and parameters to minimize variability in the assay. In this stage, we found the concentration range that allowed for evaluating non-linear and linear responses. Additionally, we evaluated the effect of only Transferon® on the proliferation of Jurkat cells as a control for the assay. The proliferation percentage (%) was calculated by dividing the O.D. of the cells treated with Transferon® by the O.D. of the untreated cells with and without exposure to azathioprine.

3.5. Method Validation

3.5.1. Precision

Precision was evaluated at the level of repeatability and IP. Repeatability was estimated through the %CV between three independent replicates during an analytic run. The IP was measured through the %CV between two analysts, two instruments, and two independent analytical runs. Five concentration levels with independent triplicates were included in all the assays. The established acceptance criterion was a CV ≤ 25% for each dilution level.

3.5.2. Accuracy

Accuracy was evaluated as the dilutional linearity at dilution levels of 60, 70, 100, 130, and 140% for the dose–response curve. Relative potency was calculated with PLA analysis using the Softmax Pro 7.0.3 GxP software (Molecular Devices, San Jose, CA, USA), and the potency was relative at the 100% linearity level. The acceptance criterion for linearity was $r^2 \geq 0.80$ between the nominal and the measured values.

3.5.3. Specificity

Specificity was evaluated by comparing the biological response of Transferon® with respect to other products composed of a complex mixture of peptides, including glatiramer acetate (Copaxone®) and hydrolyzed collagen (Colagenart®). Additionally, the obtained response was compared to the vehicle control (water for injection). The established acceptance criterion was the expected value for the characteristic biological response with Transferon® while complex mixtures of peptides or the vehicle control did not show biological effect.

3.5.4. System Suitability

System suitability was established according to the linear model and precision. The acceptance criteria were: linear response ($r^2 \geq 0.8$); ratio (Δ) between the maximum response and control response ≥ 2, using at least four points in the construction of the straight line; and CV ≤ 25%.

3.6. Batch-to-Batch Consitency

Relative potency was determined in eight Transferon® batches using PLA analysis and an F-test to compare slopes. A reference standard batch was used to calculate the relative potency. The acceptance criteria were: relative potency between 80–125% and 95% confidence intervals (C.I.) between 74–136%.

3.7. Statistical Analysis

The fitting of raw data to the linear model and relative potency analysis were performed using the Sofmax Pro 7.0.3 GxP software. An analysis of covariance (ANCOVA) with the F distribution was used to test for equality of slopes. The analysis was performed using the Graph Pad Prism 6.0 software (GraphPad Software, San Diego, La Jolla CA, USA).

4. Conclusions

The validation of the bioassay according to international guidelines for pharmaceutical products showed that it was suitable to evaluate the biological activity of DLEs and to determine the relative potency. In addition, we confirmed that this bioassay was also suitable to determine the relative potency among different batches of Transferon®, which confirmed the consistency of the quality attributes. The collective information from this study will allow for the establishment of relative potency as a critical attribute of Transferon®, along with the rapid implementation of this assay in a quality control laboratory as batch release analysis.

Supplementary Materials: The following are available online, Figure S1: Determination of repeatability (P) and intermediate precision (IP). (A) Inter-analysts %CV. (B) Inter-instruments %CV between different instruments (Microplate Reader MR). (C) Inter-analytical runs %CV.

Author Contributions: Conceptualization, G.C.-U., S.M.P.-T. and E.M.-R.; methodology, G.C.-U. and J.E.L.-T.; validation, G.C.-U. and J.E.L.-T.; formal analysis, G.C.-U.; resources, S.M.P.-T. and E.M.-R.; data curation, G.C.-U., J.E.L.-T., C.A.L.-M. and E.M.-R.; writing—original draft preparation, G.C.-U., J.E.L.-T., G.M.-S., C.A.L.-M. and E.M.-R.; writing—review and editing, G.C.-U., J.E.L.-T., G.M.-S., C.A.L.-M., S.E.-P., M.V.-V., L.P., S.M.P.-T. and E.M.-R.; supervision, G.M.-S., C.A.L.-M., L.P., S.M.P.-T. and E.M.-R.

Funding: This work was supported by UDIBI.

Acknowledgments: The authors thank CONACYT, who granted resources for our laboratory through "Laboratorio Nacional para Servicios Especializados de Investigación, Desarrollo e Innovación (I+D+i) para Farmoquímicos y Biotecnológicos" (LANSEIDI-FarBiotec-CONACyT).

Conflicts of Interest: Carballo-Uicab G, Linares-Trejo JE, Mellado-Sánchez G, López-Morales CA, Estrada-Parra S, Pérez-Tapia SM, and Medina-Rivero E have participated at different stages of the development of Transferon®. Pavón L and Velasco-Velázquez M declare no conflict of interest.

References

1. Hernandez-Esquivel, M.A.; Perez-Torres, A.; Romero-Romero, L.; Reyes-Matute, A.; Loaiza, B.; Mellado-Sanchez, G.; Pavon, L.; Medina-Rivero, E.; Pestell, R.G.; Perez-Tapia, S.M.; et al. The dialyzable leukocyte extract Transferon (™) inhibits tumor growth and brain metastasis in a murine model of prostate cancer. *Biomed. Pharmacother.* **2018**, *101*, 938–944. [CrossRef] [PubMed]
2. Jimenez-Uribe, A.P.; Valencia-Martinez, H.; Carballo-Uicab, G.; Vallejo-Castillo, L.; Medina-Rivero, E.; Chacon-Salinas, R.; Pavon, L.; Velasco-Velazquez, M.A.; Mellado-Sanchez, G.; Estrada-Parra, S.; et al. CD80 Expression Correlates with IL-6 Production in THP-1-Like Macrophages Costimulated with LPS and Dialyzable Leukocyte Extract (Transferon®). *J. Immunol. Res.* **2019**, *2019*, 2198508. [CrossRef] [PubMed]
3. Medina-Rivero, E.; Merchand-Reyes, G.; Pavon, L.; Vazquez-Leyva, S.; Perez-Sanchez, G.; Salinas-Jazmin, N.; Estrada-Parra, S.; Velasco-Velazquez, M.; Perez-Tapia, S.M. Batch-to-batch reproducibility of Transferon. *J. Pharm. Biomed. Anal.* **2014**, *88*, 289–294. [CrossRef] [PubMed]
4. Xiong, H.; Yu, L.X.; Qu, H. Batch-to-batch quality consistency evaluation of botanical drug products using multivariate statistical analysis of the chromatographic fingerprint. *AAPS PharmSciTech* **2013**, *14*, 802–810. [CrossRef] [PubMed]
5. Guideline, I.H.T. Validation of Analytical Procedures: Text and methodology Q2 (R1) version 4. In Proceedings of the International Conference for Harmonization, Geneva, Switzerland, November 2005.
6. WHO. *Guidelines on Evaluation of Similar Biotherapeutic Products (SBPs)*; Annex 2; Technical Report Series No. 977; WHO: Geneva, Switzerland, 2009; pp. 64–65.

7. Hussaarts, L.; Muhlebach, S.; Shah, V.P.; McNeil, S.; Borchard, G.; Fluhmann, B.; Weinstein, V.; Neervannan, S.; Griffiths, E.; Jiang, W.; et al. Equivalence of complex drug products: Advances in and challenges for current regulatory frameworks. *Ann. N. Y. Acad. Sci.* **2017**, *1407*, 39–49. [CrossRef] [PubMed]
8. *USP chapter <1032> Development and Design of Bioassays*; USP 35-NF-30; USP Pharmacopeical Convention: Rockville, MD, USA, 2017.
9. Lopez-Morales, C.A.; Vazquez-Leyva, S.; Vallejo-Castillo, L.; Carballo-Uicab, G.; Munoz-Garcia, L.; Herbert-Pucheta, J.E.; Zepeda-Vallejo, L.G.; Velasco-Velazquez, M.; Pavon, L.; Perez-Tapia, S.M.; et al. Determination of Peptide Profile Consistency and Safety of Collagen Hydrolysates as Quality Attributes. *J. Food Sci.* **2019**, *84*, 430–439. [CrossRef] [PubMed]
10. Ramirez-Ramirez, D.; Vadillo, E.; Arriaga-Pizano, L.A.; Mayani, H.; Estrada-Parra, S.; Velasco-Velazquez, M.A.; Perez-Tapia, S.M.; Pelayo, R. Early Differentiation of Human CD11c(+)NK Cells with gammadelta T Cell Activation Properties Is Promoted by Dialyzable Leukocyte Extracts. *J. Immunol. Res.* **2016**, *2016*, 4097642. [CrossRef] [PubMed]
11. Salinas-Jazmin, N.; Estrada-Parra, S.; Becerril-Garcia, M.A.; Limon-Flores, A.Y.; Vazquez-Leyva, S.; Medina-Rivero, E.; Pavon, L.; Velasco-Velazquez, M.A.; Perez-Tapia, S.M. Herpes murine model as a biological assay to test dialyzable leukocyte extracts activity. *J. Immunol. Res.* **2015**, *2015*, 146305. [CrossRef] [PubMed]
12. Hernandez, M.E.; Mendieta, D.; Perez-Tapia, M.; Bojalil, R.; Estrada-Garcia, I.; Estrada-Parra, S.; Pavon, L. Effect of selective serotonin reuptake inhibitors and immunomodulator on cytokines levels: An alternative therapy for patients with major depressive disorder. *Clin. Dev. Immunol.* **2013**, *2013*, 267871. [CrossRef] [PubMed]
13. Berron-Perez, R.; Chavez-Sanchez, R.; Estrada-Garcia, I.; Espinosa-Padilla, S.; Cortez-Gomez, R.; Serrano-Miranda, E.; Ondarza-Aguilera, R.; Perez-Tapia, M.; Olvera, B.P.; Mdel, C.J.-M.; et al. Indications, usage, and dosage of the transfer factor. *Rev. Alerg. Mex.* **2007**, *54*, 134–139. [PubMed]
14. Castrejón-Vázquez, M.I.; Reséndiz-Albor, A.A.; Ynga-Durand, M.A.; Arciniega-Martínez, I.M.; Orellana-Villazon, V.I.; García-López, C.A.; Laue-Noguera, M.L.; Vargas-Camaño, M.E. Dialyzable Leukocyte Extract (Transferon) administration in Sepsis: Experience from a single referral pediatric intensive care unit. *BioMed. Res. Int.* **2019**, in press.
15. Estrada-Parra, S.; Nagaya, A.; Serrano, E.; Rodriguez, O.; Santamaria, V.; Ondarza, R.; Chavez, R.; Correa, B.; Monges, A.; Cabezas, R.; et al. Comparative study of transfer factor and acyclovir in the treatment of herpes zoster. *Int. J. Immunopharmacol.* **1998**, *20*, 521–535. [CrossRef]
16. Cardoso, F.M.; Tomkova, M.; Petrovajova, D.; Bubanova, M.; Ragac, O.; Hornakova, T. New and cost effective cell-based assay for Dialyzed Leukocyte Extract (DLE)-induced Jurkat cells proliferation under azathioprine treatment. *J. Pharm. Biomed. Anal.* **2017**, *138*, 100–108. [CrossRef] [PubMed]
17. Chapter 5.3, Statistical Analysis of Results of Biological Assays and Test. In *European Pharmacopia 6.0*, 5th ed.; The Stationery Office: London, UK, 2005.
18. *USP Chapter <1034> Analysis of Biological Assays*; USP 35-NF-30; USP Pharmacopeical Convention: Rockville, MD, USA, 2013.
19. *USP Chapter <1033> Biological Assay Validation*; USP 35-NF-30; USP Pharmacopeical Convention: Rockville, MD, USA, 2017.
20. Maltzman, J.S.; Koretzky, G.A. Azathioprine: Old drug, new actions. *J. Clin. Investig.* **2003**, *111*, 1122–1124. [CrossRef] [PubMed]
21. Fleetwood, K.; Bursa, F.; Yellowlees, A. Parallelism in practice: Approaches to parallelism in bioassays. *PDA J. Pharm. Sci. Technol.* **2015**, *69*, 248–263. [CrossRef] [PubMed]
22. Food Drug and Administration. Bioanalytical Method Validation. In *Guidance for Industry*; Biopharmaceutics, Ed.; Food Drug and Administration: White Oak, MD, USA, 2018; pp. 1–35.

Sample Availability: Samples of Transferon® are available from the authors.

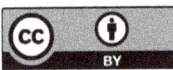

© 2019 by the authors. Licensee MDPI, Basel, Switzerland. This article is an open access article distributed under the terms and conditions of the Creative Commons Attribution (CC BY) license (http://creativecommons.org/licenses/by/4.0/).

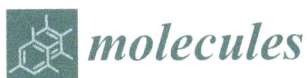

Article

Development of an Oriental Medicine Discrimination Method through Analysis of Steroidal Saponins in *Dioscorea nipponica* Makino and Their Anti-Osteosarcoma Effects

Joo Tae Hwang, Ki-Sun Park, Jin Ah Ryuk, Hye Jin Kim and Byoung Seob Ko *

Korea Institute of Oriental Medicine, Daejeon 34054, Korea; jthwang@kiom.re.kr (J.T.H.); kisunpark@kiom.re.kr (K.-S.P.); yukjinah@kiom.re.kr (J.A.R.); kimhyejin43@kiom.re.kr (H.J.K.)
* Correspondence: bsko@kiom.re.kr; Tel.: +82-42-868-9542; Fax: +82-42-868-9537

Received: 7 October 2019; Accepted: 5 November 2019; Published: 6 November 2019

Abstract: To prevent confusing *Dioscorea nipponica* (DN), an Oriental medicine, with *Dioscorea quinquelobata* (DQ) and *Dioscorea septemloba* (DS), a simple and accurate quantitative analysis method using HPLC combined with ultraviolet (UV) detection was developed and verified with UPLC-QTOF/MS through identification of five saponin glycosides: protodioscin (**1**), protogracillin (**2**), pseudoprotodioscin (**3**), dioscin (**4**), and gracillin (**5**). The newly developed analysis method showed sufficient reproducibility (<1.91%) and accuracy (92.1%–102.6%) and was able to identify DN based on the presence of compound **3** (13.821 ± 0.037 mg/mL) and the absence of **5**. Compound **1**, which is present in DN at a relatively high level (159.983 ± 0.064 mg/mL), was also an important marker for identification. Among the three species, DN showed the strongest activation of apoptotic signaling in osteosarcoma cells, while the four compounds detected in DN showed IC_{50} values of 6.43 (**1**), 10.61 (**2**), 10.48 (**3**), and 6.90 (**4**). In conclusion, the strong inhibitory effect of DN against osteosarcoma was confirmed to be associated with **1** and **4**, which is also related to the quantitative results. Therefore, the results of this study might provide important information for quality control related to Oriental medicine.

Keywords: *Dioscorea nipponica* Makino; steroidal saponin; HPLC-UV; UPLC-QTOF/MS; validation; osteosarcoma; apoptosis

---

Academic Editors: In-Soo Yoon and Hyun-Jong Cho

1. Introduction

Among the various *Dioscorea* families, *Dioscorea nipponica* (DN) is a wild perennial species that is widely distributed in the Korean peninsula, Japan, and China, along with *Dioscorea tokoro*, *Dioscorea japonica*, *Dioscorea tenuipes*, *Dioscorea quinquelobata* (DQ), and *Dioscorea septemloba* (DS). DN, the dried roots and stems of which are used for medicinal purposes in Oriental medicine, is known as Cheon-san-ryong. This medicine has traditionally been prescribed for the treatment of rheumatism, asthma, and bronchitis; alleviating pain; and improving blood circulation. Additionally, the origin of the species specified in the standard medicines of North Korea [1] and China [2] is designated as DN. In China, which is a major producer of DN, approximately 49 species of the genus *Dioscorea* are found, and two of these species, DN and *Dioscorea panthaica*, are systematically managed by the Chinese Pharmacopeia Committee (CHD) as raw medicine materials [3]. However, in the private sector in South Korea, this medicine is not explicitly distinguished from DQ and DS, which are homogeneous and morphologically similar to DN [4]. Thus, a scientific and systematic approach to clearly identify the origin of DN is absolutely necessary, but no relevant research has been carried out to date. Additionally, quality control of raw materials is always necessary for commercial development, and the development of chemical analysis methods is key to quality control.

As part of this study, previously reported compounds from the *Dioscorea* family, including DQ and DS, were searched. In previous studies, steroidal saponins have mainly been found in members of the genus *Dioscoreaceae*, and the identified active components are steroidal saponins, including furostanol saponins and isospirostanol saponins [5]. Among the identified compounds, the steroidal saponins of three furostanol derivatives, protodioscin (**1**), protogracillin (**2**), and pseudoprotodioscin (**3**), and two spirostanol derivatives, dioscin (**4**), and gracillin (**5**), could be utilized as important indicators for development of an analytical method (Figure 1). Due to their biological activities, members of the genus *Dioscoreaceae* are being studied by numerous researchers to achieve efficient separation and purification of one of the steroids, diosgenin, and its steroidal saponin, dioscin [6]. For example, a recent study reported the optimized extraction of these compounds, with the highest extract content when 50% acetonitrile (ACN) was used for 60 minutes in ultrasonic extraction. However, compared with the yield of individual compounds, protodioscin had the best extraction efficiency at 50% ACN, whereas for dioscin, 70% ACN was more efficient [7]. Several analytical methods for determination of the above compounds have been reported previously. Although these analyses primarily used LC-ESI-MS or MS/MS, the development of analysis methods using HPLC is also frequently reported [8–10]. However, these analytical methods could not be fully verified because there were not sufficient indicator components to clearly distinguish the origin of the drug from similar species, and the steroidal saponins of *Dioscorea* have been tentatively confirmed by MS fragmentation analyses. Additionally, in the case of steroidal saponins, ultraviolet (UV) detection is generally less sensitive, and thus, it is natural to use ELSD (evaporative scattering detection) detectors, including for MS analysis, frequently. These detectors can be a powerful detection method but limit analysis options. Therefore, it is also very important to develop an analysis method that is reliable and exhibits sufficient sensitivity using UV detectors for a wide range of sample extract analyses.

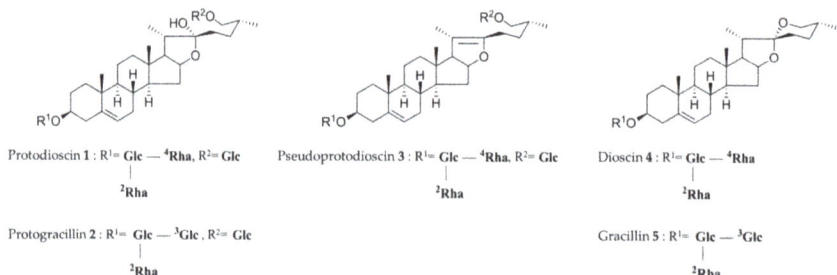

Figure 1. Chemical structures of the standards for HPLC validations (Glc = β-D-glucopyranosyl, Rha = α-L-rhamnopyranosyl).

Saponins show potential as anticancer agents. As previously reported, wild species of *Dioscorea* families, including DN, were found to contain at least 10 to 20 times more dioscin, a major pharmacological component and a saponin exhibiting strong anticancer activity, than cultivated species, such as *Dioscorea opposita* or *Dioscorea batatas* [11]. This finding shows that DN is a very attractive material for commercialization, which can be realized through further research. Recently, the positive effects of steroidal saponins as a treatment for osteosarcoma, which is known to have a poor prognosis, have been reported. The cause of osteosarcoma is unclear, and in most cases, it appears to be sporadic, especially in people in their teens, where it is associated with increased growth. Currently, surgery and chemotherapy are combined to treat osteosarcoma, and efforts are being made to develop new natural products for effective chemotherapy. Therefore, it is necessary to investigate the possibility of treating osteosarcoma with DS, DQ, and DN that contain steroidal saponins and to examine the most effective extracts [12–20].

Thus, here, an accurate and reproducible HPLC/UV analysis method was developed to isolate five steroid saponins that were identified in the *Dioscorea* families. This method was then applied to traditional medicines and allowed differentiation of raw materials originating from similar but different species. Quadrupole time-of-flight MS (QTOF/MS) combined with ultra-performance liquid chromatography (UPLC) was used to confirm the steroidal saponins in the samples. In addition, the bioactive compounds in raw plants were quantified, and the ability of these compounds to inhibit osteosarcoma was tested to identify new pharmacological activities of DN and its active components.

2. Results and Discussion

2.1. Optimization of Chromatographic Conditions

Generally, HPLC/UV analysis is not recommended for steroidal saponins because they lack a chromophore suitable for UV detection [3]. This challenge is a good motivator for studying whether the target compounds can be detected accurately without being influenced by impurities; although ELSD [21] or ESI-MS [22,23] detectors have been used in previous studies, low-wavelength UV offers superior sensitivity. The main focus of this study was to develop reliable analysis methods that are more efficient and generally easy for users to analyze rather than to develop powerful but less frequently used and costly analyses using various MS or MS/MS, such as the above mentioned. This is a very important factor in the industrialization of materials in the future. Clearly, however, there is a limit to determining the individual peaks accurately just by retention time through the DAD-UV wavelength. On the other hand, more reliable data can be obtained using the MS detector. In this study, to compensate for these defects, verification experiments were conducted on five compounds detected through an analysis developed with HPLC/UV using one of the most powerful MS, UHPLC-QTOF/MS. In the same manner, further results of validation tests under the ICH Guide (International Conference on Harmonization) have become an important factor in verifying the developed HPLC/UV analysis method. In addition, validation studies including quantitative analysis of steroid compounds in DN through QTOF/MS analysis had already been reported [3], but the results of the recovery rate were found to be 72.79% to 118.31%, and showed significant differences in accuracy and recoveries when compared with the results of this study using UV detector.

Therefore, the photodiode array (PDA) spectrum (190–800 nm) was used to determine the maximum absorbance of each compound, and a wavelength of 200 nm was chosen as the optimum wavelength for analysis. Reviews of UV/VIS analyses of several previously reported protodioscins have shown that the maximum absorbance of the compound is approximately 1.6 times greater at 200 nm [11], although a number of studies primarily selected wavelengths of 205 nm [8,24,25], possibly to reduce the effect of baseline signals from solvents or impurities. However, using a wavelength of 200 nm, the limit of detection (LOD) and limit of quantitation (LOQ) were determined by analyzing standards at various concentrations to evaluate whether this wavelength is suitable for developing an analysis method based on UV detection.

To optimize the conditions for analysis of steroidal saponins derived from *Dioscorea*, sufficient baseline separation between structurally similar compounds, between dioscin and gracillin and between protodioscin and protogracillin had to be achieved. Preliminary experiments were conducted using a variety of columns to improve peak resolution. Finally, these steroid glucoside compounds could be conveniently separated using a Triart C18 PFP resin column, which has lower polarity and higher hydrophobicity than a standard C18 column. Meanwhile, a previous study reported the optimal analysis conditions for compounds **1**, **2**, **4**, and **5** in DN and the resolutions of three different stationary phases (Hypersil GOLD C18, Unison UK-C18, and Kinetex C18 column) and temperatures (15 °C to 45 °C), and the Kinetex C18 column presented the most efficient separation when analysis was performed at 15 °C [26]. However, although the conditions in this previous study allowed more rapid analysis than those used in this study, the previous analysis did not include compound **3**.

Furthermore, with the selected column, the sample was eluted under gradient conditions using a mixture of acetonitrile (A) and triple-distilled water (B). The compounds were not stable when a methanolic eluent was used, as previously reported [4,8,9], because protodioscin (furanol saponin) is rapidly converted to methyl protodioscin, its 22-O-methyl analogue, under high pH or methanol conditions. In terms of the solvent gradient program and column temperature, gradient elution with A/B = 23/77 to 33/67 (0–25 min), 33/67 to 34/66 (25–50 min), and 34/66 to 100/0 (5–65 min) at a flow rate of 1 mL/min and at 40 °C provided the optimal separation performance. Under these HPLC conditions, all compounds were detected without interference from impurities, and their retention times were 12.4 (**1**), 13.5 (**2**), 22.9 (**3**), 56.3 (**4**), and 57.2 (**5**) min (Figure 2). Further, based on the analysis results at 200 nm for the five types of compounds present in each sample (DN, DS, and DQ) under the conditions set above, UV spectra with a wavelength range of 190 to 800 nm were evaluated to examine the peaks for each compound according to retention time, and a total purity of 95% was verified.

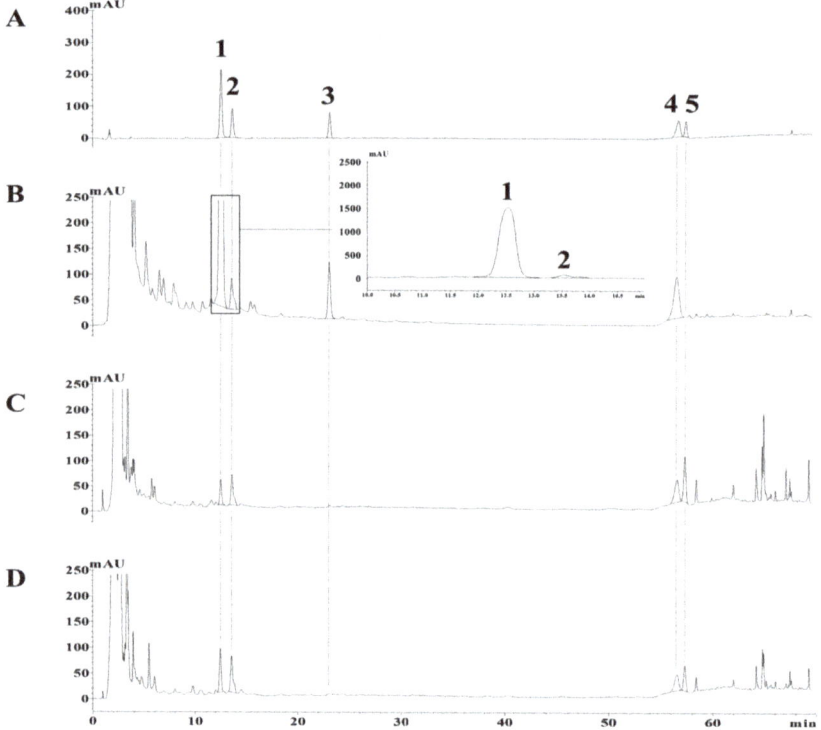

Figure 2. HPLC chromatograms of five standards (**A**, 1 mg/mL); and the DN (**B**, 40 mg/mL), DQ (**C**, 40 mg/mL) and DS (**D**, 40 mg/mL) samples. DN: *Dioscorea nipponica*; DQ: *Dioscorea quinquelobata*. DS: *Dioscorea septemloba*.

2.2. Assay Validation

2.2.1. Linearity

A linearity test was conducted to validate the calibration curve produced by the developed method. Between 7 and 12 sequentially diluted solutions of the test compounds at different concentrations (i.e., 0.01, 0.02, 0.03, 0.05, 0.1, 0.2, 0.3, 0.5, 0.7, 1, 2, and 4 mg/mL) were analyzed in triplicate. The calibration curves of the five tested compounds showed sufficient linearity with r^2 values of 0.9992 (**1**), 0.9998 (**2**), 0.9995 (**3**), 0.9990 (**4**), and 0.9999 (**5**) (Table 1).

Table 1. Linearity, LOD, and LOQ of the standard compounds.

Compounds	t_R (min)	Equation (Linear Model)[a]	Linear Range (mg/mL)	r^{2} [b]	LOD [c] (mg/mL)	LOQ [d] (mg/mL)
1	12.4	y = 3,442,356x − 8492	0.02–4	0.9992	0.0009	0.0026
2	13.5	y = 1,353,127x + 13,963	0.02–4	0.9998	0.0022	0.0065
3	22.9	y = 1,269,657x − 23,913	0.02–4	0.9995	0.0007	0.0020
4	56.3	y = 1,528,845x + 2521	0.03–0.7	0.9990	0.0132	0.0400
5	57.2	y = 1,462,227x − 826	0.01–0.3	0.9999	0.0027	0.0081

[a] y: peak area at 200 nm; x: standard concentration (mg/mL). [b] r^2: coefficient of determination with 7–12 indicated points in the calibration curves. [c] LOD: limit of detection; S/N = 3 (n = 5). [d] LOQ: limit of quantification; S/N = 10 (n = 5).

2.2.2. Precision and Accuracy

The accuracy and precision were tested using two different samples, DN and DQ, because they contained different proportions of the target compounds. As shown in Figure 2, the chromatograph of DS was similar to that of DQ, and they had the same chemical component composition. Thus, DQ, which is more important, was used for subsequent accuracy and precision experiments.

To verify the accuracy of the analysis method, recovery experiments were conducted, and the average recoveries of the DN samples after being spiked with compounds **1, 2, 3,** and **4** at three different concentrations were found to be 92.1% to 100.9% (**1**), 100.0% to 100.6% (**2**), 100.2% to 100.3% (**3**), and 100.1% to 102.6% (**4**). In the case of DQ, the recoveries of compounds **1, 2, 4,** and **5** were found to be 93.7% to 101.0% (**1**), 98.3% to 106.2% (**2**), 96.4% to 100.8% (**4**), and 93.8% to 104.5% (**5**).

To assess the precision reliability of the analysis method, the RSD (relative standard deviation) values (%) of intra- and interday experiments were determined. In the intraday variability test, the RSD values for compounds **1, 2, 3,** and **4** in DN ranged from 0.03 to 0.05 (**1**), 0.14 to 0.22 (**2**), 0.04 to 0.16 (**3**), and 0.14 to 0.22 (**4**), and in DQ, the RSD values of compounds **1, 2, 4** and **5** were identified as 1.91 (**1**), 0.31 to 1.15 (**2**), 0.26 to 0.44 (**4**), and 0.27 to 0.82 (**5**). The RSD (%) of interday analyses conducted on three consecutive days for precision verification ranged from 0.01 to 0.01 (**1**), 0.12 to 0.01 (**2**), 0.03 to 0.10 (**3**), and 0.10 to 1.48 (**4**) for DN. As with accuracy, the precision was also verified for DQ, and the RSD (%) values of the compounds ranged between 0.15 and 0.55 (**1**), 0.48 and 0.73 (**2**), 0.38 and 0.75 (**4**), and 0.29 and 0.70 (**5**). These results indicate that the precision and accuracy of the method are sufficient to ensure that simultaneous analysis of the five compounds in DN and DQ is reliable and accurate (Tables 2 and 3)

Table 2. Accuracy, intraday and interday precision of the standard compounds in DS.

Compound	Spiked Amount (mg/mL)	Content (mg/mL)		Recovery Test (%, n = 5)	Precision Test (n = 5)	
		Un-Spiked	Measured		Intra-Day RSD[a] (%)	Inter-Day RSD (%)
1	0.03	3.229654	3.227270	92.1	0.05	0.01
	0.1	3.299654	3.300564	100.9	0.03	0.01
	0.3	3.499654	3.502000	100.8	0.03	0.01
2	0.03	0.115008	0.115157	100.5	0.22	0.31
	0.1	0.185008	0.185613	100.6	0.17	0.23
	0.3	0.385008	0.384965	100.0	0.14	0.12
3	0.03	0.306423	0.306506	100.3	0.04	0.10
	0.1	0.376423	0.376691	100.3	0.08	0.06
	0.3	0.576423	0.576923	100.2	0.16	0.03
4	0.03	0.489984	0.490762	102.6	0.20	0.15
	0.1	0.559984	0.561044	101.1	0.14	1.48
	0.3	0.759984	0.760324	100.1	0.22	0.10

[a] RSD: relative standard deviation.

Table 3. Accuracy, intra- and interday precision of the standard compounds in DQ.

Compound	Spiked Amount (mg/mL)	Content (mg/mL)		Recovery Test (%, n = 5)	Precision Test (n = 5)	
		Un-Spiked	Measured		Intra-Day RSD^a(%)	Inter-Day RSD (%)
1	0.012	0.081910	0.0820287	101.0	0.24	0.55
	0.04	0.109910	0.1073792	93.7	1.91	0.15
	0.12	0.189910	0.188932	99.2	0.62	0.28
2	0.012	0.130902	0.1316462	106.2	0.31	0.73
	0.04	0.158902	0.1582045	98.3	0.75	0.50
	0.12	0.238902	0.2368625	98.3	1.15	0.48
4	0.012	0.212048	0.2116199	96.4	0.41	0.38
	0.04	0.240048	0.2400817	100.1	0.44	0.75
	0.12	0.320048	0.3210118	100.8	0.26	0.52
5	0.012	0.192213	0.1918098	96.6	0.27	0.29
	0.04	0.220213	0.2220230	104.5	0.67	0.70
	0.12	0.300213	0.2928230	93.8	0.82	0.33

^{a} RSD: relative standard deviation.

2.2.3. Limit of Detection (LOD) and Quantification (LOQ)

The LOD and LOQ were calculated based on the standard deviation of the response and the slope of the calibration curve. Thus, the average SD value ($n = 5$) obtained by analyzing each of the five low-concentration compounds was substituted for the regression curve obtained from at least five low-concentration solutions, each of which was diluted sequentially as follows: 0.0005 ~ 0.005 mg/mL for 1, 0.001 ~ 0.01 mg/mL for 2 and 3, and 0.005 ~ 0.02 mg/mL for 4 and 5. From these results, the LOD was calculated by multiplying the LOD by 3.3 and the LOQ by 10. As a result, the LOD was determined to be 0.0009 mg/mL for compound **1**, 0.0022 mg/mL for compound **2**, 0.0007 mg/mL for compound **3**, 0.0132 for compound **4**, and 0.0027 for compound **5**. Previous studies detected protodioscin (**1**) at values up to approximately 0.0016 or 0.0039 mg/mL (LOD) [27,28], and these research results also showed that the LOD was 0.0009 mg/mL, although there was a difference in the analysis wavelength. The above results show that the analysis method developed for steroidal saponins provides sufficient sensitivity, likely due to mechanical and engineering advances in analytical systems and detectors (Table 1).

2.3. Quantitation of Compounds 1–5

Using the developed analysis method, the reproducibility and accuracy of which were confirmed through HPLC validation, protodioscin (**1**), protogracillin (**2**), pseudoprotodioscin (**3**), dioscin (**4**), and gracillin (**5**) were successfully determined in DN, DQ, and DS. In DN, except for gracillin (**5**), the quantities of the four compounds tested were confirmed as 159.983 ± 0.064 mg/g for **1**, 4.250 ± 0.024 mg/g for **2**, 13.821 ± 0.037 mg/g for **3**, and 22.999 ± 0.121 mg/g for **4**. Pseudoprotodioscin (**3**) was not detected in DQ or DS, and the other compounds, protodioscin (**1**), protogracillin (**2**), dioscin (**4**), and gracillin (**5**), were found in DQ at levels of 3.496 ± 0.018 mg/g for **1**, 5.945 ± 0.020 mg/g for **2**, 10.002 ± 0.051 mg/g for **4**, and 9.011 ± 0.098 mg/g for **5**. In DS, the content of **1**, **2**, **4**, and **5** was 8.959 ± 0.014 mg/g, 9.902 ± 0.061 mg/g, 9.822 ± 0.014 mg/g, and 7.123 ± 0.031 mg/g, respectively. To summarize the above results, DN, DQ, and DS can be confirmed as the plants of origin based on the presence of pseudoprotodioscin and gracillin, and in the case of DN, the content of protodioscin is exceptionally high; thus, this component is expected to play a very important role in future activity and toxicity studies (Table 4).

Table 4. Content of compounds in the three different samples (mg/g).

Compound	Content ($n = 4$)		
	DN	DQ	DS
1	159.983 ± 0.064 [a]	3.496 ± 0.018	8.959 ± 0.014
2	4.250 ± 0.024	5.945 ± 0.020	9.902 ± 0.061
3	13.821 ± 0.037	N.D.	N.D.
4	22.999 ± 0.121	10.002 ± 0.051	9.822 ± 0.014
5	N.D.	9.011 ± 0.098	7.123 ± 0.031

[a] Standard error (mg/g).

2.4. Identification of Compound 1–5 in DN and DQ Using UHPLC-QTOF/MS

In the above experiments, using the developed method, a quantitative analysis of five compounds from DN and DQ was performed. However, to more accurately identify the compounds in the samples, a qualitative analysis using UHPLC-QTOF/MS was performed next. The total ion chromatograms (TICs) of DN and DQ were obtained, as shown in Figure 3, and compounds **1**, **2**, **3**, and **4** in DN and **1**, **2**, **4**, and **5** in DQ were observed, similar to the HPLC analysis results. In addition, based on the molecular formula of each compound, their MS/MS fragmentation data were compared, and their structures were inferred from these data. The retention times of the detected peaks were then checked, and the compounds were found to have lost two rhamnose moieties at ^{1}Glc→^{2}Rha and ^{1}Glc→^{4}Rha based on the MS/MS spectrum of the peak at 5.859 min (peak **1**), and these signals were identified as m/z 901.4789 [M-(rhamnose-H$_2$O)-H]$^-$ and 755.4203 [M-2(rhamnose-H$_2$O)-H]$^-$. Similar to peak **1**, peaks **3** and **4**, which were observed at 7.021 and 9.950 min, were also found to have lost two rhamnose moieties in the MS/MS spectrum; peak **3** showed m/z values of 883.4679 [M-(rhamnose-H$_2$O)-H]$^-$ and 737.4108 [M-2(rhamnose-H$_2$O)-H]$^-$, while peak **4** showed m/z values of 721.4151 [M-(rhamnose-H$_2$O)-H]$^-$ and 575.3580 [M-2(rhamnose-H$_2$O)-H]$^-$. On the other hand, unlike peaks **1**, **3**, and **4**, peaks **2** and **5** showed losses of glucose (^{1}Glc→^{3}Glc) and rhamnose (^{1}Glc→^{2}Rha). The MS/MS data showed fragment ions of 901.4789 [M-(glucose-H$_2$O)-H]$^-$ and 755.4210 m/z [M-(glucose-H$_2$O)-(rhamnose-H$_2$O)-H]$^-$ for peak **2** and 721.4148 [M-(glucose-H$_2$O)-H]$^-$ and 575.3566 m/z [M-(glucose-H$_2$O)-(rhamnose-H$_2$O)-H]$^-$ for peak **5**. Therefore, based on the above data and the existing literature [3,9], the structures of compounds **1**, **2**, **3**, **4**, and **5** in DN and DQ were confirmed as protodioscin (**1**), protogracillin (**2**), pseudoprotodioscin (**3**), dioscin (**4**), and gracillin (**5**) (Figure 3).

Meanwhile, the unidentified peaks (*a* to *k*) detected in the TCIs in Figure 3 were derived from the mass values of the parent molecule and fragmentation obtained through the auto MS/MS mode analysis using the Waters UNIFI software (Waters, Milford, MA, USA), and they are believed to be the most suitable compounds stored in the database library (Table 5).

Among these, *h*, the largest peak, was estimated to represent ophiopogonin B, a glycoside of the spirostane type found in *Dioscorea tokoro*, and it has a molecular weight of 722.4237 [29]. Additionally, a comparison of the ms/ms values of the product ions in the literature [30] showed values of 573.36 and 145.05 m/z, including 721.42 m/z [M-H]$^-$. The peak *d* is steroid saponin, with a molecular weight of 884.4736, and compared with the MS value in the literature, we identified ion fragments of 883.47 and 737.41 m/z, which were estimated to represent spiroconazole A, which was isolated from *Dioscorea bulbifera* [31]. Similarly, peak *e* was estimated to be a compound reported as 2,7,2′-trihydroxy-4,4′,7′-trimethoxy-1,1′-biphenanthrene, derived from the leaves of DN [32]. Peak *g* was predicted as trillin, and it has primarily been reported in *Dioscorea zingiberensis*, but was also isolated from DN [33]. Additionally, prosapogenin A of dioscin (peak *i*) was previously detected in *Dioscorea zingiberensis* using QTOF/MS [34].

On the other hand, polyphylin V has been previously detected in DN using UPLC–qTOF–MS [3], although this study identified a similar derivative, polyphylin D, at peak *a*. Peak *f* was also predicted to be blumenol C glucoside, a component related to blumenol A, which has been previously isolated from

DN [35]. Peak *k* was predicted to be neohecogenin-3-*O*-β-D-glucopyranoside, which is not a component reported in *Dioscorea* families, although hecogenin, which is dissociated from the sugar, was long ago reported as a major substance in *Dioscorea bernoulliana* [36].

The remaining peaks *b*, *c*, and *j* are considered to represent components that have not been discovered or reported thus far in *Dioscorea* families, including DN. These remaining unidentified peaks were carefully and tentatively identified, although the findings cannot be verified, using their MS/MS data as a reference. As a result, peaks *b* and *c* were identified as Timosaponin AIII [37] and Sanleng acid [38], respectively, based on the literature. Although the identity of the compound responsible for peak *j* at 6.14 min could not be inferred from the literature, it was presumed to be mutongsaponin C or akebia saponin F, according to the library program.

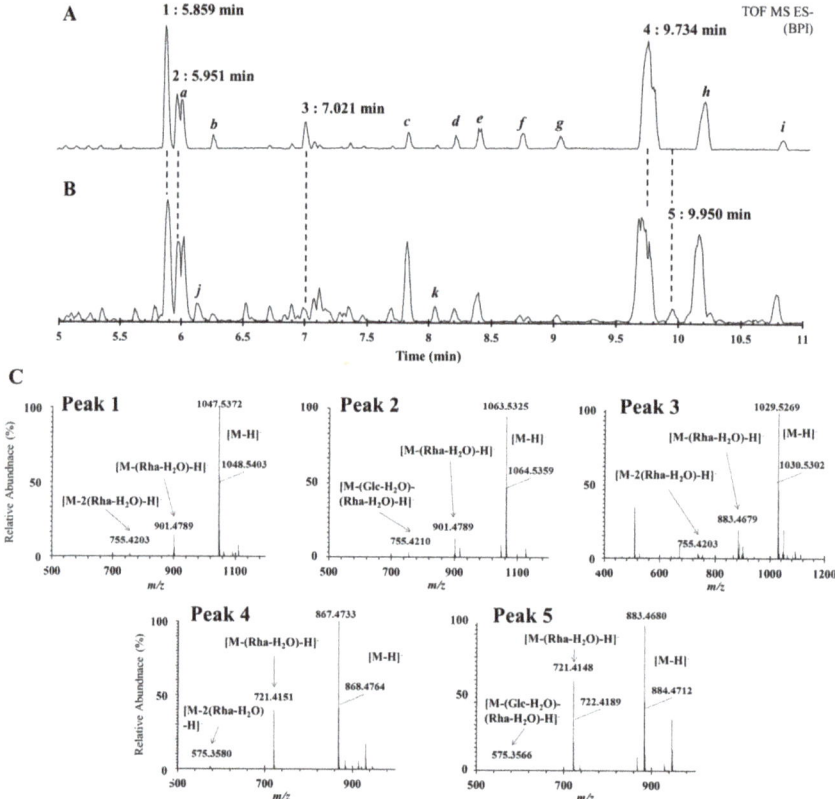

Figure 3. (**A**): Representative base peak intensity (BPI) chromatogram of DN and (**B**): DQ. (**C**): MS/MS spectrum of peak **1** (5.859 min), peak **2** (5.859 min), peak **3** (5.859 min), peak **4** (5.859 min), and peak **5** (5.859 min).

Table 5. Estimates of unidentified peaks based on the MS/MS database library.

Sample	Peak	t_R (min)	Observed (Neutral)	Observed (m/z)	Mass Error (ppm)	Tentative Identification
DN (A)	a	6.03	854.4643	899.4625 [+HCOO]	−2.3	Polyphyllin D
	b	6.25	740.4350	785.4332 [+HCOO]	0.3	Timosaponin AIII
	c	7.85	330.2406	329.2334 [-H]	0.1	Sanleng acid
	d	8.18	884.4736	929.4718 [+HCOO]	−3.6	Spiroconazole A
	e	8.39	492.1566	537.1548 [+HCOO]	−1.3	2,7,2′-Trihydroxy-4,4′,7′-trimethoxy-1,1′-biphenanthrene
	f	8.73	372.2139	417.2121 [+HCOO]	−2.1	Blumenol C glucoside
	g	9.02	576.3642	621.3624 [+HCOO]	−3.2	Trillin
	h	10.06	722.4237	767.4219 [+HCOO, -H]	−0.5	Ophiopogonin B
	i	10.76	722.4236	767.4218 [+HCOO]	−0.7	Prosapogenin A of dioscin
DQ (B)	j	6.14	1090.5550	1135.5530 [+HCOO, -H]	−1.2	Mutongsaponin C or Akebia saponin F
	k	8.03	592.3596	637.3578 [+HCOO]	−2.4	Neohecogenin-3-O-β-D-glucopyranoside

2.5. Anti-Osteosarcoma Effects of the Samples

Saponins demonstrate various pharmacological effects that can improve blood circulation, immune control, and antiviral effects. In addition, recent studies have reported that steroidal saponins exert effective anticancer activities, such as anti-invasion, anti-metastasis, and anti-angiogenic effects through various mechanisms, such as inhibition of cell proliferation and promotion of cell differentiation.

Based on the characteristics of the samples analyzed above, the biological effects of DN, DQ, and DS were investigated. The steroidal saponins present in each sample exert their potential anticancer effects by activating apoptotic signaling. In particular, DN might have a stronger apoptotic effect because it has a higher steroidal saponins content relative to the other two extracts. Since these compounds are reported to have various pharmacological activities, such as anti-obesity activity [8], anti-inflammatory activity [39], protective effects against hyperlipidemia and oxidative stress [36], and anti-tumor activity [40], information on the composition and content of the steroidal saponin present in herbal medicines is important for future research. To verify their anticancer effects, a western blotting assay to confirm the expression levels of the apoptosis markers cleaved-Cas3 and cleaved-PARP in U2OS osteosarcoma cells was attempted. As expected, DN had a more powerful apoptosis-inducing effect than DQ and DS. Furthermore, to find the individual compound responsible for the pro-apoptotic effect of DN, we examined the levels of the apoptotic markers in the presence of the four major compounds, **1**, **2**, **3**, and **4**. The IC_{50} values of **1** and **4** were 6.43 µM and 6.90 µM, respectively, while those of **3** and **4** were 10.84 µM and 10.61 µM, respectively. Based on these results, we predicted that protodioscin (**1**) and dioscin (**4**) could be important in the mechanism underlying the pro-apoptosis effect of DN against osteosarcoma cells. To verify this hypothesis, the levels of apoptosis markers were evaluated after treatment of U2OS cells with the individual compounds at the same concentrations. Interestingly, **4** showed the most potent anticancer effect, and the other compounds were less effective than **4**. Dioscin (**4**) has already been shown to inhibit the growth of colon, ovarian, and lung cancer and to be effective in apoptosis of cancer cells [41–43]. The anticancer effect caused by **4** examines whether the anticancer effect of osteosarcoma also uses the mitochondria signal pathway. Thus, we would like to emphasize the importance of natural medicine in that the strong anticancer effect of **4** can be obtained from DN. Taken together, the powerful anticancer effect of DN can be attributed to its high dioscin (**4**) content, suggesting that it might be useful for osteosarcoma treatment (Figure 4).

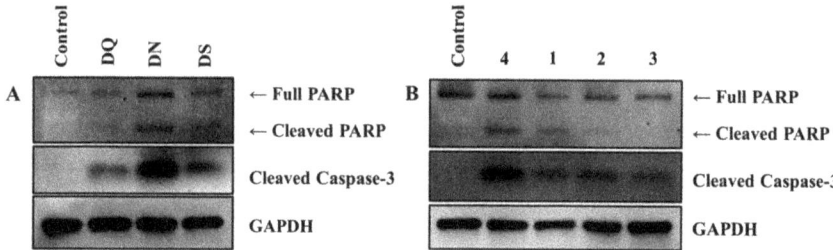

Figure 4. Effectiveness of DN against U2OS osteosarcoma cells. (**A**): U2OS cells treated with vehicle or 100 μg/mL extracts for 48 h. Apoptosis indexes (Cleaved Caspase-3 and PARP) were detected via western blotting. GAPDH served as the internal control. (**B**): U2OS cells treated with vehicle or 5 μM of each compound for 24 h.

3. Experimental

3.1. Reagents and Standards

Analytical-grade acetonitrile (ACN) and triple-distilled water were purchased from J. T. Baker (Philipsburg, NJ, USA). Standards of protodioscin (**1**), protogracillin (**2**), pseudoprotodioscin (**3**), dioscin (**4**), and gracillin (**5**) were purchased from ChemFaces (Wuhan, China), and these compounds (**1–5**) had purities of ≥98%. Stock solutions of the five reference compounds were prepared at concentrations of 5 mg/mL in 70% ACN and 30% water. The working solutions were prepared by serial dilution with 70% ACN to obtain a final concentration of 0.0005 mg/mL, and the solutions were stored at 4 °C until analysis.

3.2. Sample Preparation and Extraction

To secure the standard samples, experts from the Korea Institute of Oriental Medicine were consulted three times on collection of the samples. Ten different batches of DN raw material were collected from the regions of Eumseong and Yeongwol counties (Chungcheongbuk-do and Gangwon-do, Korea) in July 2018. Ten different batches of DQ and DS were collected from the regions of Aewol-eup (Jeju Island, Korea) in June 2018. The plant materials were identified again by an inspection committee of herbal medicines from the Korea Institute of Oriental Medicine (KIOM). Furthermore, a portion of all the collected samples were subjected to genetic DNA sequencing and HPLC analysis, and the 10 samples in each of the three groups were confirmed to be genetically and chemically identical to the other group members (data not shown). Then, all the raw materials and extracts were deposited at the KIOM (KIOM R 1803051-1 to 5).

Samples from all three groups were cleaned and dried at 50 °C for seven days in a drying oven. The dried samples were powdered, and 300 g of each sample was extracted twice for three hours using 2 L of 70% ethanol at 70 °C via reflux extraction. The extracts of the samples were concentrated at 40 °C to approximately one-quarter of their initial volume using a vacuum evaporator. Ethanol was removed from the residues by freeze-drying for 7 days, and the residual material was used for subsequent experiments.

To prepare samples for HPLC analysis, 40 mg of the extracted and dried material was dissolved in 2 mL of 70% ACN by sonication for 10 min. After centrifugation for 10 min at 4000× g, the supernatant was filtered through a disposable syringe filter (0.22 μm, 25 mm, CA syringe filter), obtained from Futecs Co., Ltd. (Daejeon, Korea), prior to injection into the HPLC system. The chromatographic peaks of the sample solution were identified by comparing their retention times and PDA spectra with those of standards.

3.3. HPLC Conditions

The HPLC analysis was conducted with a Shimadzu LC-20A Prominence Series system (Shimadzu Corporation, Kyoto, Japan) equipped with a quaternary pump (LC-20AD), vacuum degasser (DGU-20A3R), autosampler (SIL-20A), column oven (CTO-20A), and photodiode-array detector (SPD-M20A). Chromatographic data were interpreted using LabSolutions Multi PDA software. Chromatographic separation was performed on a YMC Triart C18 PFP column (4.6 × 250 mm i.d., 5 μm). The column oven was maintained at 40 °C, detection was conducted at λ = 200 nm, and online UV absorption spectra were recorded in a range from 190 to 400 nm. A gradient elution system was implemented as follows: mobile phase A, acetonitrile/B, triple-distilled water = 23/77 to 33/67 (0–25 min), 33/67 to 34/66 (25–50 min), and 34/66 to 100/0 (50–65 min) at a 1 mL/min flow rate at 40 °C, with an injection volume of 10 μL.

3.4. Validation Method for HPLC

The HPLC analysis method was validated in terms of linearity, accuracy, precision, LOD, and LOQ following the guidelines set by the International Conference on Harmonization (ICH). The linearity was established by evaluating the value of r^2 (correlation coefficient) for the calibration curve prepared from ten serially diluted solutions. The precision of the analysis method was examined using the intermediate evaluation method by measuring the intra- and interday variability. The intraday variability was determined by analyzing the sample solution on one of the study days (24 h), while the interday variability was determined by injecting the sample solutions five times per day on four different days. The relative standard deviation (RSD) values were calculated for both the retention time and peak area from these five experiments. The RSD is considered a measure of precision. Recovery tests using a sample solution spiked with each standard compound were performed to evaluate accuracy. Recovery rates were determined by calculating the mean recovery (%) of the standards from the spiked extract solutions vs. the recovery from the nonspiked extract. The LOD and LOQ were calculated based on the standard deviation of the response and the slope of the calibration curve; an S/N ratio of 3 was used for the LOD, and an S/N ratio of 10 was used for the LOQ.

3.5. UHPLC-QTOF/MS Analysis

An unbiased metabolomics analysis was performed using a UPLC system (Waters, Milford, USA). The chromatographic separation was carried out using an ACQUITY UPLC HSS T3 column (100 mm × 2.1 mm, 1.8 μm, Waters) with a column temperature of 40 °C and a flow rate of 0.5 mL/min. The mobile phase contained solvent A (water + 0.1% formic acid) and solvent B (acetonitrile + 0.1% formic acid). The metabolites were eluted using the following gradient elution conditions: 97% phase A for 0–1 min; 3%–100% linear gradient phase B for 5–16 min; 100% phase B for 16–17 min; 100%–3% reverse linear gradient phase B for 17–19 min; 97% phase A for 19–25 min. The injection volume was 5 μL. The metabolites in the eluate were detected with a high-resolution tandem mass spectrometer (SYNAPT G2 Si HDMS QTOF, Waters) in positive and negative ion modes. In positive ion mode, the capillary voltage and the cone voltage were 2 kV and 40 V, respectively. In negative ion mode, they were 1 kV and 40 V, respectively. Centroid MS^E mode was used to collect the mass spectrometry data. The primary scan ranged from 50 to 1200 Da, and the scanning time was 0.2 s. All the parent ions were fragmented using 20–40 eV. All the fragment data were collected, and the time was 0.2 s. In the data acquisition process, the signal of leucine enkephalin (LE) was obtained every 3 s for real-time quality correction. For accurate mass acquisition, LE at a flow rate of 10 μL min^{-1} was used as a lock mass with a lock spray interface to monitor both positive ($[M + H]^+$ = 556.2771) and negative ($[M - H]^-$ = 554.2615) ion modes. Data acquisition and analysis were controlled by Waters UNIFI V1.71 software. The MS and MS/MS scanning ranges were 50–1200 *m/z*.

3.6. Cell Culture

Human osteosarcoma U2OS cells were obtained from American Type Culture Collection (ATCC). The U2OS cells were cultured in Dulbecco's modified Eagle's medium (DMEM; Gibco, Grand Island, NY, USA) supplemented with 10% fetal bovine serum (FBS) and 1% penicillin/streptomycin at 37 °C in a 5% CO_2 incubator.

3.7. Western Blot Analysis

Western blotting was performed according to the manufacturer's instructions. Antibodies against PARP (1:1000, #9542, Cell Signaling), cleaved caspase-3 (1:1000, #9661, Cell Signaling), and GAPDH (1:3000, #5174, Cell Signaling) were used.

3.8. Cell Viability Assay

For cell viability assays, DN, DQ, and DS extract powders were dissolved in distilled water and then filtered through a membrane with a pore size of 0.2 µm. Each of the individual component compounds were dissolved separately in dimethyl sulfoxide and then filtered through the 0.2 µm membrane. A total of 1×10^3 cells were plated in 96-well plates and exposed to the extracts (DN, DQ and DS) and individual compounds (protodioscin, dioscin, pseudoprotodioscin, and protogracillin) at different concentrations at a final volume of 100 µL. After 48 h, MTS (Promega) solution was added to the wells at 10 µL/well. The cells were incubated for an additional 1 h, and then, the absorbance at 490 nm was recorded with a 96-well plate reader.

4. Conclusions

In this study, a method was developed to chemically distinguish five steroidal saponins, protodioscin (1), protogracillin (2), pseudoprotodioscin (3), dioscin (4), and gracillin (5), using HPLC-UV analysis, and this method could be used to distinguish DN, which is used as an Oriental medicine, from DQ and related species. The HPLC analysis method developed above was validated based on linearity ($r^2 > 0.999$), accuracy (92.1%–106.2%), precision (<1.91%), LOD (<0.0132 mg/mL), and LOQ (<0.04 mg/mL). In addition, a UHPLC-QTOF/MS analysis confirmed that the five steroidal saponins quantified by HPLC-UV were present in the samples, and their structures were predicted based on the loss of one or two sugars (rhamnose or glucose fragment ions), which were visible in the MS/MS spectra. Above all, the UHPLC-QTOF/MS results showed that the composition of the compounds in each of the different DN samples (1, 2, 3, and 4) and in each of the DQ samples (1, 2, 4, and 5) was consistent based on the HPLC-UV data. To the best of our knowledge, this method, which is based on five compounds, is the most accurate and straightforward system developed to date to identify DN. In addition, unlike many previous studies, DQ and DS, which are genetically and morphologically similar, can be compared using the approach developed here, and this information is important for future research or commercial development. Finally, based on the results of the anti-osteosarcoma activity tests and quantitative analysis of DN and its compounds, 1 and 4 were more abundant in DN than in DQ or DS, endowing DN with the strongest activity. Therefore, the strong activity of DN was due to the presence of protodioscin (1) and dioscin (4). We concluded that DN, which has been correctly determined through the above analyses, is a powerful and useful anti-osteosarcoma herbal remedy, and we are in the process of conducting a mechanistic study and in vivo experiments to further elucidate its pharmacological activity.

Author Contributions: Conceptualization, J.A.R. and B.S.K.; Data curation, J.T.H. and K.-S.P.; Formal analysis, J.T.H. and K.-S.P.; Methodology, J.T.H. and K.-S.P.; Project administration, B.S.K.; Resources, J.T.H., J.A.R., and B.S.K.; Supervision, B.S.K.; Validation, J.T.H. and H.J.K.; Writing – original draft, J.T.H. and K.-S.P.; Writing – reviewing and editing, J.T.H., K.-S.P., H.J.K., and B.S.K.

Funding: This work was supported by a grant from the National Research Council of Science & Technology (NST) provided by the Korea government (MSIT) (no. CAP-16-07-KIOM).

Conflicts of Interest: The authors declare no conflicts of interest.

References

1. The Pharmacopoeia of Democratic People's Republic of Korea. *Democratic People's Republic of Korea Pharmacopoeia Commission*, 7th ed.; Medical Science Publishing House: Pyeongyang, Democratic People's Republic of Korea, 2011; p. 385.
2. National Pharmacopoeia Commission. *Chinese Pharmacopoeia*, Pharmacopoeia of the People's Republic of China 2010 ed.; China Medico Pharmaceutical Science & Technology Publishing House: Beijing, China, 2010; Volume I, p. 251.
3. Tang, Y.; Yi, T.; Chen, H.; Zhao, Z.; Liang, Z.; Chen, H. Quantitative Comparison of Multiple Components in *Dioscorea nipponica* and *D. panthaica* by Ultra-High Performance Liquid Chromatography Coupled with Quadrupole Time-of-Flight Mass Spectrometry. *Phytochem. Anal.* **2013**, *24*, 413–422. [CrossRef] [PubMed]
4. Kang, Y.; Choi, G.; Jin, W.; Kim, H.; Kim, D. Characterization of morphological and analytical keys in *Dioscoreae nipponicae* rhizoma (*Dioscorea nipponica* Makino) and *Dioscoreae quinquelobatae* rhizoma (*Dioscorea quinquelobata* Thunb.) as Korean herbal medicines. *Korean Herb. Med. Inf.* **2014**, *2*, 7–14.
5. Ou-yang, S.; Jiang, T.; Zhu, L.; Yi, T. *Dioscorea nipponica* Makino: A systematic review on its ethnobotany, phytochemical and pharmacological profiles. *Chem. Cent. J.* **2018**, *12*, 57. [CrossRef] [PubMed]
6. Kwon, C.; Sohn, H.Y.; Kim, S.H.; Kim, J.H.; Son, K.H.; Lee, J.S.; Lim, J.K.; Kim, J. Anti-obesity effect of *Dioscorea nipponica* Makino with lipase-inhibitory activity in rodents. *Biosci. Biotechnol. Biochem.* **2014**, *67*, 1451–1456. [CrossRef]
7. Sarvin, B.; Fedorova, E.; Shpigun, O.; Titova, M.; Nikitin, M.; Kochkin, D.; Rodin, I.; Stavrianidi, A. LC-MS determination of steroidal glycosides from *Dioscorea deltoidea* Wall cell suspension culture: Optimization of pre-LC-MS procedure parameters by Latin Square design. *J. Chromatogr. B.* **2018**, *1080*, 64–70. [CrossRef]
8. Lin, S.; Wang, D.; Yang, D.; Yao, J.; Tong, Y.; Chen, J. Characterization of steroidal saponins in crude extract from *Dioscorea nipponica* Makino by liquid chromatography tandem multi-stage mass spectrometry. *Anal. Chim. Acta.* **2007**, *599*, 98–106. [CrossRef]
9. Kang, K.B.; Ryu, J.; Cho, Y.; Choi, S.; Son, M.; Sung, S.H. Combined Application of UHPLC-QTOF/MS, HPLC-ELSD and ^{1}H–NMR Spectroscopy for Quality Assessment of DA-9801, A Standardised *Dioscorea* Extract. *Phytochem. Anal.* **2017**, *28*, 185–194. [CrossRef]
10. Ko, B.; Lee, H.Y.; Kim, D.S.; Kang, S.; Ryuk, J.A. Supplementing with *Opuntia ficus-indica* Mill and *Dioscorea nipponica* Makino extracts synergistically attenuates menopausal symptoms in estrogen-deficient rats. *J. Ethnopharmacol.* **2014**, *155*, 267–276. [CrossRef]
11. Kim, K.; Kang, M.; Kim, J.; Kim, G.; Choi, S. Physicochemical Composition and Antioxidant Activities of Korean Dioscorea Species. *J. East Asian Soc. Diet. Life* **2015**, *25*, 880–886. [CrossRef]
12. Durfee, R.A.; Mohammed, M.; Luu, H.H. Review of Osteosarcoma and Current Management. *Rheumatol. Ther.* **2016**, *3*, 221–243. [CrossRef] [PubMed]
13. Nie, Z.; Peng, H. Osteosarcoma in patients below 25 years of age: An observational study of incidence, metastasis, treatment and outcomes. *Oncol. Lett.* **2018**, *16*, 6502–6514. [CrossRef] [PubMed]
14. Ferguson, A.S.; Goorin, A.M. Current treatment of osteosarcoma. *Cancer Invest.* **2001**, *19*, 292–315. [CrossRef] [PubMed]
15. Wagner, E.R.; Luther, G.; Zhu, G.; Luo, Q.; Shi, Q.; Kim, S.H.; Gao, J.; Huang, E.; Gao, Y.; Yang, K.; et al. Defective Osteogenic Differentiation in the Development of Osteosarcoma. *Sarcoma* **2011**, *2011*, 12. [CrossRef] [PubMed]
16. Jaffe, N.; Puri, A.; Gelderblom, H. Osteosarcoma: Evolution of Treatment Paradigms. *Sarcoma* **2013**, *2013*, 7. [CrossRef] [PubMed]
17. Demain, A.; Vaishnav, P. Natural products for cancer chemotherapy. *Microb Biotechnol.* **2011**, *4*, 687–699. [CrossRef]
18. Man, S.; Gao, W.; Zhang, Y.; Huang, L.; Liu, C. Chemical study and medical application of saponins as anti-cancer agents. *Fitoterapia* **2010**, *81*, 703–714. [CrossRef]
19. Ma, B.; Zhu, J.; Zhang, J.; Wang, Y.; Zhang, L.; Zhang, Q. Raddeanin A, a natural triterpenoid saponin compound, exerts anticancer effect on human osteosarcoma via the ROS/JNK and NF-κB signal pathway. *Toxicol. Appl. Pharm.* **2018**, *353*, 87–101. [CrossRef]

20. Cheng, G.; Gao, F.; Sun, X.; Bi, H.; Zhu, Y. Paris saponin VII suppresses osteosarcoma cell migration and invasion by inhibiting MMP-2/9 production via the p38 MAPK signaling pathway. *Mol. Med. Rep.* **2016**, *14*, 3199–3205. [CrossRef]
21. Tenon, M.; Feuillère, N.; Roller, M.; Birtic', S. Rapid, cost-effective and accurate quantification of *Yucca schidigera* Roezl. steroidal saponins using HPLC-ELSD method. *Food Chem.* **2017**, *221*, 1245–1252. [CrossRef]
22. Mateos, R.; Baeza, G.; Martínez-López, S.; Sarriá, B.; Bravo, L. LC–MS$_n$ characterization of saponins in mate (Ilex paraguariens, St. Hil) and their quantification by HPLC-DAD. *J. Food Compos. Anal.* **2017**, *63*, 164–170. [CrossRef]
23. Ahn, M.; Kim, J. Identification and Quantification of Steroidal Saponins in *Polygonatum* Species by HPLC/ESI/MS. *Arch Pharm Res.* **2005**, *5*, 592–597. [CrossRef] [PubMed]
24. Bardarov, V.; Dinchev, D.; Bardarov, K. Study of the chromatographic behavior of protodioscin on a C8 CORE-SHELL 2.6 μm short (5 cm) column and its determination with UV/ELSD detection. *J. Chem. Technol. Metall.* **2013**, *48*, 4, 341–346.
25. Yi, T.G.; Yeoung, Y.R.; Choi, I.; Park, N. Transcriptome analysis of *Asparagus officinalis* reveals genes involved in the biosynthesis of rutin and protodioscin. *PLoS ONE* **2019**, *14*. [CrossRef] [PubMed]
26. Kwon, H.; Choi, S.; Yoo, C.; Choi, H.; Lee, S.; Park, Y. Development of an analytical method for yam saponins using HPLC with pulsed amperometric detection at different column temperatures. *J. Sep. Sci.* **2013**, *36*, 690–698. [CrossRef]
27. Lee, E.J.; Yoo, K.S.; Patil, B.S. Development of a Rapid HPLC-UV Method for Simultaneous Quantification of Protodioscin and Rutin in White and Green Asparagus Spears. *J. Food Sci.* **2010**, *75*, 9. [CrossRef]
28. Shishovska, M.; Arsova-Sarafinovska, Z.; Memeti, S. A Simple Method for Determination of Protodioscin in *Tribulus Terrestris*, L. and Pharmaceuticals by High-Performance Liquid Chromatography Using Diode-Array Detection. *J. Chem. Eng. Res. Updates.* **2015**, *2*, 12–21.
29. Tada, A.; Shoji, J. Studies on the constituents of Ophiopogonis Tuber. II. on the structure of ophiopogonin B. *Chem. Pharm. Bull.* **1972**, *20*, 1729–1734. [CrossRef]
30. Zhenzhen, L.; Kuang, W.; Xu, X.; Li, D.; Zhu, W.; Lan, Z.; Zhang, X. Putative identification of components in Zengye Decoction and their effects on glucose consumption and lipogenesis in insulin-induced insulin-resistant HepG2 cells. *J. Chromatogr. B.* **2018**, *1073*, 145–153.
31. Teponno, R.T.; Tapondjou, A.L.; Djoukeng, D.; Abou-Mansour, E.; Tabacci, R.; Tane, P.; Lontsi, D.; Park, H. Isolation and NMR assignment of a pennogenin glycoside from *Dioscorea bulbifera* L. var *sativa*. *Nat. Prod. Sci.* **2006**, *12*, 62–66.
32. Lu, D.; Liu, J.; Li, H.; Li, P. Phenanthrene derivatives from the stems and leaves of *Dioscorea nipponica* Makino. *J. Asian. Nat. Prod. Res.* **2010**, *12*, 1–6. [CrossRef] [PubMed]
33. Wang, T.; Choi, R.C.Y.; Li, J.; Bi, C.W.C.; Ran, W.; Chen, X.; Dong, T.T.X.; Bi, K.; Tsim, K.W.K. Trillin, a steroidal saponin isolated from the rhizomes of *Dioscorea nipponica*, exerts protective effects against hyperlipidemia and oxidative stress. *J. Ethnopharmacol.* **2012**, *139*, 214–220. [CrossRef] [PubMed]
34. Yang, J.; Zhu, L.; Zhao, Y.; Xu, Y.; Sun, Q.; Liu, S.; Liu, C.; Ma, B. Separation of furostanol saponins by supercritical fluidchromatography. *J. Pharmaceut. Biomed.* **2017**, *145*, 71–78. [CrossRef] [PubMed]
35. Kim, K.H.; Kim, M.A.; Moon, E.; Kim, S.Y.; Choi, S.Z.; Son, M.W.; Lee, K.R. Furostanol saponins from the rhizomes of Dioscorea japonica and their effects on NGF induction. *Bioorg. Med. Chem. Lett.* **2011**, *21*, 2075–2078. [CrossRef] [PubMed]
36. Kadkade, P.G.; Ramiréz, M.A.; Madrid, T.R. Studies on the steroidal sapogenins of the subcellular organelles of *Dioscorea bernoulliana* tubers. *Biochem. Physiol. Pflanzen.* **1979**, *174*, 357–362. [CrossRef]
37. Ma, C.; Fan, M.; Tang, Y.; Li, Z.; Sun, Z.; Ye, G.; Huang, C. Identification of major alkaloids and steroidal saponins in rat serum by HPLC-diode array detection-MS/MS following oral administration of Huangbai-Zhimu herb-pair Extract. *Biomed. Chromatogr.* **2008**, *22*, 835–850. [CrossRef] [PubMed]
38. Lin, H.; Zhu, H.; Tan, J.; Wang, H.; Wang, Z.; Li, P.; Zhao, C.; Liu, J. Comparative analysis of chemical constituents of *Moringa oleifera* leaves from China and India by ultra-performance liquid chromatography coupled with quadrupole-time-of-flight mass spectrometry. *Molecules* **2019**, *24*, 942. [CrossRef]
39. Yu, H.; Zheng, L.; Yin, L.; Xu, L.; Qi, Y.; Han, X.; Xu, Y.; Liu, K.; Peng, J. Protective effects of the total saponins from *Dioscorea nipponica* Makino against carbon tetrachloride-induced liver injury in mice through suppression of apoptosis and inflammation. *Int. Immunopharmcol.* **2014**, *19*, 233–244. [CrossRef]

40. Chien, M.J.; Ying, T.H.; Hsieh, Y.S.; Chang, Y.C.; Yeh, C.M.; Ko, J.L.; Lee, W.S.; Chang, J.H.; Yang, S.F. *Dioscorea nipponica* Makino inhibits migration and invasion of human oral cancer HSC-3 cells by transcriptional inhibition of matrix metalloproteinase-2 through modulation of CREB and AP-1 activity. *Food. Chem. Toxicol.* **2012**, *50*, 558–566. [CrossRef]
41. Li, S.; Cheng, B.; Hou, L.; Huang, L.; Cui, Y.; Xu, D.; Shen, X.; Li, S. Dioscin inhibits colon cancer cells' growth by reactive oxygen species-mediated mitochondrial dysfunction and p38 and JNK pathways. *Anti-Cancer Drug.* **2018**, *29*, 234–242. [CrossRef]
42. Guo, X.; Ding, X. Dioscin suppresses the viability of ovarian cancer cells by regulating the VEGFR2 and PI3K/AKT/MAPK signaling pathways. *Oncol. Lett.* **2018**, *15*, 9537–9542. [CrossRef] [PubMed]
43. Wei, Y.; Xu, Y.; Han, X.; Qi, Y.; Xu, L.; Xu, Y.; Yin, L.; Sun, H.; Liu, K.; Peng, J. Anti-cancer effects of dioscin on three kinds of human lung cancer cell lines through inducing DNA damage and activating mitochondrial signal pathway. *Food Chem. Toxicol.* **2013**, *59*, 118–128. [CrossRef] [PubMed]

Sample Availability: Samples of the compounds are available from the authors.

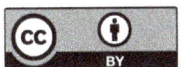

© 2019 by the authors. Licensee MDPI, Basel, Switzerland. This article is an open access article distributed under the terms and conditions of the Creative Commons Attribution (CC BY) license (http://creativecommons.org/licenses/by/4.0/).

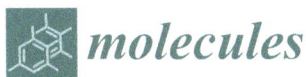

Article

Pharmacokinetic Comparison of Epinastine Using Developed Human Plasma Assays

Seung-Hyun Jeong [1], Ji-Hun Jang [1], Hea-Young Cho [2] and Yong-Bok Lee [1,*]

[1] College of Pharmacy, Chonnam National University, 77 Yongbong-ro, Buk-Gu, Gwangju 61186, Korea; rhdqn95@naver.com (S.-H.J.); jangji0121@naver.com (J.-H.J.)
[2] College of Pharmacy, CHA University, 335 Pangyo-ro, Bundang-gu, Seongnam-si, Gyeonggi-Do 13488, Korea; hycho@cha.ac.kr
* Correspondence: leeyb@chonnam.ac.kr; Tel.: +82-62-530-2931; Fax: +82-62-530-0106

Academic Editors: In-Soo Yoon and Hyun-Jong Cho
Received: 9 December 2019; Accepted: 1 January 2020; Published: 3 January 2020

Abstract: The purpose of the study was to develop two new methods, HPLC-UV and UPLC-MS/MS, for quantifying epinastine in human plasma and to compare pharmacokinetic (PK) parameters obtained using them. Even in the same sample, there may be a difference in the quantitative value of drug depending on the assay, so that minor changes in PK parameter values may affect drug dose and usage settings. Therefore, selection and establishment of analytical methods are very important in PK studies of drugs, and a comparison of PK parameters according to analytical methods will be vital. For this study of PK parameter change, we newly developed two methods, HPLC-UV and UPLC-MS/MS, which are most commonly used to quantify epinastine concentrations in human plasma. All developed methods satisfied the international guidelines and criteria for successful application to PK study of 20 mg epinastine hydrochloride tablets after oral administration to twenty-six humans. A comparison of these two methods for in vivo analysis of epinastine was performed for the first time. This comparison study confirmed that different dose and usage settings might be possible based on PK parameters calculated using other analyses. Such changes in calculated PK parameters according to analytical methods would be crucial in the clinic.

Keywords: epinastine; pharmacokinetics; HPLC-UV; UPLC-MS/MS; comparison

1. Introduction

Epinastine is a histamine H_1 receptor antagonist with high receptor selectivity. Epinastine cannot cross the blood-brain barrier in the body and may be classified as a second-generation antihistamine [1]. Based on its polarity and cationic charge at physiological pH, it cannot easily diffuse into the central nervous system (CNS) [2]. Thus, these physicochemical properties distinguish epinastine as a non-sedative antihistamine, and unlike other first-generation antihistamines acting on the CNS, it does not cause side effects, such as drowsiness or sedation [3]. Epinastine has multiple effects that inhibit the allergic response in three ways: (1) stabilizes mast cells by preventing mast cell degranulation to control the allergic response, (2) prevents histamine binding to both the H_1- and H_2-receptors to stop itching and provide lasting protection, and (3) prevents the release of pro-inflammatory chemical mediators from the blood vessel to halt progression of the allergic response [4]. In addition, Oshima et al. [5] reported that epinastine suppresses the immune responses of Th-2 cell through functional modulation of dendritic cells, which play an essential role in the development of allergic immune responses, and thus has the results in favorable modification of the clinical status of allergic diseases. Epinastine has been used in the form of eye drops primarily in association with allergic conjunctivitis. In this regard, various safety information has been established through previous preclinical and clinical trials. Brar et al. [6] reported that no significant ocular and systemic toxicity was observed in white rabbits and cynomolgus monkeys treated with 0.05–0.5% epinastine hydrochloride ophthalmic solution for 6 months. Yu et al. [7] reported that epinastine rapidly reached high levels on the ocular surface without unwanted systemic side effects when 0.05% epinastine hydrochloride ophthalmic solution was administered to allergic conjunctivitis patients for 7 days. In addition to its use as eye drops, during the last 10–15 years, tablets of epinastine hydrochloride have been used for clinical application in asthma and urticaria, and patients are prescribed at a dose of 10–20 mg once daily. In vivo metabolism of epinastine occurs mainly in the liver, but the degree of metabolism is reported to be very low. That is, most of the epinastine administered into the body is excreted in the unchanged form [8].

Analytical and pharmacokinetic (PK) reports of epinastine have been performed in the past. However, the reported methods had limitations and needed improvement. Most of all, there have been no reports on how PK characteristics can differ by analytical methods, and which PK parameters are significantly affected. Even in the same sample, there may be differences in the quantitative values depending on the analytical method, which may cause differences in the PK parameter values. Drug dose and usage settings based on the individual parameters for which the difference occurred may produce different results in the clinic. Therefore, in this study, we tried to identify the changes in PK parameters of the drug according to the analytical methods. For this study, epinastine hydrochloride tablets of 20 mg were orally administered to humans, and the subsequently collected plasma samples were analyzed by two newly developed assays (HPLC-UV and UPLC-MS/MS), which are most commonly used for quantification in biological samples. Our study also focused on comparing the performances of newly developed UPLC-MS/MS and HPLC-UV methods for the determination of epinastine in human plasma. All methods were fully validated according to international bioanalytical method guidelines and represent a useful tool for the characterization of PKs of 20 mg epinastine hydrochloride tablets in Korean subjects.

2. Results

2.1. Method Development

2.1.1. UPLC-MS/MS Method

In this study, an improved accurate and sensitive UPLC–MS/MS method was newly developed for determining epinastine in human plasma. The product ion mass spectra of epinastine were obtained by scanning the individual standard solution into the mass spectrometer. Epinastine generated protonated molecular ion as $[M+H]^+$ in positive-ion mode. Internal standard (IS) was also performed in scan mode similarly and generated a protonated molecule ion of $[M+H]^+$, such as epinastine. The most abundant fragment ion for multiple reaction monitoring (MRM) was m/z 249.8 → 193.1 for epinastine and m/z 367.9 → 294.2 for the IS, respectively. The mass spectra results of epinastine were the same as those of Do et al. [9] and Bae et al. [10]. Figure 1 presents the relevant mass spectra. Other ionization parameters that optimized the quantification of epinastine were desolvation temperature of 250 °C, collision energy of −36 eV, nebulizing nitrogen gas flow of 3 L/min, and drying nitrogen gas flow of 15 L/min.

A mobile phase with various organic solvents (including precipitation and extraction solvents), pH, and different columns was tested to yield high resolution and adequate sensitivity. The Acquity UPLC® BEH C_{18}, HALO-C_{18}, and Phenomenex KINETEX core-shell C_{18} column using acetonitrile (ACN) and 0.1% (v/v) aqueous formic acid containing 1% (v/v) of 5 mM ammonium formate (pH 3.0) buffer by gradient elution at a flow rate of 0.3 mL/min were tested to obtain an optimum chromatogram. Although the three columns mentioned above have the same chemical structure (octadecyl, C_{18}) as the stationary phase, the charging technique differs slightly from each manufacturer and also varies in particle size. Finally, the Phenomenex KINETEX core-shell C_{18} column (50 × 2.1 mm, 1.7 μm particle size) was selected because it showed relatively good symmetric peak shapes, selectivity, and sensitivity for epinastine quantification. We used a mobile phase with ACN and water containing 0.05% (v/v) trifluoracetic acid [11] or 0.3% (v/v) triethylamine [12] with Phenomenex KINETEX core-shell C_{18}

column at a flow rate of 0.3 mL/min by gradient elution for epinastine quantification. However, these results were unsatisfactory for chromatograms of epinastine due to low sensitivity and incomplete peak symmetry. To overcome these problems, we additionally tested with 1% (*v/v*) of 5 mM ammonium formate (pH 3.0) buffers of varying pH, which included 0.1% acetic acid in water (final pH 2.9), 0.01% formic acid in water (final pH 2.7), and 0.05% formic acid in water (final pH 2.5), as well as 0.1% formic acid in water (final pH 2.3), which displayed the best resolution and highest intensity. In addition, ACN as mobile phase B showed a better resolution and a higher sensitive response than the mobile phase containing methanol reported in other studies [12]. As a result, water containing 0.1% formic acid containing 1% (*v/v*) of 5 mM ammonium formate (pH 3.0) buffer (mobile phase A, pH 2.3) and ACN (mobile phase B) were selected as mobile phases using gradient elution program. The gradient elution was satisfactory regarding the retention time, peak shape, and interference peaks separating epinastine. In addition, 1% (*v/v*) of 5 mM ammonium formate buffer (pH 3.0) maintained the retention time of epinastine constant. Figure 2A presents a representative MRM chromatogram with moderate retention times of 2.07 min for epinastine and 1.99 min for the IS.

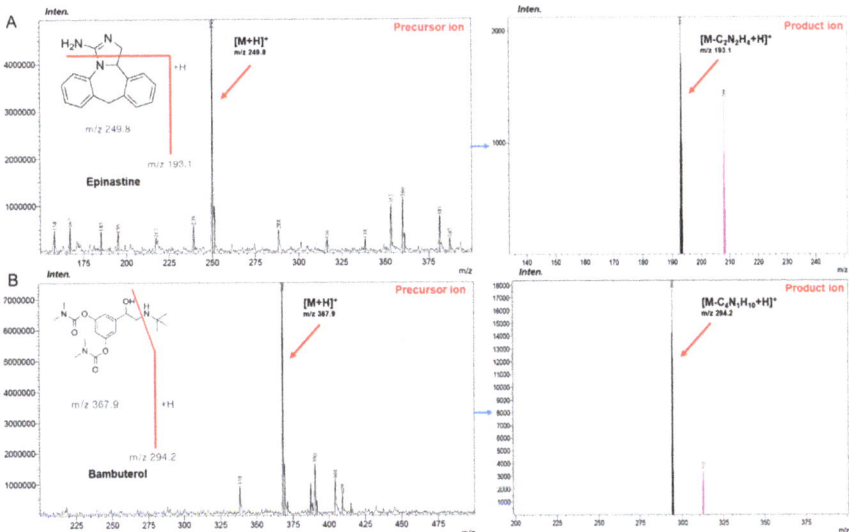

Figure 1. Positive product ion mass spectra in UPLC-MS/MS quantification; (**A**) epinastine; (**B**) bambuterol (IS). IS: internal standard.

Protein precipitation (PP) and liquid-liquid extraction (LLE) methods for sample extraction were tested. For the LLE method, di-ethyl ether, ethyl acetate, methylene chloride, and methyl tert-butyl ether (MTBE) were used for extraction from the sample. For epinastine, ethyl acetate showed much better extraction efficiency than methylene chloride, di-ethyl ether, and MTBE. Furthermore, the PP method using ACN and methanol was also tested. Methanol showed a lower noise and higher sensitive response than ACN and was finally selected as precipitation solvent for the PP method. Therefore, the PP method with methanol and the LLE method with ethyl acetate were optimized for the determination of epinastine in human plasma samples. In addition, the supernatant after extraction was evaporated to dryness under a gentle nitrogen stream at 35 °C to improve the sensitivity of epinastine in this UPLC-MS/MS method. This newly developed UPLC-MS/MS method provided higher sensitivity compared with the previous study in which the lower limit of quantitation (LLOQ) value was 1 ng/mL [10], with an LLOQ of 0.02 ng/mL.

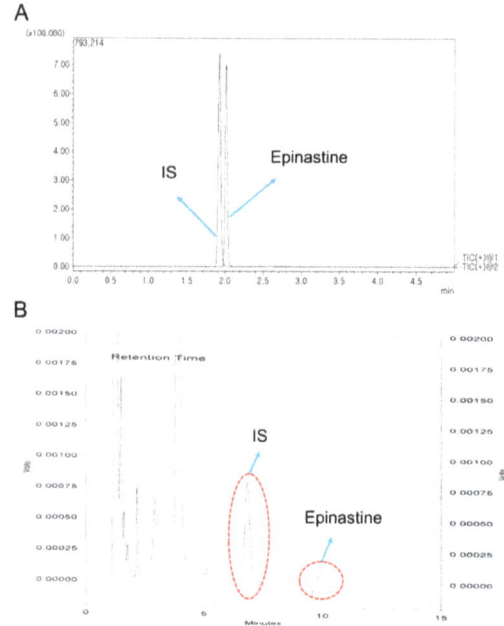

Figure 2. Representative chromatograms of epinastine and IS in MRM (multiple reaction monitoring) positive mode of UPLC-MS/MS (**A**) and HPLC-UV (**B**) method in human plasma.

2.1.2. HPLC-UV Method

A reversed-phase Nova-Pak C_{18} column (150 × 3.9 mm, 4 µm particle size) was used in the HPLC-UV method. The peak symmetry, selectivity, and shape of epinastine in the mobile phase, consisting of 20 mM phosphate (pH 5.6) buffer and methanol mixed with a small amount of ACN (64/30/6, *v/v/v*) at a flow rate of 0.8 mL/min, were observed. Figure 2B presents representative HPLC chromatograms with moderate retention times of 6.82 min for the IS and 9.91 min for epinastine. The HPLC-UV method was conducted using the isocratic elution, and the total run time was 15 min per sample. Bambuterol was selected as the IS based on peak shape and retention time in the selected column and extraction efficiency in human plasma. Only the LLE method with dichloromethane was optimized for quantification of epinastine in the sample preparation process, based on a reference related to epinastine analysis [13]. In this process, epinastine was a weakly basic substance and existed as cation at the biological pH. Thus, the plasma sample was treated with 500 µL of 0.1 M sodium carbonate to increase the extraction efficiency to the organic layer. The back-extraction process of epinastine into the aqueous layer was carried out using a 200 µL of 25 mM sulfuric acid solution. The HPLC-UV method used centrifuged upper layer directly without concentrating the decompression evaporation method using nitrogen, unlike the UPLC-MS/MS method. As a result, the time and steps required for sample preparation were reduced.

2.2. Quantitative Method Validation

2.2.1. Selectivity

Selectivity was shown in the response of the blank human plasma (Figure 3A,E), zero plasma containing the IS (Figure 3B,F), blank plasma containing LLOQ epinastine and IS (Figure 3C,G), and the plasma sample at 2 h after oral administration of epinastine hydrochloride tablet (Figure 3D,H). The representative chromatograms are presented in Figure 3, indicating no significant interferences from the endogenous substances around the retention times of analytes in blank plasma in both methods.

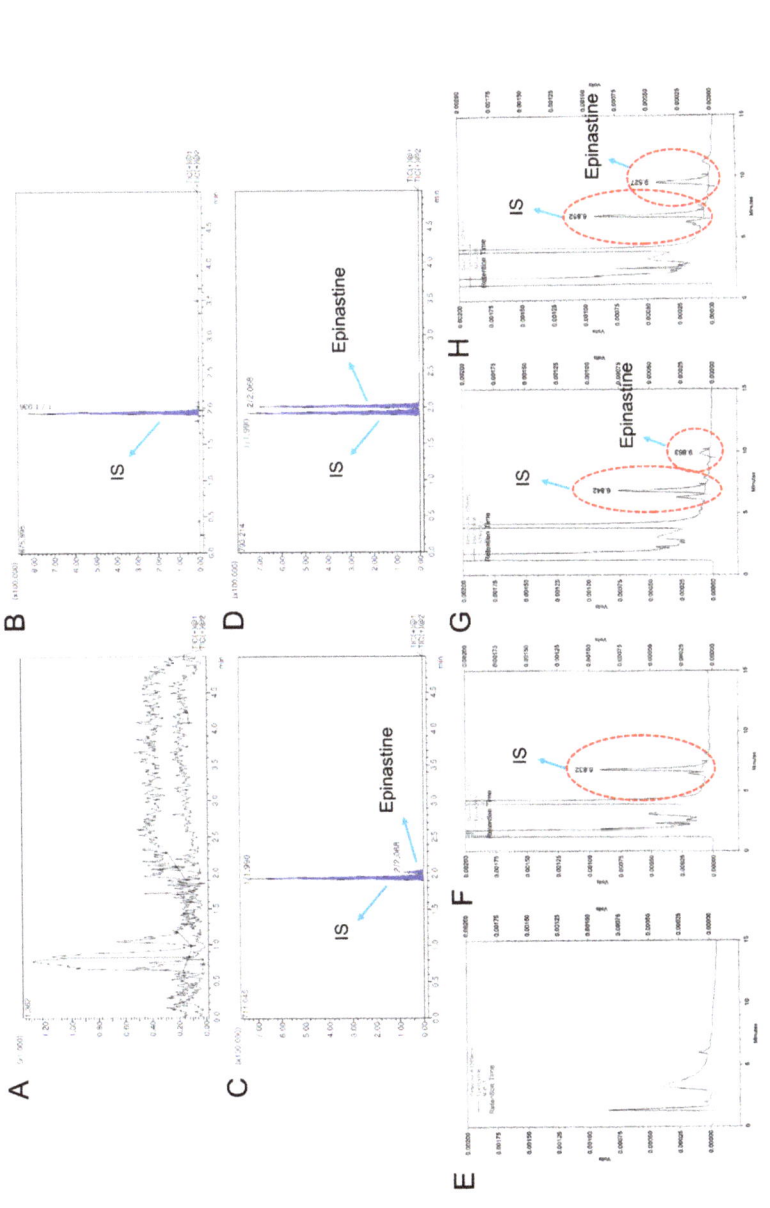

Figure 3. Chromatograms of blank plasma (**A** and **E**), zero plasma containing IS (**B** and **F**), blank plasma containing LLOQ (lower limit of quantitation) of epinastine and IS (**C** and **G**), the plasma sample at 2 h after oral administration of 20 mg epinastine hydrochloride tablet (**D** and **H**): A–D, UPLC-MS/MS; E–H, HPLC-UV.

2.2.2. Calibration Curves

Linearity for epinastine in human plasma was excellent over the concentration range of 1–100 ng/mL for HPLC-UV, and 0.02–100 ng/mL for UPLC-MS/MS. All calibration curves fitted well, with the correlation coefficient (r^2) of 0.99 or more. The linear regression equations of epinastine in human plasma were as follows: $y = (0.0262 \pm 0.0083)x + (0.00299 \pm 0.00095)$ for HPLC-UV, and $y = (0.1478 \pm 0.0307)x + (0.00263 \pm 0.00058)$ for UPLC-MS/MS with y as peak-area ratio of epinastine-to-IS and x (ng/mL) as plasma concentration of epinastine. Calibration curves for epinastine in human plasma are shown in Figure S1. The HPLC-UV and UPLC-MS/MS assays yielded LLOQs of 1 ng/mL and 0.02 ng/mL, respectively, suitable for PK study after oral administration of epinastine hydrochloride tablets in humans. The previously conducted HPLC-UV analysis [12] showed that the maximum plasma concentration (C_{max}) value of epinastine was not high (approximately mean 10 ng/mL), and was quantified below LLOQ in specific samples that corresponded to the early phase of drug absorption and terminal phase of elimination. Thus, lowering LLOQ was required for identifying a clear PK pattern in the body. The most sensitive LC-MS/MS method reported until now showed an LLOQ of about 1 ng/mL [10]. In comparison, our method had at least 50 times lower LLOQ than the previous method [10].

2.2.3. Accuracy and Precision

During the validation process of the newly developed method, excellent performance with consistent accuracy and low deviation was observed from four quality control (QC) samples. Table 1 describes the inter- and intra-batch accuracy and precision for epinastine. The intra-batch accuracy ranged from 95.15%–110.23% with a precision (coefficient of variation, CV) of <12.52% in both methods. In addition, the inter-batch accuracy ranged from 93.93%–114.47% with a precision (CV) of <8.23% in both analyses. All accuracies were within the range of 93.93% to 114.47%, and CV values for epinastine ranged from 1.32% to 12.52%. As a result, these indicated that both HPLC-UV and UPLC-MS/MS methods were reproducible and accurate for the quantification of epinastine in human plasma.

Table 1. Precision and accuracy of UPLC-MS/MS and HPLC-UV analysis for the determination of epinastine in human plasma (Mean ± SD, $n = 5$).

Method	Spiked Conc. (ng/mL)	Intra-Batch ($n = 5$)			Inter-Batch ($n = 5$)		
		Measured Conc. (ng/mL, Mean ± SD)	Precision (CV, %)	Accuracy (%)	Measured Conc. (ng/mL, Mean ± SD)	Precision (CV, %)	Accuracy (%)
UPLC-MS/MS	QC 0.02	0.020 ± 0.001	4.90	102.00	0.019 ± 0.001	5.07	94.50
	QC 5	4.918 ± 0.067	1.32	98.36	5.115 ± 0.085	1.66	102.30
	QC 20	19.386 ± 0.924	4.48	96.93	18.976 ± 1.373	6.53	94.88
	QC 80	82.029 ± 4.285	5.22	102.54	84.281 ± 5.249	6.23	105.35
HPLC-UV	QC 1	1.108 ± 0.107	11.63	110.23	1.036 ± 0.113	4.04	114.47
	QC 5	4.866 ± 0.533	12.52	95.64	5.158 ± 0.114	2.67	106.23
	QC 20	21.043 ± 1.001	3.16	105.07	18.863 ± 1.961	6.09	93.93
	QC 80	76.121 ± 7.473	9.34	95.15	82.421 ± 6.582	8.23	103.03

CV, coefficient of variation; QC, quality control.

2.2.4. Matrix Effect and Recovery

Table 2 presents the matrix effect and/or recoveries for epinastine in HPLC-UV and UPLC-MS/MS method. The extraction recoveries of epinastine from human plasma were 91.58–94.36% and 95.93–97.62%. The recoveries of IS were 96.94 ± 4.73% and 99.46 ± 3.54% in HPLC-UV and UPLC-MS/MS analysis, respectively. Significant matrix effects were not seen in the quantification of epinastine (95.28–96.63% with UPLC-MS/MS) or IS (97.35 ± 3.16% with UPLC-MS/MS). The results suggested that the recoveries of the analyte were reproducible, consistent, and precise. The simple LLE and/or PP methods optimized for extracting epinastine from human plasma were successfully applied to the determination of epinastine in human plasma.

Table 2. Recovery and matrix effect for the determination of epinastine in human plasma via UPLC-MS/MS and HPLC-UV methods (Mean ± SD, n = 5).

Method	Spiked Conc. (ng/mL)	Measured Conc. (ng/mL, Mean ± SD)	Recovery (%)	Measured Conc. (ng/mL, Mean ± SD)	Matrix Effect (%)
UPLC-MS/MS	QC 5	4.88 ± 0.16	97.62 ± 3.14	4.76 ± 0.07	95.28 ± 1.42
	QC 20	19.19 ± 0.57	95.93 ± 2.85	19.33 ± 0.49	96.63 ± 2.44
	QC 80	76.99 ± 3.46	96.24 ± 4.33	76.57 ± 1.68	95.71 ± 2.10
	IS (bambuterol) 10	9.95 ± 0.35	99.46 ± 3.54	9.74 ± 0.32	97.35 ± 3.16
HPLC-UV	QC 5	4.58 ± 0.26	91.58 ± 5.11	-	-
	QC 20	18.48 ± 1.05	92.40 ± 5.27	-	-
	QC 80	75.49 ± 5.11	94.36 ± 6.39	-	-
	IS (bambuterol) 10	9.69 ± 0.47	96.94 ± 4.73	-	-

IS, internal standard.

2.2.5. Stabilities

In both methods, the stability for epinastine was evaluated using two different levels of QC samples under various conditions. The stabilities were examined as freeze-thaw, short-term, and long-term stability. The results are presented in Table 3. Epinastine was stable in human plasma for 24 h at 25 °C without any significant degradation (range of 97.91–100.35% in both methods). In the long-term stability test for 4 weeks at −80 °C, epinastine was also stable, which guaranteed the quality of quantification after sample collection within 4 weeks (range of 98.42–101.53% in both methods). All analytes were stable after three cycles (range of 96.04–101.62% in both methods) in the freeze-thaw cycle test. Furthermore, epinastine was stable for 24 h at 25 °C ranged from 98.13–101.91% in the HPLC-UV method and stable for 24 h at 15 °C ranged from 99.33–102.09% in UPLC-MS/MS method as post-preparative stability. These ranges were within the limits of the Food and Drug Administration (FDA) guidelines (±15%) in all stability tests. In addition, the stock solutions for IS and epinastine were stable in the storage concentration for 4 weeks at −20 °C. The stability of the epinastine stock solution was 100.14 ± 2.06%, and the stability of the IS stock solution was 98.72 ± 3.38%. All these results suggested the stability of epinastine under various storage conditions.

Table 3. Stabilities of epinastine under various conditions of UPLC-MS/MS and HPLC-UV quantification methods (Mean ± SD, n = 5).

Method	Spiked Conc. (ng/mL)	Short-Term Stability (24 h)	Long-Term Stability (4 weeks)	Freeze-Thaw Stability (3 cycles)	Post-Preparative Stability (24 h)
UPLC-MS/MS	QC 5	99.44 ± 3.11	101.53 ± 1.49	101.62 ± 2.66	99.33 ± 4.02
	QC 80	98.21 ± 5.22	98.51 ± 0.99	98.11 ± 3.32	102.09 ± 1.48
HPLC-UV	QC 5	97.91 ± 4.02	98.42 ± 3.84	100.10 ± 4.35	98.13 ± 2.62
	QC 80	100.35 ± 4.83	99.55 ± 3.67	96.04 ± 4.93	101.91 ± 3.17

2.2.6. Carryover

As presented in Figure 3A,E, after injecting the highest concentration (epinastine of 100 ng/mL) sample of the standard curve, no peak of the analytes was shown in the blank plasma sample. It was validated that the carryover had no effect on the analysis.

2.2.7. Incurred Sample Reanalysis

Thirty-two (10% of the total analyzed samples) human plasma samples were examined to evaluate incurred sample reanalysis (ISR). The variability of all samples was within 20% between the value of initial analysis and that of reanalysis in both methods. In addition, twenty-five samples were within 10% in HPLC-UV, and twenty-eight samples were within 10% in UPLC-MS/MS. As a result, the newly developed method showed the reproducibility of the initial analysis results.

2.3. Methods Comparison

Individual HPLC-UV and UPLC-MS/MS methods were developed for the quantification of epinastine in human plasma. Table 4 summarizes the information for both methods. The obtained plasma concentration-time profiles (Figure 4) and calculated PK parameter values (Table 5) for epinastine showed similar findings in HPLC-UV and UPLC-MS/MS methods.

Table 4. Summary of information on UPLC-MS/MS and HPLC-UV methods developed in this study.

	UPLC-MS/MS	HPLC-UV
LLOQ	0.02 ng/mL	1 ng/mL
LOD	0.007 ng/mL	0.3 ng/mL
Calibration range	0.02–100 ng/mL	1–100 ng/mL
Run time	5 min	15 min
Sample extraction	LLE with ethyl acetate and PP with methanol	LLE with dichloromethane
Sample volume	100 μL	500 μL
Column type and size	KINETEX core-shell C_{18} (50 × 2.1 mm, 1.7 μm particle size; Phenomenex, USA)	Nova-Pak C_{18} (150 × 3.9 mm, 4 μm particle size; Waters, USA)
Mobile phase	0.1% aqueous formic acid:5 mM ammonium formate:ACN (1/1/4, $v/v/v$)	20 mM phosphate buffer:methanol:ACN (64/30/6, $v/v/v$)
Flow rate	0.3 mL/min	0.8 mL/min
Injection volume	5 μL	50 μL
Internal standard	Bambuterol (10 ng/mL)	Bambuterol (10 ng/mL)
Results	All plasma samples were quantified in the range (even in the 24 h samples).	Some plasma samples were not quantified within the range and showed values below LLOQ (at 0.5 h of initial absorption of some samples and 24 h of post-elimination).

LLOQ, lower limit of quantitation; LOD, limit of detection; LLE, liquid-liquid extraction; PP, protein precipitation.

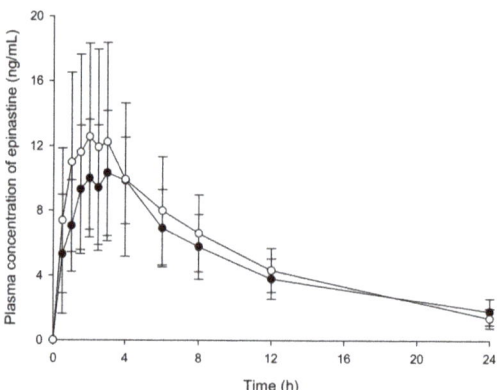

Figure 4. Mean plasma concentration-time profiles of epinastine after oral administration of 20 mg epinastine hydrochloride tablet based on UPLC-MS/MS (-○-) and HPLC-UV (-●-) methods. Vertical bars represent the standard deviation of the mean (n = 26).

Table 5. Pharmacokinetic parameters of epinastine in humans after oral administration of 20 mg epinastine hydrochloride tablet in UPLC-MS/MS and HPLC-UV quantification methods (Mean ± SD).

Parameter	UPLC-MS/MS	HPLC-UV	p-Value	Ratio ($\frac{UPLC-MS/MS}{HPLC-UV}$)
$AUC_{0-\infty}$ (h·ng/mL)	144.88 ± 45.86	143.01 ± 44.43	0.98	1.01 ± 0.32
AUC_{0-t} (h·ng/mL)	129.84 ± 39.21	115.21 ± 34.30	0.78	1.13 ± 0.36
CL/F (L/h)	150.99 ± 46.05	156.72 ± 65.34	0.92	0.96 ± 0.33
V_d/F (L)	1519.50 ± 546.31	2091.30 ± 588.22	0.45	0.73 ± 0.26
C_{max} (ng/mL)	14.82 ± 6.06	11.62 ± 3.63	0.47	1.27 ± 0.50
T_{max} (h)	2.13 ± 1.20	2.71 ± 1.27	0.52	0.79 ± 0.37
$t_{1/2}$ (h)	7.08 ± 1.80	9.95 ± 3.00	0.41	0.72 ± 0.21

$AUC_{0-\infty}$, area under the curve; AUC_{0-t}, area to final measured concentration; CL/F, clearance; V_d/F, volume of distribution; C_{max}, the maximum plasma concentration; T_{max}, the time to reach C_{max}; $t_{1/2}$, half-life.

Figure 5A depicts a two-dimensional graph of parameters derived from the same human samples. The linear regression line of the graph was as follows: y = 0.99824x + 0.59482. The slope of the regression line was close to one, and the correlation coefficient (r^2) was 0.84, indicating a strong and reliable correlation. Twenty-two samples (7.05% of total) were measured below LLOQ in HPLC-UV, while they were all quantified in UPLC-MS/MS. These results were plotted on the graph as points on the y-axis ranging from 0.07–5, with the x-axis being 0. Among the total 312 points, 297 were within the 95% prediction interval (PI), corresponding to a statistical value of 95.19%. Figure 5B shows the difference between the two analytical methods (UPLC-MS/MS-HPLC-UV), depending on the concentrations measured by HPLC-UV. The linear regression line of the graph was as follows: y = 0.0355x + 0.0926. The slope of the regression line was close to 0, indicating that the difference between the two methods was not significant. At concentrations above 15 ng/mL quantified by HPLC-UV, there were no points where the difference between the two methods exceeded the 95% PI. All points outside the 95% PI were observed at less than 15 ng/mL. These results meant that the difference between the two analytical values was greater at lower concentrations than at higher concentrations.

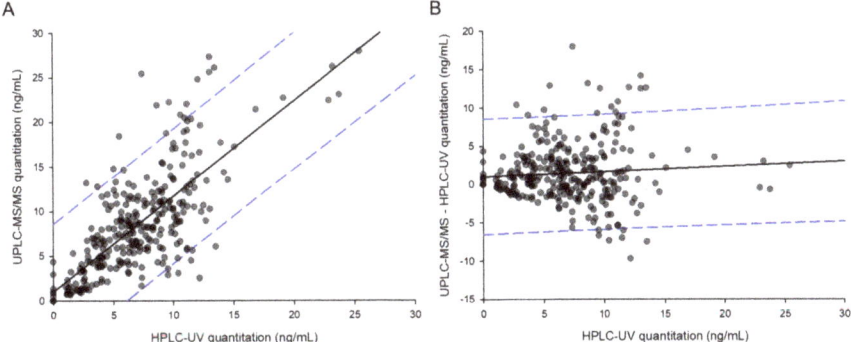

Figure 5. Comparative analysis of samples using HPLC-UV (x-axis) and UPLC-MS/MS (y-axis) (**A**), and correlation of the method differences between HPLC-UV (x-axis) and UPLC-MS/MS – HPLC-UV (y-axis) (**B**). The straight line represents the linear regression line, and the dashed line shows a 95% prediction interval line.

2.4. Pharmacokinetic Studies

The newly developed HPLC-UV and UPLC-MS/MS methods were supported in the PK study of epinastine after oral administration of 20 mg epinastine to twenty-six healthy Korean subjects. The concentration-time curves of epinastine in humans using HPLC-UV and UPLC-MS/MS quantification methods are displayed in Figure 4. After oral administration of epinastine hydrochloride tablets, the time to reach C_{max} (T_{max}) of epinastine was defined as 2–3 h. Epinastine was rapidly absorbed into the blood and was slowly removed from the blood, which could be detected even 24 h after administration. In addition, the C_{max} was relatively low on the average of 10–20 ng/mL. This might be related to reports that the absolute oral bioavailability of epinastine was as low as about 40%, and that a significant amount of orally administered epinastine was detected in feces rather than urine [1,14]. The estimated PK parameters, including area under the curve ($AUC_{0-\infty}$), half-life ($t_{1/2}$), clearance (CL/F), area to final measured concentration (AUC_{0-t}), T_{max}, C_{max}, and volume of distribution (V_d/F), are presented in Table 5. The $t_{1/2}$ of epinastine reported by Li et al. [15] was 7.79–10.68 h, and the T_{max} was 1.88–2.3 h. The $t_{1/2}$ of epinastine reported by Shi et al. [16] was 8.8–10.4 h, and the T_{max} was 2.0–2.7 h. These were similar to our PK results. The remaining reported PK results were limited for comparison with our results, as they were either in rats or administration of eye drops to the ocular pathway.

2.5. Pharmacokinetic Parameters Comparison

The student's t-test was applied to compare the differences between the PK parameters determined by quantification methods of HPLC-UV and UPLC-MS/MS. As a result, the PK parameters calculated by HPLC-UV and UPLC-MS/MS methods were not statistically different ($p > 0.05$). The ratios of $AUC_{0-\infty}$ (including AUC_{0-t}) and CL/F were close to one between HPLC-UV and UPLC-MS/MS method, whereas the ratios of $t_{1/2}$ and V_d/F varied depending on the method probably due to the low concentration of the results included in the PK regression process. The ratios of T_{max} and C_{max} were 0.79 ± 0.37 and 1.27 ± 0.50, respectively, probably related to the 2–3 h plasma concentration plateau without significant change.

In addition, we simulated epinastine plasma concentrations at multiple doses based on single-dose data from each assay. This simulation assumed that 20 mg of epinastine hydrochloride was administered at 24 h intervals, similar to clinical dosing of once-daily (mentioned in the Section 1 Introduction), and the WinNonlin® software (version 8.1, Pharsight®, a Certara™ Company, Princeton, NJ, USA) was used for multiple simulations. Figure 6 is a simulation (mean) graph of multiple doses based on single-dose data of epinastine hydrochloride obtained using HPLC-UV and UPLC-MS/MS, respectively. Steady-state (mean) plasma concentrations predicted by each assay were approximately 5.96–6.04 ng/mL with little difference. However, as shown in Table 6, the (mean) predicted $t_{1/2}$ of epinastine at steady-state was 7.35 h (by UPLC-MS/MS method) and 11.35 h (by HPLC-UV method), which were quite different between the predicted values. The predicted steady-state C_{max} (mean) was 15.69 ng/mL and 13.27 ng/mL in UPLC-MS/MS and HPLC-UV method, respectively. The predicted steady-state minimum plasma concentration (C_{min}) (mean) was 1.55 and 2.28 in UPLC-MS/MS and HPLC-UV analysis, respectively. There was no statistically significant difference ($p > 0.05$) in both C_{max} and C_{min} estimated from the two analytical methods. However, there was a significant difference ($p < 0.05$) in the ratio of C_{max}/C_{min} to 10.12 (mean) and 5.82 (mean) for UPLC-MS/MS and HPLC-UV methods, respectively.

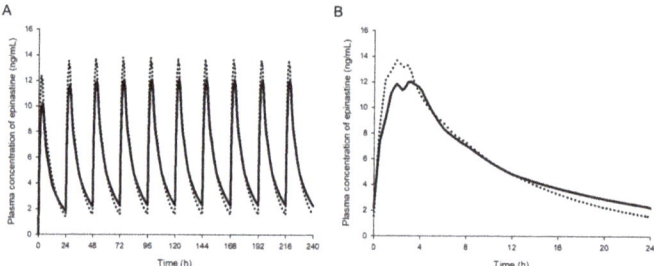

Figure 6. Simulation (mean value) graphs of multiple doses based on single-dose (mean) data of epinastine hydrochloride obtained using HPLC-UV (straight line) and UPLC-MS/MS (dashed line); (**A**) multiple simulation graph pattern; (**B**) estimated PK (pharmacokinetic) graph from 0 to 24 h at steady-state.

Table 6. Estimated pharmacokinetic parameters of epinastine in humans at steady-state after oral multiple administration of 20 mg epinastine hydrochloride tablet in UPLC-MS/MS and HPLC-UV quantification methods (Mean ± SD).

Parameter	UPLC-MS/MS	HPLC-UV	p-value	Ratio ($\frac{UPLC-MS/MS}{HPLC-UV}$)
$AUC_{0-\infty}$ (h·ng/mL)	157.38 ± 56.89	181.18 ± 68.22	0.77	0.87 ± 0.31
AUC_{0-t} (h·ng/mL)	139.75 ± 45.15	139.80 ± 43.56	0.99	1.00 ± 0.32
CL/F (L/h)	141.10 ± 44.41	131.69 ± 71.45	0.88	1.07 ± 0.33
V_d/F (L)	1457.58 ± 484.22	1878.28 ± 486.91	0.51	0.78 ± 0.26
C_{max} (ng/mL)	15.69 ± 6.17	13.27 ± 3.89	0.62	1.18 ± 0.46
C_{min} (ng/mL)	1.55 ± 0.83	2.28 ± 1.08	0.35	0.68 ± 0.36
C_{max}/C_{min}	10.12 ± 3.98	5.82 ± 1.71*	0.01	1.74
T_{max} (h)	2.02 ± 1.16	2.65 ± 1.28	0.46	0.76 ± 0.43
$t_{1/2}$ (h)	7.35 ± 1.78	11.35 ± 4.33*	0.04	0.65 ± 0.16

* $p < 0.05$, compared with calculated parameters by UPLC-MS/MS method.

3. Discussion

Until now, few studies investigated PKs of epinastine, and analytical methods with limited validation information have been proposed. Some articles have reported bioanalytical methods for epinastine based on HPLC or specific analytical conditions [14–16]. However, validation information could not be confirmed in those reports. Oiwa et al. [14] reported that after oral and intravenous (IV) administration of ^{14}C-epinastine hydrochloride in rats, there was dose-linearity, no gender difference on PKs, the largest distribution in the gastrointestinal tract, and a small amount excretion into the milk. Li et al. [15] revealed that there was no difference in PKs between healthy Chinese and Tibetans after a single oral administration of 20 mg of epinastine hydrochloride tablets using an HPLC-UV method. Shi et al. [16] also reported that test tablets had little difference in PK pattern from reference tablets in a bioequivalence study of epinastine hydrochloride in healthy Chinese subjects.

Several studies have used HPLC method for analysis of bulk drug [11], formulation [17], or dietary supplements [9], but are rarely used for biological sample analysis. In addition, the LLOQ values they presented were so high that it was very limited for application in quantifying biological samples. Although some researchers analyzed epinastine in rat plasma using HPLC-UV, there were common limitations of high LLOQ and long run time [12,13]. Ahirrao et al. [11] reported an HPLC-UV analysis of epinastine in bulk drug, and its LLOQ and limit of detection (LOD) were as high as 180 and 50 ng/mL, respectively. The HPLC-UV analysis of epinastine reported by Malakar et al. [17] was also for the pharmaceutical dosage form, and the LLOQ was very high as 2 µg/mL. Do et al. [9] reported the simultaneous analysis of 20 antihistamines, including epinastine, in dietary supplements, but it was very limited to be directly applied for the analysis of biological samples in consideration of different sample preparation and assay validation and long analysis time per sample. In addition, LLOQ was as high as 90 ng/mL and was not suitable for the analysis of biological samples. An HPLC-UV method, which analyzed rat plasma samples administered with 5–20 mg/kg epinastine, was introduced. However, the LLOQ of epinastine was very high, at 10 ng/mL [12]. Also, the amount of organic solvent required for preparation per sample was more than 5 mL, and the required time was very long (more than 30 min). There was also a report of rat plasma analysis, although the LLOQ value was also as high as 20 ng/mL [13]. The run-time per sample was very long, more than 16 min, and there was no assay validation, including stability, carry-over, etc.

There have also been some studies on human sample analysis using LC-MS/MS. However, they had limitations, such as high LLOQ [10], lack of detailed information on methodology [18], and much time and solvent [19]. Bae et al. [10] reported the LC-MS/MS method for epinastine in abstract form, but the LLOQ value was as high as 1 ng/mL, and specific experimental methods were lacked. In addition, Yu et al. [18] also measured epinastine concentrations in tear samples after topical ophthalmic administration of epinastine eyedrops to humans. However, due to the lack of detailed description and validation information of the assay, it was limited to apply for epinastine analysis in other biological samples. Although the analytical method reported by Shi et al. [19] was sensitive to 0.1 ng/mL of LLOQ, the required time for the analysis was very long, and the consumption of solvents was large due to HPLC method. Those previously reported contents on epinastine assay are summarized in Table S1.

Because of the clinical importance and wide application of epinastine, studies on various analytical methods and pharmacological effects have been reported from the past to the present. However, as mentioned above, there were limitations in reported epinastine assays, and so we have been working to develop UPLC-MS/MS and HPLC-UV methods that complement these limitations. As shown in our previous report [20], epinastine showed a very low C_{max} of 10–20 ng/mL. Therefore, it is essential to develop highly accurate and sensitive assay methods to obtain definite PK results, including the absorption and elimination phase, in drugs, such as epinastine.

The use of UPLC columns, optimizing the mobile phase, the use of gradient elution program, enhancing the extraction efficiency and removing impurities through appropriate sample preparation, and sample concentration through evaporation could greatly improve the sensitivity than the previously reported methods. Our results demonstrated that the developed methods were reproducible, selective, precise, accurate, and relatively impervious to endogenous interference. UPLC-MS/MS was found to be 50 times more sensitive than HPLC-UV for the determination of epinastine. Therefore, UPLC-MS/MS method was more adequate for the analysis of clinical samples where the dosages were lower. Highly sensitive UPLC-MS/MS was required in vivo in order to quantify substantially low levels of analytes in large numbers of biological samples. Thus, we quantified epinastine concentration in plasma samples obtained from all individuals. As a result, the PK profile, showing the elimination and the absorption phases, was determined accurately. In addition, UPLC-MS/MS required substantially less organic solvent and less sample volume for sample preparation. Furthermore, the required time for the total sample analysis was significantly reduced. It has, therefore, a more economical modality and is environmentally friendly. However, UPLC-MS/MS is associated with a high operating cost and is more expensive than HPLC-UV. Therefore, HPLC-UV analysis is more economical if the PK differences in HPLC-UV and UPLC-MS/MS quantification results are not as large as determined in the epinastine quantitative assay. Although the run time was 15 min, and the HPLC-UV method lasted three times longer, the HPLC-UV method was shorter than the UPLC-MS/MS method in sample preparation, suggesting that HPLC-UV method was more economical for the analysis of a small number of total samples. Our results illustrated the fact that UPLC-MS/MS could be very sensitive in comparison with HPLC-UV, which typically goes down to 1 ng/mL (LLOQ of developed HPLC-UV method). However, for general clinical studies, HPLC-UV analysis could be used, and an adequate PK profile could be obtained with a method validated between 1 and 100 ng/mL. The developed methods could be applied to the analysis of epinastine in plasma, as well as other biological samples. The reason for the difference in plasma sample preparation between UPLC-MS/MS and HPLC-UV methods is that the extraction solvent composition for each analytical instrument was developed and applied. Extraction solvents applied to HPLC-UV suspected significant matrix effects in UPLC-MS/MS, and the recovery was not satisfactory. In other words, it was optimized and applied to UPLC-MS/MS with an extraction solvent different from HPLC-UV in consideration of the matrix effect and recovery in UPLC-MS/MS.

The ratios ($\frac{UPLC-MS/MS}{HPLC-UV}$) presented in Table 5 have a very important meaning. As mentioned above (in the Section 4.5.3 Accuracy and precision), the accuracy and precision of analysis typically allowed for variability within ±15%. Variability within ±20% was allowed at the LLOQ. Nevertheless, the average ratio of V_d/F, C_{max}, T_{max}, and $t_{1/2}$ showed a difference of more than 20%. In other words, when comparing only the mean values of parameters (V_d/F, C_{max}, T_{max}, and $t_{1/2}$), they were out of 15% or 20% (usual tolerance in analysis). In the case of V_d/F, the mean value of epinastine after a single oral dose could be calculated as low as 27% when analyzing plasma samples using UPLC-MS/MS and as short as 28% as for $t_{1/2}$. There also could be a difference in the accumulation index as 1.117 (by UPLC-MS/MS method) and 1.301 (by HPLC-UV method), when estimating the accumulation index by the following equation: $1/1-e^{-k \cdot \tau}$, where τ is the 24 h as dosing interval. This might affect the dosing and use of epinastine in relation to a cumulative evaluation in the body at multiple doses. In the case of C_{max}, the mean value of epinastine after a single oral dose could be determined as high as 27% when analyzing plasma samples using UPLC-MS/MS and as short as 21% for T_{max}. This might affect the dosing and use of epinastine with regard to drug effects and toxicity. In addition, as shown in Figure 6 and Table 6, the results can be different when multiple-dose simulations are performed with single-dose PK parameters calculated based on data obtained by different assays. This could greatly affect PK evaluation. As shown in Table 6, the ratio of C_{max}/C_{min} at steady-state was about 2 times greater in UPLC-MS/MS than HPLC-UV. This means that if we choose the HPLC-UV method for the calculation of epinastine PK parameters, we would be apt to underestimate the safety or toxicity of epinastine. Using the UPLC-MS/MS method, we could quantify the concentration of the epinastine terminal phase in the blood, resulting in shorter $t_{1/2}$ (than HPLC-UV), large clearance (than HPLC-UV), and large estimation of the difference between steady-state C_{max} and C_{min} in multiple-dose simulations. In other words, the LLOQ reduction in the analysis by UPLC-MS/MS caused some differences in the estimation of PK parameters compared to HPLC-UV by quantifying epinastine elimination phases that were not accurately quantified by HPLC-UV. Our findings suggested that the choice of the assay for biosamples is critical for PK analysis and clinical dose and regimen settings. Previously reported literature [21,22] has emphasized that there are differences in the results of an assay for tacrolimus concentrations in the blood by different analytical methods. In particular, the difference between the results of microparticle enzyme immunoassay (MEIA) and LC-MS/MS was significant at low concentrations and suggested that it could significantly affect the treatment of patients [21]. In the study of Braun et al. [22], the same patient samples (tacrolimus administered) were analyzed by various analytical methods. As a result, the drug concentrations were measured differently at 10.5, 7.92, and 2.93 ng/mL in MEIA, enzyme-linked immune-sorbent assay, and LC-MS/MS. In other words, when one sample is analyzed by LC-MS/MS, the concentration is measured to be low, and the administration dose should be increased. On the other hand, when the MEIA method is used, the concentration could be over-estimated, indicating that dose adjustment is not necessary. This suggests that inappropriate treatment may have been performed. Although the therapeutic range of epinastine is not as narrow as that of tacrolimus, dose adjustment of epinastine due to differences in assays should be carefully considered in the treatment of patients, as with tacrolimus.

4. Materials and Methods

4.1. Reagents and Chemicals

Epinastine hydrochloride (purity ≥ 99%) was obtained from Heumann Pharma GmbH & Co. Generica KG (Nuremberg, Germany), and bambuterol (purity ≥ 99%) was purchased from Sigma-Aldrich (St. Louis, MO, USA). Bambuterol was used as an IS in both methods (HPLC-UV and UPLC-MS/MS). Figure 7 presents the structures of epinastine and bambuterol. LC-MS/MS grade water (18.2 mΩ), methanol, ACN, and HPLC grade ethyl acetate were obtained from Fisher Scientific (Hampton, NH, USA). LC-MS/MS grade formic acid was purchased from DUKSAN Inc. (Ansan, Korea). All chemicals used in this study met the highest HPLC grade or quality available.

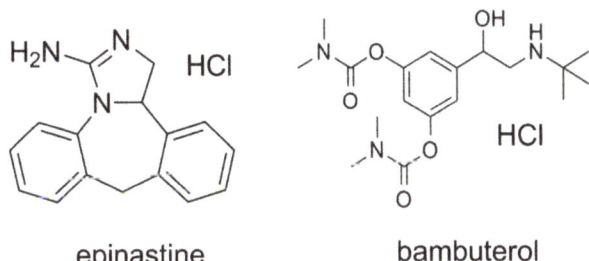

Figure 7. Chemical structures of epinastine hydrochloride and bambuterol hydrochloride (internal standard).

4.2. Chromatographic Conditions and Instrumentation

4.2.1. UPLC-MS/MS Method

The UPLC-MS/MS method was conducted using an LC-30AD of Shimadzu Nexera X2 Series UPLC system (Shimadzu, Kyoto, Japan) coupled with a SIL-30AC autosampler and DGU-20A degassing unit with Shimadzu-8040 mass spectrometer. In order to obtain an optimum chromatogram, various condition tests were carried out on the mobile phase pH (0.01% formic acid in water (pH 2.7), 0.1% formic acid in water (pH 2.3), 0.05% formic acid in water (pH 2.5), 0.1% acetic acid in water (pH 2.9), 0.05% trifluoracetic acid in water (pH 2.1), and 0.3% triethylamine in water (pH 4.5), v/v), containing 1% (v/v) of 5 mM ammonium formate (pH 3.0) buffer, and column (Acquity UPLC® BEH C_{18} (50 mm × 2.1 mm, 1.7 μm), HALO-C_{18} (100 mm × 2.1 mm, 2.7 μm), and Phenomenex KINETEX core-shell C_{18} (50 mm × 2.1 mm, 1.7 μm) column). The optimized chromatographic separation of epinastine was obtained on a Phenomenex KINETEX core-shell C_{18} column at an oven temperature of 40 °C. The mobile phase configuration was ACN (mobile phase B) and 0.1% aqueous formic acid, containing 1% (v/v) of 5 mM ammonium formate (pH 3.0) buffer (mobile phase A, pH 2.3), with gradient elution and a flow rate of 0.3 mL/min. The gradient elution program was as follows: 0–0.5 min (20% B), 0.5–1.5 min (20–80% B), 1.5–3.5 min (80% B), 3.5–3.51 min (80–20% B), and 3.51–5.0 min (20% B). All analytical procedures were conducted with positive electrospray ionization, and quantification was achieved using MRM modes at m/z 249.80 → 193.10 for epinastine and at m/z 367.90 → 294.20 for IS, respectively. Acquisition and analysis of data were achieved using a LabSolutions program. The injection volume was 5 µL, and the collision energies of epinastine and IS were −36 and −20 eV, respectively.

4.2.2. HPLC-UV Method

The HPLC system consisted of a Shimadzu LC 10 AD series (Shimadzu, Kyoto, Japan) equipped with a photodiode array detector with LabSolutions software. A Nova-Pak C_{18} column (150 × 3.9 mm, 4 µm particle size) from Waters Inc. (Milford, MA, USA) was applied as a stationary phase, and the oven temperature was maintained at 40 °C. The mobile phase consisted of 20 mM phosphate buffer (pH 3.5) and methanol mixed with a small amount of ACN (64/30/6, v/v/v) at a flow rate of 0.8 mL/min. Chromatographic separation was conducted using an isocratic elution. The total run time was 15 min per sample. Injection volume was 50 µL using the Rheodyne injector, and the detection wavelength was 220 nm. Peaks were assigned by spiking the samples with standard compounds and comparison of the retention times and UV spectra.

4.3. Preparation of Standard Solutions

Epinastine and IS stock solutions were prepared as follows: each of epinastine hydrochloride and IS was accurately weighed and dissolved in methanol at a concentration of 1 mg/mL as epinastine prior to obtaining working solutions. All stock solutions were stored at −20 °C. The standard working solutions of epinastine (10, 20, 50, 100, 200, 500, and 1000 ng/mL in HPLC-UV analytical procedure; 0.2, 1, 10, 50, 100, 500, and 1000 ng/mL in UPLC-MS/MS analytical procedure) and the IS (100 ng/mL) were diluted stepwise with 100% methanol from the standard stock solutions. In addition, calibration standards were determined by adding each diluted working solution into a blank human plasma to obtain the final concentrations of epinastine ranging from 1–100 ng/mL in HPLC-UV analytical method and 0.02–100 ng/mL in UPLC-MS/MS analytical method. In order to examine the accuracy and precision of the developed method, QC samples of four concentration levels (1, 5, 20, and 80 ng/mL in HPLC-UV; 0.02, 5, 20, and 80 ng/mL in UPLC-MS/MS) were prepared in a similar way. Preparation of QC samples and calibration curves were performed on the same day of analysis in both methods.

4.4. Sample Extraction

In the HPLC-UV analytical method, epinastine was extracted from human plasma by employing the LLE method. A total of 500 µL of human plasma samples were added to a 50 µL of the IS solution (100 ng/mL of bambuterol in 100% methanol), and 500 µL of 0.1 M sodium carbonate was added to human plasma samples. Then, 4 mL of dichloromethane was added to the mixed sample and vortexed for 7 min and centrifuged at 6000× g for 20 min. The supernatant was removed, and the organic layer was transferred to another test tube. A 200 µL of 25 mM sulfuric acid solution was added, and the mixture was back-extracted for 1 min and centrifuged at 6000 rpm for 5 min. A 150 µL of the upper layer was transferred to an Eppendorf tube (Axygen Scientific Inc., Union City, CA, USA), and an aliquot (50 µL) of this final sample solution was taken and injected into the HPLC-UV system. In UPLC-MS/MS analytical method, the sample extraction for epinastine was extensively tested using the PP method with ACN and methanol, as well as the LLE method using di-ethyl ether, ethyl acetate, methylene chloride, and MTBE. As a result, the samples were extracted by LLE using ethyl acetate, and the protein was precipitated by PP using methanol. A total of 100 µL of human plasma samples were added to a 10 µL of the IS solution (100 ng/mL of bambuterol in 100% methanol). Then, 1000 µL of ethyl acetate-methanol (1/2, v/v) was added to the mixed samples and vortexed for 6 min and centrifuged at 13,000× g for 6 min. Then, 1000 µL of the supernatant corresponding to the organic layer was dried gently with a centrifugal vacuum evaporator of the CVE-3000 model (EYELA Co., Tokyo, Japan) under nitrogen gas at 35 °C for 4 h. The dried matter was reconstituted with 50 µL of 100% methanol and vortexed for 6 min. After centrifugation for 6 min at 13,000× g, 5 µL of aliquots were injected into the UPLC-MS/MS system.

4.5. Method Validation

The validation of newly developed methods was performed in accordance with the Guidance for Industry: Bioanalytical Method Validation issued by the United States FDA [23], in terms of recovery, accuracy, precision, selectivity, linearity, sensitivity, matrix effect, carryover, stability, and ISR.

4.5.1. Selectivity and Sensitivity

Selectivity was evaluated to ensure the effect of endogenous substances located in the closed retention time of the analytes. Therefore, the blank plasma, zero plasma, plasma spiked with epinastine hydrochloride of LLOQ level, and real plasma samples collected after oral administration of two tablets of epinastine (epinastine hydrochloride 20 mg) to Korean subjects were used to prove and demonstrate selectivity. The used blank plasma was collected from six different individuals. The sensitivity of the method was expressed as LLOQ, LLOQ and LOD were determined as the lowest concentration of the standard samples within the range of quantification with a signal-to-noise ratio of at least 10:1 and 3:1, respectively, with an acceptable precision of less than 20% and accuracy within ±20%. All of these were evaluated using five replicate samples.

4.5.2. Linearity

Calibration curves were determined using the seven calibration points by linear regression with the weighting factor of 1/concentration^2. The linearity of the calibration curve was conducted by plotting the epinastine/IS peak area versus the theoretical concentration of epinastine. A correlation coefficient (r^2) value with its linear calibration equation was obtained.

4.5.3. Accuracy and Precision

Both intra-day accuracy and precision were assessed by analyzing the QC samples at five different times on the same day. In addition, inter-day evaluations were similarly conducted on five consecutive days. The concentration of each QC sample was quantified using the calibration standards prepared on that day. The precision was assessed by determining the CV value for the analysis of QC samples. The CV value at each concentration level was not allowed to deviate by more than ±15%. However, it was limited to 20% in LLOQ. The accuracy was determined based on the criteria, which are the mean value, not exceeding 15% of the nominal concentration. As with precision standards, it was limited to 20% in LLOQ.

4.5.4. Matrix Effect and Recovery

The recovery efficiencies of epinastine were assessed for the QC samples at low, medium, and high concentrations in five replicates. In addition, the recovery efficiency of the IS was determined. The extraction recovery of the assay from human plasma was evaluated by comparing the detector (UV and MS/MS) response of extracted samples (A) with those of the samples added at the same concentration after extracting the blank plasma (B). In addition, the matrix effect for UPLC-MS/MS method was assessed by comparing the peak area of analyte post-extraction (B) from blank plasma with the absolute standard (C) of the same analyte. The matrix effect and recovery efficiency were determined by the following formula: Recovery = (A)/(B) × 100%; Matrix effect = (B)/(C) × 100%.

4.5.5. Stabilities

The stabilities of epinastine in human plasma were assessed under various conditions, including freeze-thaw, long-term, and short-term stability. Two different levels of QC samples, low (5 ng/mL) and high (80 ng/mL) concentrations, were used for all stability tests. The short-term stability test was conducted by maintaining the QC samples for 24 h at 25 °C, and the long-term stability was determined by analysis of QC samples frozen for 4 weeks at −80 °C. The QC samples were stored for 24 h at −80 °C and then thawed completely at 25 °C for the freeze and thaw stability test. This cycle was repeated in succession, and analysis was conducted after the third cycle. Stabilities of epinastine and IS stock solution were measured after storage for 4 weeks at −20 °C. In addition, for post-preparative stability, the processed QC samples were placed in autosampler for 24 h at 15 °C (at UPLC-MS/MS method), and on the table for 24 h at 25 °C (at HPLC-UV method). Stabilities were determined as the % ratio of measured epinastine concentration to initial epinastine concentration (n = 5). Samples were considered stable if the test values at each level were within ±15% of the sample nominal concentration, and the precision was less than 15%.

4.5.6. Carryover

The carryover test was conducted by injecting a blank sample after injecting the sample with the highest concentration (100 ng/mL for epinastine) in the standard curve. The acceptance criterion of the carryover is that the peak in the blank sample should be less than 20% of the peak in the LLOQ sample.

4.5.7. Incurred Sample Reanalysis

ISR was conducted to ensure the reproducibility of newly developed methods for the analysis of epinastine. Sample selection (10% of the analyzed samples) was accomplished using a computerized random method for ISR. The selection criterion involved samples near the elimination phase in the PK profile of epinastine and C_{max}. Thirty-two human plasma samples were selected and compared with initial analyzed values. The results satisfied the acceptable criteria that the variability between the mean value of the initial analysis and that of the reanalysis was within ±15%. In addition, reanalysis values for 67% of all samples were within 20% of their initial values.

4.6. Pharmacokinetic Studies

Twenty-six healthy males of Korean subjects (22–25 years of age, bodyweight 60–85 kg, height 165–195 cm) were recruited for a clinical trial (as bioequivalence test). The Institutional Review Board of the Institute of Bioequivalence and Bridging Study (Chonnam National University, Gwangju, Korea) approved this study protocol (Bioequivalence Test No. 324; 02.04.2005). The clinical trial was conducted according to the revised Declaration of Helsinki for biomedical research involving human subjects and the rules of Good Clinical Practice. The written consent was obtained prior to participating from all participants. In addition, all participants received laboratory, physical, and medical tests prior to a clinical trial. As a result, this study included only well-healthy participants. All the participants fasted more than 10 h before receiving 20 mg epinastine hydrochloride tablets followed by fasting for 4 h. In addition, they avoided drinks or foods containing caffeine or xanthine ingredients during this study. All participants received two tablets of epinastine (epinastine hydrochloride 20 mg) with water of 240 mL. The blood samples were taken from the forearm vein before the administration (0 h) and 0.5, 1, 1.5, 2, 2.5, 3, 4, 6, 8, 12, and 24 h after oral administration. The blood samples were transferred into Vacutainer® tube (Becton, Dickinson and Company, Franklin Lakes, NJ, USA) of 10 mL capacity and were centrifuged (10,000 × *g*) immediately for 10 min at 4 °C. The supernatant plasma samples were transferred to polyethylene tube and stored at −80 °C until further analysis. T_{max}, C_{max}, and C_{min} were determined using the plasma drug concentration curve over time. The $AUC_{0-\infty}$ was integrated by a linear trapezoidal rule to the final measured concentration (C_{last}) and extrapolated to infinity by adding the area from C_{last} (AUC_{0-t}) to infinity (C_{last}/k); k means the elimination rate constant at terminal phase. The CL/F was determined by dividing the dose of epinastine by the $AUC_{0-\infty}$, where F is the bioavailability of oral administration. The $t_{1/2}$ was determined as $0.693/k$ and V_d/F as dose/k·$AUC_{0-\infty}$. All PK parameters were determined via noncompartmental analysis using the WinNonlin® software (version 8.1, Pharsight®, a Certara™ Company, Princeton, NJ, USA).

4.7. Pharmacokinetic Parameters Comparison

In addition to those mentioned (in the Section 4.8 Statistical analysis) to compare the differences in PK parameter values according to the analytical methods, the parameter values calculated using HPLC-UV and UPLC-MS/MS were divided as follows: $\frac{PK\ parameters\ by\ UPLC-MS/MS}{PK\ parameters\ by\ HPLC-UV}$. Closer values to 1 mean that there is little effect on the PK parameters between the two methods.

4.8. Statistical Analysis

Statistical analysis was performed using the Statistical Package for the Social Sciences (SPSS) software version 23 (IBM, Armonk, NY, USA) on the PK parameters calculated by HPLC-UV and UPLC-MS/MS methods. In other words, all PK parameters determined by each quantification method were analyzed for statistical significance by Student's t-test with $p < 0.05$, indicating a significant difference.

5. Conclusions

The purposes of this study were to compare the PK parameter values of epinastine obtained using the two methods and to discuss their meanings, as mentioned in the introduction. In this study, we provided the newly developed analysis methods—UPLC-MS/MS and HPLC-UV. Our study focused on comparing the performances of newly developed UPLC-MS/MS and HPLC-UV methods for the determination of epinastine in human plasma.

No published report has compared the differences in analytical methods, such as HPLC-UV and UPLC-MS/MS, in biosamples for epinastine. Generally, UPLC-MS/MS methods show higher throughput, selectivity, and sensitivity compared to HPLC-UV methods [24]. However, because MS detectors are expensive, analyzing biosamples using relatively less expensive UV detectors would be a great economic advantage. Numerous studies comparing LC-MS and LC-UV methods in the analysis of biosamples for other drugs have been reported from the past [24–30]. The purpose of the inter-comparison of these methods is perhaps to ensure that the results are identical even if one of the two methods is used. In other words, by choosing the appropriate analytical method for a specific situation, it would be possible to derive the optimal PK result. In general, the use of LC-UV is more appropriate where rapid turn round of data is not required, and plasma concentrations are high. However, if sensitivity is an issue, limited amounts of plasma are available, and/or where tight deadlines are pivotal, LC-MS is the method of choice [30].

Both methods were fully validated according to international bioanalytical method guidelines and represented a useful tool for the characterization of PKs of 20 mg epinastine hydrochloride tablets in Korean subjects. Furthermore, comparison (especially focused on PK parameters) of two commonly used analytical methods (HPLC-UV and UPLC-MS/MS) for in vivo analysis of epinastine was performed for the first time. As a result, this method comparison study confirmed that different dose and usage settings might be possible based on PK parameters calculated by other methods. Therefore, if careful consideration is required for dose and regimen settings of drugs, it may be necessary to consider differences in interpretation of PKs according to the assays reported in this study. Finally, our conclusion was that the choice of the assay was very important for the analysis of biological samples (especially where the concentration of drug in the plasma sample is relatively low, as in this study). The UPLC-MS/MS method, which could provide a lower LLOQ than the HPLC-UV method, quantified the concentrations of the drug's initial absorption and elimination phases in the blood, resulting in more clear PK profiles in case of epinastine. However, this conclusion could not be generalized for some drugs. Due to the presence of the matrix effect or the reduction of ionization sites, there might be some drugs that are more sensitively quantified in LC-UV than LC-MS/MS. These results might affect the calculation of PK parameters (such as $t_{1/2}$ and clearance) and simulation results at multiple doses, although there were no significant differences in concentration values. In the case of drugs requiring tight therapeutic drug monitoring (TDM), very careful attention should be paid to the dosage and regimen based on these PK parameters. As a result, this study suggested that UPLC-MS/MS was better for PK studies on substances with low plasma concentrations despite the maximum daily dose of the drug, such as epinastine. Our findings are very new and have not been reported previously and are expected to be very important data for PK studies and interpretation of results.

Supplementary Materials: The following are available online at http://www.mdpi.com/1420-3049/25/1/209/s1, Figure S1: Calibration curves of epinastine in human plasma by HPLC-UV (A) and UPLC-MS/MS methods (B). The linear straight line refers to the regression line and the vertical bars represent the standard deviation of the mean (n = 5)., Table S1: Summary of previously reported epinastine assays.

Author Contributions: Conceptualization, S.-H.J. and Y.-B.L.; methodology, J.-H.J. and S.-H.J.; validation, S.-H.J. and H.-Y.C.; investigation, J.-H.J. and S.-H.J.; data curation, S.-H.J.; writing—original draft preparation, S.-H.J.; writing—review and editing, J.-H.J., S.-H.J., H.-Y.C., and Y.-B.L.; supervision, Y.-B.L. All authors have read and agreed to the published version of the manuscript.

Funding: This research was financially supported by Chonnam National University (Grant number: 2018–3362), Korea.

Conflicts of Interest: The authors declare no conflict of interest.

References

1. González, M.A.; Estes, K.S. Pharmacokinetic overview of oral second-generation H1 antihistamines. *Int. J. Clin. Pharm. Ther.* **1998**, *36*, 292–300.
2. Sarashina, A.; Tatami, S.; Yamamura, N.; Tsuda, Y.; Igarashi, T. Population pharmacokinetics of epinastine, a histamine H1 receptor antagonist, in adults and children. *Br. J. Clin. Pharmacol.* **2005**, *59*, 43–53. [CrossRef]
3. Kishimoto, W.; Hiroi, T.; Sakai, K.; Funae, Y.; Igarashi, T. Metabolism of epinastine, a histamine H1 receptor antagonist, in human liver microsomes in comparison with that of terfenadine. *Res. Commun. Mol. Pathol. Pharmacol.* **1997**, *98*, 273–292.
4. El-Bagary, R.; Boshra, A.; El-Hakeem, M.M.; Abdelra'oof, A.M. Three analytical methods for determination of epinastine hydrochloride in bulk and in ophthalmic solutions. *J. Chem. Pharm. Res.* **2012**, *4*, 1361–1369.
5. Oshima, K.-Z.; Asano, K.; Kanai, K.-I.; Suzuki, M.; Suzaki, H. Influence of epinastine hydrochloride, an H1-receptor antagonist, on the function of mite allergen-pulsed murine bone marrow-derived dendritic cells in vitro and in vivo. *Mediat. Inflamm.* **2009**, *2009*. [CrossRef] [PubMed]
6. Brar, B.; Vangyi, C.; Tarlo, K.; Short, B. Preclinical safety of ophthalmic epinastine in rabbits and monkeys. *Invest. Ophthalmol. Vis. Sci.* **2002**, *43*, 108.
7. Yu, D.; Ghosh, P.; Tang-Liu, D. Pharmacokinetic and safety profile of epinastine after ocular administration in patients with allergic conjunctivitis. *J. Allergy Clin. Immunol.* **2003**, *111*, S237. [CrossRef]
8. Fraunfelder, F.W. Epinastine hydrochloride for atopic disease. *Drugs Today* **2004**, *40*, 677–684. [CrossRef] [PubMed]
9. Do, J.-A.; Kim, J.Y.; Choi, J.Y.; Lee, J.H.; Kim, H.J.; Noh, E.; Cho, S.-H.; Yoon, C.-Y.; Kim, W.-S. Development of a LC–MS/MS method for simultaneous analysis of 20 antihistamines in dietary supplements. *Anal. Sci. Technol.* **2015**, *28*, 86–97. [CrossRef]
10. Bae, H.J.; Joung, S.K.; Cho, K.H.; Lee, H.J. Validated LC-MS/MS Method for Determination of Epinastine in Human Plasma. In Proceedings of the Fall Conference of The Korean Society of Analytical Sciences, Jeju, Korea, 15–17 November 2009; The Korean Society of Analytical Sciences: Jeju, Korea, 2009.
11. Ahirrao, V.; Pawar, R. Stability-indicating LC Method for the determination of epinastine in bulk drug and in pharmaceutical dosage form. *Res. J. Recent Sci.* **2012**, *1*, 281–288.

12. Ogiso, T.; Kasutani, M.; Tanaka, H.; Iwaki, M.; Tanino, T. Pharmacokinetics of epinastine and a possible mechanism for double peaks in oral plasma concentration profiles. *Biol. Pharm. Bull* **2001**, *24*, 790–794. [CrossRef] [PubMed]
13. Ohtani, H.; Kotaki, H.; Sawada, Y.; Iga, T. Quantitative determination of epinastine in plasma by high-performance liquid chromatography. *J. Chromatogr. B* **1996**, *683*, 281–284. [CrossRef]
14. Oiwa, Y.; Shibata, T.; Kobayashi, O.; Matsumura, R.; Kohei, H.; Momose, Y.; Shigematsu, A. Pharmacokinetic studies on 14C-epinastine hydrochloride (WAL 801 Cl)(I). *Jpn. Pharmacol. Ther.* **1992**, *20*, 483–506.
15. Li, Z.; Wang, X.; Zhang, Z.; Xi, R. Study on pharmacokinetics of epinastine hydrochloride tablets in Chinese Han and Tibetan healthy volunteers. *Pharm. Care Res.* **2011**, *11*, 373–376. [CrossRef]
16. Shi, S.-J.; Li, Z.-F.; Chen, H.-T.; Zeng, F.-D. Pharmacokinetics and bioequivalence of epinastine hydrochloride, a histamine H1 receptor antagonist, in healthy Chinese volunteers. *Chin. J. Clin. Pharmacol. Ther.* **2007**, *12*, 214–218.
17. Malakar, A.; Bokshi, B. Development and validation of stability indicating RP-HPLC method for the determination of epinastine hydrochloride in pharmaceutical dosage form. *Int. Curr. Pharm. J.* **2012**, *1*, 50–55. [CrossRef]
18. Yu, D.; Tang-Liu, D. Analyses of tear concentrations of epinastine after topical ophthalmic administration. *J. Allergy Clin. Immunol.* **2005**, *115*, S130. [CrossRef]
19. Shi, L.; Chen, X.; Zhang, Y.; Wei, C.; Geng, C.; Gao, M.; Shaikh, A.S.; Wang, B.; Guo, R. A more rapid, simple and sensitive HPLC-MS/MS method for determination of epinastine in human plasma and application to a bioequivalence study. *Lat. Am. J. Pharm.* **2016**, *35*, 1314–1320.
20. Kang, H.-A.; Cho, H.-Y.; Yoon, H.; Kim, S.-M.; Kim, D.-H.; Park, S.; Kim, H.-H.; Lee, Y.-B. Bioequivalence of S-napine tablet 10 mg to Alesion tablet (epinastine HCl 10 mg). *J. Pharm. Investig.* **2006**, *36*, 405–411.
21. Kim, E.-Y.; Kang, W.; Gwak, H.-S. Comparison of analytical methods of tacrolimus in plasma and population pharmacokinetics in liver transplant recipients. *Korean J. Clin. Pharm.* **2008**, *18*, 60–67.
22. Braun, F.; Lorf, T.; Schütz, E.; Christians, U.; Grupp, C.; Sattler, B.; Canelo, R.; Sewing, K.F.; Armstrong, V.W.; Oellerich, M.; et al. Clinical relevance of monitoring tacrolimus: Comparison of microparticle enzyme immunoassay, enzyme-linked immunosorbent assay, and liquid chromatography mass spectrometry in renal transplant recipients converted from cyclosporine to tacrolimus. *Transplant. Proc.* **1996**, *28*, 3175–3176. [PubMed]
23. FDA. *Guidance for Industry: Bioanalytical Method Validation*; US Department of Health and Human Services, Food and Drug Administration, Center for Drug Evaluation and Research (CDER), Center for Veterinary Medicine (CVM): Rockville, MD, USA, 2018. Available online: https://www.fda.gov/files/drugs/published/Bioanalytical-Method-Validation-Guidance-for-Industry.pdf (accessed on 1 December 2019).
24. Georgiță, C.; Sora, I.; Albu, F.; Monciu, C.M. Comparison of a LC/MS method with a LC/UV method for the determination of metformin in plasma samples. *Farmacia* **2010**, *58*, 158–169.
25. Roth, O.; Spreux-Varoquaux, O.; Bouchet, S.; Rousselot, P.; Castaigne, S.; Rigaudeau, S.; Raggueneau, V.; Therond, P.; Devillier, P.; Molimard, M. Imatinib assay by HPLC with photodiode-array UV detection in plasma from patients with chronic myeloid leukemia: Comparison with LC-MS/MS. *Clin. Chim. Acta* **2010**, *411*, 140–146. [CrossRef] [PubMed]
26. Sallustio, B.C.; Noll, B.D.; Morris, R.G. Comparison of blood sirolimus, tacrolimus and everolimus concentrations measured by LC-MS/MS, HPLC-UV and immunoassay methods. *Clin. Biochem.* **2011**, *44*, 231–236. [CrossRef]
27. Suneetha, A.; Raja, R.K. Comparison of LC-UV and LC-MS methods for simultaneous determination of teriflunomide, dimethyl fumarate and fampridine in human plasma: Application to rat pharmacokinetic study. *Biomed. Chromatogr.* **2016**, *30*, 1371–1377. [CrossRef]
28. Bedor, D.; Goncalves, T.; Ferreira, M.; De Sousa, C.; Menezes, A.; Oliveira, E.; De Santana, D. Simultaneous determination of sulfamethoxazole and trimethoprim in biological fluids for high-throughput analysis: Comparison of HPLC with ultraviolet and tandem mass spectrometric detection. *J. Chromatogr. B* **2008**, *863*, 46–54. [CrossRef]

29. Jang, J.-H.; Jeong, S.-H.; Cho, H.-Y.; Lee, Y.-B. Comparison of UPLC-MS/MS and HPLC-UV methods for the determination of zaltoprofen in human plasma. *J. Pharm. Investig.* **2019**, *49*, 613–624. [CrossRef]
30. Baldrey, S.; Brodie, R.; Morris, G.; Jenkins, E.; Brookes, S. Comparison of LC-UV and LC-MS-MS for the determination of taxol. *Chromatographia* **2002**, *55*, S187–S192. [CrossRef]

Sample Availability: Samples are available from the authors.

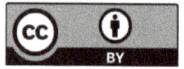

© 2020 by the authors. Licensee MDPI, Basel, Switzerland. This article is an open access article distributed under the terms and conditions of the Creative Commons Attribution (CC BY) license (http://creativecommons.org/licenses/by/4.0/).

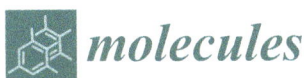

Article

Development and Validation of Analytical Method for SH-1242 in the Rat and Mouse Plasma by Liquid Chromatography/Tandem Mass Spectrometry

Yoo-Seong Jeong [1], Minjeong Baek [1], Seungbeom Lee [1,2], Min-Soo Kim [1], Han-Joo Maeng [3], Jong-Hwa Lee [4], Young-Ger Suh [1,2] and Suk-Jae Chung [1,*]

1. College of Pharmacy and Research Institute of Pharmaceutical Sciences, Seoul National University, 1 Gwanak-ro, Gwanak-gu, Seoul 08826, Korea; jus2401@snu.ac.kr (Y.-S.J.); jormungand@snu.ac.kr (M.B.); lastchaos21c@snu.ac.kr (S.L.); misol@snu.ac.kr (M.-S.K.); ygsuh@cha.ac.kr (Y.-G.S.)
2. College of Pharmacy, CHA University, 120 Haeryong-ro, Pocheon-si, Gyeonggi-do 11160, Korea
3. College of Pharmacy, Gachon University, 191 Hambakmoei-ro, Yeonsu-gu, Incheon 21936, Korea; hjmaeng@gachon.ac.kr
4. Korea Institute of Toxicology, 141 Gajeong-ro, Yuseong-gu, Daejeon 34114, Korea; jhl@kitox.re.kr
* Correspondence: sukjae@snu.ac.kr; Tel.: +82-2-880-9176

Received: 20 December 2019; Accepted: 20 January 2020; Published: 25 January 2020

Abstract: SH-1242, a novel inhibitor of heat shock protein 90 (HSP90), is a synthetic analog of deguelin: It was previously reported that the treatment of SH-1242 led to a strong suppression of hypoxia-mediated retinal neovascularization and vascular leakage in diabetic retinas by inhibiting the hypoxia-induced upregulation of expression in hypoxia-inducible factor 1α (HIF-1α) and vascular endothelial growth factor (VEGF). In this study, an analytical method for the quantification of SH-1242 in biological samples from rats and mice was developed/validated for application in pharmacokinetic studies. SH-1242 and deguelin, an internal standard of the assay, in plasma samples from the rodents were extracted with methanol containing 0.1% formic acid and analyzed at m/z transition values of 368.9→151.0 and 395.0→213.0, respectively. The method was validated in terms of accuracy, precision, dilution, matrix effects, recovery, and stability and shown to comply with validation guidelines when it was used in the concentration ranges of 1–1000 ng/mL for rat plasma and of 2–1000 ng/mL for mouse plasma. SH-1242 levels in plasma samples were readily determined using the developed method for up to 480 min after the intravenous administration of 0.1 mg/kg SH-1242 to rats and for up to 120 min to mice. These findings suggested that the current method was practical and reliable for pharmacokinetic studies on SH-1242 in preclinical animal species.

Keywords: SH-1242; 2-(3,4-dimethoxyphenyl)-1-(5-methoxy-2,2-dimethyl-2H-chromen-6-yl)ethanone; pharmacokinetics; HPLC-MS/MS

1. Introduction

Heat shock protein 90 (HSP90) is a chaperone protein that plays a vital role in the regulation of its target proteins via stabilizing them under cellular stresses, post-translational folding, and degrading damaged proteins [1]. Hypoxia-inducible factor 1 (HIF-1), one of the client proteins of HSP90, is a transcription factor that is associated with the promotion of angiogenesis in regions of vascular dysfunction, e.g., hypoxic cancer environments. HIF-1 has also been reported to facilitate the expression of vascular endothelial growth factor (VEGF) [2,3] and to be pathologically related to diabetic retinopathy and age-related macular degeneration, as well as cancers [4,5]. Deguelin is a naturally occurring rotenoid, a flavonoid, and has been shown to inhibit HSP90's function [6]. Although its underlying mechanism has not been fully delineated, this inhibition appears to be related to the attenuation of the binding of clients to ATP-binding pocket of HSP90 by deguelin and to the accelerated decomposition of HIF-1 [6]. Previously, a variety of deguelin analogs were synthesized and screened for HSP90 inhibition [7,8]. In particular, we noted that SH-1242 (2-(3,4-dimethoxyphenyl)-1-(5-methoxy-2,2-dimethyl-2H-chromen-6-yl)ethanone) possessed a potent anti-proliferative activity against human cancer cells [9] and suppressed hypoxia-mediated retinal neovascularization/vascular leakage in diabetic retinas [10]. Furthermore, potent antitumor effects of SH-1242 were also found in various cancer cell lines and in vivo animal models with significantly reduced neurotoxicity [11], suggesting SH-1242 is a reasonable candidate as an experimental inhibitor of HSP90.

Since SH-1242 was found to exhibit a strong antiangiogenic activity in the low nM range (e.g., an effective concentration of approximately down to 10 nM in in vitro model of hypoxia-mediated angiogenesis) [10], a sensitive/robust quantification method for SH-1242, especially in complex biological matrices (e.g., plasma samples), is required for the further development of SH-1242 as a new drug. However, previous attempts to develop methodologies for the analyses of deguelin analogs have primarily focused on the determination of rotenoid levels in natural sources [12–15]. In particular, an analytical method capable of quantifying deguelin analogs in the nano-molar range in biological matrices from animal species used for preclinical study settings was not reported. Therefore, the objective of this study was to develop and validate an analytical method for the determination of SH-1242 in plasma samples of rats and mice in accordance with the U.S. Food and Drug Administration (US FDA) guidance [16]. We were particularly interested in developing the assay capable of measuring the rotenoid analogs at the lower limit of quantification (LLOQ) down to low ng/mL range for the application of the devised method to pharmacokinetic studies in the preclinical animal species.

2. Results and Discussion

2.1. Mass Spectrometry and Chromatography

Based on the chemical structures and product-ion spectra of SH-1242 and internal standard (IS) (Figure 1), m/z transition values were set at 368.9→151.0 for SH-1242 and 395.0→213.0 for the IS (deguelin). For the IS, this m/z transition value was comparable to the fragmentation pattern found in the literature [12,17]. Isocratic flow with the run time of 3 min per sample resulted in adequate chromatographic separations for SH-1242 and IS without any apparent interfering peaks (Supplementary Figure S1). SH-1242 and the IS were adequately resolved with the retention times of 1 min for SH-1242 and 0.96 min for IS. These observations indicated that the analytical method in this study allowed adequate throughput for the chromatographic separation of SH-1242 with a reasonable resolution. Therefore, the chromatographic conditions were used for subsequent analyses.

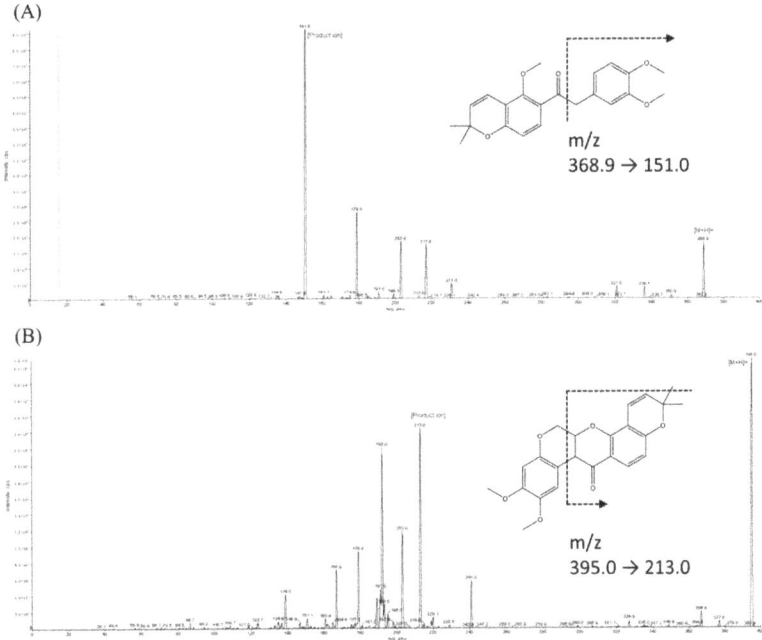

Figure 1. The product-ion scan spectra and proposed multiple reaction monitoring (MRM) transitions of (**A**) SH-1242 and (**B**) deguelin, (the internal standard).

2.2. Selectivity

Representative ion chromatograms of double blanks, zero blanks, and lower limit of quantification (LLOQ) samples are shown in Supplementary Figure S1. The results obtained from six replicates of double blank, zero blank, and LLOQ samples showed that no appreciable interfering peak was evident in the vicinity of the retention times for the analyte and IS peaks (Table 1). At the LLOQ level (1 ng/mL for rat plasma and 2 ng/mL for mouse plasma), the precision of the peak area was found to be 5.15% and 10.5% for rat and mouse plasma, respectively. Taken together, these observations showed that the current HPLC-MS/MS assay provided adequate selectivity for the analysis of SH-1242 in rat and mouse plasma samples.

Table 1. The specificity of SH-1242 in rat and mouse plasma.

MATRIX LOT	Response (Peak Area)							
	Rat Plasma				Mouse Plasma			
	Double Blank [a]	Zero Blank [b]	LLOQ (1 ng/mL)	HQC (800 ng/mL)	Double Blank	Zero Blank	LLOQ (2 ng/mL)	HQC (800 ng/mL)
1	0	0	209	71,500	0	0	150	23,800
2	0	0	214	80,700	0	0	137	24,500
3	0	0	212	77,100	0	0	121	22,100
4	0	0	225	78,000	0	0	119	22,400
5	0	0	238	77,600	0	0	114	23,700
6	0	0	211	77,200	0	0	134	24,400
Mean	0	0	218	77,000	0	0	129	23,500
CV(%) [c]	0	0	5.15	3.91	0	0	10.5	4.30

[a] Double blank: sample containing no analyte or IS. [b] Zero blank: sample containing only IS. [c] Coefficient of variation (CV%) = (standard deviation/mean) × 100. IS: internal standard, LLOQ: lower limit of quantification, HQC: high QC.

2.3. LLOQ and Linearity

The concentration levels of SH-1242 at which the signal-to-noise ratio was consistently 10 or more with acceptable precision (i.e., less than 20% CV) was found to be 1 ng/mL for rat plasma and 2 ng/mL for mouse plasma. Calibration curves (Supplementary Figure S2), including the LLOQ, were apparently linear over the specified concentration ranges for rat and mouse plasma (Table 2). Consistent with this statement, the correlation coefficients (i.e., R values with the weighting factor of $1/x^2$) of the calibration curves ranged from 0.995 to 0.999, with all the calibrators found to be within the acceptance criterion of 15% (20% at LLOQ).

Table 2. Calibration curves for SH-1242 in rat and mouse plasma.

Run	Rat Plasma			Mouse Plasma		
	Slope	Intercept	R	Slope	Intercept	R
1	0.00349	0.00340	0.999	0.00633	0.00982	0.995
2	0.00329	0.00281	0.999	0.00450	0.00679	0.999
3	0.00339	0.00227	0.998	0.00515	0.00378	0.999
4	0.00335	0.00402	0.999	0.00583	0.00897	0.996
5	0.00337	0.00417	0.999	0.00616	0.00194	0.998
Mean	0.00338	0.00333	0.999	0.00559	0.00626	0.997
CV(%) [a]	2.16	-	-	13.6	-	-

[a] Coefficient of variation (CV%) = (standard deviation/mean) × 100.

2.4. Accuracy, Precision, and Dilution Integrity

The accuracies and precisions of QC samples of SH-1242 in rat and mouse plasma are summarized in Table 3. Intra-day (inter-day) precisions of QC samples ranged from 3.85% to 12.7% (2.84% to 12.8%) and from 2.55% to 3.09% (3.57% to 6.72%) for the rat and mouse plasma, respectively; the intra-day (inter-day) accuracies (as a relative error, RE%) of QC samples ranged from −5.15% to 4.83% (−2.83% to 4.63%) in rat plasma and −6.02% to 1.42% (−2.53% to 1.63%) in mouse plasma. In addition, when SH-1242 samples of concentration of 8000 ng/mL (i.e., exceeding the ULOQ of 1000 ng/mL) were 10-fold diluted, calculated mean intra-day (inter-day) concentrations were 764 ng/mL (743 ng/mL) with a CV value of 1.39% (2.84%) for rats and 757 ng/mL (782 ng/mL) with a CV value of 4.47% (6.72%) for mice, indicating that plasma samples with SH-1242 concentrations exceeding ULOQ could be diluted for analysis. Taken together, these results indicated that the current assay was accurate and precise for the estimation of SH-1242 concentration in plasma samples obtained from rats or mice.

Table 3. Accuracy and precision of SH-1242 determinations in rat and mouse quality control (QC) samples.

Batch	Rat Plasma Theoretical Concentration (ng/mL)					Mouse Plasma Theoretical Concentration (ng/mL)				
	LLOQ	LQC	MQC	HQC	HQC [a]	LLOQ	LQC	MQC	HQC	HQC [a]
	1	2	40	800	800	2	4	40	800	800
	Intra-day ($n = 6$)									
Mean	1	1.98	41.9	759	764	1.95	4.06	39.7	752	757
Precision (CV%) [b]	12.7	4.64	4.41	3.85	1.39	2.56	2.55	2.96	3.09	4.47
Accuracy (RE%) [c]	0.38	−0.83	4.83	−5.15	−4.48	−2.42	1.42	−0.83	−6.02	−5.35
	Inter-day ($n = 30$)									
Mean	1.04	2.04	41.9	777	743	1.99	4.04	40.7	780	782
Precision (CV%) [b]	12.8	5.04	5.03	4.24	2.84	5.87	4.43	3.57	5.27	6.72
Accuracy (RE%) [c]	3.95	2.22	4.63	−2.83	−7.15	−0.73	0.91	1.63	−2.53	−2.30

[a] Analyzed after a ten-fold dilution with blank plasma. [b] CV(%) = (standard deviation/mean) × 100. [c] RE(%) = [(calculated concentration − theoretical concentration)/theoretical concentration] × 100. RE: relative error, LQC and MQC: low and mid QC.

2.5. Matrix Effect, Extraction Efficiency, and Recovery

Matrix effect, recovery, and extraction efficiency for SH-1242 in rat and mouse plasma samples are summarized (Table 4). The mean extraction efficiencies ranged from 107% to 119% for rat plasma and from 91.1% to 107% for mouse plasma, indicating that the loss of the analyte through the extraction process was not significant in both matrices. However, the matrix effect of SH-1242 ranged from 82.2% to 92.8% for rat plasma and from 44.7% to 48.0% for mouse plasma. For rats, the recovery (or IS-normalized recovery) of SH-1242 ranged from 91.3% to 108% (103% to 118%). In line with this, the recovery of other rotenoids from human serum (e.g., rotenone, rotenolone, and deguelin) was reported to be in a range from 92.3% to 115% [17]. In contrast, the recovery of SH-1242 after the extraction from mouse plasma was ranged from 43.7% to 47.8% (Table 4). Collectively, these observations indicated that there were distinct differences in the matrix effects and IS-normalized recoveries of rotenoid compounds in biological matrices between human/rat and mouse. These discrepancies might be related to the different SH-1242 LLOQ values observed for the two matrices (i.e., 1 ng/mL for rat plasma vs. 2 ng/mL for mouse plasma): It is possible that factors influencing the detection process of the rotenoids (e.g., electrospray ionization in HPLC-MS/MS interface) [18,19] are different between the matrices. Nevertheless, variabilities in peak responses used for the calculation of the recovery parameters were consistently less than 15% (Table 4) for rat and mouse plasma. In addition, no appreciable difference was found on essential assay parameters for the two matrices (e.g., accuracies and precisions). Therefore, despite the differences in the matrix effect/recovery in both biological matrices, we assumed that the devised assay was still applicable for pharmacokinetic studies involving the animal species and the applicability subsequently tested.

Table 4. Matrix effect, extraction efficiency, and recovery of the assay for SH-1242 determination in rat and mouse plasma samples.

Nominal Concentration (ng/mL)	Matrix Effect (%) [a]	Extraction Efficiency (%) [b]	Recovery (%) [c]	IS-Normalized Recovery (%) [c]	CV (%) [d]			
					Analyte		IS	
					Set 1	Set 2	Set 1	Set 2
Rat plasma								
2	92.8	107	99	110	9.08	2.92	5.95	2.13
40	90.4	119	108	118	7.11	6.05	2.96	2.01
800	82.2	111	91.3	103	2.31	6.72	3.12	1.95
Mouse plasma								
2	45.9	101	46.3	74.4	6.38	2.92	6.77	2.13
40	44.7	107	47.8	74.3	7.10	6.05	2.65	2.01
800	48	91.1	43.7	73.4	10.5	6.72	7.52	1.95

[a] Matrix effect was calculated by expressing the ratio of the mean peak area of the analyte added after extraction to the mean peak area of neat standard solution (Set 2) of the analyte multiplied by 100. [b] Extraction efficiency was calculated by dividing the mean peak area of the analyte added before extraction (Set 1) by the mean peak area of the analyte added after extraction multiplied by 100. [c] Recovery (IS-normalized recovery) was calculated by the ratio of the mean peak area of the analyte (normalized by IS peak area) added before extraction (Set 1) to the mean peak area of a neat standard solution of the analyte (normalized by IS peak area) (Set 2) multiplied by 100. [d] CV was calculated as a standard deviation of the peak area divided by the mean peak area multiplied by 100.

2.6. Stability

The stability of SH-1242 and IS in stock solutions was studied at concentrations of 1 mg/mL and 500 ng/mL, respectively, under different storage conditions. As summarized in Table 5, the relative responses of SH-1242 and IS stock solutions compared to those at time zero (i.e., the reference value) were ranged from 85.2% to 109% and from 86.2% to 105%, respectively. In addition, when QC samples, containing SH-1242 at three different concentration levels for rat or mouse plasma, were subjected to various handling and storage conditions (Table 6), we found that benchtop stability at room temperature for 24 h, autosampler stability at 4 °C for 3 days, stability after three freeze-thaw cycles, and long term stability at 4 °C for 2 weeks were all acceptable with CV and RE values ranging from 0.825% to 8.54% and −8.71% to 4.92% for rat plasma, and from 0.699% to 12% and −4.08% to 12% for mouse plasma, respectively. Collectively, these observations suggested that SH-1242 and deguelin were adequately stable in rat and mouse plasma under various handling and storage conditions.

Table 5. Stability of SH-1242 and IS in stock solutions under typical storage conditions.

Batch (n = 3)	Response (Peak Area)					
	Initial (0 h)	Room Temp. (6 h)	Refrigerated (4 °C, 24 h)	Refrigerated (4 °C, 2 Weeks)	Refrigerated (−20 °C, 2 Weeks)	Refrigerated (−80 °C, 2 Weeks)
			SH-1242 [a]			
Mean	18,000	19,700	19,000	15,400	16,100	16,400
CV(%) [b]	3.93	13.5	11.1	9.14	5.44	3.01
Relative conc. (%) [c]	100	109	105	85.2	89.1	90.8
			IS			
Mean	19,100	19,200	20,000	17,600	17,400	16,400
CV(%)	4.27	6.20	0.762	4.65	8.36	1.53
Relative conc. (%)	100	101	105	92.3	91.4	86.2

[a] Stock solutions of SH-1242 were diluted to 50 ng/mL prior to analysis. [b] CV(%) = (standard deviation/mean) × 100. [c] Relative concentrations (%) were obtained by dividing measured values by initial values. IS: internal standard

Table 6. Stability of SH-1242 QC samples under typical storage conditions.

Batch	Rat Plasma Theoretical Concentration (ng/mL)			Mouse Plasma Theoretical Concentration (ng/mL)		
	LQC 2	MQC 40	HQC 800	LQC 4	MQC 40	HQC 800
	Benchtop stability at room temperature (25 °C) for 24 h (n = 3)					
Mean	1.87	37.3	737	4.21	41.7	810
Precision (CV%) [a]	6.95	4.35	2.62	9.47	4.38	5.57
Accuracy (RE%) [b]	−6.33	−6.83	−7.88	5.25	4.25	1.25
	Autosampler stability at 4 °C for 3 days (n = 3)					
Mean	2.00	38.9	773	4.19	42.6	863
Precision (CV%)	8.27	6.05	3.16	4.90	5.15	0.699
Accuracy (RE%)	−0.167	−2.75	−3.33	4.67	6.50	7.83
	Freeze-thaw stability (3 cycles, n = 3)					
Mean	1.84	41.97	780	4.45	42.4	840
Precision (CV%)	3.85	4.20	3.57	2.00	4.32	1.33
Accuracy (RE%)	−7.83	4.92	−2.50	11.3	6.00	5.00
	Long term stability at 4 °C for 2 weeks (n = 3)					
Mean	2.02	37.3	730	3.84	44.8	865
Precision (CV%)	8.54	2.56	0.825	12.0	1.77	4.37
Accuracy (RE%)	0.833	−6.75	−8.71	−4.08	12.0	8.08

[a] CV(%) = (standard deviation/mean) × 100. [b] RE(%) = [(calculated concentration − theoretical concentration)/theoretical concentration] × 100.

2.7. Applicability of the Assay to Pharmacokinetic Studies

To determine whether the current assay could be applied to pharmacokinetic studies on SH-1242 in preclinical animal species, SH-1242 was intravenously administered to rats or mice at a dose of 0.1 mg/kg. Concentration-time profiles of SH-1242 in rats and mice are shown in Figure 2, and calculated pharmacokinetic parameters, including $T_{1/2}$, CL, area under the curve from time zero to infinity (AUC_{inf}), mean residence time (MRT), and V_{ss}, are listed in Table 7. For rats, AUC_{inf}, CL, V_{ss}, and $T_{1/2}$ values of SH-1242 were 3350 ± 573 ng·min/mL, 30.5 ± 4.49 mL/min/kg, 4380 ± 716 mL/kg, and 146 ± 59 min, respectively. Interestingly, SH-1242 appeared to have lower systemic clearance and relatively limited distribution space, compared to those of deguelin, a model rotenoid, in rats (e.g., CL value of 72.7 mL/min/kg, and V_{ss} value of 30.5 L/kg) [20]. In mice, AUC_{inf}, CL, V_{ss}, and $T_{1/2}$ values of SH-1242 were 1440 ng·min/mL, 69.4 mL/min/kg, 2060 mL/kg, and 26.3 min, respectively. In general,

SH-1242 concentrations were readily measurable in all plasma samples in both animals at up to 8 h after the intravenous administration, indicating that the developed method could be readily applicable for the characterization of the pharmacokinetics of SH-1242 in preclinical study settings.

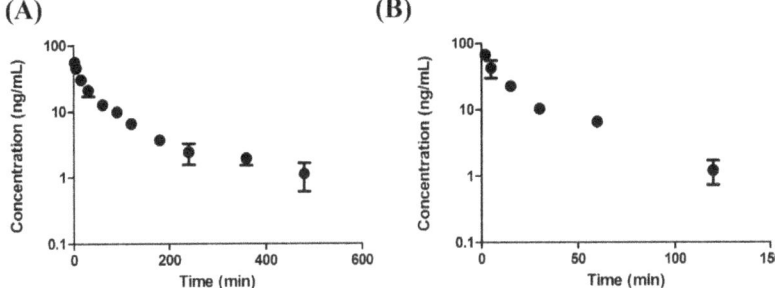

Figure 2. Mean concentration-time profiles of SH-1242 after (**A**) an intravenous injection of 0.1 mg/kg SH-1242 ($n = 4$) to rats and (**B**) an intravenous injection of 0.1 mg/kg SH-1242 ($n = 3$ for each time point) to mice. Results are presented as means ± standard deviations.

Table 7. Pharmacokinetic parameters of SH-1242 after a single intravenous administration at a dose of 0.1 mg/kg to rats and mice.

Pharmacokinetic Parameters (Units)	Rats	Mice
	Mean ± S.D.	Representative [a]
$T_{1/2}$ (min)	146 ± 59	26.3
CL (mL/min/kg)	30.5 ± 4.49	69.4
AUC_{inf} (ng·min/mL)	3350 ± 573	1440
MRT (min)	149 ± 46.9	29.6
V_{ss} (mL/kg)	4380 ± 716	2060

[a] Because of the study design (i.e., one-time point sample per mouse), the calculation of the standard deviation was not possible for pharmacokinetic parameters in mice.

3. Materials and Methods

3.1. Chemicals, Reagents, and Experimental Animals

SH-1242 (purity of >99%) and deguelin (purity of >99%, IS of this study) were synthesized, as previously described [9]. Methanol and acetonitrile (high-performance liquid chromatography (HPLC) grade) were purchased from Fisher Scientific (Pittsburgh, PA, USA). Double-distilled water (DDW) was prepared in-house using a Millipore Simplicity water purification system (Millipore, Bedford, MA, USA). Formic acid (FA) was purchased from Sigma-Aldrich (St. Louis, MO, USA). Blank rat and mouse plasma samples were collected from animals provided by Orient Bio Inc. (Gyeonggi-do, Korea). Experimental protocols involving animals used in this study were carefully reviewed by the Seoul National University Institutional Animal Care and Use Committee (IACUC), in accordance with the 'Principles of Laboratory Animal Care' guideline, published by the National Institutes of Health publication number 85-23, revised 1985 (SNU-170303-1 and SNU-170120-4-4).

3.2. HPLC Conditions

A Waters e2695 HPLC system (Milford, MA, USA) consisting of a binary pump, an online degasser, an autosampler, a column heater, and a reversed-phase HPLC column (Poroshell 120 EC-C18 2.7 µm (4.6 mm × 50 mm, Agilent, Santa Clara, CA, USA)) was used for chromatographic separations. The mobile phase was composed of 0.1% FA in acetonitrile and 0.1% FA in DDW in a ratio of 80:20 and was isocratically delivered at a flow rate of 1 mL/min. Throughout the assay, the temperatures of analytical samples and the column were maintained at 4 °C and 25 °C, respectively, and the run time was 3 min for each sample.

3.3. Mass Spectrometer Conditions

In this study, mass spectrometric detection was conducted using API 3200 Qtrap® (Applied Biosystems, Foster City, CA, USA), equipped with an electrospray ionization (ESI) source in the positive ion mode. Multiple reaction monitoring (MRM) method was used to quantify the analytes: m/z transitions were monitored at 368.9→151.0 for SH-1242 and 395.0→213.0 for IS. After a series of optimization studies to secure a sensitive and robust response of the signal, conditions, such as ion spray voltage, source temperature, and the three source gas pressure values (i.e., curtain gas pressure, ion source gas 1 and 2), were determined to be 5000 V, 200 °C, and 50 psi, respectively (Supplementary Figure S3). In addition, using the quantitative optimization mode built-in Analyst^{TM} software (version 1.4.2, Applied Biosystems, Waltham, MA, USA), the following factors were obtained: Declustering potentials for SH-1242 and IS were 41 V and 61 V, respectively, and entrance potentials were 4.5 V and 7 V, collision energies were 27 V and 29 V, and the collision cell exit potential was 4 V for both analytes. In this study, the Analyst^{TM} software was used for data acquisition and quantification.

3.4. Standards and Quality Control (QC) Samples

Stock solutions of SH-1242 and IS were prepared at the concentrations of 1 mg/mL and 500 ng/mL in methanol, respectively. A serial dilution of the SH-1242 stock solution with methanol was carried out to obtain a set of SH-1242 standard solutions, and 5 µL aliquots of these standard solutions were added to 45 µL of blank plasma to prepare SH-1242 calibration standards at concentrations of 1, 2, 5, 10, 20, 50, 100, 200, 500, and 1000 ng/mL for rat plasma and 2, 5, 10, 20, 50, 100, 200, 500, and 1000 ng/mL for mouse plasma. Using similar dilution protocol, a batch of QC samples for SH-1242 was prepared at concentrations of 1 (LLOQ), 2 (low QC), 40 (mid QC), and 800 ng/mL (high QC) for rat plasma and 2 (LLOQ), 4 (low QC), 40 (mid QC), and 800 ng/mL (high QC) for mouse plasma. Samples were then processed according to the procedure described in Section 3.5.

3.5. Sample Preparation

A total of 50 µL aliquots of plasma samples, calibration standards, or QC samples were transferred to Safeseal Microcentrifuge Tubes (Sorenson BioScience, Murray, UT, USA), followed by the addition of 200 µL of IS stock solution. Mixtures were vortex-mixed for 5 min and centrifuged at 16,100 g for 5 min at 4 °C. Supernatants were subsequently transferred to fresh analysis vials (MicroSolv Technology Corporation, Leland, NC, USA), and 50 µL aliquots were injected onto the HPLC-MS/MS system. In this study, the injection volume (i.e., 50 µL) was less than 10% of the void volume of the column of 830 µL (i.e., 4.6 mm of inner diameter and 50 mm of length) and did not appear to have any appreciable impact on the performance of the instrument (e.g., analyte peak width, retention time, and carryover) [21].

3.6. Method Validation

3.6.1. Selectivity

Six lots of pooled rat and mouse plasma samples were used to evaluate assay selectivity. The presence of any interfering peak in double blank samples (i.e., blank plasma without SH-1242 or IS), zero blank samples (i.e., blank plasma with IS only), and LLOQ samples was carefully monitored. In this study, assay selectivity was assumed adequate when no apparent interfering peaks were observed in the vicinities of the analyte peaks.

3.6.2. LLOQ and Linearity

The LLOQ of SH-1242 was determined to be the minimum concentration, with a signal-to-noise ratio being consistently greater than 10. Throughout our preliminary studies, LLOQ values of SH-1242 in the rat and mouse plasma were determined to be 1 ng/mL and 2 ng/mL, respectively, and these concentrations were subsequently used in the development of the assay. Various concentrations of SH-1242, ranging from 1 ng/mL to 1000 ng/mL for rat plasma (ten concentration levels) and 2 ng/mL to 1000 ng/mL for mouse plasma (nine concentration levels), were used to determine the linearity of the assay. A calibration curve was constructed by plotting SH-1242-to-IS peak area ratios against nominal SH-1242 concentrations. The linear least-square regression method with a weighting factor of $1/x^2$ was used to determine the slope and y-intercept.

3.6.3. Precision, Accuracy, and Dilution Integrity

Accuracy and precision within and between runs were assessed using five separate batches of QC samples. Each batch consisted of six replicates of QC samples at four concentration levels (LLOQ, 2 or 4 ng/mL, 40 ng/mL, and 800 ng/mL, in rat or mouse plasma, respectively). The accuracy of the assay was determined by calculating the percent differences between the calculated and theoretical concentrations, and the precision of the method was defined as the coefficient of variation (CV) percentage at each concentration. The method was considered accurate when the calculated concentrations of QC samples were within 15% of nominal concentrations. In addition, the assay was considered precise when the CV of calculated concentrations of QC samples was 15% or less (viz, 20% CV for LLOQ samples).

When it was necessary to study dilution integrity of the assay, a fresh batch of six-replicate samples (50 µL) was first prepared in rat or mouse plasma at an SH-1242 concentration of 8000 ng/mL (i.e., at a concentration exceeding the upper limit of quantification (ULOQ)). Samples were then diluted 10-fold with blank plasma (with 450 µL) to have the expected plasma concentration of 800 ng/mL and to bring the final concentration within the calibration range. Diluted samples were then processed and analyzed, as described in Section 3.5.

3.6.4. Matrix Effect, Extraction Efficiency, and Recovery

The extent of matrix effect, extraction efficiency, and recovery of SH-1242 in the rat and mouse plasma was evaluated by analyzing three sets of plasma standards at three different concentration levels (2 ng/mL, 40 ng/mL, and 800 ng/mL) [22,23]. Pre-spiked extracted samples (Set 1; extracted after the addition of analyte to blank plasma) were prepared according to the procedure described in Section 3.5. Similarly, post-spiked extracted samples were prepared by processing blank plasma and then adding SH-1242 to have the prescribed concentrations. Extraction efficiency was determined by dividing the mean peak areas of pre-spiked extracted samples (Set 1) by those of post-spiked extracted samples. Mean peak areas of the pre- and post-spiked extraction samples were divided by the mean peak areas of neat standard solutions of the analyte in methanol containing 0.1% FA (Set 2) to determine the recovery and matrix effect, respectively.

3.6.5. Stability

The stability of SH-1242 and IS was evaluated under various storage and handling conditions. Stock solutions of SH-1242 and IS at concentrations of 1 mg/mL and 500 ng/mL, respectively, were stored at room temperature (25 °C) for 6 h, under refrigerated conditions (4 °C) for 24 h or 2 weeks, or under two different frozen conditions (−20 °C and −80 °C) for 2 weeks. Solutions of SH-1242 were diluted to 50 ng/mL prior to analysis. In addition, QC samples at three different concentrations (2 or 4 ng/mL, 40 ng/mL, and 800 ng/mL) were prepared and processed. The samples were then placed in various handling conditions (i.e., standing in an autosampler (4 °C for 3 days) or under bench-top condition (25 °C for 24 h), or subjected to three freeze-thaw cycles, or long-term refrigeration (4 °C for 2 weeks)). Mean peak areas of stock solutions were compared with those of fresh stock solutions. For QC samples, the results were compared with nominal concentrations. In this study, analytes were considered stable under test conditions when accuracies at each concentration were within 15% of nominal concentration.

3.7. Application of the Assay to Pharmacokinetic Studies of SH-1242

To test the applicability of the current assay to pharmacokinetic studies, in preclinical animal species, male Sprague-Dawley rats (weighing 250–270 g) or ICR mice (weighing 18–20 g) were used. Prior to the experiment, animals fasted for 12 h with free access to water. SH-1242 was dissolved in a dosing vehicle consisting of dimethyl sulfoxide, PEG400 (Sigma-Aldrich, St. Louis, MO, USA), and normal saline in a ratio of 1:6:3 ($v/v/v\%$), and intravenously bolus-injected to the right femoral vein at 2 mL/kg for rats or to the tail vein at 5 mL/kg for mice. In this study, the intravenous dose of SH-1242 was set at 0.1 mg/kg for both species. Blood samples (approximately 150 µL each) were collected in heparinized tubes via the right femoral artery at 2, 5, 15, 30, 60, 90, 120, 180, 240, 360, and 480 min after the administration to rats ($n = 4$) and via the retro-orbital plexus at 2, 5, 15, 30, 60, or 120 min after the administration to mice ($n = 3$ for each time point). For the mouse study, a blood sample was obtained once from each animal, and the animal was sacrificed after collection. Plasma was obtained by centrifuging blood samples at 16,100 g for 5 min at 4 °C and then processed, as described in Section 3.5. The plasma concentration versus time data was analyzed using the non-compartmental method in the WinNonlin software (WinNonlin Professional 5.0.1.; Pharsight, Mountain View, CA, USA) to calculate essential kinetic parameters, such as terminal phase half-life ($T_{1/2}$), systemic clearance (CL), and steady-state volume of distribution (V_{ss}).

4. Conclusions

A straightforward and rapid HPLC-MS/MS assay was developed and validated for the quantification of SH-1242 in rat and mouse plasma. The method was validated in terms of its selectivity, linearity, accuracy, precision, dilution, matrix effects, recovery, and stability. Assay parameters were found to comply with the acceptance criteria described in U.S. FDA guidelines. The developed assay was found to be suitable for pharmacokinetic studies on SH-1242, involving rats and mice.

Supplementary Materials: The following are available online. Figure S1: Multiple reaction monitoring (MRM) chromatograms of (A) double blank rat plasma, (B) zero blank rat plasma containing 500 ng/mL IS, (C) rat plasma containing SH-1242 at LLOQ (1 ng/mL) and IS, (D) double blank mouse plasma, (E) zero blank mouse plasma containing 500 ng/mL IS, and (F) mouse plasma containing SH-1242 at LLOQ (2 ng/mL) and IS. Figure S2: Calibration curves for the LC-MS/MS analysis of SH-1242 in (A) the rat and (B) mouse plasma (i.e., 5 separate runs). Data are presented as means ± standard deviations. Slopes and intercepts of linear regression lines are showed in Table 2. Figure S3: Dependency of variables related to source/gas on the signal intensity in turbo VTM ion spray ionization mode. Closed circles and error bars represent the mean and upper/lower response of the signal during 1 min infusion of SH-1242 solution at 1 µg/mL (in 50% methanolic solution containing 0.1% FA).

Author Contributions: Conceptualization, Y.-S.J and S.-J.C.; data curation, Y.-S.J., M.B., and M.-S.K.; funding acquisition, H.-J.M. and S.-J.C.; methodology and validation, Y.-S.J., M.B., M.-S.K., H.-J.M., J.-H.L., and S.-J.C.; resources, S.L. and Y.-G.S.; writing-original draft, Y.-S.J., M.B., and S.-J.C.; investigation and writing-review and editing, Y.-S.J., M.B., S.L., M.-S.K., H.-J.M., J.-H.L., Y.-G.S., and S.-J.C.; supervision, S.-J.C. All authors have read and agreed to the published version of the manuscript.

Funding: This research was supported by a grant of the National Research Foundation of Korea (NRF) funded by the Korean government (MSIP) (No. 2009-0083533). In addition, this research was supported by the Basic Science Research Program through the National Research Foundation of Korea (NRF) grant funded by the Korea government (MSIT) (NRF-2019R1F1A1058103).

Conflicts of Interest: The authors declare no conflict of interest.

References

1. Pearl, L.H.; Prodromou, C.; Workman, P. The Hsp90 molecular chaperone: An open and shut case for treatment. *Biochem. J.* **2008**, *410*, 439–453. [CrossRef]
2. Ke, Q.; Costa, M. Hypoxia-inducible factor-1 (HIF-1). *Mol. Pharmacol.* **2006**, *70*, 1469–1480. [CrossRef] [PubMed]
3. Volm, M.; Koomägi, R. Hypoxia-inducible factor (HIF-1) and its relationship to apoptosis and proliferation in lung cancer. *Anticancer Res.* **2000**, *20*, 1527–1533.

4. Lin, M.; Chen, Y.; Jin, J.; Hu, Y.; Zhou, K.; Zhu, M.; Le, Y.-Z.; Ge, J.; Johnson, R.; Ma, J.-X. Ischaemia-induced retinal neovascularisation and diabetic retinopathy in mice with conditional knockout of hypoxia-inducible factor-1 in retinal Müller cells. *Diabetologia* **2011**, *54*, 1554–1566. [CrossRef]
5. Krishna Vadlapatla, R.; Dutt Vadlapudi, A.; Mitra, A.K. Hypoxia-inducible factor-1 (HIF-1): A potential target for intervention in ocular neovascular diseases. *Curr. Drug Targets* **2013**, *14*, 919–935. [CrossRef]
6. Oh, S.H.; Woo, J.K.; Yazici, Y.D.; Myers, J.N.; Kim, W.-Y.; Jin, Q.; Hong, S.S.; Park, H.-J.; Suh, Y.-G.; Kim, K.-W. Structural basis for depletion of heat shock protein 90 client proteins by deguelin. *J. Natl. Cancer Inst.* **2007**, *99*, 949–961. [CrossRef]
7. Kim, H.S.; Hong, M.; Ann, J.; Yoon, S.; Nguyen, C.-T.; Lee, S.-C.; Lee, H.-Y.; Suh, Y.-G.; Seo, J.H.; Choi, H. Synthesis and biological evaluation of C-ring truncated deguelin derivatives as heat shock protein 90 (HSP90) inhibitors. *Bioorg. Med. Chem.* **2016**, *24*, 6082–6093. [CrossRef]
8. Kim, H.S.; Hong, M.; Lee, S.-C.; Lee, H.-Y.; Suh, Y.-G.; Oh, D.-C.; Seo, J.H.; Choi, H.; Kim, J.Y.; Kim, K.-W. Ring-truncated deguelin derivatives as potent Hypoxia Inducible Factor-1α (HIF-1α) inhibitors. *Eur. J. Med. Chem.* **2015**, *104*, 157–164. [CrossRef]
9. Chang, D.-J.; An, H.; Kim, K.-s.; Kim, H.H.; Jung, J.; Lee, J.M.; Kim, N.-J.; Han, Y.T.; Yun, H.; Lee, S. Design, synthesis, and biological evaluation of novel deguelin-based heat shock protein 90 (HSP90) inhibitors targeting proliferation and angiogenesis. *J. Med. Chem.* **2012**, *55*, 10863–10884. [CrossRef] [PubMed]
10. Jo, D.H.; An, H.; Chang, D.-J.; Baek, Y.-Y.; Cho, C.S.; Jun, H.O.; Park, S.-J.; Kim, J.H.; Lee, H.-Y.; Kim, K.-W. Hypoxia-mediated retinal neovascularization and vascular leakage in diabetic retina is suppressed by HIF-1α destabilization by SH-1242 and SH-1280, novel hsp90 inhibitors. *J. Mol. Med. (Heidelberg, Ger.)* **2014**, *92*, 1083–1092. [CrossRef] [PubMed]
11. Lee, S.-C.; Min, H.-Y.; Choi, H.; Bae, S.Y.; Park, K.H.; Hyun, S.Y.; Lee, H.J.; Moon, J.; Park, S.-H.; Kim, J.Y. Deguelin analogue SH-1242 inhibits Hsp90 activity and exerts potent anticancer efficacy with limited neurotoxicity. *Cancer Res.* **2016**, *76*, 686–699. [CrossRef] [PubMed]
12. Prestes, O.D.; Padilla-Sánchez, J.A.; Romero-González, R.; Grio, S.L.; Frenich, A.G.; Martínez-Vidal, J.L. Comparison of several extraction procedures for the determination of biopesticides in soil samples by ultrahigh pressure LC-MS/MS. *J. Sep. Sci.* **2012**, *35*, 861–868. [CrossRef] [PubMed]
13. Caboni, P.; Sarais, G.; Angioni, A.; Garau, V.L.; Cabras, P. Fast and versatile multiresidue method for the analysis of botanical insecticides on fruits and vegetables by HPLC/DAD/MS. *J. Agric. Food Chem.* **2005**, *53*, 8644–8649. [CrossRef] [PubMed]
14. Dos Santos Pereira, A.; Serrano, M.A.A.; De Aquino Neto, F.R.; Da Cunha Pinto, A.; Texeira, D.F.; Gilbert, B. Analysis and quantitation of rotenoids and flavonoids in Derris (Lonchocarpus urucu) by high-temperature high-resolution gas chromatography. *J. Chromatogr. Sci.* **2000**, *38*, 174–180. [CrossRef]
15. Ye, H.; Chen, L.; Li, Y.; Peng, A.; Fu, A.; Song, H.; Tang, M.; Luo, H.; Luo, Y.; Xu, Y. Preparative isolation and purification of three rotenoids and one isoflavone from the seeds of Millettia pachycarpa Benth by high-speed counter-current chromatography. *J. Chromatogr. A* **2008**, *1178*, 101–107. [CrossRef]
16. FDA. *Guidance for Industry: Bioanalytical Method Validation*; US Department of Heath and Human Services Food and Drug Administration: Rockville, MD, USA, 2018.
17. Caboni, P.; Sarais, G.; Vargiu, S.; De Luca, M.A.; Garau, V.L.; Ibba, A.; Cabras, P. LC–MS–MS determination of rotenone, deguelin, and rotenolone in human serum. *Chromatographia* **2008**, *68*, 739–745. [CrossRef]
18. Jacobson, B.-M.; Olsson, A.; Fakt, C.; Öhman, D. The use of human plasma as matrix for calibration standards in pre-clinical LC–MS/MS methods—A way to reduce animal use. *J. Pharm. Biomed. Anal.* **2011**, *54*, 826–829. [CrossRef]
19. Matuszewski, B.; Constanzer, M.; Chavez-Eng, C. Strategies for the assessment of matrix effect in quantitative bioanalytical methods based on HPLC– MS/MS. *Anal. Chem.* **2003**, *75*, 3019–3030. [CrossRef]
20. Udeani, G.O.; Zhao, G.-M.; Shin, Y.G.; Kosmeder Ii, J.W.; Beecher, C.W.; Kinghorn, A.D.; Moriarty, R.M.; Moon, R.C.; Pezzuto, J.M. Pharmacokinetics of deguelin, a cancer chemopreventive agent in rats. *Cancer Chemother. Pharmacol.* **2001**, *47*, 263–268. [CrossRef]
21. Kromidas, S. *More practical problem solving in HPLC*; John Wiley & Sons: Weinheim, Germany, 2008.
22. Lee, J.H.; Woo, Y.A.; Hwang, I.C.; Kim, C.Y.; Kim, D.D.; Shim, C.K.; Chung, S.J. Quantification of CKD-501, lobeglitazone, in rat plasma using a liquid-chromatography/tandem mass spectrometry method and its applications to pharmacokinetic studies. *J. Pharm. Biomed. Anal.* **2009**, *50*, 872–877. [CrossRef]

23. Lee, M.; Kim, D.; Shin, J.; Lee, H.-Y.; Park, S.; Lee, H.-S.; Kang, J.-H.; Chung, S.-J. Quantification of IDP-73152, a novel antibiotic, in plasma from mice, rats and humans using an ultra-high performance liquid chromatography/tandem mass spectrometry method for use in pharmacokinetic studies. *J. Pharm. Biomed. Anal.* **2017**, *145*, 364–371. [CrossRef] [PubMed]

Sample Availability: Samples are available from the authors.

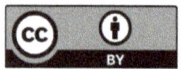 © 2020 by the authors. Licensee MDPI, Basel, Switzerland. This article is an open access article distributed under the terms and conditions of the Creative Commons Attribution (CC BY) license (http://creativecommons.org/licenses/by/4.0/).

MDPI
St. Alban-Anlage 66
4052 Basel
Switzerland
Tel. +41 61 683 77 34
Fax +41 61 302 89 18
www.mdpi.com

Molecules Editorial Office
E-mail: molecules@mdpi.com
www.mdpi.com/journal/molecules

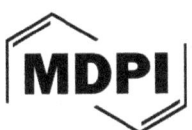

www.ingramcontent.com/pod-product-compliance
Lightning Source LLC
LaVergne TN
LVHW070210100526
838202LV00015B/2026

9 783036 563305